W9-BJH-470

Compliments of

GlaxoWellcome
Oncology/HIV

Handbook of Cancer Chemotherapy

Fourth Edition

Roland T. Skeel, M.D.

Professor of Medicine, and Chief of Hematology and Oncology, Medical College of Ohio; Attending Physician, Internal Medicine Service, Medical College of Ohio Hospital, Toledo, Ohio

Neil A. Lachant, M.D.

Associate Professor of Medicine, Medical College of Ohio; Attending Physician and Hematologist, Internal Medicine Service, Medical College of Ohio Hospital, Toledo, Ohio

Little, Brown and Company
Boston   New York   Toronto   London

Copyright © 1995 by Roland T. Skeel

Fourth Edition

Previous editions copyright © 1987, 1991 by Roland T. Skeel

First edition titled *Manual of Cancer Chemotherapy* © 1982 by Little, Brown and Company (Inc.)

All rights reserved. No part of this book may be reproduced in any form or by any electronic or mechanical means, including information storage and retrieval systems, without permission in writing from the publisher, except by a reviewer who may quote brief passages in a review.

Library of Congress Cataloging-in-Publication Data

Handbook of cancer chemotherapy / [edited by] Roland T. Skeel, Neil A. Lachant.—4th ed.
    p.   cm.
  Includes bibliographical references and index.
  ISBN 0-316-79575-5
  1. Cancer—Chemotherapy—Handbooks, manuals, etc. I. Skeel, Roland T. II. Lachant, Neil A.
  [DNLM: 1. Neoplasms—drug therapy—handbooks. QZ 39 H2355 1995]
RC271.C5H36 1995
616.99′4061—dc20
DNLM/DLC
for Library of Congress   95-6680
                                     CIP

Printed in the United States of America

RRD-VA

Editorial: Nancy Megley
Production Editor: Marie A. Salter
Copyeditor: Mary Babcock
Indexer: Alexandra Nickerson
Production Supervisor: Louis C. Bruno, Jr.
Cover Designer: Louis C. Bruno, Jr.

Contents

Contributing Authors

Jane B. Alavi, M.D.
Associate Professor of Medicine, University of
Pennsylvania School of Medicine and Hospital
of the University of Pennsylvania, Philadelphia

Robert S. Benjamin, M.D.
Professor of Medicine and Chairman, Department of
Melanoma/Sarcoma Medical Oncology, University of
Texas M. D. Anderson Cancer Center, Houston

Eduardo D. Bruera, M.D.
Professor of Oncology, and Alberta Cancer Foundation
Chair in Palliative Medicine, University of Alberta
Faculty of Medicine; Director, Palliative Care Program,
Edmonton General Hospital, Edmonton, Alberta, Canada

David F. Cella, Ph.D.
Associate Professor of Psychology and Social Sciences,
Rush Medical College of Rush University; Director,
Division of Psychosocial Oncology, Rush Cancer
Institute, Rush-Presbyterian-St. Luke's Medical Center,
Chicago

Charles S. Cleeland, Ph.D.
Professor of Neurology, University of Wisconsin Medical
School, Madison, Wisconsin

Ronald C. DeConti, M.D.
Professor of Medicine, University of South Florida
College of Medicine; Attending Physician, Department of
Medical Oncology, H. Lee Moffitt Cancer Center, Tampa,
Florida

Ralph R. Dobelbower, M.D., Ph.D.
Professor and Chairman, Department of Radiation
Therapy, and Professor of Neurological Surgery, Medical
College of Ohio; Chief of Radiation Therapy Service,
Medical College of Ohio Hospital, Toledo, Ohio

Kathy S. N. Franco-Bronson, M.D.
Section Head, Consultation-Liaison Service, Department
of Psychiatry and Psychology, Cleveland Clinic
Foundation, Cleveland

Roberto Franco-Saenz, M.D.
Professor of Medicine, and Chief of Endocrinology and
Metabolism, Department of Medicine, Medical College of
Ohio; Attending Physician, Internal Medicine Service,
Medical College of Ohio Hospital, Toledo, Ohio

Walter H. Gajewski, M.D.
Assistant Professor, Department of Obstetrics and
Gynecology and Gynecologic Oncology, Brown University
School of Medicine; Associate Director of Gynecologic
Oncology, Program in Oncology, Women and Infants
Hospital, Providence, Rhode Island

Patricia A. Ganz, M.D.
Professor of Medicine and Health Services, University of
California, Los Angeles, UCLA Schools of Medicine and
Public Health; Director, Division of Cancer Prevention
and Control Research, Jonsson Comprehensive Cancer
Center, Los Angeles

C. O. Granai, M.D.
Associate Professor and Director of Gynecologic Oncology,
Department of Obstetrics and Gynecology and
Gynecologic Oncology, Brown University School of
Medicine; Director of Gynecologic Oncology, Program in
Oncology, Women and Infants Hospital, Providence,
Rhode Island

Lynne Jahnke, M.D.
Former Fellow, Division of Hematology and Oncology,
Northwestern University Medical School, Chicago;
Attending Physician, Division of Hematology and
Oncology, Kaiser-Permanente Hospital, South
San Francisco, California

Samir N. Khleif, M.D.
Senior Clinical Investigator, NCI-Navy Medical Oncology
Branch, National Cancer Institute; Assistant Professor of
Medicine, Uniformed University of the Health Sciences,
F. Edward Hébert School of Medicine, Bethesda,
Maryland

Neil A. Lachant, M.D.
Associate Professor of Medicine, Medical College of Ohio;
Attending Physician and Hematologist, Internal
Medicine Service, Medical College of Ohio Hospital,
Toledo, Ohio

Rodger D. MacArthur, M.D.
Associate Professor of Medicine, Division of Infectious
Diseases, Wayne State University School of Medicine;
Director of HIV/AIDS Clinical Research, Harper Hospital
and Detroit Medical Center, Detroit

John C. Marsh, M.D.
Professor of Medicine and Lecturer in Pharmacology,
Yale University School of Medicine; Attending Physician,
Division of Internal Medicine (Medical Oncology), Yale-
New Haven Hospital, New Haven, Connecticut

Hollis W. Merrick, M.D., C.M.
Professor of Surgery, Medical College of Ohio; Attending
Surgeon, Medical College of Ohio Hospital, Toledo, Ohio

Larry Nathanson, M.D.
Professor of Medicine, State University of New York at
Stony Brook Health Sciences School of Medicine, Stony
Brook, New York; Chief, Division of Oncology/
Hematology, Winthrop-University Hospital, Mineola,
New York

James A. Neidhart, M.D.
Professor of Medicine, University of New Mexico School of Medicine; Director, University of New Mexico Cancer Center, University of New Mexico Medical Center, Albuquerque, New Mexico

Craig R. Nichols, M.D.
Associate Professor of Medicine, Indiana University School of Medicine, Indianapolis

Martin M. Oken, M.D.
Director, Virginia Piper Cancer Institute, Abbott Northwestern Hospital, Minneapolis

Carol S. Palackdharry, M.D., M.S.
Associate Professor of Medicine, Medical College of Ohio; Attending Physician, Internal Medicine Service, Medical College of Ohio Hospital, Toledo, Ohio

David R. Parkinson, M.D.
Chief, Investigational Drug Branch, Cancer Therapy Evaluation Program, Division of Cancer Treatment, National Cancer Institute, Bethesda, Maryland

Walter D. Y. Quan, Jr., M.D.
Attending Physician, Department of Medicine, Saint Luke's Medical Center, Cleveland, Ohio

Scott B. Saxman, M.D.
Assistant Professor of Medicine, Indiana University School of Medicine, Indianapolis

David J. Schifeling, M.D.
Assistant Professor of Internal Medicine, University of Tennessee, Memphis, College of Medicine, Memphis, Tennessee

Joan H. Schiller, M.D.
Associate Professor, Department of Human Oncology, University of Wisconsin Medical School; Chief of Medical Oncology, William S. Middleton Veterans Administration Hospital, Madison, Wisconsin

Joy D. Skeel, M.Div.
Associate Professor, Departments of Psychiatry and Medicine, Medical College of Ohio; Director of Medical Humanities and Ethics, Medical College of Ohio Hospital, Toledo, Ohio

Roland T. Skeel, M.D.
Professor of Medicine, and Chief of Hematology and Oncology, Medical College of Ohio; Attending Physician, Internal Medicine Service, Medical College of Ohio Hospital, Toledo, Ohio

Mary R. Smith, M.D.
Professor of Clinical Medicine and Pathology, and Associate Dean for Medical Education, Medical College of Ohio; Attending Physician, Internal Medicine and Pathology Services, Medical College of Ohio Hospital, Toledo, Ohio

Richard S. Stein, M.D.
Associate Professor of Medicine, Vanderbilt University School of Medicine, Nashville, Tennessee

Janelle M. Tipton, M.S.N., R.N., O.C.N.
Adjunct Instructor, School of Nursing, Medical College of Ohio; Oncology Nurse Specialist, Department of Nursing Resources, Medical College of Ohio Hospital, Toledo, Ohio

Jamie H. Von Roenn, M.D.
Associate Professor of Medicine, Northwestern University Medical School, Chicago

Peter White, M.D.
Professor of Medicine, and Associate Dean for Academic Affairs, Medical College of Ohio; Attending Physician, Internal Medicine Service, Medical College of Ohio Hospital, Toledo, Ohio

Preface

Cure of cancer with chemotherapy or other systemic treatment has been a long-term aspiration for many people: for those engaged in cancer research, for physicians who are daily faced with patients who have cancer, and for others in the health professions; it has also been a fervent hope of patients and their families. While cure is possible for a small percentage of some common tumors, particularly when there is only micrometastasis, and for some more advanced tumors such as lymphomas, for most patients chemotherapy remains, at best.

The hope for more specific, radically improved medical treatment for cancer has been stimulated by the tremendous recent increase in information on the molecular basis of cancer development and the natural mechanisms of cell growth and death. While this new knowledge offers the potential for more specific and effective therapy of cancer by interference with oncogenes and oncogene products, or by manipulation of tumor suppressor genes or their products, its practical value in the treatment of patients remains unrealized. In contrast, continuing research into (1) ways to enhance inherent biologic responses of the host to cancer, and (2) support of patients undergoing the rigors of cancer treatment, has resulted in improved therapy in several cancers, though cures are still uncommonly seen. Current trials that combine the biologic therapies with each other and with chemotherapy offer a realistic expectation of continued progress in treatment during the second half of this decade. During the past several years, we have witnessed the introduction of new chemotherapeutic and biologic agents, more effective combinations of drugs, and better ways of using older agents either alone or in conjunction with surgery, radiotherapy, or biologic therapy, each of which has resulted in cures of selected cancers and better palliation in many others.

Several new chapters have been added to this edition of the *Handbook of Cancer Chemotherapy*. Bone marrow transplantation following high-dose chemotherapy with or without radiotherapy has been used experimentally for many years, particularly in the leukemias and lymphomas. In recent years, high-dose chemotherapy with progenitor cell or cytokine support has become a standard of care for a few cancers, particularly following failure after using primary treatment, and offers the potential of improved survival for some patients. Because this technology is widely available and one that all those caring for patients with cancer should understand, we have added a chapter on high-dose chemotherapy and the role of progenitor cell and cytokine support. Quality-of-life considerations and cost-utility assessments in cancer treatment decisions are two related areas that have recently assumed increasing importance in cancer clinical trials, health policy decisions, and individual patient care recommendations. A chapter covering these areas has been added to the first section of the book, which covers basic principles and considerations of rational chemotherapy. Finally, in the supportive care section we have added an important new chapter that addresses issues of cancer survivorship: insurance, employment, and psychosocial factors. Several chapters have undergone major revision, including the chapters on HIV-associated malignancies, myeloproliferative and myelodysplastic syndromes, gynecologic cancer, urologic and male genital malignancies, carcinoma of the lung, critical care issues in oncology, and managing cancer pain.

The *Handbook* continues to be a practical pocket reference with a wealth of information for oncology specialists, nononcology physicians, house officers, oncology nurses, pharmacists, and medical students. It can even be read and understood by many patients and their families, who want to be able to find practical information about their cancer and its treatment. Unlike most other books, the *Handbook* combines in one place the rationale and the specific details necessary to safely administer chemotherapy for most adult cancers. We believe that with the additions and revisions in this edition, the *Handbook* will continue to be a valuable resource for physicians, nurses, students, and others.

R.T.S.
N.A.L.

Basic Principles
and Considerations
of Rational Chemotherapy

Notice. The indications and dosages of all drugs in this book have been recommended in the medical literature and conform to the practices of the general medical community. The medications described do not necessarily have specific approval by the Food and Drug Administration for use in the diseases and dosages for which they are recommended. The package insert for each drug should be consulted for use and dosage as approved by the FDA. Because standards for usage change, it is advisable to keep abreast of revised recommendations, particularly those concerning new drugs.

Biologic and Pharmacologic Basis of Cancer Chemotherapy

Roland T. Skeel

I. **General mechanisms by which chemotherapeutic agents control cancer.** The purpose of treating cancer with chemotherapeutic agents is to prevent cancer cells from multiplying, invading, metastasizing, and ultimately killing the host (patient). Most agents currently in use appear to exert their effect primarily on cell multiplication and tumor growth. Because cell multiplication is a characteristic of many normal cells as well as cancer cells, most cancer chemotherapeutic agents also have toxic effects on normal cells, particularly those with a rapid rate of turnover, such as bone marrow and mucous membrane cells. The goal in selecting an effective drug, therefore, is to find an agent that has marked growth inhibitory or controlling effect on the cancer cell with minimal toxic effect on the host. In the most effective chemotherapeutic regimens, the drugs are capable not only of inhibiting but also of completely eradicating all neoplastic cells while sufficiently preserving normal marrow and other target organs to allow a return to normal, or at least satisfactory, function.

Ideally, the pharmacologist or medicinal chemist would like to look at the cancer cell, discover how it differs from the normal host cell, and then design a chemotherapeutic agent to capitalize on that difference. In practice, often less rational means are used. The effectiveness of agents is discovered by treating either animal or human neoplasms, after which the pharmacologist attempts to discover why the agent works as well as it does. With few exceptions, the reasons chemotherapeutic agents are more effective against cancer cells than normal cells are poorly understood.

Inhibition of cell multiplication and tumor growth can take place at several levels within the cell.

1. Macromolecular synthesis and function
2. Cytoplasmic organization
3. Cell membrane synthesis function

A. **Standard agents.** Most agents currently in use or under investigation, with the exception of immunotherapeutic agents and other biologic response modifiers (BRMs), appear to have their primary effect on either macromolecular synthesis or function. This effect means that they interfere with either the synthesis of DNA, RNA, or proteins or the appropriate functioning of the preformed molecule. When interference in the macromolecular synthesis or function in the neoplastic cell population is sufficiently great, a proportion of the cells die. Some cells die because of the direct effect of the chemotherapeutic agent. In other instances, the chemotherapy may trigger differentiation, senescence, or apoptosis, the cell's own mechanism of programmed death. The

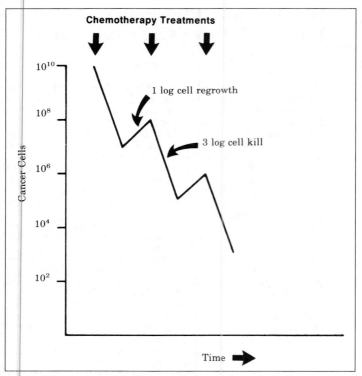

Fig. 1-1. Effect of chemotherapy on cancer cell numbers. In an ideal system, chemotherapy kills a constant proportion of the remaining cancer cells with each dose. Between doses, cell regrowth occurs. When therapy is successful, cell killing is greater than cell growth.

interrelationship between p53 mutations and resistance to the cytotoxic effects of radiotherapy and several chemotherapeutic agents, when better understood, may further our understanding of resistance and provide new therapeutic strategies. Cell death may or may not take place at the time of exposure to the drug. Often a cell must undergo several divisions before the lethal event that took place earlier finally results in the death of the cell. Because only a proportion of the cells die with a given treatment, repeated doses of chemotherapy must be used to continue to reduce the cell number (Fig. 1-1). In an ideal system, each time the dose is repeated the same *proportion* of cells—not the same absolute number—is killed. In the example shown in Figure 1-1, 99.9% (3 logs) of the cancer cells are killed with each treatment, and there is a 10-fold (1 log) growth between treatments for a net reduction of 2 logs with each treatment. Starting at 10^{10} cells (about 10 gm or 10 cm^3 leukemia cells), it would take five treatments to reach fewer than 10^0, or one, cell. Such a model makes certain assumptions that rarely are strictly true in clinical practice.

1. All cells in a tumor population are equally sensitive to a drug.
2. Drug accessibility and cell sensitivity are independent of the location of the cells within the host and independent of local host factors, such as blood supply or surrounding fibrosis.
3. Cell sensitivity does not change during the course of therapy.

The lack of curability of most initially sensitive tumors is probably a reflection of the degree to which these assumptions do not hold true.

B. Biologic response modifiers. Within individual cells and cell populations there are intricate interrelated mechanisms that promote or suppress cell growth, lead to cell differentiation, or set the cell on the path to inevitable death (apoptosis). These activities appear to be controlled in large part by normal and mutated promoter genes, tumor suppressor genes, and their products. Included in these products are a host of cell growth factors. Many of these factors have been biosynthesized and are now used in standard and investigational therapy. They are discussed more fully in Chapter 3.

The recent expansion of understanding of the biologic control of normal cells and tumor growth at the molecular level has not yet led to improved therapy for cancer, though it has helped to explain differences in response among populations of patients. Further understanding holds a great potential for providing a powerful, selective means to control neoplastic cell growth and may lead to effective cancer treatments in the next decade.

II. Tumor cell kinetics and chemotherapy. Cancer cells, unlike other body cells, are characterized by a growth process whereby their sensitivity to normal controlling factors has been partially or completely lost. As a result of this uncontrolled growth, it was once thought that cancer cells grew or multiplied faster than normal cells, and that this growth rate was responsible for their sensitivity to chemotherapy. It now is known that most cancer cells grow less rapidly than the more active, normal cells, such as bone marrow. Thus although the growth rate of many cancers is faster than that of normal surrounding tissues, growth rate alone cannot explain the greater sensitivity of cancer cells to chemotherapy.

A. Tumor growth. The growth of a tumor depends on several interrelated factors.

1. **Cell cycle time,** or the average time for a cell that has just completed mitosis to grow and again divide and pass through mitosis, determines the maximum growth rate for a tumor but probably does not determine drug sensitivity. The relative proportion of cell cycle time taken up by the DNA synthesis phase may

relate to drug sensitivity of some types (S-phase-specific) of chemotherapeutic agents.

2. **Growth fraction,** or the fraction of cells undergoing cell division, represents the portion of cells that are sensitive to drugs whose major effect is exerted on cells that are actively dividing. If the growth fraction approaches 1 and the cell death rate is low, the *tumor doubling time* approximates the cell cycle time.

3. **Total number of cells in the population** (determined at some arbitrary time at which the growth measurement is started) is clinically important because it is an index of how advanced is the cancer; it frequently correlates with normal organ dysfunction. As the total number of cells increases, so does the number of resistant cells, which in turn leads to decreased curability. Large tumors may also have greater compromise of blood supply and oxygenation, which can impair drug delivery to the tumor cells and impair sensitivity to both chemotherapy and radiotherapy.

4. **Intrinsic cell death rate** of tumors is difficult to measure in patients but probably makes a major contribution by slowing the growth rate of many solid tumors.

B. **Cell cycle.** The cell cycle of cancer cells is qualitatively the same as that of normal cells (Fig. 1-2). Each cell begins its growth during a postmitotic period, a phase called G_1, during which enzymes necessary for DNA production, other proteins, and RNA are produced. G_1 is followed by a period of DNA *synthesis* (S) in which essentially all DNA synthesis for a given cycle takes place. When DNA synthesis is complete, the cell enters a *premitotic period* (G_2) during which further protein and RNA synthesis occur. This gap is followed immediately by *mitosis* (M), at the end of which actual physical division takes place, two daughter cells are formed, and each again enters G_1. The G_1 phase is in equilibrium with a *resting state* called G_0. Cells in G_0 are relatively inactive with respect to macromolecular synthesis and are consequently insensitive to many chemotherapeutic agents, particularly those that affect macromolecular synthesis.

C. **Phase and cell cycle specificity.** Most chemotherapeutic agents can be grouped according to whether they depend on cells being in cycle (i.e., not in G_0) and, if they depend on the cell being in cycle, whether their activity is greater when the cell is in a specific phase of the cycle. It is important to note that most agents cannot be assigned to one category exclusively. Nonetheless, these classifications can be helpful for understanding drug activity.

1. **Phase-specific drugs.** Those agents most active against cells that are in a specific phase of the cell cycle are called *cell cycle phase-specific drugs*. A partial list of these drugs is shown in Table 1-1.

a. **Implications of phase-specific drugs.** Phase

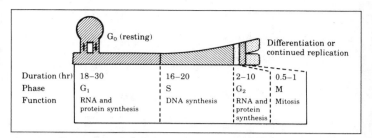

Fig. 1-2. Cell cycle time for human tissues has a wide range (16–260 hours), with marked differences among normal and tumor tissues. Normal marrow and gastrointestinal-lining cells have cell cycle times of 24–48 hours. Representative durations and the kinetic or synthetic activity are indicated for each phase.

specificity has important implications for cancer chemotherapy.

(1) **Limitation to single-exposure cell kill.** With a phase-specific agent there is a limit to the number of cells that can be killed by a single instantaneous (or very short) drug exposure because only those cells in the sensitive phase are killed. A higher dose kills no more cells.

(2) **Increasing cell kill by prolonged exposure.** For more cells to be killed requires either prolonged exposure to, or repeated doses of, the drug to allow more cells to enter the sensitive phase of the cycle. Theoretically, all cells could be killed if the blood level, or more importantly the intracellular concentration, of the drug remains sufficiently high while all cells in the target population pass through one complete cell cycle. This theory assumes that the drug does not prevent the passage of cells from one (insensitive) phase to another (sensitive) phase.

(3) **Recruitment.** A higher number of cells could be killed by a phase-specific drug if the proportion of cells in the sensitive phase could be increased (recruited).

b. **Cytarabine.** One of the best examples of a phase-specific agent is cytarabine (ara-C), which is an inhibitor of DNA synthesis and thus is active only in the S phase (at standard doses). Ara-C is rapidly deaminated in vivo to an inactive compound, ara-U; and rapid injections result in very short, effective levels of ara-C. As a result, single doses of ara-C are nontoxic to the normal hematopoietic system and are generally ineffective for treating leukemia. If the drug is given as a daily rapid injection, some patients with leu-

Table 1-1. Cell cycle phase-specific chemotherapeutic agents

Phase of greatest activity	Class	Type	Characteristic agents
Gap 1 (G$_1$)	Natural product	Enzyme	Asparaginase
	Hormone	Corticosteroid	Prednisone
G$_1$/S junction	Antimetabolite	Purine analog	Cladribine
DNA synthesis (S)	Antimetabolite	Pyrimidine analog	Cytarabine, fluorouracil
	Antimetabolite	Folic acid analog	Methotrexate
	Antimetabolite	Purine analog	Thioguanine, fludarabine
	Miscellaneous	Substituted urea	Hydroxyurea
Gap 2 (G$_2$)	Natural product	Antibiotic	Bleomycin
	Natural product	Topoisomerase II inhibitor	Etoposide
	Natural product	Microtubule polymerization and stabilization	Paclitaxel (Taxol)
Mitosis (M)	Natural product	Mitotic inhibitor	Vinblastine, vincristine, vindesine

kemia respond well but not nearly as well as when ara-C is given on an every-12-hour schedule. The apparent reason for the greater effectiveness of the 12-hour schedule is that the S phase (DNA synthesis) of human acute nonlymphocytic leukemia cells lasts about 18–20 hours. If the drug is given every 24 hours, some cells that have not entered the S phase when the drug is first administered would not be sensitive to its effect. Therefore these cells could pass all the way through the S phase before the next dose is administered and would completely escape any cytotoxic effect. However, when the drug is given every 12 hours, no cell that was "in cycle" would be able to escape exposure to ara-C, as none would be able to get through one complete S phase without the drug being present.

If all cells were in active cycle, i.e., if none were resting in a prolonged G_1 or G_0 phase, it would be theoretically possible to kill any cells in a population by a continuous or scheduled exposure equivalent to one complete cell cycle. Experiments with patients who have acute leukemia have shown that if tritiated thymidine is used to label cells as they enter DNA synthesis, it may be 7–10 days before the maximum number of leukemia cells have passed through the S phase. This factor means that, barring permutations caused by itself or other drugs, for ara-C to have a maximum effect on the leukemia the repeated exposure must be continued for a 7–10-day period. Clinically, continuous infusion or every-12-hour dosing of ara-C for 5 days or more appears to be most effective for treating newly diagnosed patients with acute nonlymphocytic leukemia. Even with such prolonged exposure, however, a few of the cells appear not to have passed through the S phase.

2. **Cell cycle-specific drugs.** Agents that are effective while cells are actively in cycle but are not dependent on the cell being in a particular phase are called *cell cycle-specific drugs (phase-nonspecific)*. This group includes most of the alkylating agents, antitumor antibiotics, and some miscellaneous agents, examples of which are shown in Table 1-2. Some agents in this group are not totally phase-nonspecific; they may have greater activity in one phase than in another but not to the degree of the phase-specific agents. Many agents also appear to have some activity in cells that are not in cycle, although not as much as when the cells are rapidly dividing.

3. **Cell cycle-nonspecific drugs.** A third group of drugs appears to be effective whether cancer cells are in cycle or are resting. In this respect, these agents are similar to photon irradiation. Drugs in this category are called *cell cycle-nonspecific* and in-

Table 1-2. Cell cycle-specific and cell cycle-nonspecific chemotherapeutic agents

Class	Type	Characteristic agents
Cell cycle-specific		
Alkylating agent	Nitrogen mustard	Chlorambucil, cyclophosphamide, melphalan
	Alkyl sulfonate	Busulfan
	Triazine	Dacarbazine
	Metal salt	Cisplatin, carboplatin
Natural product	Antibiotic	Dactinomycin, daunorubicin, doxorubicin, idarubicin
Cell cycle-nonspecific		
Alkylating agent	Nitrogen mustard	Mechlorethamine
	Nitrosourea	Carmustine, lomustine

clude mechlorethamine (nitrogen mustard) and the nitrosoureas (see Table 1-2).

D. Changes in tumor cell kinetics and therapy implications. As cancer cells grow from a few cells to a lethal tumor burden, certain changes occur in the growth rate of the population and affect the strategies of chemotherapy. These changes have been determined by observing the characteristics of experimental tumors in animals and neoplastic cells growing in tissue culture. Such model systems readily permit accurate cell number determinations to be made and growth rates to be determined. (Because tumor cells cannot be injected or implanted into humans and permitted to grow, studies of growth rates of intact tumors in humans must largely be limited to observing the growth rate of macroscopic tumors.)

    1. Stages of tumor growth. Immediately after inoculating a tissue culture or an experimental animal with tumor cells, there is a *lag phase* during which there is little tumor growth. Presumably, the cells in this phase are becoming accustomed to the new environment and are preparing to enter into cycle. The lag phase is followed by a period of rapid growth called *log phase,* during which there are repeated doublings of the cell number. In populations in which the growth fraction approaches 100% and the cell death rate is low, the population doubles within a period approximating the cell cycle time. As the cell number or tumor size becomes macroscopic, the doubling time of the tumor cell population becomes prolonged and levels off (*plateau phase*). Most clinically measurable human cancers are probably in the plateau phase, which may account, in part, for the slow doubling time observed in many human cancers (30–300 days). Because the rate of change in the slope of the growth curve during the premeasurable period is unknown for most human cancers, extrapolation from two points when the mass is measurable to estimate the onset of the growth of the malignancy is subject to considerable error. The prolongation in tumor doubling time in the plateau phase may be due to a smaller growth fraction, a change in the cell cycle time, an increased intrinsic death rate, or a combination of these factors. Factors responsible for these changes include decreased nutrients or growth promotion factors, increased inhibitory metabolites or inhibitory growth factors, and inhibition of growth by other cell–cell interactions, as briefly discussed in sec. **I.B.**

2. **Growth rate and effectiveness of chemotherapy.** Chemotherapeutic agents are most effective during the period of logarithmic growth. As might be expected, this result is particularly true for the antimetabolites, which are largely S-phase-specific. As a result, when human tumors become macroscopic, the effectiveness of many chemotherapeutic agents is reduced because only part of the cell population is actively dividing. Theoretically, if the cell population could be reduced sufficiently by other means, such as surgery or radiotherapy, chemotherapy would be more effective because a higher fraction of the remaining cells would be in logarithmic growth. The validity of this theoretical premise is supported by varying degrees of success of surgery plus chemotherapy or radiotherapy plus chemotherapy for breast cancer, colon cancer, Wilms' tumor, ovarian cancer, small-cell anaplastic cell carcinoma of the lung, non-small-cell carcinoma of the lung, head and neck cancers, and osteosarcomas.

III. **Combination chemotherapy.** Combinations of drugs are frequently more effective in producing responses and prolonging life than the same drugs used sequentially. There are several reasons combinations are likely to be more effective than single agents.

A. **Reasons for effectiveness of combinations**

1. **Prevention of resistant clones.** If 1 in 10^5 cells is resistant to drug A and 1 in 10^5 is resistant to drug B, it is likely that treating a macroscopic tumor (which generally would have more than 10^9 cells) with either agent alone would result in several clones of cells that are resistant to that drug. Once a resistant clone has grown to macroscopic size, and if the same mutant frequency persists for drug B, resistance to that agent would also emerge. If both drugs are used at the outset of therapy or in close sequence, however, the likelihood of a cell being resistant to both drugs (excluding for a moment the situation of pleiotropic drug resistance) is only 1 in 10^{10}.

Thus the combination confers considerable advantage against the emergence of resistant clones. Compounding the problem of preexisting resistant clones is the resistance that develops through spontaneous mutation in the absence of drug exposure. The use of multiple drugs with independent mechanisms of action or alternating non-cross-resistant combinations (as well as the use of surgery or radiotherapy to eliminate macroscopic tumor) theoretically minimizes the chances for outgrowth of resistant clones and increases the likelihood of remission or cure.

2. **Cytotoxicity to resting and dividing cells.** The combination of a drug that is cell cycle-specific (phase-nonspecific) or cell cycle-nonspecific with a drug that is cell cycle phase-specific can kill cells that are slowly dividing as well as those that are actively dividing. The use of cell cycle-nonspecific drugs can also help recruit cells into a more actively dividing state, which results in their being more sensitive to the cell cycle phase-specific agents.

3. **Biochemical enhancement of effect**

   a. **Combinations of individually effective drugs** that affect different biochemical pathways or steps in a single pathway can enhance each other.

   b. **Combinations of an active agent with an inactive agent** potentially can result in beneficial effects by several mechanisms.

      (1) **An intracellular increase** in the drug or its active metabolites, by either increasing influx or decreasing efflux (e.g., calcium channel inhibitors with multiple agents affected by multidrug resistance due to P-glycoprotein overexpression).

      (2) **Reduced metabolic inactivation** of the drug (e.g., inhibition of cytidine deaminase inactivation of ara-C with tetrahydrouridine or inhibition of 5′-nucleotidase inactivation of arabinosyl cytosine monophosphate (ara-CMP) with etidronate).

      (3) **Cooperative inhibition** of a single enzyme or reaction (e.g., leucovorin enhancement of fluorouracil inhibition of thymidylate synthetase).

      (4) **Enhancement of drug action** by inhibition of competing metabolites (e.g., N-phosphonacetyl-L-aspartic acid [PALA] inhibition of de novo pyrimidine synthesis with resultant increased incorporation of 5-fluorouridine triphosphate [5FUTP] into RNA).

4. **Sanctuary access.** Combinations can be used to provide access to sanctuary sites for reasons such as drug solubility or affinity of specific tissues for a particular drug type.

5. **Rescue.** Combinations can be used in which one agent rescues the host from the toxic effects of

another drug (e.g., leucovorin following high-dose methotrexate).

B. Principles of agent selection. When selecting appropriate agents for use in a combination, the following principles should be observed.

    1. Choose individually active drugs. Do not use a combination in which one agent is inactive when used alone unless there is a clear, specific biochemical or pharmacologic reason to do so, e.g., high-dose methotrexate followed by leucovorin rescue or leucovorin followed by fluorouracil. *This principle is not applicable to the combined use of BRMs and chemotherapeutic agents,* as cooperativity of BRMs and chemotherapy may not depend on independent cytotoxic effect of the BRMs.

    2. When possible, choose drugs in which the dose-limiting toxicities differ qualitatively or in time of occurrence. Often, however, two or more agents that have marrow toxicity must be used, and the selection of a safe dose of each is critical. As a starting point, two drugs in combination can usually be given at two-thirds of the dose used when the drugs are given alone. Whenever a new drug combination is tried, a careful evaluation for both expected and unanticipated toxicities must be carried out.

    3. Select agents for a combination for which there is a biochemical or pharmacologic rationale. Preferably this rationale has been tested in an animal tumor system and in the appropriate model system and has been found to be better than either agent alone.

    4. Be cautious when attempting to improve on a successful two-drug combination by adding a third, fourth, and fifth drug simultaneously. Although this approach may be beneficial, two undesirable results may be seen:

        a. An intolerable level of toxicity that leads to excessive morbidity and mortality.

        b. Unchanged or reduced antitumor effect because of the necessity to reduce the dose of the most effective drugs to a level below which antitumor responses are not seen, despite the theoretical advantages of the combination. Therefore the addition of each new agent to a combination must be carefully considered, the principles of combination therapy closely followed, and controlled clinical trials carried out to compare the efficacy of any new regimen with a more established (standard) treatment program.

C. Clinical effectiveness of combinations. Combinations of drugs have been clearly demonstrated to be better than single agents for treating many, but not all, human cancers. The benefit of combinations of drugs compared with the same drugs used sequentially has been marked in diseases such as acute lymphocytic and acute nonlymphocytic leukemia, Hodgkin's lymphoma, non-Hodgkin's lymphomas with more aggressive behavior (intermediate and high-grade), breast carcinoma, anaplastic small-cell carcinoma of the lung, and testicular carcinoma. The benefit is less clear in cancers such as non-small-cell carcinoma of the lung, non-Hodgkin's lymphomas with favorable prognoses, ovarian carcinoma, head and neck carcinomas, melanoma, and colorectal carcinomas, although reports exist for each of these tumors in which combinations are better in one respect or another than single agents.

IV. **Resistance to antineoplastic agents.** Resistance to antineoplastic chemotherapy is a combined characteristic of a specific drug, a specific tumor, and a specific host whereby the drug is ineffective in controlling the tumor without excessive toxicity. Resistance of a tumor to a drug is the reciprocal of selectivity of that drug for that tumor. The problem for the medical oncologist or pharmacologist is not simply to find an agent that is cytotoxic but to find one that selectively kills neoplastic cells while preserving the essential host cells and their function. Were it not for the problem of resistance of human cancer to antineoplastic agents or, conversely, the lack of selectivity of those agents, cancer chemotherapy would be similar to antibacterial chemotherapy in which complete eradication of infection is regularly observed. Such a utopian state of cancer chemotherapy has not yet been achieved for most human cancers. The problem of resistance and ways to overcome or even exploit it remains an area of major interest for the chemotherapist.

Resistance to antineoplastic chemotherapeutic agents may be either natural or acquired. *Natural resistance* refers to the initial unresponsiveness of a tumor to a given drug, and *acquired resistance* refers to the unresponsiveness that emerges after initially successful treatment. There are three basic categories of resistance to chemotherapy: kinetic, biochemical, and pharmacologic.

A. **Cell kinetics and resistance.** Resistance based on cell population kinetics relates to cycle and phase specificity, growth fractions and the implications of these factors for responsiveness to specific agents, and schedules of drug administration. A particular problem with many human tumors is that they are in a plateau growth phase with a small growth fraction. This factor renders many of the cells insensitive to the antimetabolites and relatively unresponsive to many of the other chemotherapeutic agents. Strategies to overcome resistance due to cell kinetics include the following.

1. Reducing tumor bulk with surgery or radiotherapy
2. Using combinations to include drugs that affect resting populations (with many G_0 cells)
3. Scheduling of drugs to prevent phase escape or to synchronize cell populations and increase cell kill

B. **Biochemical causes of resistance.** Resistance can occur for biochemical reasons, including the inability of a tumor to convert a drug to its active form, ability of a tumor to inactivate a drug, or the location of a tumor at a site where substrates are present that bypass an otherwise lethal blockade. How cells become resistant is only partially understood. In one pre-B cell leukemia cell line; bcl-2 overexpression rendered cells resistant to several chemotherapeutic agents. Because bcl-2 blocks apoptosis, it has been proposed that the overexpression blocked chemotherapy-induced apoptosis.

Multidrug resistance (MDR), also called pleiotropic drug resistance, is a phenomenon whereby treatment with one agent confers resistance not only to that drug and others of its class but also to several other unrelated agents. MDR is commonly mediated by an enhanced energy-dependent drug efflux mechanism that results in lower intracellular drug concentrations. With this type of MDR, overexpression of a membrane transport protein called P-glycoprotein is commonly observed. Combination chemotherapy can overcome biochemical resistance by increasing the amount of active drug intracellularly as a result of biochemical interactions or effects on drug transport across the cell membrane. Calcium channel blockers, antiarrhythmics, cyclosporin A, and other agents have been found to modulate the MDR effect in vitro, and some beneficial effects have been clinically observed.

The use of a second agent to rescue normal cells may also permit the use of high doses of the first agent, which can overcome the resistance caused by a low rate of conversion to the active metabolite or a high rate of inactivation. Another way to overcome resistance is to follow marrow-lethal doses of chemotherapy by posttherapy infusion of stem cells obtained from the peripheral blood or bone marrow. This experimental technique shows some promise for treatment of lymphomas, chronic granulocytic leukemia, and a few other cancers. A more widely applicable technique may be to combine high-dose chemotherapy with blood cell growth factors, e.g., granulocyte colony-stimulating factor and granulocyte-macrophage colony-stimulating factor. These and other marrow protective and stimulating agents are being increasingly used and may enhance the effectiveness of chemotherapy on several cancers. High-dose therapy is discussed more extensively in Chapter 2.

C. **Pharmacologic causes of resistance.** Apparent resistance to cancer chemotherapy can result from poor or erratic absorption, increased excretion or catabolism, and drug interactions, all leading to inadequate blood levels of the drug. Strictly speaking, this result is not true resistance; but to the degree that the insufficient blood levels are not appreciated by the clinician, resistance appears to be present. The variation from patient to patient at the highest tolerated dose has led to dose-modification schemes that permit dose escalation when the toxicities of the chemotherapy regimen are minimal or nonexistent, as well as dose reduction when toxicities are great. This regulation is particularly important for some chemotherapeutic agents for which the dose–response curve is steep. Selection of the appropriate dose on the basis of predicted pharmacologic behavior is essential not only to avoid serious toxicity for some agents but also to optimize effectiveness. This has been applied successfully to dose selection of carboplatin by predicting the area under the curve (AUC, i.e., time × concentration) using creatinine clearance.

True pharmacologic resistance is caused by the poor transport of agents into certain body tissues and tumor cells. For example, the central nervous system (CNS) is a site many drugs do not reach well. Several drug characteristics favor transport into the CNS, including high lipid solubility and low molecular weight. For tumors that originate in the CNS or metastasize there, drugs of choice should be those that achieve effective antitumor concentration in brain tissue and are effective against the tumor cell type being treated.

D. Nonselectivity and resistance. Nonselectivity is not a mechanism for resistance but rather an acknowledgment that for most cancers and most drugs the reasons for resistance and selectivity are only partially understood, at best.

Given a limited understanding of the biochemical differences between normal and malignant cells, it is gratifying that chemotherapy is successful as frequently as it is. It is to be hoped that in 20 years we will view current chemotherapy as a crude beginning, and that many more tumor target-directed agents will have been found that have a high potential for curing the human cancers that now defy treatment.

Selected Readings

Baguley, B. C., Holdaway, K. M., and Fray, L. M. Design of DNA intercolators to overcome topoisomerase II-mediated multidrug resistance. *J. Natl. Cancer Inst.* 82:398, 1990.

Baserga, R. The cell cycle. *N. Engl. J. Med.* 304:453, 1981.

Clarkson, B., et al. Studies of cellular proliferation in human leukemia. *Cancer* 25:1237, 1970.

Dalton, W. S., et al. Drug resistance in multiple myeloma and non-Hodgkin's lymphoma: detection of P-glycoprotein and potential circumvention by addition of verapamil to chemotherapy. *J. Clin. Oncol.* 7:415, 1989.

Endicott, J. A., and Ling, U. The biochemistry of P-glycoprotein-median multidrug resistance. *Annu. Rev. Biochem.* 58:137, 1989.

Friedland, M. L. Combination Chemotherapy. In M. C. Perry (ed.), *The Chemotherapy Source Book.* Baltimore: Williams & Wilkins, 1992. Pp. 90–95.

Goldie, J. H. Drug Resistance. In M. C. Perry (ed.), *The Chemotherapy Source Book.* Baltimore: Williams & Wilkins, 1992. Pp. 54–66.

Goldie, J. H., and Coldman, A. J. A mathematical model for

relating drug sensitivity of tumors to their spontaneous mutation rate. *Cancer Treat. Rep.* 63:1727, 1979.

Kinzler, K. W., and Vogelstein, B. Cancer therapy meets p53. *N. Engl. J. Med.* 331:49, 1994.

Morrow, C. S., and Cowan, K. H. Drug Resistance and Its Clinical Circumvention. In J. F. Holland et al. (eds.), *Cancer Medicine* (3rd ed.). Philadelphia: Lea & Febiger, 1993. Pp. 618–630.

Norton, L., and Surbone, A. Cytokinetics. In J. F. Holland et al. (eds.), *Cancer Medicine* (3rd ed.). Philadelphia: Lea & Febiger, 1993. Pp. 598–617.

Schabel, F. M., Jr. The use of tumor growth kinetics in planning "curative" chemotherapy of advanced solid tumors. *Cancer Res.* 29:2384, 1969.

Sikic, B. I. Modulation of multidrug resistance: at the threshold. *J. Clin. Oncol.* 11:1629, 1993.

Yarbro, J. W. The Scientific Basis of Cancer Chemotherapy. In M. C. Perry (ed.), *The Chemotherapy Source Book*. Baltimore: Williams & Wilkins, 1992. Pp. 2–14.

High-Dose Chemotherapy and the Role of Progenitor Cell and Cytokine Support

James A. Neidhart

Intensification of the doses of chemotherapeutic agents is a therapeutic strategy that stems from pioneering preclinical studies in animal models where curability of tumors was usually dependent on delivery of the maximum sublethal dose. A decade ago the clinical translation of this principle was to ensure that the dose of chemotherapy given a patient produced definite but safe side effects. Such doses were and still are considered "standard." In selected patients such a dosing approach can produce cures. In most it does not. This fact led to clinical attempts to escalate doses even further, often producing life-threatening toxicities.

Dose escalation is a nascent and evolving technology. Modern supportive modalities, including antibiotics, anti-emetic agents, transfusion of progenitor cells, and hemato-poietic cytokines, have allowed multifold escalations of the dose of chemotherapeutic agents to levels that would have been lethal in the past. There is considerable and legitimate controversy regarding the value of such dose intensification and which dose-intensified regimens are optimal. Many questions remain and therefore the discussion in this chapter must be interpreted in the context of uncertainty and evolution.

Even the nomenclature is not standardized and is confusing. Modest dose escalations do not produce a better clinical outcome. Several recent randomized trials in lung cancer, lymphoma, and breast cancer demonstrated that dosages high enough to routinely produce marked but non-life-threatening cytopenia for several days do not produce higher complete remission rates or better survival. The terms *high dose* and *dose intensification* are often used to describe these regimens, although dosing levels are sever-alfold below those usually given in the most aggressive pro-grams. The line representing log kill of malignant cells re-mains linear or slightly curvilinear through up to 10-fold dose escalations for many chemotherapeutic agents and particularly for the alkylating agents. Patients with cancer probably have from 8–12 logs of cancer cell burden at the time of initiation of chemotherapy. If the goal of treatment is to attempt to cure, then the additional logs of kill ob-tained with marked as opposed to modest dose escalations may be critical.

For the purposes of this chapter, *dose intensification* and *high-dose therapy* are defined as regimens that always pro-duce life-threatening granulocytopenia, thrombocytopenia, or both of at least a week's duration. The term *preparative regimen* is often used to describe the dose-intensified che-motherapeutic regimen given shortly before the reinfusion of progenitor cells. This suggests that the purpose of the chemotherapy is to prevent graft rejection through immunosuppression. While it certainly may accomplish that end, the primary purpose of the chemotherapy is antitumor effect. At this time there are minimal data supporting an immunotherapeutic effect (graft versus tumor) of the progenitor cell infusion except perhaps in patients with acute myelocytic leukemia. In the discussion that follows, I treat the progenitor cell infusion as a supportive and not a therapeutic procedure and focus on the intensified chemotherapy as the therapeutic modality.

I. Rationale. The cytocidal effect of chemotherapy in cell culture and animal models follows first-order kinetics. Each treatment kills a set fraction of cancer cells irrespective of the starting number, as long as other conditions are uniform. The degree of fractional kill in these experimental systems is dose-dependent. Alkylating agents have the steepest dose-response curves, usually have myelosuppression as their dose-limiting toxicity, and are not cell cycle–specific; therefore, they are the foundation of most dose-intensive regimens. A modest escalation in the dose may result in a much higher fractional kill of tumor cells. The effect of chemotherapy is also highly dependent on tumor characteristics. Large tumors have a lower fraction of actively dividing cells and are more heterogeneous with a higher likelihood of containing chemotherapy-resistant cells. Sublethal chemotherapy also selects for and encourages the development of resistant cells. The use of several chemotherapeutic agents with different mechanisms of action inhibits the development of resistance.

Translating these preclinical observations to the clinic suggests that the optimum treatments would be those using the highest possible doses of agents with a steep dose-response curve as early as possible in patients with previously untreated metastatic tumor. Retrospective analysis of clinical trials for relationships of dose and response suggests that the rate of partial responses increases with increasing dosage. More recent randomized trials, particularly in breast cancer, convincingly documented lower response and survival rates when doses were reduced below those usually given but beg the question of the value of increasing doses substantially above those usually administered.

Dose intensity, therefore, remains an approach based on sound preclinical principles but without convincing clinical justification in most tumor types. The goal of dose-intensive therapy is generally cure or substantially improved survival. Eradication of tumor (cure) in the clinical setting usually means an 8–12 log kill of cancer cells. A complete clinical remission can be obtained with as little as a 4 log cell kill and a partial response (50% tumor reduction) with as little as a 1 or 2 log kill. Less than a complete clinical remission is of little value in this setting and improvement in overall or disease-free survival is the important final end point. Complete clinical remissions are the surrogate short-term markers of potentially successful therapy.

II. **Chemotherapeutic agents and regimens useful in dose-intensive strategies.** Agents are chosen for dose intensification based on the steepness and linearity of their dose-response curves; the absence of nonhematologic toxicities that prevent dose escalation; and when in combination, a synergistic antitumor effect with a minimum of overlapping nonhematologic toxicity. There have been few randomized studies of the various agents to date so the choice of agents and regimens is largely anecdotal and a matter of comfort and personal experience.

A. **Alkylating agents (alkylators)**

1. **Cyclophosphamide** is probably the most widely used chemotherapeutic agent for intensification. Total doses of 5000–7000 mg/m^2 are given over 1–4 days. Aggressive hydration and diuresis and/or administration of mesna are necessary to prevent hemorrhagic cystitis. The nonhematologic dose-limiting toxicities are cardiac or pulmonary. The cardiac effect is a potentially fatal hemorrhagic vascular injury that manifests clinically in up to 25% of patients, within 3–4 weeks of treatment, as heart failure or pericardial effusions. The risk of cardiac toxicity is not cumulative, with repeated doses being tolerated in the patients who recover. The pulmonary toxicity of cyclophosphamide consists of proliferation of atypical type II pneumocytes with fibrosis. It usually manifests clinically within a month of therapy as dyspnea with interstitial x-ray changes and often pleural effusions. Its antitumor effect as a single agent is limited although it is used for enhancing the numbers of circulating progenitor cells for collection by apheresis. Cyclophosphamide spares marrow stem cells and can be used at high doses without progenitor replacement. Cyclophosphamide requires activation in the liver, but there is no evidence that the P-450 system necessary for that activation is saturated at doses used in intensification. Clearance of cyclophosphamide increases quickly following the first dose and there is considerable interpatient variability in plasma concentrations with repeated dosing. Bone marrow–purging programs have used 4-hydroperoxycyclophosphamide, a synthetic analog of the active metabolite of cyclophosphamide that does not require activation for its activity and thus is effective in vitro.

2. **Ifosfamide** is an isomer of cyclophosphamide that is less widely used in intensification regimens. It also requires hydroxylation to an active metabolite. It has been used in total doses of 8–16 gm/m^2 given over 3–4 days. The higher doses saturate activation systems and large amounts of drug can be excreted unchanged (inactive) in the urine. The elimination half-life of the drug is also prolonged at the higher doses. No definite antitumor advantage has yet been established for ifosfamide versus cyclophosphamide

in intensive dosing regimens. Mesna is required to prevent hemorrhagic cystitis and should be given as a continuous infusion and continued for 6–8 hours after the last dose of ifosfamide. As with other alkylating agents, hematologic toxicity is prominent. Central nervous system toxicity manifested by lethargy, confusion, seizures, or stupor may be seen with high doses of ifosfamide. Renal and hepatotoxicity may also be seen.

3. **Thiotepa** and its oxymetabolite triethylenephosphoramide (TEPA) have antitumor activity. Thiotepa penetrates the blood-brain barrier better than most alkylating agents and has bone marrow suppression as its limiting toxicity, with mucositis and central nervous system toxicity only at very high doses. It has one of the steeper dose-response curves and is not cross-resistant with cyclophosphamide. It therefore has been included in many different dose-intensive regimens including the *bialkylator* or *trialkylator* regimens such as those using the combination of cyclophosphamide, thiotepa, and carboplatin. Doses of up to 1100 mg/m^2 have been used but generally a total dose of 700–750 mg/m^2 is given over 3 days. It may increase the risk of hepatic venoocclusive disease when used with other agents known to have that toxicity. TEPA is largely protein-bound and its metabolism may be altered in patients who have hypoproteinemia.

4. **Carmustine (BCNU)** hydrolyses in vivo to form two metabolites active by alkylation or carbamoylation. Due to poor solubility, it is formulated in a 10% alcohol solution, which may account for the hypotension seen during or shortly following administration. BCNU, which undergoes spontaneous hydrolysis, should be used soon after reconstitution, should be protected from light, and is usually given as a 2-hour infusion. The dose for intensive therapy programs is about three times the standard dose, with the most common dose being 600 mg/m^2. Nonhematologic toxicities are delayed and cumulative. Hematologic toxicity is delayed and prolonged. Nonhematologic toxicities consist of venoocclusive disease of the liver, pulmonary toxicity, renal toxicity, and cardiac toxicity. Liver and pulmonary toxicities can be severe and life-threatening.

5. **Busulfan** is a bifunctional alkylating agent that is available only in oral formulation but commonly is used in dose-intensive regimens primarily for leukemia. The elimination half-life is about 3.0 hours in adults and 2.0 hours in children, with considerable interpatient variability in pharmacokinetics. The usual transplant regimen is 1 mg/kg orally every 6 hours over 4 days for a total dose of 16 mg/kg. The major nonhematologic toxicities are venoocclusive disease of the liver and interstitial pneumonitis with fibrosis.

6. **Cisplatin** is an alkylating agent used in dose-intensive regimens primarily because of non-cross-reactive toxicities, synergism with other alkylators, and its broad range of antitumor activity. The dose of cisplatin can be escalated only about twofold to threefold, however, due to renal and neurologic toxicity. The usual dosage in intensive regimens is 150–160 mg/m^2 given over 3 days although doses of 200 mg/m^2 have been used. Cisplatin must be reconstituted in a chloride-containing solution to minimize spontaneous hydrolysis. Aggressive hydration and diuresis are required to avoid renal tubular toxicity. Magnesium wasting due to cisplatin commonly leads to secondary hypocalcemia and hypokalemia so administration of these electrolytes with cisplatin is worthwhile. Peripheral neuropathy and high-frequency hearing loss from cisplatin are long-term side effects and on occasion can be bothersome. These side effects are one reason why cisplatin is not commonly used in dose-intensive regimens for children. Renal toxicity is unusual if careful attention is paid to hydration and to dose modification for underlying renal disease.

7. **Carboplatin** has been explored in dose-intensive regimens as an alternative for cisplatin that might avoid the neurologic and renal toxicities. The hematologic toxicity of carboplatin is substantial when doses are escalated and becomes limiting in dose-intensive regimens that do not use progenitor cell replacement. Carboplatin may exacerbate the hepatic toxicity seen with several agents used in dose-intensive regimens. Doses for intensive therapy range from 800–1600 mg/m^2 usually divided over 5 days. Mucositis and diarrhea may be severe and limiting but are not clearly dose-related. Neurologic side effects can be severe at higher doses and range from cognitive dysfunction to seizures.

B. **Nonalkylating and less commonly used agents**

1. **Etoposide** is a topoisomerase II inhibitor that shows synergism with cisplatin. Its primary nonhematologic toxicities are mucositis at doses above about 1500 mg/m^2 and hypotension from the lipid formulation. It is well tolerated in dose-intensive regimens and while doses of up to 5000 mg/m^2 have been given, the usual dose in escalated regimens is 1200–1600 mg/m^2, which represents a threefold to sixfold increase over standard doses. It has good single-agent activity against lung and germ-cell cancers, leukemia, and lymphoma and is commonly used in dose-intensive regimens.

2. **Other chemotherapeutic agents** may be useful in dose-intensive regimens but either are less commonly used, do not have a wide spectrum of potential applications, or have been incompletely developed at this time. Cytarabine (cytosine arabinoside) is used in high doses for treatment of acute leukemia and in

some regimens for non-Hodgkin's lymphoma but has not been used and is probably of little use in other diseases. Methotrexate and fluorouracil are antimetabolites that were some of the earliest agents used in intensive dosing but can be quite toxic and were never convincingly shown to have substantially greater antitumor effect at the higher doses. Melphalan is an alkylating agent available in the United States only in oral formulation although there is wider use in other countries where an intravenous formulation is available. Mitoxantrone is an anthraquinone that induces breakage of DNA strands, perhaps through an effect on topoisomerase II. To date it has one of the steepest dose-response curves documented in certain in vitro culture systems, although it has not yet been shown to be of greater value in high doses in the clinic. Its dose can be escalated eightfold to 10-fold above standard doses (to about 80 mg/m^2) with minimal nonhematologic toxicity and without inducing irreversible myelosuppression. Paclitaxel (Taxol) stabilizes microtubules leading to mitotic arrest and thus has a mechanism of action different from that of most chemotherapeutic agents. It does not have a steep dose-response curve and neurotoxicity limits dose escalation, but it currently is being explored as a component of dose-intensive regimens.

3. **Total body irradiation (TBI)** has been used since the earliest days of bone marrow transplantation programs for both immunosuppression (prevention of allograft rejection) and antitumor effect. The usual dosage of TBI is 10–12 Gy given as six fractions over 3 days. Fractionation substantially decreases the risk of both interstitial pneumonitis and venoocclusive disease of the liver. Above that dose, pulmonary, hepatic, and gastrointestinal toxicities become limiting and life-threatening with little therapeutic gain. Currently TBI is used to a limited extent and almost exclusively in marrow transplantation programs for leukemia or lymphoma.

C. **Regimens.** The many regimens used for dose intensification are largely empiric and few have been compared in randomized trials. Important issues such as optimum combinations or doses, the benefit of an "induction" regimen before intensification, and the benefit of repeated cycles of dose intensity have not been addressed. Generally single agents given in doses high enough to produce life-threatening toxicities have not produced a better and more durable antitumor effect and thus have a poor therapeutic ratio. More fundamentally, to date there have been no reported randomized trials of true dose-intensive regimens compared to standard regimens or to regimens with modestly escalated doses. The common themes of dose-intensive regimens at present are reliance on alkylating agents or agents such as topoisomerase inhibitors that might act synergistically with alkylators. Selected regimens that are used more commonly or demonstrate current directions are listed here, with references provided in Selected Readings, not as an endorsement but for information only.

1. **CPB** is a trialkylator regimen popularized at Duke University by Peters and used primarily for the treatment of advanced or high-risk breast cancer. An induction regimen of four cycles of cyclophosphamide, doxorubicin, and fluorouracil (CAF) is followed by dose-intensive therapy with cyclophosphamide at 1875 mg/m^2/day for 3 days, cisplatin at 55 mg/m^2/day as a continuous 72-hour infusion (same days as cyclophosphamide), and carmustine at 600 mg/m^2 as a single dose given on the day after cyclophosphamide and cisplatin are given. All patients receive progenitor cell replacement, with bone marrow, peripheral blood stem cells (PBSCs), or both collected during the phase of induction therapy. Patients also receive either filgrastim (granulocyte colony-stimulating factor [G-CSF]) or sargramostim (granulocyte-macrophage colony-stimulating factor [GM-CSF]) and locoregional radiation therapy. In a recent report, serious toxicities consisted of documented sepsis (19%), pulmonary toxicity 1–6 months following treatment (31%), and hemolytic-uremic syndrome (8%). Treatment-related mortality was 11.7% (10 of 85 patients). Fifty-four percent of patients with metastatic breast cancer obtained a complete clinical response with this intensification regimen and one-fourth of those remained free of disease at follow-up of up to 7 years. Seventy-two percent of patients with high-risk breast cancer treated in the adjuvant setting remained free of disease at 2.5 years compared with historical control subjects in whom only 52% of patients remained free of disease at this time point.

2. **CTCb** as most recently used at the Dana Farber Cancer Institute combines four alkylating agents and two progenitor cell rescues for treatment of metastatic breast cancer. Patients receive three to four induction cycles of cyclophosphamide at 1200 mg/m^2 and doxorubicin at 75 mg/m^2 followed by two cycles of doxorubicin at 75 mg/m^2 and fluorouracil at 1500 mg/m^2. Marrow and peripheral blood progenitor cells (PBPCs) are harvested following the first and second regimens, respectively. Melphalan is given at a dose of 140–180 mg/m^2 followed by PBPCs. Patients then receive cyclophosphamide at 6000 mg/m^2, thiotepa at 500 mg/m^2, and carboplatin at 800 mg/m^2 with marrow, PBPCs, and G-CSF. Cytopenic fever developed in most patients receiving this regimen and documented sepsis or infection occurred in about 20%. Severe stomatitis was seen with 35–45% of the intensification cycles. The average length of hospitalization was 31 days for the two cycles. There were no treatment-related deaths. The complete remission (CR) rate in patients with metastatic but previously

untreated breast cancer was 35%, with a progression-free survival rate of 52% at 15 months.

3. **CEP or DICEP** uses two alkylators and a topoisomerase inhibitor given for two or three cycles with or without progenitor cell replacement. The CEP regimen uses an average of four cycles of standard induction therapy followed by two cycles of intensification with or without marrow transplantation. The DICEP regimen starts with intensification and is given for three cycles to responding patients. Neither induction treatment nor progenitor cell replacement are used. Cyclophosphamide doses are 5000–5250 mg/m^2; etoposide, 1200–1500 mg/m^2; and cisplatin, 150–180 mg/m^2. Treatment-related mortality is about 8–9%. Severe nonhematologic toxicities occur from less than 20% of cycles and are usually fatigue, vomiting, or mucositis. For metastatic breast cancer, the CR rates for both regimens are about 50%, with overlapping survival curves and a 45% survival rate at about 60 months of follow-up. The CEP regimen now has updated follow-up: 16% of patients remain disease-free for up to 5.5 years. There do not seem to be major differences in hematologic recovery between use or nonuse of progenitor cell replacement for two cycles. Neither is there any definite difference in response rate or durability when three rather than two cycles are used or when an induction regimen is used, although these two regimens have not been directly compared.

4. **BUSCY** is a bialkylator regimen reported almost exclusively for the treatment of leukemia and believed to require progenitor replacement. Cyclophosphamide is given at a dose of 120 mg/kg (4800 mg/m^2) and busulfan, at 16 mg/kg in divided doses over 4 days. This regimen is usually supported with an allogeneic transplant so graft-versus-host disease is the primary toxicity, with up to a 27% treatment-related mortality. This is the only dose-intensive regimen that has been directly compared to another in a randomized study. (See sec. **II.C.5**.)

5. **CyTBI** is the original "preparative regimen" used for marrow transplantation and today is used primarily for the treatment of leukemia or lymphoma in certain institutions. Cyclophosphamide is commonly given at 4800 mg/m^2 (120 mg/kg) divided in two or more doses over 2 days, while TBI is given at the doses and schedule such as are outlined in the previous section (**II.B.3**). CyTBI was better than BUSCY in a randomized trial entering patients with acute myelogenous leukemia in their first CR. Mortality was lower (3 versus 27%) and the disease-free survival rate was better at 3 years (73 versus 49%).

6. **CBV** is a variant of the CPB regimen with a substitution of moderate-dose etoposide (750 mg/m^2) for the cisplatin and a lower dose of carmustine (300 mg/m^2). Not surprisingly, the toxicities are less and the

regimen is fairly well tolerated. This regimen was developed at the M.D. Anderson Cancer Center and popularized for use in lymphomas at the University of Nebraska. A variant of CBV with higher doses of cyclophosphamide (7.2 gm/m^2), carmustine (600 mg/m^2), and etoposide (2400 mg/m^2) was reported to have higher CR rates but also three times the mortality (21 versus 7%).

III. **Progenitor cell replacement** became a possibility over four decades ago with the observation that lethally irradiated mice survived after marrow replacement. Sporadic attempts at bone marrow transplantation in humans occurred over the next 20 years but only in the last 15 years has there been intensive laboratory and clinical investigation. The hematopoietic stem cell has now been characterized in humans to the extent it can be isolated and expanded in vitro. Technology now allows molecular tagging and tracking of both normal and malignant cells found in the marrow or peripheral blood. Evolving issues and technologies at this time relate to the use of marrow or peripheral blood as a source of progenitor cells and contamination of marrow or blood by malignant cells with the possibility of subsequent growth of transfused malignant cells.

Hematopoietic recovery following transplantation is believed to occur in two waves, with committed progenitor cells repopulating the marrow within the first month and the true pluripotent stem cell responsible for the delayed but durable component of hematologic recovery. Techniques of marrow harvest and apheresis are not discussed in detail here. The exact number of nucleated cells required for marrow reconstitution has not been established but the usual number of cells administered is 1–3 × 10^8/kg of weight of the recipient or a ½ to 1 liter of donor marrow. Processing of marrow or peripheral blood is not complicated and is within the capabilities of most institutions with large oncology programs. Basically the nucleated cells are enriched by differential centrifugation; cryopreserved slowly, usually with dimethylsulfoxide; then rapidly thawed at the bedside; and infused intravenously approximately 36–48 hours after the last dose of intensive chemotherapy.

A. **Allogeneic marrow transplants** are used mostly for the treatment of leukemia (73%) or marrow insufficiency syndromes such as aplastic anemia or thalassemia major. Only 10% are for lymphoma or other malignancy, according to figures from the International Bone Marrow Transplant Registry (IBMTR). Most allogeneic transplantations are and should be done at institutions that perform at least five per year. Approximately 350 institutions worldwide were known to have active allotransplantation programs in 1990, with about 90 in the United States. Twins (syngeneic transplant) or human leukocyte antigen (HLA)–identical siblings are the preferred donors although nonrelated but matched donors can now be obtained through international donor registry programs. Still, finding a donor is often a problem and only 10% of allogeneic transplants are from unrelated donors, leaving most patients who might benefit without a donor. Graft-versus-host disease is the most common cause of treatment-related mortality. Treatment-related deaths occur in 3–10% of recipients of transplants from a twin and in 21–34% of recipients of transplants from an HLA-identical sibling for leukemia. A lower relapse rate in patients receiving marrow from an HLA-matched sibling than in those receiving marrow from a twin is the strongest evidence for a graft-versus-leukemia effect, although the higher mortality in the former group results in comparable overall survival rates.

B. **Autologous bone marrow transplants (ABMTs)** are available in most patients but have the problem of contamination by malignant cells. Tumor cells commonly are found in the marrow of patients with breast cancer, even in the early stages. About one-fourth of patients with advanced breast cancer have detectable cells in the peripheral circulation and this number increases to 100% following techniques for mobilization of stem cells. Similar findings but with lower rates of contamination have been reported for lymphoma and lung cancer. There is no doubt that malignant cells contaminating progenitor cell collections repopulate the donor and cause relapse, even after purging. Molecular marking techniques recently have been used to confirm that the source of leukemic relapse in children following dose-intensive therapy with transplantation was the transplanted leukemic cell. This has led to a considerable effort to purge the progenitor cells of tumor contamination by a variety of techniques ranging from in vitro chemotherapy to immunologic separation. Purging has never been shown to be of value in humans although it has in animal models. An alternative to purging is positive selection of stem cells. This is currently a more realistic possibility with commercial development of columns that retain stem cells on an immunologic basis while discarding tumor and more mature hematopoietic cells. The latter techniques are still investigational.

C. **Peripheral blood stem cells (PBSCs)** may be used as the source of progenitor cells in addition to or in place of bone marrow. While bone marrow transplantation is the traditional means of replacing progenitor cells, PBSCs have many potential and proven advantages and may become the preferred method in the near future. The advantages of bone marrow include less time for collection, although hospitalization and anesthesia are required, and the theoretical argument that marrow may contain a larger proportion of long-term repopulating stem cells and therefore produce more durable marrow reconstitution. In nonrandomized studies, PBSCs produced a shorter time to granulocyte recovery, which has been attributed to a larger number of more mature and committed progenitors in PBSCs than in marrow. Data regarding the relative time to recovery of platelet counts following marrow or PBSC transplantation are still conflicting, although there is no apparent disadvantage to using PBSCs. Chemotherapy, hematopoietic cytokines, or both can be used to mobilize progenitor cells from the marrow, increase the yield of progenitor cells with each pheresis, and therefore decrease the number of phereses and time required to collect PBSCs. Unfortunately, mobilization techniques also seem to increase the frequency and number of circulating tumor cells. Chemotherapeutic agents used for mobilization include high-dose cyclophosphamide, cytosine arabinoside, fluorouracil, carboplatin, or even combinations such as CEP. Both GM-CSF and G-CSF are effective in mobilization but use in combination with chemotherapy increases the yield of progenitor cells. The most effective means of removing tumor from progenitor collections seems to be *positive selection of progenitors* using CD-34 monoclonal antibodies for immunoabsorption, which can decrease tumor contamination by 1 to 4 logs. This technique is experimental at this time.

D. Hematopoietic cytokines shorten the time to granulocyte recovery following either bone marrow or PBSC replacement or following dose-intensive chemotherapy without progenitor replacement. Time to platelet recovery is not substantially improved with the cytokines presently available clinically. GM-CSF (sargramostin) usually has been given intravenously as a continuous 1- or 2-hour infusion when used with transplantation programs or as a once- or twice-daily subcutaneous injection with dose-intensive regimens not using progenitor replacement. Doses are usually in the $250-500\text{-}\mu g/m^2$ range, although no convincing comparisons of dose, route, or schedule have been done. G-CSF (filgrastim) has been less widely used in dose-intensive regimens but seems to provide comparable times to recovery as those seen with GM-CSF. Doses range from $10-60$ $\mu g/kg$ ($400-2400$ $\mu g/m^2$) but the optimum dosing schema has not been demonstrated yet. Hematopoietic cytokines are generally started the day of or following progenitor replacement or about 3 to 4 days after chemotherapy. They are usually started the day following chemotherapy in dose-intensive regimens not using progenitor replacement. When used at the usual doses in conjunction with intensive chemotherapy regimens, cytokines do not contribute to overall toxicity and may alleviate some nonhematologic toxicities such as stomatitis. Several new hematopoietic cytokines IL-3, PIXY 321, IL-6, IL-11, stem cell factor) are presently in trial, with the goal of shortening the time to platelet recovery.

E. Dose-intensive therapy given without progenitor cell replacement offers several theoretical and practical advantages. The original motivation for regimens such as DICEP was to develop a dose-intensive chemotherapy that could be given repeatedly, thus theoretically maximizing log kill of malignant cells. Whether the inability to utilize certain agents such as BCNU in these regimens will decrease the rate or durability of response remains to be seen. This approach is obviously the least costly and most sure in terms of avoiding reinfusion of tumor cells with progenitor cells and avoiding the need for purging or progenitor selection. The most effective cytokine support regimen in our hands has been a sequence of GM-CSF at 7.5 μg/kg (300 μg/m^2) daily from the day following chemotherapy (day 4) for 10 days followed by G-CSF at 5 μg/kg (200 μg/m^2) until the granulocyte count reaches 1000/μl. Both cytokines are given as divided twice-daily subcutaneous injections. This is primarily an outpatient regimen. Historically controlled and randomized studies demonstrated that progenitor cells do not hasten recovery with DICEP for the first two cycles. Recovery after the third cycle may be delayed.

IV. Toxicities of dose-intensive therapies can be formidable and life-threatening. They vary considerably with different regimens and the practicing oncologist should be thoroughly familiar with a particular regimen before using it. There is no standard supportive approach to patients receiving dose-intensive therapy. Bacterial and fungal sepsis can be effectively prevented or treated with current antibiotic therapies, and most intensive regimens include an approach to prophylactic antibiotic use. Stomatitis and esophagitis can be severe with some regimens. Hepatic and renal failure or pulmonary toxicities can occur in 20–30% of patients. Cytomegalovirus infections and less commonly, *Pneumocystis carinii* infections can complicate any transplant regimen and can be confused with alkylating agent–related pulmonary toxicity, which can be delayed. In an occasional patient, an acute respiratory distress syndrome that responds to steroid therapy may develop during granulocyte recovery. Transfusion requirements and complications require ready availability of an expert transfusion medicine team. Recommended guidelines for the care of patients are included in the Selected Readings at the end of this chapter.

V. Response and long-term outcomes. The goal of therapy with dose-intensive regimens is to cure or substantially prolong (e.g., by 2–3 years) good-quality survival. The short-term surrogate marker for improved survival or cure is complete clinical disappearance of disease (CR). Partial remissions rarely translate into important increases in survival and represent only a 1–3 log kill of malignant cells. Therefore, partial remission rates have little meaning in dose-intensive regimens except as a hint of activity in refractory patients, and rarely translate to important clinical benefit. As early data accumulate, it also appears that substantially less than one-half rather than a majority of patients with advanced malignancy will obtain durable remissions with current dose-intensive regimens. This might mean that median survival rates will not change but the percentage of patients free of disease at 2 or 3 years may increase. The role of dose intensity is covered in disease-related chapters and is presented only in summary form here.

A. Leukemia

1. **Acute nonlymphocytic leukemia (ANLL)** (also called acute myelocytic leukemia) is curable with initial standard therapy in approximately 30–40% of adult patients under the age of 50 years. These patients cannot be cured with standard therapy after the first relapse. Ten percent of patients with refractory ANLL remain free of disease 10 years after an allogeneic transplantation and few of these experience relapse over the next 10 years. Forty to 75% of patients who received transplants during their first CR remain leukemia-free for up to 10 years. This percentage drops to less than 50% when patients receive transplants during their second CR and to less than 25% when they are treated in later stages. I am aware of no randomized but many nonrandomized comparisons of standard treatment with bone marrow transplantation in patients during their first CR of ANLL. While many investigators argue for use of bone marrow transplantation during first CR, their studies at best showed a collective trend toward improved survival with transplantation, and I believe the question of the best and proper use of bone marrow transplantation in ANLL remains unsettled. The mortality rates of patients who receive allogeneic transplants are high, and the availability of transplants is low. Autologous transplants recently have been used, but the relapse rates with reinfusion of leukemic cells are high and purging techniques imperfect at present. A conservative approach would be to follow patients closely and offer bone marrow transplantation at the earliest relapse or during second CR as secondary standard reinduction regimens improve. Potential donors of allogeneic marrow could be sought before the patient relapses. The graft-versus-leukemia effect is important and a closely matched sibling donor is best if available.

2. **Acute lymphocytic leukemia (ALL)** is curable with standard therapy in the majority of affected children. Even in high-risk patients, there does not seem to be an advantage to early transplantation. Patients who experience relapse and who have an HLA-compatible sibling donor may be considered candidates for transplantation, although there is no definite advantage over aggressive standard therapy. The cure rate for adult patients with ALL is 25–35% with standard therapy, with reports of 40–70% durable remission rate following transplantation during first CR, although again there is controversy and no definite advantage to transplantation.

3. **Chronic myelogenous leukemia** is one of the few noncontroversial indications for allogeneic bone marrow transplantation. Patients with an HLA-compatible sibling donor should undergo transplan-

tation in the first chronic phase of the disease, preferably within the first year of diagnosis. The leukemia-free survival rate at 5 years is 80–90% and is highly dependent on a graft-versus-host (leukemia) effect and the development of donor chimerism. Due to transplant-related mortality, the overall survival rate is about 50% but transplantation is the only potentially curable alternative for these patients. Waiting for the first accelerated phase to develop before performing a transplant results in a 10–20% loss in the leukemia-free and overall survival rates. Patients who experience relapse following allogeneic transplantation may enter a second complete clinical and cytogenetic remission with infusion of donor white blood cells. Due to the mortality rate of allogeneic transplantation and the limited availability of donors, the use of autologous marrow for transplantation has been explored but at this time should still be considered an unproven alternative and used only in the investigational setting.

B. Lymphoma

1. **Hodgkin's disease** is often curable with initial standard therapy but approximately a third of patients still experience relapse or fail to enter a first CR. Second-line standard therapies are not curative in the majority of patients. The CR rate following dose-intensive therapy and transplantation for relapsed Hodgkin's disease is about 50%, with half of these remissions being durable. Patients who undergo transplantation during their first sensitive relapse (obtaining a CR to a standard salvage chemotherapy regimen) have about a 40% chance of remaining free of disease at 10 years. A variety of different chemotherapeutic regimens have been used, with none showing a definite advantage in terms of disease-free survival, although the more aggressive regimens often have a higher response rate initially with a trade-off of higher mortality. There is no survival advantage to allogeneic versus autologous transplants although there is some evidence for a graft-versus-lymphoma effect. The most commonly used regimen in this country is probably CBV while BEAM (BCNU, etoposide, cytarabine, melphalan) is most widely used in Europe.

2. **Non-Hodgkin's lymphoma** initially was treated with dose-intensive regimens when patients experienced relapse and were refractory to secondary standard therapy. In this setting the survival rate was only about 20% and the CR rate about 25%. Patients who failed to achieve even a first CR with standard therapy did not do well with transplantation. The ability to administer repeated cycles of dose-intensive therapy does seem to improve outcome in this setting, with a CR rate of 50% and a 5-year survival rate of about 50% following three cycles of DICEP

without progenitor replacement. Patients with earlier and more chemosensitive disease do better with dose-intensive treatment than do those with refractory disease. The results of DICEP are similar to those of ABMT, since the progression-free survival rate for patients treated while in an untreated relapse or a chemosensitive relapse is also about 50% after a single-cycle dose-intensive therapy followed by ABMT. Repeated cycles of DICEP in this setting have not yet been reported. There is no regimen proved best for lymphoma nor is there an advantage to use of allogeneic rather than autologous transplants. There has not yet been a randomized comparison of dose-intensive therapy versus standard therapy in high-risk lymphoma, of various transplant regimens against each other, or of repeated cycles of dose intensity (e.g., DICEP) versus single cycles. The use of dose-intensive therapies and transplantation has now become accepted in this country, primarily due to the lack of a good alternative therapy and a proven long-term disease-free survival rate with intensive therapy.

C. **Breast cancer** remains a very controversial disease in terms of the value of ABMT or dose intensity in general. The CR rates following intensive combination chemotherapy are in the range of 50%, compared to 5–10% following standard therapy. Unfortunately, most of these CRs are not durable, with about 20% of patients alive and free of disease at 6–7 years, although the overall survival rate seems to be in the range of 40–50%, which is better than the 20% five-year survival rate that would be expected with standard therapy. Pending completion of a randomized trial in metastatic disease, this controversy will probably not be laid to rest in the medical literature. There is no dose-intensive regimen that is clearly the best, although the CPB, CEP, and DICEP regimens have the longest follow-up times and are comparable in terms of outcome. Several randomized trials currently are evaluating the use of dose-intensive therapy in the adjuvant setting.

D. **Other malignancies** have been treated with dose-intensive regimens and transplantation, but in a preliminary way without convincing evidence of benefit. In some diseases such as testicular cancer, myeloma, and ovarian cancers, these therapies have shown encouraging results in early studies and clearly should be evaluated further. In others such as renal cancer, malignant melanoma, colon cancer, and arguably sarcoma, there has been no tendency to an improved CR or survival rate with dose-intensive therapies although the patient numbers are generally small. Results for small-cell cancer of the lung have been disappointing, with high CR rates but no improvement in survival. There are few reported studies on non-small-cell lung cancer, cervical cancer, and oropharyngeal cancers, particularly in combination with other therapies in early disease.

Selected Readings

Armitage, J. O. Bone marrow transplantation. *N. Engl. J. Med.* 330:827, 1994.

Ayash, L. J., et al. Double dose-intensive chemotherapy with autologous marrow and peripheral-blood progenitor-cell support for metastatic breast cancer: a feasibility study. *J. Clin. Oncol.* 12:37, 1994.

Dunphy, F. R., et al. Treatment of estrogen receptor-negative or hormonally refractory breast cancer with double high-dose chemotherapy intensification and bone marrow support. *J. Clin. Oncol.* 8:1207, 1990.

Eddy, D. M. High-dose chemotherapy with autologous bone marrow transplantation for the treatment of metastatic breast cancer. *J. Clin. Oncol.* 10:657, 1992.

Gale, R. P., et al. Identical-twin bone marrow transplants for leukemia. *Ann. Intern. Med.* 120:646, 1994.

Neidhart, J., et al. Multiple cycles of dose-intensive cyclophosphamide, etoposide, and cisplatin (DICEP) produce durable responses in refractory non-Hodgkin's lymphoma. *Cancer Invest.* 12:1, 1994.

Peters, W. P., et al. High-dose chemotherapy and autologous bone marrow support as consolidation after standard-dose adjuvant therapy for high-risk primary breast cancer. *J. Clin. Oncol.* 11:1132, 1993.

Rowe, J. M., et al. Recommended guidelines for the management of autologous and allogenic bone marrow transplantation. *Ann. Intern. Med.* 120:143, 1994.

Principles of Therapy with Biologic Response Modifiers and Their Role in Cancer Management

David R. Parkinson

I. **Definition of biologic therapy.** The term *biologic therapy* describes a variety of agents and therapeutic approaches that have evolved from advanced understanding of the biology of the immune system, the nature of tumor cells, and the relation between them. The description of cellular antitumor mechanisms, isolation and production in pharmacologic amounts of the proteins that regulate the activity of these cells, and development of monoclonal antibody (MoAb) technology have permitted clinical applications in humans that were derived from preclinical studies in animal tumor models.

II. **Biologic agents.** A series of proteins are responsible for the growth and development of cells of the hematopoietic and lymphoid systems. The nomenclature is confusing and misleading. A *cytokine* is a protein produced and secreted by a cell; therefore a *lymphokine* is a cytokine produced by a lymphocyte. Although many of these regulatory proteins stimulate the growth of certain cells expressing their specific cell surface receptors, they may have other widespread biologic effects as well, including antiproliferative, differentiation-inducing, or functional activation effects. These properties expand the possible applications of these proteins, but they also complicate their study and are responsible for some of the pleiotropic side effects noted when these cytokines are administered as drugs.

   A. **Cytokines.** Several of the central regulatory cytokines have been isolated, and some, e.g., interferon alpha (IFN-α), are now in general clinical use. Others are still under study for their possible roles in cancer medicine.

      1. **Interleukin-1 (IL-1).** The two forms of IL-1 (alpha and beta) are produced by a wide range of cells after stimulation. These cytokines, which bind to a common receptor, are among the most pleiotropic with regard to their biologic properties. IL-1 plays an important role in inflammation, inducing fever and acute-phase reactant release, and it may play a role in tissue repair following injury. Furthermore, IL-1 has immunostimulatory properties that help to activate T lymphocytes and to induce the production of other cytokines. It both induces and is a cofactor for hematopoietic growth factors such as granulocyte and monocyte colony-stimulating factors. Experimentally, IL-1 is both a chemoprotector and a radioprotector, protecting animals against otherwise lethal myelosuppressive doses of cytotoxic agents. For

these reasons, IL-1 has been studied in wound healing, as an adjuvant in vaccine trials, and for use in association with chemotherapy and irradiation.

2. **Interleukin-2.** Originally termed T cell growth factor, IL-2 is a lymphokine product of activated T cells that binds to a specific cell surface receptor on activated T lymphocytes; the protein is central to T cell proliferation but also activates natural killer (NK) cells. Because of its powerful immunostimulatory properties, IL-2 has been widely studied for its antitumor properties. In animals IL-2 is active as a single agent in a dose- and schedule-dependent manner. For a given IL-2 treatment schedule, antitumor activity can be enhanced by the addition of other cytokines, e.g., IFN-α and tumor necrosis factor-alpha (TNF-α), or by the concomitant use of activated antitumor lymphocytes or monoclonal antibodies directed against the tumor.

IL-2 has been extensively studied in clinical trials in patients. It has single-agent activity against renal cell carcinoma and malignant melanoma. The greatest antitumor effects have been observed with high-dose IL-2 therapy. Single-agent, bolus IL-2 administered intravenously at a dose of 600,000 or 720,000 IU every 8 hours for up to 5 days has received U.S. Food and Drug Administration (FDA) approval for the treatment of metastatic renal cell carcinoma. Such intensive treatment can be administered only to patients carefully selected for cardiopulmonary status. Nevertheless, this therapy is associated with significant toxicity and should only be administered by physicians experienced in its use. IL-2 also forms the basis for adoptive cellular treatment approaches and will be studied together with administration of cancer vaccines.

3. **Interleukin-4.** IL-4 is stimulatory for B cells and together with IL-2 is a growth factor for cytotoxic T cells. This wide range of immunostimulatory properties has led to its study in cancer therapy.

4. **Interleukin-6.** The IL-6 molecule possesses widespread biologic effects. In addition to playing a central role in the induction of the acute-phase response, it is important in B cell growth and differentiation and may interact with IL-2 in T cell differentiation. For these reasons and because it is active as a single agent in tumor models and may serve as an autocrine growth factor in myeloma, both IL-6 and anti-IL-6 treatment strategies are being studied in patients with malignancy.

5. **Interleukin-7 and interleukin-12.** Growth factors for early lymphoid progenitors, these cytokines are important in T cell activation; IL-12 will be studied as a cancer vaccine adjuvant.

6. **Interferon alpha.** Described initially for their antiviral properties, the alpha and beta interferons, the "type I" interferons, subserve a wide variety of bio-

logic effects, some of which have proved useful in cancer therapy. IFN-α has been most widely studied. Its immunomodulatory effect includes activation of NK cells, modulation of antibody production by B lymphocytes, and induction on the tumor cell surface of major histocompatibility complex (MHC) antigens, making the tumor more susceptible to immune-mediated killing. However, the principal antitumor effects of this interferon are probably related to its direct antiproliferative effects.

IFN-α is an active agent in hairy-cell leukemia (for which it is approved) and in the early phase of chronic myelogenous leukemia. It has activity as well in low-grade non-Hodgkin's lymphoma, multiple myeloma, and cutaneous T cell lymphoma. Some solid tumors, principally melanoma and renal cell carcinoma, but also some squamous cell and basal cell carcinomas of the skin, have responded to interferon. Other clinical indications for the use of IFN-α include chronic infection with hepatitis C, condyloma acuminatum, and juvenile laryngeal carcinomatosis.

7. **Interferon gamma.** This interferon has weaker antiviral and a wider range of immunobiologic properties than IFN-α. It activates monocytes and macrophages, thereby upregulating Fc receptors, enhancing phagocytosis, and killing intracellular organisms. It increases the surface expression of MHC and tumor-associated antigens. IFN-γ has been disappointing as an antitumor agent when used alone, and it is now being studied in combination with other biologic agents. It is effective in chronic granulomatous disease where its prophylactic use decreases the incidence and severity of infections.

8. **Tumor necrosis factor.** Originally named for their antitumor effects in animal models, TNF-α and TNF-β ("lymphotoxin") are the products of activated macrophages, share a common receptor, and subserve a wide variety of biologic effects. They serve as growth factors for fibroblasts, have some antiviral activity, activate procoagulase activity on endothelial cells, and activate osteoclasts. Immunomodulatory effects include the induction of surface MHC antigens and interaction with other cytokines such as IL-2, but TNF is directly cytotoxic to some cells, possibly through the induction of oxygen radicals. TNF may play a role in tumor cachexia. It has been shown to inhibit the enzyme lipoprotein lipase. Acute intravenous administration of TNF leads to decreased systemic vascular resistance mediated through the induction of nitric oxide in endothelial cells. The TNF generated during gram-negative shock may be responsible for the lethality of these infections, and strategies for the treatment of this condition involve blocking the effects of TNF. As a single agent, TNF has been inactive systemically in cancer therapy

in humans, perhaps because toxicity, principally hypotension, has limited the doses that can be administered systemically. It has been used more successfully in the treatment of recurrent extremity melanoma, when administered by isolated limb perfusion together with melphalan.

B. Hematopoietic growth factors

1. **Erythropoietin.** Erythropoietin promotes the proliferation and differentiation of committed erythroid precursors. This factor may decrease transfusion requirements during chemotherapy and may be studied together with other factors in bone marrow failure states.

2. **Granulocyte colony-stimulating factor (G-CSF)** is a growth factor with proliferative activity for bone marrow progenitors committed to the neutrophil line.

3. **Granulocyte-macrophage colony-stimulating factor (GM-CSF).** Much more than G-CSF, GM-CSF exhibits its predominant proliferative effects on multipotential stem cells. However, this protein also inhibits neutrophil migration, potentiates the functions of neutrophils and macrophages, and results in production of a spectrum of cytokines from these activated cells; therefore it has been studied for its ability to reconstitute bone marrow and to activate macrophages.

4. **Interleukin-3.** Also known as "multi-CSF," IL-3 stimulates early multipotent marrow stem cells. The effects of both IL-3 and GM-CSF on these early stem cells can be enhanced by IL-1 and IL-6, suggesting that in the future these agents may be used in combination.

5. **Macrophage colony-stimulating factor.** Also known as colony-stimulating factor 1 (CSF-1), this growth factor is relatively lineage-specific. It is responsible for the proliferation and activation of monocytes.

6. **Thrombopoietin (TPO).** This recently isolated factor enhances megakaryocyte development and will enter clinical trials for prevention and treatment of thrombocytopenia.

C. Other growth factors and regulatory proteins

1. **Transforming growth factors (TGFs).** This group of regulatory molecules has profound effects on growth and differentiation. TGF-α is related to epidermal growth factor (EGF) and binds to the EGF receptor. TGF-β, an immunosuppressive protein, also enhances wound healing. It is being studied clinically for this use and for possible prevention or treatment of chemotherapy-associated mucositis.

2. **Other growth and differentiation factors.** It is becoming increasingly clear that a spectrum of proteins important in the control of growth, differentiation, and function exists for all organ systems. Further understanding of these proteins and their receptors will allow greater understanding of their

roles in normal and disordered biology. Some of these proteins or their receptors may ultimately find a role in therapeutics.

D. Monoclonal antibodies. Antibodies binding to tumor-associated cell surface antigens can result in the destruction of tumor cells through a number of possible mechanisms, including activation of complement and antibody-dependent cell-mediated cytotoxicity (ADCC). Furthermore, these antibodies may be useful as means of targeting cytotoxic radioisotopes, toxins, or drugs to tumors, enhancing their delivery to tumors while minimizing systemic exposure. MoAb technology has made important contributions to cancer medicine by allowing the study of differentiation-associated antigens and the phenotypic characterization of both hematopoietic and solid tumors. Antigens expressed with relative specificity on tumor cell surfaces have been defined and have served as targets for diagnostic and therapeutic applications of antibodies.

1. **Murine MoAb.** The first MoAbs used in vivo diagnostically and therapeutically were murine. Studies have pointed out the ability of particular MoAbs to bind selectively to tumors, but have also revealed the complexities involved in the clinical use of these agents. Relative distribution and densities of antigen on normal and malignant tissues, the affinity of the antibody for the antigen, and the behavior of the antigen after antibody binding all have effects on the success of this approach. The internal modulation of antigen from the cell surface after antibody binding is an impediment for treatment strategies using antibody alone, a necessity for immunotoxins or chemoimmune conjugates, and irrelevant to radioisotope therapeutic strategies.

   Murine antibodies are weak activators of the human immune system, and when used alone against T or B cell lymphoid malignancies, they have generally exhibited only transient antitumor activity. The antibodies against solid tumors have been largely inactive when studied in clinical trials. A problem with the repeated use of murine MoAbs has been the development of human anti-mouse antibodies (HAMAs).

2. **Human MoAbs.** Although human antibodies have the theoretical advantage of less immunogenicity, longer half-life, and greater immunologic activity, they have been difficult to generate in pharmacologic quantities.

3. **Chimeric and humanized MoAbs.** A solution to the problems just described has been the generation of genetically engineered antibodies, which combine the antigen-binding properties of the murine antibodies with the advantages of a human antibody backbone (chimeric antibody) or which have had mouse-specific sequences altered (humanized antibody) to decrease immunogenicity.

   4. Antibody fragments. Small antigen-binding proteins, either antibody fragments such as $F(ab')_2$, or single-chain antigen-binding proteins, may have shorter half-lives, greater access to tumor, and advantages as targeting agents.

   E. Antiangiogenesis agents. A number of agents are now being studied clinically for their ability to interfere with tumor new blood vessel formation. Several interfere with the production or binding of either basic fibroblast growth factor (bFGF) or vascular endothelial-derived growth factor (VEGF), two important angiogenic polypeptides. IFN-α, analogs of the antibiotic fumagillin, and platelet factor-4 are all being studied in this regard.

III. Biologic strategies in cancer therapy

   A. Single-agent therapy. As noted already, some cytokines, principally IFN-α and IL-2, have been active as single agents in cancer therapy. In the case of IFN-α, the doses necessary for an antitumor effect range from the very low doses necessary for hairy-cell leukemia (as low as 2–5 MU given subcutaneously daily of either IFN-α_{2a} or IFN-α_{2b}) to the higher doses necessary for melanoma (as it was used in adjuvant melanoma trials conducted by the Eastern Cooperative Oncology Group), which are associated with significant side effects. This problem is even more of an issue with IL-2, as noted already, where the doses necessary for an antitumor effect may be associated with life-threatening toxicity. Current treatment strategies are designed to understand mechanisms of both antitumor effects and toxic effects in the expectation of developing less morbid, more effective therapy. One long-discussed but unproven tenet of biologic therapy is that since the optimal immunobiologic effects ("optimal biologic dose") observed with an agent may be significantly less than the maximally tolerated dose (MTD), clinically useful effects may be observed at low, nontoxic doses. However, the validity of this concept can be tested only through clinical trials. At least with IL-2, the MTD appears to be associated with the greatest clinical activity.

   B. Combination therapy. Since preclinical models suggest that combinations of biologic agents have greater therapeutic effects than single agents, clinical trials have studied the effects of immunostimulatory cytokines such as IL-2 administered together with MoAbs or with activated antitumor lymphocytes such as lymphokine activated killer (LAK) cells or cells generated from the tumor itself.

   Preclinical studies suggest that certain combinations of biologic and cytotoxic agents may be synergistic. TNF, for example, is both a radiosensitizer and an enhancer of the antitumor effects of topoisomerase inhibitors such as etoposide. Interferon similarly enhances the antitumor activity of cisplatin and fluorouracil, and these combinations have been studied extensively in clinical trials.

C. Adoptive cellular therapy, gene therapy, and cancer vaccines. This treatment strategy involves the transfer of antitumor effective cells to the tumor-bearing host. To date, these cells have principally been either LAK cells generated by in vitro activation of peripheral blood lymphocytes with IL-2 or expanded populations of lymphocytes generated from the patient's own tumor. In some cases these tumor-infiltrating lymphocytes (TILs) can be shown to exhibit specific cytotoxicity against the autologous tumor. While this treatment approach is still experimental, it has allowed the isolation and characterization of human melanoma antigens recognized by T cells, including MAGE-1 and -3, MART-1, gp100, and tyrosinase. Cloned antigens have been used in the creation of vaccines involving peptides or vaccinia virus. Alternatively, gene transfer techniques have been used to increase the immunogenicity of autologous tumor cells, for use in vaccination strategies.

D. Targeted therapy. As noted already, tumor-associated surface structures, either tumor-associated antigens or receptors, can be used for targeted therapy.

    1. Immunotoxins. Conjugates of plant toxins, such as ricin or *Pseudomonas* exotoxin to MoAbs, have been used in therapeutic approaches, with responses noted in non-Hodgkin's lymphoma and chronic lymphocytic leukemia. Disadvantages of this strategy include the fact that target antigens must be internalized after antibody binding, antigen-negative cells can escape, and the plant toxin may be immunogenic.

    2. Chimeric toxins. Fusion genes composed of the cytotoxic portions of bacterial genes (e.g., diphtheria toxin or *Pseudomonas* exotoxin) and targeting ligands (e.g., the cytokines IL-2 or TGF-α) can be used to produce cytotoxic chimeric proteins that target specifically to cells expressing the respective high-affinity receptor. IL-2/diphtheria toxin fusion protein has been active in the clinic against IL-2 receptor-expressing malignancies, including chronic lymphocytic leukemia and mycosis fungoides.

    3. Radioimmunotherapy. The selective targeting of radioisotopes to tumor presents many theoretical advantages over external beam radiation with regard to therapeutic index. In addition, owing to the bystander effect, even antigen-negative cells may be killed in this approach, and antibody need not be internalized for the therapy to be effective. Difficulties to date have included the necessity of developing more stable linker chemistry for the attachment of isotopes other than iodine, the poor radiation characteristics of the iodine isotopes used in the initial studies, and the limitation of dose escalation by myelosuppression using the initial radioimmune conjugates. Nevertheless, radioiodinated MoAbs against B cell antigens have been used successfully in the treatment of chemotherapy-refractory non-Hodgkin's lymphoma. Conjugates using isotopes such as yttrium 90 are under development; and together with dose fractionation and hematopoietic growth factors, they may permit delivery of therapeutic doses of radiation to solid tumors.

4. **Chemoimmunotherapy.** This potential therapeutic strategy has been hindered by a lack of good conjugation technology and appropriate chemotherapeutic agents. Doxorubicin-antibody constructs are being studied clinically.

E. **Reduction of chemotherapy or irradiation toxicity.** The hematopoietic growth factors have been studied extensively with regard to their ability to decrease the length of myelosuppression, the depth of the neutrophil nadir, the number of febrile events, and the incidence of mucositis following administration of cytotoxic drugs or radiation. There are several settings in which these factors have been utilized in association with myelosuppressive chemotherapy. The American Society of Clinical Oncology has produced a set of guidelines for the clinical use of G-CSF and GM-CSF, the two approved hematopoietic growth factors in the United States, which were published in the *Journal of Clinical Oncology* in November 1994. Use of these factors is recommended for the following:

1. The reduction of a likelihood of first-cycle neutropenia when this likelihood is otherwise 40% or higher (primary prophylaxis)
2. In further cycles of chemotherapy after occurrence of febrile neutropenia, when maintenance of dose intensity rather than dose reduction is appropriate (secondary prophylaxis)
3. After high-dose chemotherapy followed by peripheral blood stem cell or autologous bone marrow support
4. Rarely in the treatment of established febrile neutropenia, generally only when the infection is life-threatening or is expected to require prolonged antibiotic or antifungal therapy

Recommended doses for G-CSF (filgrastim) are 5 μg/kg/day and for GM-CSF (sargramostim), 250 μg/m^2/day.

F. **Increasing the effectiveness of chemotherapy or irradiation.** Less clear than the toxicity reduction issue is whether the use of myeloid growth factors allows significant increases in dose intensity for chemotherapy, through either dose escalation or a decrease in the interval between chemotherapy cycles. The agents are also being used in conjunction with bone marrow transplantation in attempts to decrease the morbidity and mortality associated with that procedure.

G. **Differentiation therapy.** Many of the myeloid growth and immune stimulating factors described already also have differentiation-inducing properties. The hematopoietic factors, including IL-3 and GM-CSF, are being studied in disorders of bone marrow differentiation, including myelodysplasia and aplastic anemia. Similarly,

Table 3-1. Current status of biologic agents in cancer therapy

Agent	Status
Interferon alpha	FDA-approved for hairy-cell leukemia and AIDS-related Kaposi's sarcoma
	Responses also in chronic myelogenous leukemia, where 10–15% of patients with early chronic chronic phase become Philadelphia chromosome-negative
	Responses in low-grade non-Hodgkin's lymphoma, cutaneous T cell lymphomas
	Under investigation in combination with 5-fluorouracil, cisplatin, and other cytotoxic agents; also in combination with IL-2
	Activity in nonmalignant indications: condyloma acuminatum, chronic hepatitis (B and C), juvenile laryngeal papillomatosis
Interferon beta	Still investigational for use in cancer: has many properties similar to IFN-α; FDA-approved in therapy of multiple sclerosis
Interferon gamma	Active in decreasing infections in chronic granulomatous disease (FDA-approved)
	Under investigation in cancer biotherapy for macrophage-stimulating and tumor antigen-upregulating properties
Interleukin-1	Investigational: under study for wound healing and chemoprotective and radioprotective properties
Interleukin-2	Single-agent activity in metastatic renal cell carcinoma (FDA-approved indication) and malignant melanoma
Interleukin-4	Investigational: immunostimulatory agent
Interleukin-12	Investigational: in clinical trials, potential T cell-enhancing agent
Transforming growth factor-beta (TGF-β)	Potential uses to decrease chemotherapy-associated mucositis, or for myeloprotection; in clinical trial

Table 3-1. (continued)

Agent	Status
G-CSF	Decreases length of myelosuppression following cytotoxic agents; reduces length of neutropenia and incidence of febrile episodes during cytotoxic chemotherapy (FDA-approved)
GM-CSF	Marrow-restorative properties similar to G-CSF; also being studied for monocyte proliferation and activating characteristics
IL-3	Investigational: under study for myelorestorative properties; also being studied in aplastic anemia and myelodysplasia
IL-6	Investigational: under study for its platelet-stimulating activities
M-CSF (CSF-1)	Investigational: potential uses in infections and cancer applications follow from its proliferative and activating effects on monocytes
Monoclonal antibodies	Anti-CD3 approved for treatment of allograft rejection; other antibodies remain investigational for therapeutic purposes
Immunotoxins	Investigational: demonstrate antitumor activity in refractory non-Hodgkin's lymphoma and chronic lymphocytic leukemia
Fusion toxins	Investigational: anti-IL-2 toxin has produced antitumor activity in non-Hodgkin's lymphoma; other cytokine–toxic conjugates under development
Radioimmunoconjugates	Investigational: anti-B cell–iodine 131 conjugates have been active in refractory B cell lymphomas
Antiangiogenesis factors (e.g., platelet factor-4)	Investigational: interference with tumor new blood vessel formation

the interleukins may find application in certain individuals with some inherited or acquired immunodeficiency states. A group of agents active in differentiation, the retinoids, are under study for both treatment and prevention of malignancy. Tretinoin (all *trans*-retinoic acid) is active in inducing remission of acute promyelocytic leukemia. Isotretinoin (13-*cis*-retinoic acid) has induced remissions of advanced squamous cell carcinoma of the skin or cervix and cutaneous T cell lymphoma. Isotretinoin has also been shown to reduce the incidence of secondary malignancies in patients who have had squamous cell carcinoma of the head and neck. Preclinical studies suggest that these agents may be even more active when used together with some of the cytokines and growth factors discussed earlier.

IV. **Toxicities of biologic therapy.** In general, the predictable toxicities of biologic agents are dose- and schedule-related. Administration of the interferons on a daily basis is associated with systemic symptoms, e.g., fever, fatigue, and myalgia. Nonsteroidal anti-inflammatory agents and acetaminophen are useful for alleviating these symptoms, although tachyphylaxis occurs with continued therapy and these symptoms diminish over time.

The toxicities with IL-2 are dose-dependent. The importance of careful patient selection for high-dose IL-2 therapy cannot be overemphasized as the high-dose IL-2 regimens are associated with significant cardiovascular complications, including hypotension and the development of a full-blown capillary leak syndrome. Clinical manifestations include decreased serum albumin, weight gain, and development of peripheral edema in the setting of fluid support for blood pressure. This fluid overload can be associated with pulmonary compromise. Other cardiac complications of high-dose IL-2 therapy include arrhythmias, principally supraventricular, and myocardial infarction. The latter complication is largely avoided by prescreening patient candidates for the presence of ischemic heart disease.

Patients on IL-2 develop a characteristic erythematous rash that may progress to desquamation. IL-2 therapy can exacerbate preexisting psoriasis and, rarely, is associated with the development of a pemphiguslike syndrome.

Patients on IL-2 characteristically have a decreased appetite, and may develop nausea and occasional diarrhea. The development of hypothyroidism has been described in association with IL-2 therapy and rarely with interferon therapy.

Development of neuropsychiatric changes, e.g., confusion, during IL-2 therapy is an indication to halt therapy. Like other IL-2 effects, these problems are reversible, but unlike the others, the neuropsychiatric changes may continue to progress for a while after discontinuation of therapy.

Although corticosteroids prevent or attenuate most IL-2-related side effects presumably by preventing the release of such IL-2-induced cytokines as TNF and IFN-γ, concern over the potential deleterious effects on the antitumor effects of IL-2 precludes their use except in life-threatening situations.

MoAb administration has been associated with hypotension and shortness of breath. The risk of anaphylaxis, greater with repeated dosing, has led to routine administration of an intravenous test dose with anaphylactic precautions (including epinephrine, steroids, and antihistamines) on hand.

The use of ricin-conjugated immunotoxins has been associated with myalgias, elevated serum creatine phosphokinase levels, and occasional rhabdomyolysis.

V. **Current status of biologic agents in cancer therapy.** As noted in Table 3-1, biologic agents have found clinical applications in some cancer-related situations. Many more potential applications are under investigation, limited only by our understanding of the biologic characteristics of these agents and their effects on normal and malignant cells.

Selected Readings

American Society of Clinical Oncology recommendations for the use of hematopoietic colony-stimulating factors: evidence-based, clinical practice guidelines. *J. Clin. Oncol.* 12:2471, 1994.

DeVita, V. T., Jr., Hellman, S., and Rosenberg, S. A. *Cancer: Principles and Practice.* Philadelphia: Lippincott, 1993.

Sznol, M., Parkinson, D. R. Clinical applications of IL-2. *Oncology* 8:61, 1994.

Zalutsky, M. R. *Antibodies in Radiodiagnosis and Therapy.* Boca Raton, FL: CRC Press, 1989.

Principles of Surgery in Cancer Management

Hollis W. Merrick

The traditional role of surgery in cancer management has been diagnosis and treatment of the primary disease. For many years, in fact, surgery was the only curative mode of cancer treatment. Even now more cancers are cured by surgery alone than by any other modality alone or in combination. As additional forms of treatment have become more effective, the role of surgery has evolved and is now often integrated with radiotherapy and chemotherapy. Improvement in surgical techniques and greater knowledge of the cancers often allow better surgical management of the patient with cancer. Furthermore, with longer survival there are more opportunities to perform secondary and tertiary procedures. With the increasing complexity of cancer therapy, it has become apparent that it is in the patient's best interest that the various specialties evaluate the patient and integrate the benefits of their therapy forms at an early stage. However, the involvement of the surgeon remains vital to the care of the patient through all phases of the disease.

I. **Prevention.** Surgeons are frequently the principal providers of care for the patient and family with cancer. They, therefore, are responsible for educating patients about cancer etiology, incidence, and prevention. For example, families of patients with polyposis coli, familial colon cancer, or ulcerative colitis require education concerning the need for frequent examination for cancer. These patients require regular evaluation by colonoscopy and barium enema, since colectomy performed at the appropriate time can prevent the occurrence of cancer. Women with fibrocystic changes for whom there is a history of breast cancer in a mother or sister are at high risk (12 times greater than normal risk) for cancer of the breast and must be encouraged to have regular breast examinations and mammograms when they reach the age of high risk (> 35 years). Similarly, prophylactic mastectomy at the appropriate time can prevent the emergence of breast cancer. Other genetic cancers, such as medullary cancer of the thyroid in multiple endocrine neoplasia (MEN) types IIa and IIb and familial ovarian cancer, can be prevented by prophylactic surgery.

All patients should be apprised of the risks of smoking and the benefit of eating diets low in fat and high in fiber.

II. **Diagnosis.** The key to therapy of any malignant disease is accurate diagnosis. It is best gained by microscopic examination of representative tissue obtained by the surgeon by the least invasive manner possible. The diagnostic technique employed varies depending on the natural history of the tumor being investigated.

A. **Cytology.** The use of exfoliative cytology, as with a Papanicolaou smear, has been instrumental in decreasing the morbidity due to uterine disease. Cells can also be obtained by fine needle aspiration, as from a superficial lesion (e.g., a breast tumor) or from a deep body cavity, such as a lung nodule or a pancreatic mass. Biopsies of organs or sites that are not superficial can be guided under computed tomographic (CT) or ultrasonographic control. Cytologic analysis can provide a diagnosis of cancer. However, major surgical resections usually should not be undertaken on the basis of cytology alone, as the error inherent in the technique is higher than that of the standard histologic diagnosis. Techniques of making the cytologic preparation and the experience of the cytologist are critical to the reliability of this method of diagnosis.

B. **Needle biopsy.** The use of a cutting biopsy needle allows the surgeon to obtain a core of tissue from a suspected tumor that is sufficient for diagnosis of most tumor types. Lymphomas and sarcomas are exceptions for which a larger amount of tissue obtained by incisional or excisional biopsy are usually necessary for accurate and complete diagnosis.

C. **Incisional biopsy.** Incisional biopsy involves removing a wedge of tissue from a large tumor mass. It is often necessary for diagnosis of large masses before major resections and is the preferred technique for diagnosing soft tissue sarcomas. A disadvantage of this technique, however, is the opening of new tissue planes for potential contamination by tumor cells. It is important to place an incision so it is compatible with a subsequent cancer operation, particularly with an extremity or head or neck lesion. Misplacement of an incision can often compromise subsequent surgical management.

D. **Excisional biopsy.** Excision of an entire tumor with little or no margin of surrounding normal tissue may be performed. This technique is acceptable when the excision can be carried out without entering new tissue planes or interfering with subsequent surgical management.

E. **Comments.** Although the type of diagnostic biopsy performed does not directly affect survival, it is generally advisable to avoid contaminating the adjacent normal tissue or entering new tissue planes. Attention should be paid to details of the procedure. The occurrence of a hematoma after biopsy can lead to the spread of residual tumor cells. It has been documented with breast cancer that this complication can lead to an increased rate of local recurrence on the chest wall following primary biopsy. When multiple sites are being biopsied, it is essential to avoid contamination from one wound to another by either instruments or gloves.

Close cooperation with the pathologist is essential to obtain the best results. The tissue must be handled appropriately if such special studies as estrogen receptor analysis, immunohistochemistry, electron microscopy, flow cytometry, cytogenetics, molecular gene analysis, or tissue culture are required from the biopsy specimen. It is important, for example, when doing a breast biopsy to prepare immediately a frozen section of a suspicious lesion. A sample from a positive lesion can be frozen for estrogen and progesterone receptor assays. Placing the specimen in formaldehyde eliminates the possibility of these assays, which may be vitally important for subsequent management of the patient.

III. **Staging.** The need for accurate staging prior to treatment planning has become important in a wide variety of malignancies. Detection of widespread metastatic disease in patients with breast cancer, for example, renders the standard mastectomy an inappropriate procedure. Conversely, in some patients the exact extent of the disease can be determined only through surgery. Staging laparotomy is performed for Hodgkin's disease to plan accurately for more conservative treatment modalities. The requirement for accurately staging (and debulking) ovarian cancer before starting therapy has been demonstrated.

Staging during an operative procedure is also vitally important. For example, detection of positive parapancreatic nodal involvement secondary to cancer of the pancreas would preclude a Whipple resection with its associated high risk of mortality as being a futile procedure. Similarly, with a positive celiac axis biopsy for esophageal cancer, it is important to spare the patient the risk of the morbidity and mortality associated with a hazardous procedure. As a final step of intraoperative staging, placement of metallic clips to define the borders of a tumor (e.g., for cancer of the pancreas) or the level of dissection (e.g., the upper limits of an axillary dissection for breast cancer) facilitates future management planning by the radiotherapist. Care must be taken, however, to use clips that do not interfere with the quality of CT scans or preclude the use of magnetic resonance imaging (MRI).

IV. **Surgery for treatment of cancer.** Surgery is a highly effective modality for curing cancer confined to an accessible site. However, even though all visible tumor may be removed, a significant number of patients have micrometastatic disease at the time of surgery. Extension of the surgery to the regional node-bearing areas may improve survival, but positive involvement of these areas also signifies the probability of distant disease.

The development of additional forms of therapy has given hope to patients who formerly were considered incurable. Similarly, the role of surgery has expanded beyond treatment of the primary tumor to involve a wide variety of palliative, reconstructive, and rehabilitative procedures.

A. **Treatment of the primary cancer.** Appropriate treatment of local disease is vitally important in the management of the cancer patient in order to obtain the best possible control at the outset of the disease. The surgeon usually has the first (and thus the best) opportunity to exercise this control. Most solid tumors are best treated with en bloc resection of the primary tumor and the regional lymphatic drainage areas. It is important to take the appropriate amount of margin that is compatible with a low recurrence rate. For example, a margin of 5 cm from the tumor of colon cancer is compatible with a low recurrence rate. The surgeon must weigh the relative risks and benefits of the surgical procedure proposed with respect to adequate local control and acceptable risk of morbidity and mortality for the patient. A difficult clinical problem, for example, is management of cancer of the pancreas. A Whipple resection offers the best chance to cure the patient. However, only 4% of operated patients live 5 years, whereas the reported operative mortality in multiple series of patients undergoing a Whipple resection is 14%.

The surgeon must be aware of the capabilities of radiotherapy, chemotherapy, or both to improve local and systemic control of the cancer or to be the primary therapy. For example, head and neck cancers may be treated with radiotherapy in conjunction with surgery, or radiotherapy may be the preferred method for treatment of tumors in certain locations. "Neoadjuvant" chemotherapy given to individuals with bulky or initially unresectable tumors (e.g., lung cancer or head and neck cancers) may render the tumors more resectable and lead to a better long-term response and survival. Thus, the surgeon must be aware of improvements in other forms of treatment in the rapidly changing field of cancer therapy so the patient can be offered the optimal overall treatment.

B. Reduction of bulk residual disease. The idea of cytoreductive surgery has undergone much study. Resection of bulk disease for treatment of certain cancers may well lead to increased ability to control residual disease that has not been resected. For example, removing all bulk disease to a size of 2 cm or less renders ovarian cancer tumors more responsive to chemotherapy and improves survival. Therefore, there is an indication for using debulking when an additional form of effective therapy is available. However, to perform this procedure when no other effective therapy is present is of no benefit to the patient and does not extend survival. Debulking, however, is a fertile field for investigation of new modalities. The role of intraoperative radiation therapy for control of small residual bulk tumor or microscopic disease remains to be established. If this technique proves to be effective, it may offer the benefit of significant palliation for solid tumors in conjunction with surgical debulking.

In contrast to solid tumors, debulking is not of value in hematologic malignancies such as lymphoma.

C. Resection of metastatic disease with curative intent. Patients with metastatic disease as the only site of their tumor should undergo resection if it can be accomplished with acceptable morbidity. Examples are metastases to the liver, lung, and brain, which have the potential of being cured by surgery. This method is particularly valid for one to three isolated metastases of slow-growing tumors not responsive to chemotherapy, e.g., adenocarcinomas and sarcomas. Pulmonary metastases from sarcoma are not infrequently the sole site of disease. Up to 30% of patients with pulmonary metastasis can be cured with resection of single or multiple lesions. Similar control rates are found with adenocarcinomas in which the lung disease is the sole site of metastasis. Similarly, hepatic metastases, particularly from colon cancer, can be resected, leading to a long-term cure rate of approximately 25%. Although this method is by far the most effective single modality, studies combining resection and infusion of chemotherapy potentially offer the prospect of improving the survival rate. Resection of solitary brain metastases should also be considered when the brain is the only site of disease. Careful consideration of the functional defect resulting from surgery should be considered in cases of solitary brain metastases.

D. **Establishment of vascular access, infusion, and perfusion (see Chap. 40).** The use of permanent right atrial catheters permits painless, reliable access for administration of chemotherapy and nutrition. These catheters have reduced the incidence of skin complications due to extravasation of drugs and have improved adherence to drug administration scheduling by providing a reliable access site. Infusion devices that are available permit direct administration of chemotherapeutic drugs to an organ site, such as the liver. In addition, peritoneal catheters have provided ready access to the abdomen for chemotherapy of ovarian or colon cancers.

E. **Treatment of oncologic emergencies.** Emergency situations that call for surgical intervention may arise in cancer patients. They usually involve hemorrhage, perforation, and abscess formation. The cancer patient is often at risk because of bone marrow suppression due to chemotherapy or irradiation. Metastasis of tumor to the central nervous system, causing cord compression, may require emergency neurosurgical decompression and radiation therapy for preservation of function.

Selected Readings

Brandt, B., and Ehrenhaft, J. L. Surgical management of pulmonary metastases. *Curr. Probl. Cancer* 5:4, 1980.

Dupont, W. D., and Page, D. L. Risk factors for breast cancer in women with proliferative breast disease. *N. Engl. J. Med.* 313:146, 1985.

rays, gamma rays, and electron beams are the most important forms of external beam radiation therapy.

a. Electromagnetic radiation consists of x-rays and gamma rays. Although their sources differ, these photons are physically identical. X-rays are created through the interactions of electrons with matter, while gamma rays originate from the atomic nucleus during radioactive decay.

b. Particulate radiation

   (1) Electron beams for clinical irradiation are produced by accelerators (betatrons, linear accelerators, microtrons).

   (2) Other ionizing particles include **protons, neutrons, alpha particles, and negative pi mesons.** (See sec. **VIII.D.**)

2. Radiation exposure. The basic unit of radiation exposure is the Roentgen, which is defined as the sum of all electric charges on all ions of one sign produced in air when irradiated by photons divided by the mass of air irradiated by the photons. One Roentgen equals 2.58×10^{14} coulombs/kg of air.

3. Radiation dose. The international unit of absorbed dose is the Gray (Gy), which is 1 joule/kg. One Gy is equivalent to 100 rad (an older term, defined as the absorption of 100 ergs/gm of matter). In this handbook, the term *centigray* (cGy) is used rather than rad (1 cGy = 1 rad).

4. Radiation quality. Radiation quality defines the ability of radiation to penetrate matter below the surface. When considering radiation doses, it is important to know the depth-dose characteristics of the treatment beam employed. As the energy of a radiation beam increases, the more penetrating it becomes.

B. Biologic principles of radiation therapy. Factors that affect the response of malignant (and normal) cells to irradiation include radiation sensitivity, cellular repair capacity, heterogeneity of the cell population, cellular oxygenation, linear energy transfer, relative biologic effectiveness, and position in the cell cycle.

1. Radiation sensitivity is somewhat dependent on histology. In some malignancies the cells are exquisitely radiosensitive (e.g., seminoma and leukemia), whereas in others they are relatively radioresistant (e.g., melanoma and glioblastoma multiforme).

2. Cellular repair capacity for radiation damage is severely lacking in certain histologic variants (seminoma and leukemia) but seems to be enhanced in some neoplastic cells (melanoma).

3. Oxygen is a potent radiation sensitizer, presumably because of its high electronegativity and its ability to scavenge and interact with free radicals. The *oxygen enhancement ratio* (OER), defined as the ratio between the dose for anoxic cells and the dose for oxygenated cells to achieve isoeffect, is approximately

2.5–3.0 for low-energy x-rays. Thus the dose of radiation needed to achieve the same effect is 2.5–3.0 times greater for anoxic cells than for oxygenated cells. This point is important for clinical radiotherapy, as many tumors are thought to contain central hypoxic cores in which cancer cells are alive but the oxygen supply is compromised; hence these cells are radioresistant.

4. **Linear energy transfer** (LET) is defined as the density of ionizing events resulting from a specific type of radiation. Particle beams (neutrons, protons, stripped nuclei, and others) have higher LET than do x-rays or gamma rays. Ionizing events resulting from the passage of particles through tissue are closer together than for photons, and therefore more energy is deposited per unit length of beam path. Because of this increased density of energy transfer, cells are more damaged than they would be from the passage of lower LET beams.

5. **Relative biologic effectiveness** (RBE) describes the observation that different radiations produce different net cellular effects. Orthovoltage (250 kVp x-ray) is the standard for comparison. The radiation dose for a test beam and an orthovoltage beam is determined for an isoeffect level. The ratio of the two radiation doses necessary to achieve the same effect is defined as the RBE for the test beam. For example, most neutron beams employed clinically have an RBE of approximately 3.

6. **Radiosensitivity** is a function of the position of a given cell in the cell cycle. Cells in mitosis are more sensitive to radiation damage than cells in interphase. Cell sensitivity in S phase is lower than in phase G_1 or G_2. If the malignant cells within a tumor could be synchronized in the cell cycle, the response of those cells to radiation could be enhanced by irradiating when most of the cells were in a radiation-sensitive phase.

C. **Clinical principles of radiation therapy.** Radiation treatment depends on the principle of the therapeutic ratio.

$$\text{Therapeutic ratio} = \frac{\text{normal tissue complication dose}}{\text{tumoricidal dose}}$$

If the therapeutic ratio is much greater than 1 (a large normal tissue complication dose compared to the tumoricidal dose), cure without complication can be achieved. On the other hand, if the tumoricidal dose exceeds the normal tissue complication dose in any given clinical situation, the therapeutic ratio is less than 1, and cure without complication is categorically impossible. In many clinical situations, the therapeutic ratio is empirically close to 1, and radiation oncologists use many maneuvers (fractionation of dose, protraction of dose, multiple fields, brachytherapy, shaped fields, displace-

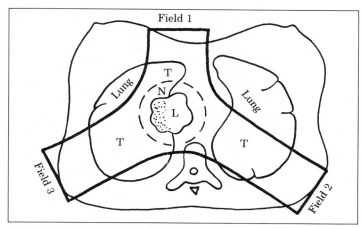

Fig. 5-1. Three-field treatment plan for a hilar lesion (*L*), illustrating the pulmonary tissue as matrix tissue (*stippled*), normal tissue (*N*) within the target volume (*broken line*), and transit tissue (*T*).

ment of normal structures, and others) to enhance the therapeutic ratio. Most of these maneuvers either relatively increase the dose to the disease or diminish the dose to the adjacent normal tissue or transit tissues.

Complications from radiation treatment come not from irradiation of tumors but from the dose to normal tissues (Fig. 5-1). Within the treatment field of any malignant tumor, there exist malignant cells and nonmalignant cells. These cells behave differently in response to irradiation, and it is this differential response that accounts for the existence of the therapeutic ratio. Furthermore, there appear to be differences in the repair of sublethal and potentially lethal radiation injury between normal cells and malignant cells. Radiation oncologists take advantage of these inherent differences by administering repeated fractions of the radiation dose, allowing sufficient time between dose increments for repair of radiation damage in the normal cell population. Protraction and fractionation of radiation dose are used to enhance the therapeutic ratio.

Radiation dose can be delivered by external beam therapy, brachytherapy (intracavitary or interstitial radioisotope therapy), or systemic radioisotope administration.

1. **External beam therapy.** Radiation treatment delivered by a source external to the body is generally referred to as external beam therapy. Superficial beams (90–120 kVp) may be used to irradiate certain superficial lesions of the skin and mucous membranes. Orthovoltage beams (140–500 kVp) may be used to treat slightly deeper lesions that tend to be

infiltrative (skin cancers about the inner canthus of the eye, the junction of the pinna with the scalp, and the nasolabial fold). Superficial and orthovoltage beams deliver maximum doses at the surface of irradiated tissue. The depth of the maximum dose and the penetration of the beam increase with increasing beam energy. Megavoltage beams may be generated by radioisotope decay (^{60}Co teletherapy) or electron accelerators (linear accelerators, betatrons, and microtrons). Electron beams produced by accelerators may be used in situations in which it is desirable to avoid a radiation dose to deeply situated structures while homogeneously irradiating more superficial structures. The effective depth of an electron beam is directly related to the energy of the electrons.

Linear accelerators and ^{60}Co teletherapy units are the most common radiotherapeutic devices in use in the United States today. Effective use of such equipment is enhanced by a radiation therapy simulator, an x-ray imaging device employed to help map out the radiation fields. Modern radiotherapy facilities today are equipped with a radiation therapy simulator, at least one megavoltage radiation therapy device, a source of electron beams, and a treatment planning computer.

2. **Brachytherapy (short-distance therapy)**
   a. **Intracavitary radioisotope therapy** is the instillation or application of radioisotope inside a body cavity. Colloidal suspensions of radioisotope (e.g., ^{32}P) may be instilled in the pleural or peritoneal cavities in situations in which pleural or peritoneal implants of disease, such as ovarian cancer, are less than 2 mm thick (because of the limited range of penetration of the ^{32}P beta emissions) and in which there is no loculation of fluid or obliteration of the anatomic space.

   More commonly, radioisotopes are temporarily brought into immediate proximity with gynecologic malignancies with the use of specially designed applicators. Remarkably high local doses of radiation can be achieved in this manner. The isotopes commonly employed for this purpose are ^{226}Ra, ^{60}Co, ^{192}Ir, and ^{137}Cs.

   b. **Interstitial radioisotope therapy.** Radioactive materials may be implanted temporarily or permanently in malignant neoplasms or in tumor beds. Isotopes commonly used for this purpose include ^{192}Ir, ^{125}I, ^{226}Ra, and ^{137}Cs. Radioactive seeds are commonly employed for permanent interstitial implants, whereas seeds, wires, and needles may be used for temporary implants; the latter procedures are best accomplished using afterloading techniques to minimize radiation exposure of hospital personnel. Interstitial implantation of radioisotope may be employed as the sole treatment modality (e.g., localized prostate cancer), as a boost dose in conjunction with external beam therapy (e.g., early breast cancer, head and neck cancers), or as an adjuvant to surgery (e.g., sarcoma resection bed).

3. **Systemic radioisotope administration.** Radioisotopes may be administered systemically in certain clinical situations (e.g., disseminated thyroid cancer or symptomatic widespread bone metastases from breast or prostate cancer). This form of treatment depends on preferential concentration of radioisotope within neoplastic tissues. In disseminated thyroid cancer, ^{131}I is the radioisotope of choice, whereas ^{89}Sr is used for osseous metastases from breast or prostate cancer. Improvements in the specificity of monoclonal antibodies may make this form of administration of radiotherapeutic agents more useful and more common.

III. **Definitive irradiation.** Radiation treatment is used as a single modality with curative intent in many diseases, including medulloblastoma, skin cancer, certain gynecologic cancers, seminoma, many head and neck cancers, regionally localized breast cancer, nonmetastatic retinoblastoma, Hodgkin's disease, and certain non-Hodgkin's lymphomas. Depending on the clinical circumstances, definitive irradiation may be delivered with external beam therapy, interstitial therapy, intracavitary therapy, and in appropriately equipped facilities with intraoperative radiation therapy. The following are examples of diseases that may be approached with definitive radiation treatment.

A. **Hodgkin's disease.** The malignant cells of Hodgkin's disease are exquisitely radiosensitive. Patients with early-stage disease (I, II, and IIIA) are effectively treated with external beam irradiation as a single modality. Patients with more advanced disease commonly undergo irradiation to areas of bulky disease after induction chemotherapy.

Above the diaphragm, mantle fields (see Fig. 26-1) are used to treat the contiguous lymph node-bearing regions from the mediastinum to the mastoid tip. An inverted-Y field (see Fig. 26-1) is often used to irradiate the contiguous node-bearing areas from the periaortic region to the femoral triangle. Local control of Hodgkin's disease is highly dose-dependent. Doses as low as 35–40 Gy result in 95% control rates for local disease. Mantle and inverted-Y fields are not commonly treated concurrently. Usually a rest period is prescribed for marrow recovery between supradiaphragmatic and infradiaphragmatic courses of radiation therapy.

B. **Laryngeal cancer.** Laryngeal carcinoma confined to the vocal cord(s) is highly curable with external beam irradiation. Small, coplanar opposed fields are used to deliver 60–70 Gy in 6–8 weeks. Wedges or compensators may be necessary to achieve uniform dose distribution within the treatment volume. Such treatment commonly results in preservation of voice that is of much higher quality than that resulting from voice-preserving surgical procedures for laryngeal cancer. For lesions confined to the vocal cord, the success rate is greater than 90%.

C. **Breast cancer.** Radiation therapy is effective treatment for early-stage breast cancer. It has been shown that local control of cancer in patients with primary lesions less than 4 cm in diameter is slightly superior in patients treated with tylectomy and primary radiation therapy compared to modified radical mastectomy; survival is equivalent. The breast is commonly treated with medial and lateral tangential fields to avoid irradiation of pulmonary and cardiac tissue. The regional lymph nodes, if not adequately excised and if not included in the tangential portals, can be treated with anterior and posterior custom-shaped fields that mate the dose profile to the patient's cervicothoracic anatomy. A dose of 45–50 Gy is administered to the breast and sometimes to the regional lymph nodes (usually depending on the findings of the axillary node dissection since extracapsular extension of disease is an indication for axillary irradiation); the tumor bed dose is commonly boosted to 60–66 Gy using (1) reduced fields of photons or electrons or (2) interstitial implantation of radioisotope. A good cosmetic result is achieved in at least 75% of patients. Cosmetic defects are strongly related to the placement of surgical scars and the extent of surgical debulking. Surgery more extensive than complete excision of the lump generally results in a less desirable cosmetic effect and does little to decrease local recurrence.

D. **Gynecologic cancer.** For early cancers of the intact uterine cervix (International Federation of Gynecology and Obstetrics (FIGO) stages I and IIA), surgery and radiation therapy are equally effective. For the more advanced stages irradiation is clearly the treatment of choice. External beam radiation therapy and intracavitary brachytherapy are integrated in the treatment of gynecologic cancer to mate the dose profile to the disease profile. Typically, the "whole pelvis" is irradiated to a dose of 40–50 Gy using external beam therapy. The anatomy of the gynecologic organs, often distorted by neoplasm, frequently returns toward normal as the tumor shrinks under the effects of fractionated ionizing external beam irradiation. This return to normal, of course, facilitates intracavitary placement of radioisotope to deliver high doses of radiation to the pelvic structures involved with tumor. Typically, the intracavitary radioisotope brachytherapy applications are planned with an interval of 10–14 days between 48-hour applications. Optimal interdigitation of intracavitary brachytherapy and external beam therapy is strongly dependent on the disease stage, individual pelvic anatomy (and its distortion by tumor), tumor response to irradiation, and the experience of the radiation therapist.

E. **Other tumors.** Many other cancers may be successfully treated with radiation therapy as a single modality, particularly in the event that patients are medically unfit for surgery or refuse it. Generally, tumors amenable to interstitial brachytherapy tend to have a better prognosis than other tumors. It remains to be seen whether intraoperative radiation therapy can produce similar results in a different spectrum of tumors.

IV. Palliative irradiation. Irradiation is an effective palliative modality for symptomatic patients in many clinical situations.

   A. Symptom prophylaxis. Local irradiation may be administered prophylactically in certain situations based on the known natural history of the disease and the anticipated morbidity thereof. For example, the brain is a known sanctuary site and area of frequent recurrence in patients with otherwise localized oat-cell carcinoma. Prophylactic cerebral irradiation may be administered in such instances. (See Chap. 12, sec. **V.F.** for discussion.) Patients with metastatic breast cancer found to have asymptomatic lesions in the femoral neck or shaft are at risk of sudden fracture with attendant high morbidity. This risk may be significantly reduced by local prophylactic irradiation.

   B. Symptom management. Bone pain, symptoms of brain metastases, bleeding, cough, hemoptysis, visceral pain, and airway obstruction are only a few of the commonly encountered symptoms of cancer that often can be relieved or prevented by local irradiation. Treatment of patients with such problems is highly individualized. The area to be irradiated, the size of the fields, and the timing and fractionation of radiation dose are functions of the extent of disease and various other individual patient factors, including anticipated survival, performance status, and especially prior treatment with radiation and antineoplastic drugs. Palliative radiation doses generally need not be as high as those required for definitive treatment and are often administered in accelerated time-dose fractionation schemes. Brachytherapy is generally reserved for definitive management of cancer but, in highly selected individual cases, may be indicated for palliation of symptoms. In such instances, the use of afterloading techniques, relatively low-energy isotopes (e.g., ^{125}I), or both is especially important from a radiation protection point of view.

   C. Radiation therapy emergencies. Certain cancer problems constitute oncologic emergencies and require the immediate attention of a radiation oncologist and other physicians.

   1. Spinal cord compression
   2. Severe airway compromise
   3. Brain metastasis with rapid or refractory neurologic decompensation
   4. Malignant cardiac tamponade
   5. Superior vena cava compression (usually not a true emergency)

   Radiation therapy consultation should never be delayed in such situations.

V. Radiation effects in normal tissues

A. Organ tolerance.
Normal organs and tissues vary considerably in the extent and type of reaction to therapeutic doses of ionizing radiation (Table 5-1). The severity of the reaction depends not only on the total radiation dose, but also on the size of individual radiation fractions, the overall time of treatment, the volume of the organ or tissue irradiated, and the presence or absence of a whole host of mitigating factors (radiosensitizing drugs, radioprotective drugs, hyperthermia, local tissue hypoxia, etc.).

Table 5-1. Radiation tolerance of normal tissues and organs

Organ	Injury	Dose (Gy) to cause 5-year complication rate of 5%	Dose (Gy) to cause 5-year complication rate of 50%	Portion of organ
I. Potentially severe or fatal radiation injury				
Bone marrow	Pancytopenia	2.5	4.5	Whole
	Aplasia	30	40	Segmental
Liver	Hepatitis	25	40	Whole
Stomach	Ulcer, hemorrhage	45	55	100 cm^2
Intestine	Ulcer, perforation	45	55	400 cm^2
Rectum	Stricture, ulcer	60	80	100 cm^2
Brain	Infarct, necrosis	60	70	Whole
Spinal cord	Infarct, myelitis, necrosis	45	55	10 cm
Heart	Pericarditis	45	55	0.6
Lung	Acute and chronic pneumonitis	30	35	100 cm^2
Kidney	Acute and chronic nephrosclerosis	15	25	Whole
Fetus	Death	2	4	Whole
II. Potentially mild to moderate radiation injury				
Bladder	Contracture	60	80	Whole
Testes	Sterilization	1	2	Whole
Ovary	Sterilization	2–3	6–12	Whole
Lens	Cataract	5	12	Whole/part
Vagina	Ulcer, fistula	90	100	Whole/part
Breast (child)	No development	10	25	Whole
Breast (adult)	Atrophy, necrosis	>50	>100	Whole

Note: Doses of radiation (Gy) needed to produce tissue or organ damage within 5 years of treatment when delivered at a standard time-dose fractionation.
Source: Modified from P. Rubin. *Clinical Oncology.* Rochester, NY: American Cancer Society, 1983.

B. The bone marrow is of particular importance to the radiation oncologist, as it is included to a greater or lesser extent in nearly every radiation therapy field. The marrow is a very sensitive tissue, and the effects of therapeutic irradiation must be monitored in every patient. Table 5-2 summarizes the distribution of active hematopoietic bone marrow in the healthy adult human and provides estimates of the percentage of the total marrow irradiated with several common radiation fields.

C. Acute, subacute, and late effects. In general, radiation effects may be classified as acute (those occurring within 3 months of a course of therapeutic irradiation), subacute (3–6 months), or late (beyond 6 months). For example, nausea and diarrhea may occur during or immediately following a course of pelvic irradiation (acute effects), while rectovaginal fistula formation, if and when it occurs, is usually a late complication of pelvic irradiation. Acute radiation effects are usually mediated via the inflammatory reaction to the physical insult of irradiation, while late effects are mediated via scar formation and contracture or via injury to the intima of small-caliber blood vessels (a late-responding tissue).

Table 5-2. Bone marrow distribution in normal adult humans by skeletal region and radiation field

Site	Marrow volume (%)
Vertebral column	
Cervical	3
Thoracic	14
Lumbar	11
Sacral	14
Total vertebral column	42
Long bones	
Humerus	1
Femur	2
Clavicle	1
Other bones	
Scapula	2
Sternum	2
Ribs (all)	8
Standard fields	
Whole brain	12
Tangential breast and chest wall	4
Mantle	28
Paraaortic	14
Inverted Y	40
Typical anteroposterior-posteroanterior whole pelvis	20
Typical four-field whole pelvis	25

Source: Extracted from R. E. Ellis. The distribution of active bone marrow in the adult. *Phys. Med. Biol.* 5:255, 1961.

The correlation between acute effects and late effects of irradiation is not high.

VI. **Hyperthermia.** There has been a reawakening of interest in heat as a treatment for cancer. Hyperthermia has been used as a sole modality for cancer treatment, but it is much more effective when combined with radiation treatment as a biologic response modifier.

The *thermal enhancement ratio* (TER) is defined as the ratio between the x-ray dose given alone and the x-ray dose given with heat necessary to produce a certain effect. The TER appears to be greatest when heat and radiation are delivered simultaneously, but this situation is often not possible. Clinically, temperatures of 42–43°C are typically employed for 40–60 minutes. Heating may be local or systemic, and it may be delivered in a number of ways, e.g., waterbath, thermal blanket, ultrasound, and microwave. Hyperthermia treatment devices are now commercially available, but the use of heat as a biologic response modifier for radiation treatment is not so common today as it was just a few years ago.

VII. **Combined-modality therapy.** Many oncologic problems are best managed by one of three treatment modalities: surgery, radiation therapy, or chemotherapy. Frequently patients with cancer present with a bulky primary lesion, macroscopically evident regional disease, and perhaps microscopic or submicroscopic systemic disease. For this reason, oncologists often adopt a multidisciplinary approach to the treatment of cancer, selecting two or perhaps three modalities of therapy for sequential or simultaneous use. This approach requires close cooperation between the surgical oncologist, radiation oncologist, and medical oncologist to provide the patient with the best treatment. Although combined-modality therapy is not effective or desirable for all kinds or stages of cancer, the regular practice of a multidisciplinary approach provides the best opportunity to exploit the advantages of each mode of treatment. Surgery and radiation therapy are local treatments. However, cancer is often not a local disease, and systemic therapy is frequently necessary to improve overall disease control.

Irradiation may be used as an adjuvant to chemotherapy or to surgery; chemotherapy may be used as an adjuvant to surgery or to irradiation; or all three modalities may be combined in a given clinical situation.

A. **Irradiation as an adjuvant to surgery.** When surgery and irradiation are used together simultaneously or sequentially, close cooperation between the surgical oncologist and the radiation oncologist is of key importance. If combined-modality therapy is anticipated, even in the form of postoperative irradiation, it is generally in the patient's best interests to obtain a radiation oncology consultation preoperatively. In situations in which the decision to administer radiation therapy postoperatively is made at the operating table, it is best to request intraoperative consultation so that the radiation oncologist can see and palpate the extent of the tumor or tumor bed that will require irradiation postoperatively. In such situations, the appropriate placement of radiopaque localizing markers is of great importance, as is histologic confirmation of cancer, even in patients with clearly unresectable disease. A detailed operative note describing the size and extent of the neoplasm, the fixation or actual invasion of adjacent structures, and the presence of involved adjacent lymph nodes and other structures is of paramount importance.

Patients who require surgical procedures in previously irradiated fields also deserve preoperative radiation oncology consultation. With use of localization films, records, previously applied fiducial marks, and the like, the radiation dose profiles can often be reestablished preoperatively. This method assists the surgical oncologist with incision placement and extent of surgery. For example, if an intestinal bypass procedure is to be performed in a previously irradiated area, it is important to know the borders of the radiation field with some precision so that nonirradiated bowel may be used for each side of the anastomosis. The skin of a previously irradiated neck tolerates J- or U-shaped incisions much better than a trifurcated incision.

Radiation therapy is an effective adjuvant to surgery for many diseases, e.g., stage II testicular seminoma, stages B2 and C rectal carcinoma, and resectable pancreatic adenocarcinoma. Radiotherapy may be delivered pre- or postoperatively, or both ("sandwich therapy"). Intraoperative irradiation is also a possibility. The advantages of preoperative, postoperative, and intraoperative irradiation are outlined in Table 5-3.

B. **Chemotherapy as an adjuvant to irradiation.** Chemotherapy may be employed before, during, or after a course of radiation treatment for malignant disease. Sandwich therapy may also be used with radiotherapy sandwiched between the preirradiation and postirradiation course of chemotherapy.

1. **Preirradiation chemotherapy.** Chemotherapy given prior to a course of definitive irradiation (or surgery) is termed *induction chemotherapy* or *neoadjuvant chemotherapy*. The biologic advantages of such an approach are as follows.

1. Unirradiated tumor vessels permit optimal drug delivery.
2. Nutrition and patient condition are generally better prior to irradiation, permitting improved tolerance to chemotherapy.
3. There is no delay in institution of systemic treatment.

The disadvantages are as follows.

1. Radiation therapy is delayed.
2. Nutrition and patient condition are generally worse after chemotherapy, often resulting in impaired tolerance of definitive radiotherapy.

Table 5-3. Advantages and disadvantages of preoperative, postoperative, and intraoperative irradiation

Preoperative irradiation		Postoperative irradiation		Intraoperative irradiation	
Advantages	Disadvantages	Advantages	Disadvantages	Advantages	Disadvantages
Undisturbed local vasculature, better tissue oxygenation before surgery; tumor more radiosensitive. Less radical surgery may be required.	Definitive surgery is delayed. Postoperative recovery may be prolonged. Increased morbidity. Surgical resection may become more difficult.	May better tailor radiation dose profile to disease profile. Accurate surgical and histopathologic staging of disease. Tissue repair and healing proceed normally.	Disturbed tumor bed vasculature; tumor may be less radiosensitive. Surgical complications may delay irradiation; tumor cells may repopulate.	Small volume of normal tissue irradiated. Dose to normal structures is minimized. Very high doses may be delivered.	Only a single fraction may be delivered. Surgical complications may be increased. Limited availability.

Unresectable tumor may become resectable.

Tumor dissemination during surgery may be decreased.

Tumor cells rendered nonviable before being surgically dislodged into circulatory system.

Apparent reduction in histopathologic stage of disease.

Apparent reduction in histopathologic stage of disease.

Higher radiation doses may be delivered to small volumes.

Scarring may trap normally mobile structures (e.g., bowel) in radiation field.

No delay between surgery and irradiation.

More accurate dose localization.

Accurate surgical staging of diseases.

> **2. Concurrent chemotherapy.** Chemotherapy administered during a course of irradiation presents the following theoretical advantages.
>
> > 1. Systemic chemotherapeutic agents (dactinomycin, doxorubicin [Adriamycin], bleomycin, cisplatin, fluorouracil, hydroxyurea, and methotrexate) may act as radiosensitizers.
> > 2. There is no delay in institution of systemic therapy.
>
> Concurrent combined-modality therapy is associated with increased treatment morbidity, and doses of radiation and drug must be scaled down appropriately.
>
> **3. Postirradiation chemotherapy.** Postirradiation chemotherapy is generally used as an adjuvant in situations in which micrometastases are suspected (e.g., breast cancer with demonstrated axillary node metastases, certain sarcomas).
>
> **4. Sandwich chemotherapy.** Employing systemic chemotherapy before and after a course of definitive irradiation combines the advantages of items **1** and **3** above. The morbidity is combined as well. Several such regimens are being tested at present.
>
> **5. Intraoperative radiation therapy.** The role of chemotherapy given prior to, during, or after intraoperative radiation therapy remains to be established by prospective study.

C. Irradiation as an adjuvant to chemotherapy. In some clinical oncologic situations in which chemotherapy is the primary treatment modality, radiation therapy can be used as an adjuvant for "consolidation." For example, the treatment of choice for advanced non-Hodgkin's lymphoma is multiple-agent chemotherapy. In this setting, the most common site of first recurrence is in areas of bulky disease, which are identified before systemic therapy is begun. With the patient in remission, such areas of bulky disease can be irradiated.

Local irradiation can be used as an adjuvant to chemotherapy to treat sanctuary sites of disease (e.g., the brain) for oat-cell carcinoma and acute lymphocytic leukemia.

D. Morbidity of combined-modality therapy. Whenever therapeutic modalities are combined in antineoplastic treatment, it must be remembered that potential morbidity is also combined. In certain situations the effect can be synergistic rather than simply additive.

> **1. Morbidity of surgery plus irradiation.** Radiation therapy, even in relatively low doses, impairs wound healing because of interference with fibroblastic proliferation. Therefore, impaired wound healing and even wound breakdown can result from combined-modality treatment. Lymph node dissections combined with local radiation therapy increase the incidence of distal lymphedema (in head, arm, and leg). Prior abdominal surgery increases the risk of intes-

tinal radiation injury, probably by partially immobilizing small bowel with postoperative adhesive disease. Previously irradiated tissues should be handled delicately during subsequent surgical procedures. Attention must be directed to vascular supply and vascular integrity when planning surgery in irradiated fields.

2. **Morbidity of chemotherapy combined with radiation therapy.** Morbidity of radiation therapy may be immediate (during or immediately after a course of treatment) or delayed (months to years after therapy). Combining chemotherapy with radiation therapy can enhance both the immediate and the delayed morbidity of irradiation.

Exacerbation of radiation reactions in mucosal or dermal tissues can occur with concomitant use of dactinomycin, bleomycin, fluorouracil, hydroxyurea, or doxorubicin. Doxorubicin and daunorubicin have been implicated in anamnestic responses to radiation therapy when given following a course of irradiation ("radiation recall"). The threshold dose for radiation pneumonitis is significantly lowered when the irradiation is administered in conjunction with doxorubicin, dactinomycin, hydroxyurea, vincristine, or procarbazine.

Leukoencephalopathy may result from combined cranial irradiation and methotrexate. Late development of leukemia and other malignant tumors can result from certain combinations of chemotherapy and irradiation. In Hodgkin's disease the risk may be as high as 10% for patients treated with extended-field irradiation and combination chemotherapy. Semustine has been implicated as an etiologic event in the late development of leukemia in patients treated with chemotherapy plus radiation therapy. Continuous monitoring of ongoing studies may elucidate additional risks of combined-modality therapy. (See also Chap. 10.)

VIII. **New directions.** The field of radiation therapy is anything but static. New modalities of treatment are constantly coming to the fore. The following are but a few examples.

A. **Dynamic radiation treatment.** Most modern megavoltage radiation therapy machines have isocentric rotational capability: The gantry of the machine can rotate the treatment head around the patient on the supporting couch while aiming the radiation beam at a given point within the patient's body. With such an arrangement, one can irradiate deeply situated tumors with relatively high doses while limiting the dose to the transit tissues to tolerable levels. With the advent of computed tomography and magnetic resonance imaging, it is now relatively easy to construct three-dimensional images of tumors (and of surrounding normal tissues). With *dynamic radiation therapy,* the shape of the radiation beam is a function of gantry rotation angle, and it is then possible to conform the radiation dose profile to the three-dimensional shape of the tumor. It requires a computer-controlled multileaf radiation beam collimator for the treatment machine. This technology is not now widely available, but it is becoming more so. As its use becomes widespread, it will enhance the radiation oncologist's ability to tailor radiation dose profiles to tumor profiles and thereby improve the therapeutic ratio.

B. **High-dose remote afterloading.** Radiation exposure of medical personnel is a problem associated with intracavitary or interstitial brachytherapy. Historically, radioactive sources were placed in body cavities or directly into tumors by the surgeon or radiation therapist with attendant significant radiation exposure. In an attempt to reduce such exposure, afterloading techniques were developed so that hollow needles, hollow plastic tubes, or other applicators were placed at the time of surgery. At a later time, radioisotopes were inserted into the tubes, needles, or applicators, reducing the overall exposure of medical personnel.

High-dose remote afterloading systems have proliferated. These radiotherapy devices generally use relatively small sources of ^{137}Cs, ^{60}Co, or ^{192}Ir, which are housed in a radioprotective safe when not in use but which can be delivered *by remote control* into appropriate applicators in various body cavities or into tumor-bearing tissues. This system eliminates radiation exposure of medical personnel. Several such devices are now commercially available, and clinical experience with this relatively new treatment modality is fairly extensive in the treatment of tumors of the prostate, bladder, cervix, lung, esophagus, breast, and head and neck. This type of therapy is now being accomplished with high-LET sources also. It is often combined with external radiation treatment and occasionally with hyperthermia. Occasionally the procedure is performed intraoperatively. The high doses employed with this therapeutic modality necessitate better understanding of altered fractionation schemes, and much clinical research remains to be done.

C. **Radiation sensitizers.** Radiation sensitizers are drugs or other agents that possess the ability to enhance the effects of ionizing radiation when administered before, during, or after radiation treatment. In this regard, they act as biologic response modifiers. Many drugs possess these properties, e.g., fluorouracil, mitomycin, cisplatin, doxorubicin, and misonidazole. The ideal radiation sensitizer is nontoxic and selectively enhances the radiosensitivity of cancer cells (but not that of normal cells). Such an ideal sensitizer, of course, has yet to be found.

With the use of radiation sensitizers, major advances have occurred in the treatment of cancers of the esophagus, anus, and bladder. As late as 1975, abdominoperineal resection was routinely used for anal cancer. Today, most such cancers can be treated effectively with radiation therapy and radiosensitizing doses of fluorouracil and mitomycin without the loss of anal function, which generally remains good to excellent.

D. Exotic radiation beams. Generating high-LET radiation beams (especially negative pi mesons and stripped nuclei) is expensive and requires elaborate high-energy equipment that is not generally available; however, a few clinical research centers are actively studying such beams in the treatment of cancer.

High-LET neutron beams are available at lower cost, but such equipment is still much more expensive than conventional radiation therapy equipment. Neutron beam therapy is at least twice as effective as conventional photon beam therapy for treating unresectable salivary gland cancers. It is clearly the treatment choice for such tumors. Neutron beam therapy also seems to be more effective than conventional x-ray treatment for locally advanced prostatic cancer. Limited availability of high-LET beams precludes widespread employment of this therapeutic modality.

Clearly, the use of exotic radiation beams and combinations thereof with conventional radiation therapy, surgery, and biologic response modifiers requires a great deal of basic and clinical investigation.

E. Photodynamic therapy. Certain light-absorbing compounds, usually hematoporphyrin derivatives, can be made to concentrate preferentially in some tumors under certain conditions. When exposed to light of appropriate energy (often generated by a ruby laser), these compounds will preferentially absorb the red-light energy. The deposition of energy in the neoplastic tissue can produce tissue necrosis, and therefore the process can be used as a form of local cancer treatment. At present this technique is entirely investigational and much basic study must be done before this exciting new modality is introduced into the clinic for routine cancer therapy. The possible future combinations of photodynamic therapy with conventional modes of antineoplastic therapy are many.

F. Stereotactic radiosurgery. Technologic advances in tumor imaging (computed tomography, magnetic resonance imaging, etc.) and radiation dose-delivery systems have stimulated the development of rigid patient immobilization systems that together permit the radiation oncology team to deposit very large radiation doses (30 Gy or more) to small volumes (up to 2.5-cm diameter) in the head with millimeter accuracy. This high-dose, small-volume treatment technique has been found useful for small, discrete intracranial disease, but is still largely investigational. Although there is a rapid proliferation of this new technology, further clinical experience will be necessary to fully define the role of stereotactic radiosurgery in the neurooncologist's therapeutic armamentarium.

G. Three-dimensional conformal irradiation. New developments in computer applications in the field of radiation oncology treatment planning now facilitate three-dimensional display of reconstructed images of tumors and adjacent critical normal tissues and organs. This permits the radiation oncologist to view and irradiate tumors from an infinite variety of conventional and unconventional perspectives. This decreases the radiation dose to the normal tissues adjacent to the tumor while, at the same time, gives higher than conventional doses to the tumor itself. This has the potential of increasing local tumor control rates while lowering radiation complication rates.

Selected Readings

Abe, M., Takahashi, M., and Sugahara, T. *Hyperthermia in Cancer Therapy*. Tokyo: Cosmos, 1985.

Anghileri, L. J., and Robert, J. *Hyperthermia in Cancer Treatment* (Vols. I, II, and III). Boca Raton, FL: CRC Press, 1986.

Brady, L. W. *Radiation Sensitizers*. New York: Masson, 1983.

Brady, L. W., and Perez, C. A. *Principles and Practice of Radiation Oncology*. Philadelphia: Lippincott, 1992.

Calvo, F. A. *Intraoperative Radiotherapy: Clinical Experiences and Results*. Heidelberg: Springer, 1992.

Catterall, M., and Bewley, D. *Fast Neutrons in the Treatment of Cancer*. Orlando, FL: Grune & Stratton, 1979.

Coia, L. R., and Moylan, D. J. *Introduction to Clinical Radiation Oncology*. Madison, WI: Medical Physics Publishing, 1991.

DeVita, V. T., Hellman, S., and Rosenberg, S. A. *Cancer Principles & Practice of Oncology*. Philadelphia: Lippincott, 1993.

Dobelbower, R. R., Jr., and Abe, M. *Intraoperative Radiation Therapy*. Boca Raton, FL: CRC Press, 1989.

Hall, E. J. *Radiobiology for the Radiologist*. Philadelphia: Lippincott, 1994.

Halperin, E. C., et al. *Pediatric Radiation Oncology*. New York: Raven Press, 1989.

Hornback, N. B. *Hyperthermia and Cancer: Human Clinical Trial Experience* (Vols. I and II). Boca Raton: CRC Press, 1984.

Mansfield, C. M. *Therapeutic Radiology*. New York: Elsevier, 1989.

Meyer, J. L., and Vaeth, J. M. *Organ Conservation in Curative Cancer Treatment: Indications, Contraindications, Methods*. Basel: Karger, 1993.

Moosa, A. R. *Comprehensive Textbook of Oncology*. Baltimore: Williams & Wilkins, 1991.

Moss, W. T., and Cox, J. D. *Radiation Oncology Rationale Technique Results*. St. Louis: Mosby, 1989.

Pierquin, B., Wison, J. F., and Chassagne, D. *Modern Brachytherapy*. New York: Masson, 1987.

Wang, C. C. *Clinical Radiation Oncology: Indications, Techniques, and Results*. Littleton, MA: PSG Publishing, 1988.

Ethical Considerations in Cancer Chemotherapy

Joy D. Skeel

Consideration of ethical principles in the practice of cancer chemotherapy presupposes the need for a high degree of sensitivity by the physician for the fears and anxieties of the patient about the seriousness of the diagnosis of cancer and the need for chemotherapy. In addition to being aware of the emotional factors involved when caring for patients who require chemotherapy, physicians should also be aware of the ethical issues involved. This chapter does not deal with the emotional aspects of the disease and its treatment; discussion is restricted to ethical principles, informed consent, refusal of treatment, and decisions at the end of life.

I. **Basic concepts**
  A. **Respect for persons.** The respect for persons is an umbrella principle in medical ethics. Other principles, rules, and concepts, such as autonomy and nonmaleficence, in medical ethics are derived from this concept.
  B. **Autonomy.** Patient autonomy means that patients are self-governing, i.e., free from controlling outside influences, when making decisions regarding their own bodies. Since the early 1960s the concept of patient autonomy has become increasingly important, ethically and legally, in the practice of medicine. Needless to say, this principle plays an important role in all areas of medicine but particularly in informed consent related to research protocols and choice of other therapies.
  C. **Nonmaleficence** means not harming the patient. This principle requires that a patient not be injured or put at serious risk of harm.
  D. **Beneficence** means doing what is perceived to be good for the patient. This principle involves actively doing good, which includes preventing harm, removing harm, and providing benefits.
  E. **Paternalism.** This concept (or attitude) is the opposite of respecting another person's autonomy. It conveys the image of the strong, domineering father who assumed he knew what was best for his children. (In medicine, physicians and patients are substituted, respectively, for fathers and children.) For many years physicians made decisions they considered to be in the best interest of their patients without involving the patients substantively in the decision-making process. Paternalism is ostensibly less prevalent today than during the pre-1970s.

II. **Informed consent.** According to Jonsen, Siegler, and Winslade, informed consent is the willing and uncoerced acceptance of a medical intervention by the patient after adequate disclosure of the nature of the intervention and its risks and benefits, as well as disclosure of alternative interventions and their risks and benefits.

A. Functions of informed consent. The functions of informed consent are the following.

1. Promote individual autonomy and rational decision making
2. Protect patients and research subjects
3. Avoid coercive practices in medicine
4. Encourage health care professionals to examine their practice of giving information to patients
5. Help to maintain trust

B. Five essential elements of informed consent. Beauchamp and Childress stated that there are five elements involved in the process for a patient to give informed consent: competence (decision-making capacity), disclosure of information, comprehension of the information disclosed, voluntariness, and authorization.

1. **Competence** refers to the ability to make reasonable decisions, usually within a specific sphere of a person's life. It is essential to note that persons may be capable of making reasonable decisions in some, but not all, areas of their lives. For example, although individuals may no longer be capable of running the family business, they may well be competent to say what they do (or do not) want done to their bodies (i.e., what treatments they will or will not accept).

   a. **Three general standards of competence** may be applied.

      1. Capacity to reach a decision based on rational reasons
      2. Capacity to reach a reasonable result through a decision
      3. Capacity to make a decision at all

   b. **Application to chemotherapy decisions.** In the context of making decisions regarding chemotherapy, the three standards just mentioned could be interpreted to mean that a patient would be able to:

      1. Decide whether to accept or refuse the chemotherapy and give the reasons for the choice
      2. Understand its potential risks and benefits
      3. Understand the purpose of the chemotherapy

   c. **Problems.** Occasionally attempts are made to label patients incompetent when they choose to refuse therapy a physician deems the treatment of choice. Although there are troublesome cases where competence to decide about therapy may be borderline, it is inappropriate to label a patient incompetent merely because he or she disagrees with the physician's recommendation(s). It is also necessary to acknowledge that patients sometimes make choices their physicians consider unwise.

(1) **Health care professional's bias.** On the surface it may appear easier for a patient to be able to consent to standard treatment because the physician (or other health care professional) may assume that standard treatment is more benign than investigational treatment—as well it may be. This assumption may not be valid, however, but merely reflects the health care professional's bias or value judgment.

(2) **Unfair assumption.** It will, in all likelihood, take more time to explain the pros and cons of investigational treatment, but the assumption that the patient should be required to show any greater capacity for decision making (competence) to consent to investigational treatment than to standard treatment is unfair. It could be argued that patients are being discriminated against and possibly losing a viable option for better treatment if they are not allowed to participate in research protocols.

2. **Disclosure of information** to the patient. The patient should be told what the planned method of treatment is, with its risks and benefits, along with the alternative possible treatments and their attendant risks and benefits. Some physicians also mention the possibility of unforeseen risks. The patient should be told the purpose of the treatment and be given the opportunity to ask questions. Three standards for disclosure have been developed.

   a. **Professional practice standard** relies heavily on what the physician thinks is appropriate for the patient to know. There are several problems with this standard, including the fact that it can be paternalistic and thus undermine the concept of patient autonomy.

   b. **Reasonable person standard** is based on what the hypothetical reasonable person, in contrast to the real individual person sitting in front of the physician, would want or need to know to make a reasonable, informed decision.

   c. **Subjective standard** incorporates the specific situation of the individual person and what he or she would want or need to know based on physical and emotional needs.

   d. **A compromise** between the reasonable person standard and the subjective standard probably offers the best solution. Physicians often do not have time to have a detailed psychologic history of their patients; thus a totally subjective standard would be difficult to apply. However, a physician can provide the information a reasonable person would want or need to know and then encourage the patient to ask additional questions.

The questions should be answered truthfully and simply, with care being taken to avoid medical jargon.

3. **Comprehension of information disclosed.** Beauchamp and Childress noted that this element may be the most important part of the informed consent process. It is sometimes difficult to assess the degree of understanding a patient possesses, but a patient should be able, at the least, to state the risks and benefits of the treatment proposed and to acknowledge if there are alternative treatments available.

4. **Voluntariness** refers to an individual's ability to make a decision free from coercion or undue influence by others.

   a. **Voluntariness includes** having adequate information regarding the options available. For example, if a patient has information only regarding therapy A and none regarding therapy B, the decision to accept therapy A is not truly voluntary.

   b. **Voluntariness is impeded** if the patient feels coerced by the physician (whether intentionally or unintentionally) to accept one therapy over another.

5. **Authorization** simply means that a person actively and autonomously authorizes a professional to perform some medical procedure or to involve the patient in a research protocol.

C. **Problems with informed consent**

   1. **Standard of disclosure.** As noted, problems occur when trying to devise a standard of disclosure that allows a patient to make an informed decision regarding treatment options. The best alternative seems to be the compromise as discussed in sec. **B.2.d.**

   2. **Abdicating patient's rights.** There are occasional (rare) circumstances when patients prefer to have the physician make decisions for them, but it ought to be the rare exception rather than the rule, as it opens the door to potential abuse.

   3. **Remote risks.** Whether to disclose the possibility of remote risks seems to depend on the severity of the risk (e.g., death versus loss of hair) and how remote it is (1:100,000 versus 1:1000). If the risk is severe, e.g., death, it might be disclosed to the patient if the incidence is approximately 1:10,000, but its remoteness ought to be emphasized.

D. **Nondisclosure** is occasionally built into research protocols. These protocols should be carefully reviewed by institutional review boards.

E. **Practical application**

   1. **Competence.** If a patient is known by the physician, assessment of the person's capacity to make decisions is usually straightforward. If the patient's ability to make decisions is in question, a mini-mental status examination may be utilized or a psychia-

try consultation requested. If it is determined that the patient's decision-making capacity is diminished and the patient is incapable of making decisions, it is necessary to identify a surrogate decision-maker, either by designating a family member or by instituting guardianship proceedings.

2. **Disclosure of information.** Simple, straightforward language is recommended for describing the proposed therapy. When a research protocol includes a lengthy consent form, it is wise to read through it slowly with the patient and provide opportunities for questions. It is sometimes helpful, if the patient agrees, to have a close family member or friend present for these discussions so informed discussion can continue after the physician leaves the room. A word of caution regarding the presence of other persons during disclosure of information: A physician should pay primary attention to the patient, as patients occasionally complain that their physician seems to find it easier to talk to their families than to them. Therefore, although family members may be included in these discussions, the patient should be the primary focus. A physician should disclose his or her role in research protocols to patients in a straightforward manner. Patients should also be informed that research protocols allow them to make a contribution to society if they choose to be involved (particularly in phase I or II trials) and provide them with the newest therapies available. At the same time, patients should not be made to feel that their physician will be angry or will abandon them if they choose not to participate.

   Cautionary note to the physician-researcher: There is a fine line between encouraging patients to participate in research protocols and (1) subtly coercing them by displays of physician disappointment if the patients choose not to participate, or (2) excessively raising patient expectations about the potential benefit to them from the protocol. When the physician finds him- or herself in the dual roles of physician and researcher, the physician's primary obligation is to benefit the patient unless it is stated otherwise to the patient.

3. **Understanding.** The most practical way for a physician or other health professional to assess patients' comprehension of information disclosed is to ask them questions about the risks and benefits of the proposed treatment. They should also be able to state what the alternative treatment(s) would be as well as their general awareness of the risks and benefits of the other options.

4. **Voluntariness.** Patients should not feel that excessive pressure is being put on them to accept one form of treatment over another. This statement is not meant to imply that physicians ought not make recommendations; because they should. However, a

physician must be cautious when filling the dual roles of researcher and physician so as not to coerce patients to participate in a research protocol when that is not truly their choice.

5. **Authorization.** A patient authorizes a physician to proceed with a specific therapy when the individual has made an autonomous choice regarding the available treatments.

III. **Refusal of treatment** by a patient and informed consent go hand in hand. Refusal of treatment, like informed consent, ought to be informed, competent, voluntary, and authorized.

   A. **Principles involved in refusal of treatment**

      1. **The issue of patient autonomy** is at the center of discussions regarding refusal of treatment by the competent patient.

      2. **The principle of nonmaleficence** is equally important for incompetent patients.

   B. **Refusals of treatment** should be respected in cases involving competent persons unless such nontreatment would cause significant harm to other persons, particularly young children. It does not mean that there should not be serious conversations to learn why a person is refusing treatment; misperceptions regarding treatment should be clarified. It is appropriate for physicians to counsel, advise, and persuade a patient to accept treatment, particularly when the patient's disease is believed to be treatable or curable. The physician is also obligated to listen—and to hear—the patient's reasons for refusing treatment. Sometimes it is reasonable to negotiate a specific time period during which treatment will be tried and then reassessed.

      Questions may be asked whether there is a difference between competence required to *refuse treatment* and competence required to *understand and accept rigors of treatment* necessary for complex and complicated chemotherapy. There are several issues here.

      1. **Issues related to understanding information presented.** So long as the patient can meet the standards of competence and understanding of options as described earlier, then one has to accept the patient's decision.

      2. **Issues related to how information is presented,** i.e., whether the physician and others involved in informing the patient present information and answer the patient's questions openly, clearly, and without jargon and whether they try to avoid forcing their values and biases on the patient. Health care professionals continually need to listen to themselves as they present information to a patient and recognize the power they have to influence a patient by their use of language. They should also try to be aware of their own values and biases as well as external influences such as economic resources, e.g., whether the patient has insurance, which affect how information is presented.

3. **Issues arising from the assumption that anyone can really know ahead of time whether she or he can tolerate consequences or effects of chemotherapy.** Accepting chemotherapy and signing a consent form does not cast the patient's decision in stone. If the patient chooses to opt out, even though supported physically and emotionally by the health care team, and after full disclosure of consequences of changing course midstream, then the patient's autonomy should be respected. If the patient decides over a period of time that his or her quality of life is so compromised by the treatment, the patient should be able to stop or change therapy. No one can fully project personal responses to serious side effects until they are experienced.

C. **Physician response**
   1. **Frustration.** This response is understandable if the physician believes the patient could benefit from the treatment being refused. Nonetheless, if autonomy is a value to be preserved, competent persons should be allowed to make their own decisions.
   2. **Paternalism.** The physician may be tempted to override the patient's refusal of treatment, but this behavior is difficult or impossible to justify when the patient is competent.
   3. **Changing physicians.** If the physician is strongly opposed to the patient's decision to refuse treatment, he or she may suggest that the patient change physicians. The physician, however, must be careful not to be perceived as abandoning the patient. If the physician is gravely concerned that the patient is making a wrong decision, a consultation may be requested from an ethicist, if there is one in the institution, or from an ethics committee.

D. **Incompetent patients.** Treatment may be refused for incompetent patients by proxy decision-makers, who are usually family members or court-appointed guardians.
   1. **The principle of nonmaleficence** requires that the best interests of these patients be protected.
   2. **Hospital ethicists or ethics committees** may be helpful in resolving disputes that arise in these circumstances, particularly when the proxy decision-maker and physician disagree as to the appropriate course of treatment.

IV. **Decisions at the end of life**
   A. **Giving information.** This time is no different from any other time in the physician–patient relationship; patients deserve to know what is occurring over the course of the illness so they can get their lives in order. However, information should be given in a compassionate manner so the patient does not feel badgered or as if all hope has been destroyed.
   B. **Decisions regarding how aggressively to treat**
      1. **Options must be presented clearly and openly.**
         a. Some patients may want to be **treated aggressively,** including intubation and perhaps even

cardiopulmonary resuscitation, even if there is only minimal hope for a meaningful quality of life.

b. Other patients may wish to be involved in **clinical research studies** to provide a contribution to society and medicine.

c. Still other patients may opt for **palliative care** and no further treatment.

2. **Palliation remains a problem,** as documented in several journals and articles that provide results of studies showing that adequate use of pain medications is not occurring, even among medical oncologists who have been viewed as skilled in the relief of pain and suffering. *Relief of pain and suffering should be a high priority even if there is a risk of hastening death when adequate analgesia is administered.*

3. **Physician-assisted suicide** is more likely to become an issue when patients fear their pain and suffering is not adequately treated. Assisted suicide is a serious issue being openly discussed in the United States. The activities of Dr. Jack Kevorkian and the frank articles and book written by Dr. Timothy Quill have generated much discussion as well as attempts to pass legislation for and against assisted suicide. Whether a physician participates in assisted suicide by prescribing medications intended to help a patient die depends on the physician's values and what kind of patient–physician relationship exists, i.e., how well the physician knows the patient. As things now stand legally, the physician's decision will also be determined by his or her willingness to take the legal risk of assisting a patient to die.

Physicians are not required to violate their sense of professional integrity; thus they are not obligated to participate in assisting a patient's death. This caveat, however, does not relieve the physician of the obligation to prescribe adequate medication to relieve a patient's pain and suffering.

4. **Options regarding where care will be provided should be discussed.**

a. Some patients prefer to die in the **hospital setting** or in an extended-care facility.

b. Others may choose to become part of a **hospice program** (where available), which may mean dying at home or in a hospice unit.

C. **Continued caring.** During this time, when aggressive treatment is usually curtailed, the patient and family need to feel cared for by the medical team. Although treatment, except for palliation, may stop, caring must not.

D. **Advance directives,** such as the Living Will, Durable Power of Attorney for Health Care, and other documents usually called medical directives provide varying degrees of assistance to health care professionals regarding patients' wishes if they are no longer able to communicate them to their physician. The states vary widely in how liberal or how restrictive the formal documents are. For example, Ohio's Durable Power of Attorney for Health Care has been modified significantly by the Living Will legislation but remains difficult to understand and cumbersome to fill out appropriately. Advance directives are meant to provide direction to physicians and other health care professionals, and *they can be best utilized if discussed in advance by patient and physician.* It means that physicians should ask patients if they have signed such a document and discuss it before it becomes necessary to use it. Once again, if the physician is concerned about the document, a consultation with the ethicist or the ethics committee may be useful. Individuals in states such as Ohio are well advised to make their wishes known via advance directives, since "nondeclarants" (those who have not executed advance directives) may be left in a state of "limbo" for a prolonged period if they become permanently unconscious.

Selected Readings

Beauchamp, T., and Childress, J. *Principles of Biomedical Ethics* (4th ed.). New York: Oxford University Press, 1994.

Cantor, N. The permanently unconscious patient. *Am. J. Law Med.* 15:381, 1989.

Emanuel, E., and Emanuel, L. Living wills: past, present, and future. *J. Clin. Ethics* 1:9, 1990; see copy of the Medical Directive, p. 17.

Jonsen, A., Siegler, M., and Winslade, W. *Clinical Ethics.* New York: Macmillan, 1982.

Lidz, C., et al. *Informed Consent: A Study in Decision-making in Psychiatry.* New York: Guilford Press, 1984.

Quill, T. E. Death and dignity. *N. Engl. J. Med.* 324:691, 1991.

Reich, W. T. (ed.), *Encyclopedia of Bioethics* (2nd ed.). New York: Free Press, 1994.

Roth, L., Meisel, A., and Lidz, C. Tests of Competency to Consent to Treatment. In R. B. Edwards (ed.), *Psychiatry and Ethics.* Buffalo: Prometheus Books, 1982. Pp. 201–211.

Solomon, M. Z., et al. Decisions near the end of life. *Am. J. Public Health* 83:14, 1993.

von Roenn, J. H., et al. Physician attitudes and practice in cancer pain management. *Ann. Intern. Med.* 119:121, 1993.

Using Quality-of-Life and Cost-Utility Assessments in Cancer Treatment Decisions

David F. Cella

The essence of medicine is providing care that improves the quality of patients' lives. On the surface, this simple clinical truth can be lost in the search for curative or time-extending treatments for cancer. However, when surveyed, most oncologists will acknowledge that their decision making with regards to treatment is driven more by consideration of quality of life than sheer quantity of life. At issue is not the degree of importance or value placed on quality-of-life considerations in cancer treatment decisions; at issue is the extent to which standardized approaches to measuring quality of life can be used sensibly by the clinician in thinking through and discussing treatment options with patients. For while virtually all medical practitioners will agree that quality of life is important, there is currently little agreement or even understanding about how quality-of-life considerations can be used systematically in decision making. Consequently, most clinical oncologists use unsystematic, idiosyncratic approaches to learn about their patients' quality of life and personal values, and then apply this knowledge to make clinical decisions. This chapter summarizes some recent work in cancer outcome evaluation research and the current thinking regarding how quality-of-life and cost-outcome data may help transform cancer treatment decision making into a more systematic exercise. While this is not an effort to create practice guidelines, such an approach clearly overlaps with that concept.

I. **Cancer Outcomes: Time, Quality, Cost.** Outcomes of cancer treatment can arguably be reduced to three types: survival time, quality of life, and cost associated with therapy. Other end points, such as disease-free interval or tumor response, are of value presumably because they are associated with improved quality of life. Survival time is highly valued by both patients and their health care providers. This is particularly true when time added by a treatment is spent in relatively good health (i.e., time spent with good quality of life). Sometimes, a cancer treatment adds time *and* quality by virtue of its reduction of tumor burden. Examples have been seen in advanced lung and breast cancer, for which life-extending chemotherapy has also promoted physical well-being and functional status that appear to outweigh the toxicity of treatment. In such a case, the decision to treat is straightforward. More often, however, time and quality are at odds with one another, or at least unrelated to one another. The third factor, cost, looms as an issue throughout all of these clinical considerations. It has become clear that not every available treatment can be given to every patient who might potentially benefit.

Whether the payer is the patient, the insurance company, the government, or the provider (in the case of uninsured, indigent patients), decisions about cost-effectiveness or cost-utility must be made.

Symptom relief is highly valued by patients, and is usually associated with improvement in general functioning and well-being (i.e., overall quality of life). However, side effects and costs of therapy also must be included in the equation in order to fully balance the treatment decision. Patients tend not to think dichotomously in terms of toxicity versus efficacy; rather they consider the aggregate of their capabilities, circumstances, and somatic sensations. In fact, they often confuse symptoms with side effects. It is therefore advisable to survey patients in terms of their symptom experience, using a valid self-report questionnaire, and help them to make decisions about treatment by estimating which deficiencies or improvements are attributable to disease versus treatment. The dialogue this requires is challenging because it can threaten the tendency patients have to protect themselves from negative feelings. Unfortunately, the consequence of avoiding this dialogue is often unnecessary treatment given with misunderstood intentions.

II. **Intentions of cancer chemotherapy.** Cancer chemotherapy is given with one of three therapeutic intentions: curative, life-extending, and palliative. Table 7-1 summarizes the purpose and trade-offs involved in each of these types of treatment. It also describes the treatment and health-related quality of life (HQL) challenge of each type of treatment. The clinical (treatment and quality of life) challenges are overlapping and interdependent, reflecting the extent to which HQL is implicitly on the mind of the decision-maker with regard to chemotherapy.

A. **Curative** treatments are given to eradicate the disease, and so there is a high degree of tolerance for acute side effects and disruption of overall quality of life, because the prospect of cure is so highly valued. When following these patients over time, it remains important to determine whether any late or delayed adverse effects (e.g., infertility, second malignancy) remain acceptable to patients in light of their earlier choice.

B. **Life-extending** treatments are given to prolong life either by shrinking tumor mass or by reversing or slowing the rate of progression. Here, the acceptability of disruption and toxicity caused by treatment must be weighed against the symptom relief and time added by the treatment. This is difficult to do on an individual basis because of the uncertainty associated with outcomes in any given case. It is conceivable that with pooled data, a decision can be made on a policy level, using confidence intervals for efficacy (time added), toxicity, and cost. However, current methods for this decision making are highly dependent on time as the end point of interest. This places treatments for people with little time to live at a disadvantage over those with more time to live.

Table 7-1. Three intentions of cancer chemotherapy

	Curative	Life-extending	Palliative
Purpose	To eradicate disease	To prolong life, presumably adding valued time	Symptom control
Trade-off	High tolerance of acute effects in exchange for better chance of cure; concern for late effects	Moderate tolerance of acute effects in exchange to add time; concern for value of added time	Low tolerance of acute effects in exchange for symptom control; concern for better quality of life
Treatment challenge	Spare or minimally treat the already cured patient	Treat when added time outweighs side effects	Treat when not treating leads to lower HQL
HQL challenge	Determine acceptable consequences to patients	Estimate trade-offs among time, symptom relief, and toxicity	Estimate trade-offs between symptom relief and toxicity

HQL = health-related quality of life.

C. **Palliation** of symptoms is a legitimate goal of chemotherapy. Careful attention must be paid to the acute side effects, because if they outweigh the symptom relief resulting from a reduction of tumor burden, the purpose of treatment has been defeated. Short-term palliation is typically of great value to the patient and family, yet if it is evaluated in a cost-utility fashion it may appear to be more expensive than it is worth. This is further illustrated by an example in section **V**.

III. **Definition of quality of life.** HQL refers to the extent to which one's usual or expected physical, emotional, and social well-being is affected by a medical condition or its treatment. Essential components of this definition are the multidimensionality and subjectivity of HQL.

A. **Multidimensionality.** HQL incorporates physical, functional, emotional, and social dimensions. The physical dimension includes symptoms of disease and side effects of treatment. The functional dimension, often driven by physical well-being, includes self-care ability and productivity in one's usual role (at work, school, or home). The emotional dimension reflects not only negative affect such as anxiety and depression, but also positive mood and well-being. The social dimension extends from intimate relationships including sexuality, into family needs and support received from friends. Ideally, considerations about treatment would factor each of these dimensions into the final decision.

B. **Subjectivity.** HQL is a highly individualized entity that cannot easily be estimated by outside observers. The difficulty that outside observers have in evaluating an individual patient's HQL is most extreme with the emotional and social dimensions, because these dimensions are less visible to the observer. Some patients with minimal actual dysfunction are extremely dissatisfied, while others seem quite able to tolerate severe impairment and may even feel fortunate to be obtaining therapy. Many decisions about treatment are best made with this knowledge. Patients' perceptions of their illness are extremely variable, and factors other than actual disability enter into that perception. For example, two patients with cancer pain may experience the same pain relief of opioid therapy very differently. One may continue with pain behaviors and remain depressed and withdrawn, despite clear improvement in sleep and functional status. The other might perceive the pain relief as a hopeful sign that has positive effects on cognition, outlook, and social contacts. These two people will report different HQL ratings and should probably be managed differently.

IV. **Approaches to measuring quality of life.** Over time, two approaches to measuring HQL have evolved: psychometric and utility. These approaches have evolved independently of one another, largely because they were developed within different scientific disciplines. Psychometric approaches derive from psychology whereas utility approaches derive from economics. Only recently have investigators considered integrating these two approaches. This remains a critical challenge in HQL measurement, one that carries some risk.

A. **Psychometric approach.** The psychometric approach includes generic health profile measurement and specific instruments intended to measure the multidimensional impact of a specific disease, treatment, or condition. An important contribution of the psychometric approach is that it provides measurement of subjective or perceived well-being. However, psychometric approaches do not typically provide enumerated personal values for the health states they measure. This poses a problem for decision making. Very often, two patients with very similar disease and treatment options will accept very different therapies. Because psychometric measures typically do not incorporate patient-specific weights for individual domains or anchor states of health to a common standard, evaluating trade-offs between quality and length of life, or between one dimension of HQL and another, is difficult. This presents a challenge in a clinical trial where the primary purpose for integrating HQL measurement is to incorporate data on the impact of treatment on both length and quality of life into conclusions about treatment efficacy. The collection of patient preferences in clinical trials would allow the effect of treatment on quality-adjusted survival as well as on conventional outcome measures to be evaluated. Further, the addition of patient preference assessments to clinical trial outcome evaluation can make it possible to distinguish patients who favor one treatment over another when both may have equivalent survival outcome. A strategy for doing this has been described by Till and colleagues (see Selected Readings).

1. **Functional Assessment of Cancer Therapy (FACT) measurement system: a sample psychometric instrument.** Table 7-2 provides an example of a psychometric HQL instrument. The FACT measurement system is a 34–50-item compilation of a generic core (34 items) and many specific subscales, which reflect symptoms or problems associated with different disease sites (e.g., breast, bladder, cervix, colon/rectum, head and neck, lung, ovary, and prostate) and human immunodeficiency virus (HIV) infection. The scales were developed using more than 200 patients with cancer and 40 oncology specialists. The scales were then validated on a sample of 630 patients with a variety of cancers at different stages. The FACT yields a total HQL score and subtest scores for physical well-being, social/family well-being, relationship with physician, emotional well-being, functional well-being, and disease-specific concerns. Version 3 of the FACT-L (lung cancer) is duplicated in Table 7-2 to demonstrate the FACT-G (general) (items 1–34), which can be given to any patient with cancer, and the lung cancer subscale

(questions 35–44), which is administered only to people with lung cancer.

Questionnaires such as the FACT-L are typically self-administered by the patient. Most patients require little if any assistance in completing them. After completion of the questionnaire, the responses can be reviewed by the physician or nurse as a means of screening for problem areas. The FACT (or other comparable HQL instrument) can be adapted easily for clinical use as an inventory of potential problem areas. It also can be administered via interactive computer such that patients can directly enter their responses into a data base and obtain immediate feedback as to their current HQL. With some further refining, these data can then be used by the clinician in consultation with the patient, to make treatment decisions based on the patient's current HQL. Frequent, even routine, use of a health status instrument such as the FACT is strongly recommended for two reasons. First, repeated use with different patients fosters a familiarity with the instrument, which eventually allows providers to become their own "yardstick" in patient assessment. Second, as health care reform demands increased accountability for outcomes of treatment as justification for continuing the treatment, quality-of-life data can be used within a practice group to monitor patients' self-perceived health and response to treatments.

There is currently very little known about the relationship between patients' HQL and their treatment preferences. Initial studies suggested that most people, regardless of age or physical health status, wish to be "as aggressive as possible," and are very dependent on the advice of their physician to determine what loss in terms of toxicity and cost is reasonable to incur in exchange for probability of clinical effect. From the patient perspective, social factors such as a good social support network in general, and having dependent children in particular, seem to contribute to a willingness to be aggressive in treatment choices.

B. **Utility approach.** In contrast to the psychometric approach, which focuses on the health status of the individual patient, the utility approach is explicitly concerned with treatment decision making, usually at a policy level. In this approach, treatments typically are evaluated as to their benefit compared in some way to their cost. The utility approach to health status measurement evolved from a tradition of cost-benefit analysis, into cost-effectiveness approaches, and most recently, cost-utility approaches. The cost-utility approach extends the cost-effectiveness approach conceptually by evaluating the HQL benefit produced by the clinical effects of a treatment, thereby including the (presumed) patient's perspective. Two general cost-utility methods

Table 7-2. The Functional Assessment of Cancer Therapy—Lung cancer (FACT-L), version 3: a health-related quality-of-life instrument

Below is a list of statements that other people with your illness have said are important. By circling one number per line, please indicate how true each statement has been for you *during the past 7 days.*

PHYSICAL WELL-BEING

	Not at all	A little bit	Some-what	Quite a bit	Very much
During the past 7 days:					
1. I have a lack of energy	0	1	2	3	4
2. I have nausea	0	1	2	3	4
3. Because of my physical condition, I have trouble meeting the needs of my family	0	1	2	3	4
4. I have pain	0	1	2	3	4
5. I am bothered by side effects of treatment	0	1	2	3	4
6. I feel sick	0	1	2	3	4
7. I am forced to spend time in bed	0	1	2	3	4

8. Looking at the above 7 questions, how much would you say your **PHYSICAL WELL-BEING** affects your quality of life?

(Circle one number)

0	1	2	3	4	5	6	7	8	9	10
Not at all										Very much so

SOCIAL/FAMILY WELL-BEING

During the past 7 days:

	Not at all	A little bit	Some-what	Quite a bit	Very much
9. I feel distant from my friends	0	1	2	3	4
10. I get emotional support from my family	0	1	2	3	4
11. I get support from my friends and neighbors	0	1	2	3	4
12. My family has accepted my illness	0	1	2	3	4
13. Family communication about my illness is poor	0	1	2	3	4
14. I feel close to my partner (or the person who is my main support)	0	1	2	3	4
15. Have you been sexually active during the past year? No ___ Yes ___ If yes: I am satisfied with my sex life	0	1	2	3	4

16. Looking at the above 7 questions, how much would you say your **SOCIAL/ FAMILY WELL-BEING** affects your quality of life?

(Circle one number)

0	1	2	3	4	5	6	7	8	9	10
Not at all										Very much so

RELATIONSHIP WITH DOCTOR

During the past 7 days:

	Not at all	A little bit	Some-what	Quite a bit	Very much
17. I have confidence in my doctor(s)	0	1	2	3	4
18. My doctor is available to answer my questions	0	1	2	3	4

19. Looking at the above 2 questions, how much would you say your **RELATIONSHIP WITH THE DOCTOR** affects your quality of life?

(Circle one number)

0	1	2	3	4	5	6	7	8	9	10
Not at all										Very much so

Table 7-2. (continued)

EMOTIONAL WELL-BEING

During the past 7 days:

	Not at all	A little bit	Some-what	Quite a bit	Very much
20. I feel sad	0	1	2	3	4
21. I am proud of how I'm coping with my illness	0	1	2	3	4
22. I am losing hope in the fight against my illness	0	1	2	3	4
23. I feel nervous	0	1	2	3	4
24. I worry about dying	0	1	2	3	4
25. I worry that my condition will get worse	0	1	2	3	4

26. Looking at the above 6 questions, how much would you say your
EMOTIONAL WELL-BEING affects your quality of life?

(Circle one number)

0　1　2　3　4　5　6　7　8　9　10

Not at all　　　　　　　　　　　**Very much so**

FUNCTIONAL WELL-BEING

During the past 7 days:

	Not at all	A little bit	Some-what	Quite a bit	Very much
27. I am able to work (include work in home)	0	1	2	3	4
28. My work (include work in home) is fulfilling	0	1	2	3	4
29. I am able to enjoy life	0	1	2	3	4
30. I have accepted my illness	0	1	2	3	4
31. I am sleeping well	0	1	2	3	4

	Not at all		A little bit		Some- what		Quite a bit		Very much so
	0	1	2	3	4	5	6	7	8 9 10

32. I am enjoying the things I usually do for fun 0 1 2 3 4 5 6 7 8 9 10
33. I am content with the quality of my life right now 0 1 2 3 4 5 6 7 8 9 10

(Circle one number)
0 1 Not at all ... 9 10 Very much so

34. Looking at the above 7 questions, how much would you say your **FUNCTIONAL WELL-BEING** affects your quality of life?

ADDITIONAL CONCERNS

During the past 7 days:

	Not at all	A little bit	Some-what	Quite a bit	Very much
	0	1	2	3	4
35. I have been short of breath	0	1	2	3	4
36. I am losing weight	0	1	2	3	4
37. My thinking is clear	0	1	2	3	4
38. I have been coughing	0	1	2	3	4
39. I have been bothered by hair loss ..	0	1	2	3	4
40. I have a good appetite	0	1	2	3	4
41. I feel tightness in my chest	0	1	2	3	4
42. Breathing is easy for me	0	1	2	3	4
43. Have you ever smoked? No ___ Yes ___ If yes: I regret my smoking	0	1	2	3	4

(Circle one number)
0 1 Not at all ... 9 10 Very much so

44. Looking at the above 9 questions, how much would you say these **ADDITIONAL CONCERNS** affect your quality of life?

are the *standard gamble approach* and the *time trade-off approach*. In the standard gamble approach, people are asked to choose between their current state of health and a "gamble" in which they have various probabilities for death or perfect health (cure). The time trade-off method is easier to perform and involves asking people how much time they would be willing to give up in order to live out their remaining life expectancy in perfect health. All utility approaches share in common the use of a single scale in which 0 = death and 1 = perfect health. In practice, most cost-utility analyses employ expert estimates of utility weights, or in some cases, weights provided by healthy members of the general public. It is often assumed that these weights are reasonable approximations of patient preferences. This assumption is currently being tested by a number of investigators.

1. **Quality-Adjusted Time Without Symptoms and Toxicity (Q-TWiST): a sample utility approach.** The only utility approach that was developed to be cancer-specific is the Quality-adjusted Time Without Symptoms and Toxicity (Q-TWiST) approach, which attempts to evaluate the effectiveness of adjuvant chemotherapy for early-stage breast cancer. In the future, there may be application of a similar method for use in evaluating palliative care. It discounts survival time by reducing it according to a predetermined utility weight (0–1 range), which accounts for the impact of disease symptoms and treatment side effects. Like other utility methods, it does not, to date, generate the utility weights from patients themselves; rather it depends on an assumed perspective. Thresholds for decision making were determined by modeling actual survival data, and judgments were made by the investigators regarding where patient preferences were likely to fall relative to these threshold values.

2. **The Q-TWiST approach with other approaches.** The Q-TWiST approach carries some advantages over other approaches in that it is inexpensive to derive and allows for adjustment of survival time with the (presumed) HQL of that time. It may be possible to integrate the Q-TWiST approach with a psychometric scale or a patient preference scaling approach that increases sensitivity of measurement from the perspective of the patient. If the relationship between psychometric data and utilities can be established, it will become possible to collect psychometric data and base utility estimates on the reports of patients rather than the best guesses of others.

C. **Summary of the two approaches.** The utility approach informs physicians about the relative value of various health states; however, because of its emphasis on a single summary score, it fails to reflect the specific problems that might emerge. The psychometric approach provides the detailed perspective of the patient, but it does not generally tell how important a given problem or set of problems is to a group of patients. An oncologist familiar with both approaches is in an exceptionally good position to integrate them clinically. Cognitively capable patients can benefit from decision making that begins by informing of the details of treatment trade-offs (e.g., symptoms versus side effects), including available probabilities of occurrence. This information would ideally come from clinical trials that employed psychometric HQL or health status instruments such as the FACT. The next step would be to pose probable outcomes in terms familiar to the patient and relevant to his or her value system. One can envision two patients with similar disease and prognosis receiving quite different treatments as a result of using this approach. A familiar example is the decision regarding lumpectomy versus mastectomy for women with early-stage breast cancer. There are many possible extensions of this in chemotherapy given with curative, life-extending, and palliative intent.

V. Cost-effectiveness and cost-utility. Cost-effectiveness studies compare the costs associated with a given treatment to its clinical benefits, usually expressed in familiar units of improvement or decline. In oncology, these units could be survival time, disease-free interval, or tumor size. Cost-utility studies take cost-effectiveness to its next logical step by comparing the costs associated with a given treatment to its clinical benefits in terms that have meaning or value to the patient. Cost-utility studies are therefore implicitly (if not explicitly) concerned with HQL because treatment benefit is expressed in terms of patients' value systems. There are many other similarities between psychometric and economic (utility) studies as they relate to cancer treatment, particularly in the clinical trials arena. These are summarized in Table 7-3. This common ground between approaches to evaluating cancer treatments lends further support to the integration of psychometric and utility approaches to cancer treatment outcome measurement.

Although previous efforts to combine psychometric and utility approaches have been relatively unsuccessful, these approaches must be integrated in order to advance the field. An integrative approach could be applied in which a well-validated HQL scale can be administered to a patient receiving palliative care. This patient's total score can be converted to a standardized score, which allows for both ease of communication and possible utility analysis. However, physicians must use caution in interpreting results with the usual economic analysis procedures. The example given in the next paragraph will illustrate.

Classic economic analyses involve setting cost as the numerator. The denominator can then be either off-setting monetary units (cost-benefit), natural units of efficacy (cost-effectiveness), or quality of life (cost-utility). Typically, this last analysis takes the form of cost per quality-adjusted

Table 7-3. Similarities between psychometric (HQL) and utility (economic) studies in cancer

	True for economic studies?	True for HQL studies?
External pressure (e.g., health care reform) has forced a marriage between social science and medicine.	Yes	Yes
Studies cannot succeed without support and input of clinicians.	Yes	Yes
Studies place a significant additional burden on clinical trial system.	Yes	Yes
Priorities for studies are determined by relevance to decision making.	Yes	Yes
Outcome is usually considered "secondary" to survival time.	Yes	Yes
Success depends on ability to bring in new, outside expertise to oncology.	Yes	Yes
Initial emphasis has been on phase III studies.	Yes	Yes
Studies demand collecting more end points without added funding.	Yes	Yes
Studies require longer-than-usual follow-up of nonsurvival data	Yes	Yes
Studies require turning directly to patients for data collection.	Yes	Yes
Patient-reported data are the "gold standard."	No	Yes
Studies usually require more patients than a typical phase III trial.	Yes	No

HQL = health-related quality of life.

life-years (QALY) gained. In other words, time, adjusted for its quality, is the valued end point. Therefore, this means that treatments associated with conditions associated with longer survival times will appear more "valuable" than those associated with conditions associated with shorter survival times. For example, assume a person lives 10 years and receives a treatment that improves the quality of those 10 years from a utility score of 0.5 up to 0.6. This person has gained 1.0 QALY, moving up from 5.0 (10 years × 0.5 untreated utility) to 6.0 (10 years × 0.6 treated utility) QALY. If that treatment cost $1000 to deliver, the incremental cost per QALY would be $1000.

Now consider how the cost per QALY would change if that same $1000 treatment produced the same increase in utility (0.5 to 0.6), except that the person only lives for 0.1 year (i.e., about 5 weeks). The same benefit, at the same cost, now posts an incremental cost per QALY of $100,000 (Table 7-4). Few would question the societal value of a treatment

Table 7-4. Is there an economic bias against palliative care?

Treatment cost	Time	Untreated utility	Untreated QALY	Treated utility	Treated QALY	$\Delta_{Cost}/\Delta_{QALY}$
$1000	10 yr	0.5	5 yr	0.6	6 yr	$1000
$1000	0.1 yr	0.5	0.05 yr	0.6	0.06 yr	$100,000

QALY = quality-adjusted life year.

that costs $1000/QALY; however, it may become difficult to defend a palliative treatment that costs $100,000/QALY.

Some quality-of-life instruments and cost-utility analyses have contributed to an understanding of the diverse costs and benefits of cancer therapies. However, more work is needed to further our understanding of the diverse risks, costs, and benefits associated with cancer chemotherapy. Because of their clinical experience and expertise, and because of their position as decision-makers to whom vulnerable patients turn, oncologists are well positioned to assume leadership in integrating HQL and cost-utility assessments into the decision-making process about cancer treatment.

Selected Readings

Cella, D. F. Quality of life: the concept. *J. Palliat. Care* 8:8, 1992.

Cella, D. F., et al: The Functional Assessment of Cancer Therapy (FACT) scale: development and validation of the general measure. *J. Clin. Oncol.* 11:570, 1993.

Coates, A., Gebski, V., and Stat, M., for the Australian-New Zealand Breast Cancer Trials Group. Improving the quality of life during chemotherapy for advanced breast cancer. *N. Engl. J. Med.* 317:1490, 1987.

Drummond, M. F., Stoddart, G. L., and Torrance, G. W. *Methods for Economic Evaluation of Health Care Programmes.* Oxford: Oxford University Press, 1987.

Ganz, P. A., et al. Estimating the quality of life in a clinical trial of patients with metastatic lung cancer using the Karnofsky Performance Status and the Functional Living Index-Cancer. *Cancer* 61:849, 1988.

Gelber, R. D., Goldhirsch, A., and Cavalli, F. Quality-of-life-adjusted evaluation of adjuvant therapies for operable breast cancer. *Ann. Intern. Med.* 114:621, 1991.

Feeny, D., LaBelle, R., and Torrance, G. W. Integrating Economic Evaluations and Assessments. In B. Spilker (ed.), *Quality of Life Assessments in Clinical Trials.* New York: Raven Press, 1990. Pp. 71–83.

Tannock, I. F. Management of Breast and Prostate Cancer: How Does Quality of Life Enter the Equation? In N. S. Tchekmedyian and D. F. Cella (eds.), *Quality of Life in Oncology Practice and Research.* Williston Park, NY: Dominus (PRR), 1991.

Tannock, I. F., et al. A randomized trial of two dose levels of cyclophosphamide, methotrexate and fluorouracil chemotherapy for patients with metastatic breast cancer. *J. Clin. Oncol.* 6:1377, 1988.

Till, J. E., Sutherland, H. J., and Meslin, E. M. Is there a role for preference assessments in research on quality of life in oncology. *Qual. Life Res.* 1:31, 1992.

Torrance, G. W. Measurement of health state utilities for economic appraisal: a review article. *J. Health Economics* 5:1, 1986.

Systematic Assessment of the Patient with Cancer and Long-Term Medical Complications of Treatment

Roland T. Skeel and Patricia A. Ganz

I. Establishing the diagnosis

A. Pathologic diagnosis is critical. Although it is a truism to state that the diagnosis of cancer must be firmly established before chemotherapy or any other treatment is administered, the critical nature of accurate diagnosis warrants a reminder. As a rule, there must be cytologic or histologic evidence of neoplastic cells, together with a clinical picture consistent with the diagnosis of the cancer under consideration.

Most commonly, patients present to their physician with a complaint such as a cough or a lump; through a logical sequence of evaluation, the presence of cancer is revealed on a cytologic or histologic specimen. Less frequently, lesions are discovered fortuitously during routine examination, systematic screening for cancer, or evaluation of an unrelated disorder. With some types of cancer, pathologists can establish the diagnosis on small amounts of material obtained from needle biopsies, aspirations, or tissue scrapings. Other cancers require larger pieces of tissue for special staining, immunohistologic evaluation, flow cytometry, examination by electron microscopy, or more sophisticated studies such as evaluation for gene rearrangement.

It is often helpful to confer with the pathologist prior to obtaining a specimen in order to determine what kind and size of specimen is adequate to establish the complete diagnosis. When a tissue diagnosis of cancer is made by the pathologist, it is incumbent on the clinician to review the material with the pathologist. Not only is this practice good medicine (and good learning), but also it helps to be able to tell the patient you have seen the cancer with your own eyes when you give the diagnosis. It also prevents the physician from administering chemotherapy without a pathologic diagnosis. The pathologist often gives a better consultation—not just a tissue diagnosis—if the clinician shows a personal interest.

B. Pathologic and clinical diagnosis must be consistent. Once the tissue diagnosis is established, the clinician must be certain that the pathologic diagnosis is consistent with the clinical findings. If the two are not consistent, a search must be made for additional information, clinical or pathologic, that allows the clinician to make a unified diagnosis. It must be remembered that a pathologic diagnosis, like a clinical diagnosis, is also an opinion with varying levels of certainty. The first part of the pathologic diagnosis—and usually the easier part—is an opinion whether the tissue examined is neoplastic. Because most pathologists rarely render a diagnosis of cancer unless the degree of certainty is high, a positive diagnosis of cancer is generally reliable. Absence of definitively diagnosed cancer in a specimen does not mean that cancer is not present, however. It only means that it could not be diagnosed on the tissue obtained, and clinical circumstances must establish if additional tissue sampling is necessary. The second part of the pathologist's diagnosis is an opinion about the type of cancer. This determination is not necessary in all circumstances but nearly always is helpful for selecting the most appropriate therapy and making a determination of prognosis.

C. Treatment without a pathologic diagnosis. There are rare circumstances in which treatment is undertaken before a pathologic diagnosis is established. Such circumstances are clearly exceptions, however, and involve fewer than 1% of all patients with cancer. Therapy is begun without a pathologic diagnosis only when:

1. Withholding prompt treatment or carrying out the procedures required to establish the diagnosis would greatly increase a patient's morbidity or risk of mortality
2. The likelihood of a benign diagnosis is remote

Two examples of such circumstances are (1) a patient with a primary tumor of the midbrain, and (2) a patient with superior vena cava syndrome with no accessible supraclavicular nodes and no endobronchial disease found on bronchoscopy in whom the risk of bleeding from mediastinoscopy is deemed greater than the risk from radiotherapy for a disease of uncertain nature.

II. Staging. Once the diagnosis of cancer is firmly established, it is important to determine the anatomic extent or stage of the disease. The steps taken for staging vary considerably among cancers because of the differing natural histories of these tumors.

A. Staging system criteria. For most cancers, a system of staging has been established based on the following.

1. Natural history and mode of spread of the cancer
2. Prognostic import for the staging parameters used
3. Value of the criteria used for decisions about therapy

B. Staging and therapy decisions. In the past, surgery and radiotherapy were used to treat patients with cancer in "early" stages, and chemotherapy was used when surgery and radiotherapy were no longer effective or when the disease was in an advanced stage at presentation. In such circumstances, chemotherapy was only palliative (except for gestational choriocarcinoma), and in the absence of exquisitely sensitive tumors or strikingly potent drugs, the likelihood of increasing the survival was low. As we have learned more about cancer growth, tumor cell kinetics, and the development of resistance, the value of early intervention with chemotherapy has been transposed from animal models to human cancers. To plan this intervention and evaluate its effectiveness, careful staging has become increasingly important. Only when the exact extent of disease has been established can the most rational plan of treatment for the individual patient be devised, whether it be surgery, radiotherapy, chemotherapy, or biologic therapy alone or in combination. While no single staging system is universally used for all cancers, the system developed jointly by the American Joint Committee on Cancer (AJCC) and the TNM Committee of the International Union Against Cancer (UICC) is most widely used for staging solid tumors. It is based on the status of the primary tumor (T), regional lymph nodes (N), and distant metastasis (M). For some cancers, tumor grade (G) also is taken into account. The stage of the tumor is based on a condensation of the total possible TNM and G categories to create relatively homogeneous stage groupings, usually stages 0, I, II, III, and IV. When relevant to the specific cancers whose chemotherapy is discussed in Part III of this *Handbook,* the staging system or systems most commonly used for that cancer are discussed.

III. **Performance status.** The performance status refers to the level of activity of which a patient is capable. It is an independent measurement (independent from the anatomic extent or histologic characteristics of the cancer) of how much the cancer or comorbid conditions have affected the patient and a prognostic indicator of how well the patient is likely to do with treatment.

   A. **Types of performance status scales.** Two performance status scales are in wide use.

      1. **Karnofsky Performance Status Scale** (Table 8-1) has 10 levels of activity. It has the advantage of allowing discrimination over a wide scale but the disadvantages of being difficult to remember easily and perhaps making discriminations that are not clinically useful.

      2. **Eastern Cooperative Oncology Group (ECOG) Performance Status Scale** (Table 8-2) has the advantages of being easy to remember and making discriminations that are clinically useful.

      3. **Using the criteria of each scale,** patients who are fully active or mildly symptomatic respond more frequently to treatment and survive longer than do patients who are less active or severely symptomatic. A clear designation of the performance status distribution of patients in therapeutic clinical trials is thus critical in determining comparability and generalizability of trials and effectiveness of the treatments used.

   B. **Use of performance status for choosing treatment.** In the individualization of therapy, the performance status is often a useful parameter for helping the clinician decide whether the patient will benefit from treatment or will be made worse. For example, unless there is some

Table 8-1. Karnofsky Performance Status Scale

Functional capability	Level of activity
Able to carry on normal activity; no special care needed	100%—normal; no complaints, no evidence of disease
	90%—able to carry on normal activity; minor signs or symptoms of disease
	80%—normal activity with effort; some signs or symptoms of disease
Unable to work; able to live at home; cares for most personal needs; varying amount of assistance needed	70%—cares for self; unable to carry on normal activity or to do active work
	60%—requires occasional assistance but is able to care for most of own needs
	50%—requires considerable assistance and frequent medical care
Unable to care for self; requires equivalent of institutional or hospital care	40%—disabled; requires special medical care and assistance
	30%—severely disabled; hospitalization indicated, although death not imminent
	20%—very sick; hospitalization necessary; active supportive treatment necessary
	10%—moribund; fatal processes progressing rapidly
	0%—dead

reason to expect a dramatic response of a cancer to chemotherapy, treatment is often withheld from patients with an ECOG performance status of 4, as responses to therapy are infrequent and toxic effects of the treatment are likely to be great.

C. **Quality of life.** A related but partially independent measure of performance status can be determined based on patients' own perceptions of their quality of life (QOL). QOL evaluations have been shown to be independent predictors of tumor response and survival in some cancers, and they are important components in a comprehensive assessment of response to therapy. The uses of QOL evaluations in cancer therapy are discussed extensively in Chapter 7.

IV. **Response to therapy.** Response to therapy may be measured by (1) survival, (2) objective change in tumor size or

Table 8-2. ECOG Performance Status Scale

Grade	Level of activity
0	Fully active, able to carry on all predisease performance without restriction (Karnofsky 90–100%)
1	Restricted in physically strenuous activity but ambulatory and able to carry out work of a light or sedentary nature, e.g., light house work, office work (Karnofsky 70–80%)
2	Ambulatory and capable of all self-care but unable to carry out any work activities; up and about more than 50% of waking hours (Karnofsky 50–60%)
3	Capable of only limited self-care, confined to bed or chair more than 50% of waking hours (Karnofsky 30–40%)
4	Completely disabled; cannot carry on any self-care; totally confined to bed or chair (Karnofsky 10–20%)

in tumor product (e.g., immunoglobulin in myeloma), and (3) subjective change.

A. Survival. One goal of cancer therapy is to allow patients to live as long and with the same QOL as they would have if they did not have the cancer. If this goal is achieved, it can be said that the patient is cured of the cancer (though biologically the cancer may still be present). From a practical standpoint we do not wait to see if patients live a normal life-span before saying that a given treatment is capable of achieving a cure, but we follow a cohort of patients to see if their survival within a given time span is different from a comparable cohort without the cancer. For the evaluation of response to adjuvant therapy (additional treatment following surgery or radiotherapy that is given to treat potential nonmeasurable, micrometastatic disease) or neoadjuvant therapy (chemotherapy or biologic therapy given as initial treatment prior to surgery or radiotherapy), survival analysis (rather than tumor response) must be used as the definitive objective measure of antineoplastic effect. With neoadjuvant therapy, tumor response and resectability are also partial determinants of effectiveness.

It is, of course, possible that a patient may be cured of the cancer but die early owing to complications associated with the treatment. Even with complications (unless they are acute ones such as bleeding or infection) survival of patients who have been cured of the cancer is likely to be longer than if the treatment had not been given though shorter than if the patient never had the cancer.

If cure is not possible, the reduced goal is to allow the patient to live longer than if the therapy under consideration were not given. It is important for physicians to know if, and with what likelihood, any given treatment will result in a longer life. Such information helps the physician to choose whether to recommend treatment and the patient to decide whether to undertake the recommended treatment program.

B. **Objective response.** Although survival is important to the individual patient, it is not easy to predict how long a patient is going to live; thus survival does not give an early measurement of treatment effectiveness. Tumor regression, on the other hand, frequently occurs early in the course of effective treatment and is therefore a readily used measurement of treatment benefit. Tumor regression can be determined by the reduced size of a tumor or the reduction of tumor products.

1. **Tumor size.** When tumor size is measured, responses are usually classified as follows.

   a. **Complete response** is the disappearance of all evidence of the cancer for at least two measurement periods separated by at least 4 weeks.

   b. **Partial response** is a decrease of 50% or more in the sum of the products of the largest diameter and the diameter perpendicular to the largest (diameter product) of all measurable lesions with no appearance of any new lesions for at least 4 weeks. When there are more than three or four measurable lesions, representative lesions are usually measured, rather than all lesions.

   c. **Stable disease** is a decrease of less than 50% to an increase of less than 25% in the diameter product of any measurable lesions.

   d. **Progression** is an increase of more than 25% in the diameter product or the appearance of any new lesions.

If survival curves of patient populations having different categories of response are compared, those patients with a complete response frequently survive longer than those with a lesser response. If a sizable number of complete responses occur with a treatment regimen, the survival rate of patients treated with that regimen is likely to be significantly greater than that of patients who are untreated. When the number of complete responders in a population rises to about 50%, the possibility of cure for a small number of patients begins to appear. With increasing percentages of complete responders, the frequency of cures is likely to increase correspondingly.

Although patients who have partial response to a treatment usually survive longer than those who have stable disease or progression, it is often not easy to demonstrate that the overall survival of the treated population is better than that of a comparable untreated group. In part, this difficulty may be due to a phenomenon of small numbers. If only

15–20% of a population respond to therapy, the median survival rate may not change at all, and the numbers may not be high enough to demonstrate a significant difference in survival duration of the longest surviving 5–10% of patients (the "tail" of the curves) for treated and untreated populations. It is also possible that the patients who achieve a partial response to therapy are those who have less aggressive disease at the outset of treatment and thus will survive longer than the nonresponders regardless of therapy. These caveats notwithstanding, most clinicians and patients welcome a partial response and are little concerned at that point with the vagaries of survival statistics.

2. **Tumor products.** For many cancers, objective tumor size changes are difficult or impossible to document. For some of these neoplasms, tumor products (hormones, antigens, antibodies) may be measurable and may provide a good, objective way to evaluate tumor response.

   Two examples of such markers are the abnormal immunoglobulins produced in multiple myeloma and the human chorionic gonadotropin (β-hCG) produced in choriocarcinoma and testicular cancer, both of which closely reflect tumor cell mass.

3. **Evaluable disease.** Other objective changes may occur but are not easily quantifiable. When these changes are not easily measurable, they may be termed *evaluable*. For example, neurologic changes secondary to primary brain tumors cannot be measured with a caliper, but they can be evaluated using neurologic testing. An arbitrary system of grading the degree of severity of the neurologic deficit can be devised to permit objective evaluation of tumor response.

4. **Performance status** changes may also be used as a measure of objective change, although in many respects the performance status is more representative of the subjective than the objective status of the disease.

C. **Subjective change and QOL considerations.** A subjective change is one that is perceived by the patient but not necessarily by the physician or others around the patient. Subjective improvement and an acceptable QOL are often of far greater importance to the patient than objective improvement: If the cancer shrinks but the patient feels worse than before treatment, he or she is not likely to believe that the treatment was worthwhile. It is not valid to look at subjective change in isolation, however, because temporary worsening in the perceived state of well-being may be necessary to achieve subsequent long-term improvement.

   This point is particularly well illustrated by the combined-modality treatment in which chemotherapy is used to treat micrometastases after surgical removal of the macroscopic tumor. In such a circumstance, the patient is likely to feel entirely well after the primary surgical procedure, but the side effects of chemotherapy increase the symptoms and make the patient feel subjectively worse for the period of treatment. The winner's stakes are valuable, however, because if the chemotherapy treatment of the micrometastases is successful, the patient will be cured of the cancer and can be expected to have a normal or near-normal life expectancy rather than dying from recurrent disease. Most patients agree that the temporary subjective worsening is not only tolerable but well worth the price if cure of the cancer is a distinct possibility. This judgment depends on the severity and duration of symptoms, functional impairment, and perceptions of illness, as well as on the expected benefit (increased likelihood of survival) anticipated as a result of the treatment.

When chemotherapy is given with a palliative intent, patients (and less often physicians) may be unwilling to tolerate significant side effects or subjective worsening. Fortunately, subjective improvement often accompanies objective improvement, so that patients in whom there is measurable improvement of the cancer also feel better. The degree of subjective worsening each patient is willing to tolerate varies, and the patient and physician together must discuss and evaluate whether the chemotherapy treatment program is worth continuing. Such discussions should include a clear presentation of the scientific facts that include objective survival and tumor response data together with whatever QOL information has been documented for the treatment proposed. Moreover the expressed desires and the social, economic, psychologic, and spiritual situation of the patient and his or her family must be sensitively considered.

V. Toxicity

A. Factors affecting toxicity.
One of the characteristics that distinguishes cancer chemotherapeutic agents from most other drugs is the frequency and severity of anticipated side effects at usual therapeutic doses. Because of the severity of the side effects, it is critical to carefully monitor the patient for adverse reactions so therapy can be modified before the toxicity becomes life-threatening. Most toxicities vary with the following.

1. Specific agent
2. Dose
3. Schedule of administration
4. Route of administration
5. Predisposing factors in the patient, which may be known and predictive for toxicity or unknown and result in unexpected toxic effects

B. Clinical testing of new drugs for toxicity.
Before the introduction of any agent into wide clinical use, the agent must undergo testing in carefully controlled clinical trials. The first set of clinical trials are called *phase I* trials. They are carried out with the express purpose of

determining toxicity in humans and establishing the maximum tolerated dose, although they are done only in patients who potentially might benefit from the drug. Such trials are undertaken only after extensive tests in animals have been completed. Many human toxicities are predicted by animal studies, but because of significant species' differences, initial doses used in human studies are several times lower than doses at which toxicity is first seen in animals. Phase I trials are carried out using several schedules, and the dose is escalated in successive groups of patients once the toxicity of the prior dose has been established.

At the completion of phase I trials, there is usually a great deal of information about the spectrum and anticipated severity of acute drug effects (toxicity). However, because patients in phase I trials often do not live long enough to undergo many months of treatment, chronic or cumulative effects may not be discovered. Discovery of these toxicities may occur only after widespread use of the drug in *phase II* trials (to establish the spectrum of effectiveness of the drug) or *phase III* trials (to compare the new drug or combination with standard therapy).

C. **Common acute toxicities.** Some toxicities are relatively common among cancer chemotherapeutic agents. Common acute toxicities include the following.

   1. Myelosuppression with leukopenia, thrombocytopenia, and anemia
   2. Nausea and vomiting
   3. Mucous membrane ulceration
   4. Alopecia

   Aside from nausea and vomiting, these toxicities occur because of the cytotoxic effects of chemotherapy on rapidly dividing normal cells of the bone marrow and epithelium (mucous membranes, skin, hair follicles).

D. **Selective toxicities.** Other toxicities are less common and are specific to individual drugs or classes of drugs. Examples of drugs and their related toxicities include the following.

   1. Vinca alkaloids: neurotoxicity
   2. Ifosfamide and cyclophosphamide: hemorrhagic cystitis
   3. Anthracyclines: cardiomyopathy
   4. Bleomycin: pulmonary fibrosis
   5. Asparaginase: anaphylaxis (allergic reaction)
   6. Cisplatin: renal toxicity, neurotoxicity
   7. Ifosfamide: central nervous system toxicity
   8. Mitomycin: hemolytic-uremic syndrome
   9. Procarbazine: food and drug interactions

E. **Recognition and evaluation of toxicity.** Anyone who administers chemotherapeutic agents *must be* familiar with the expected and the unusual toxicities of the agent the patient is receiving, be prepared to avert severe toxicity when possible, and be able to manage toxic complications when they cannot be avoided. The specific toxicities of commonly used individual chemotherapeutic agents are detailed in Chapter 10.

For the purpose of reporting toxicity in a uniform manner, *criteria* are often established *to grade the severity of the toxicity*. Table 8-3 shows the criteria used by several National Cancer Institute-supported clinical trials groups for the most common toxic manifestations.

F. Acute toxicity management. Prevention and treatment of myelosuppression and its consequences are discussed in Chapters 2, 3, 31, and 32. Management of nausea and vomiting, mucositis, and alopecia as well as diarrhea, nutrition problems, and drug extravasation are discussed in Chapter 33. Other acute toxicities are discussed with the individual drugs in Chapter 10. Long-term medical problems are a special issue and are highlighted in the section that follows.

VI. Late physical effects of cancer treatment

A. Late organ toxicities may be minimized by limiting doses when thresholds are known. In most instances, however, individual patient effects cannot be predicted. Treatment is primarily symptomatic.

1. Cardiac toxicity (e.g., congestive cardiomyopathy) is most commonly associated with high total doses of doxorubicin or daunorubicin. In addition, high-dose cyclophosphamide as used in transplant regimens may contribute to congestive cardiomyopathies. When mediastinal radiation is combined with these chemotherapeutic agents, cardiac toxicity may occur at lower doses. Although nuclear cineangiography has been useful for acutely monitoring the effects of these agents on the cardiac ejection fraction, recent studies reported late onset of congestive heart failure during pregnancy or the initiation of vigorous exercise programs in adults who were previously treated for cancer as children or young adults. The cardiac reserve in these previously treated cancer patients may be marginal. Mediastinal irradiation also may accelerate atherogenesis.

Because of the large number of women with breast cancer who are treated with doxorubicin as part of an adjuvant chemotherapy regimen, this group is of special concern and warrants ongoing clinical follow-up.

2. Pulmonary toxicity has been classically associated with high doses of bleomycin (>400 units). However, a number of other agents have been associated with pulmonary fibrosis (e.g., alkylating agents, methotrexate, nitrosoureas). Premature respiratory insufficiency, especially with exertion, may become evident with aging.

3. Nephrotoxicity is a potential toxicity of several agents (e.g., cisplatin, methotrexate, nitrosoureas). These agents can be associated with both acute and chronic toxicities. Rarely, some patients may require hemodialysis as a result of chronic toxicity.

4. **Neurotoxicity** has been particularly associated with the vinca alkaloids, cisplatin, epipodophyllotoxins, and paclitaxel. Peripheral neuropathy can cause considerable sensory and motor disability. Autonomic dysfunction may produce debilitating postural hypotension. Whole-brain radiation, with or without chemotherapy, can be a cause of progressive dementia and dysfunction in some long-term survivors. This is particularly a problem for patients with primary brain tumors and for patients with small-cell lung cancer who have received prophylactic therapy. Survivors of childhood leukemia have developed a variety of neuropsychologic abnormalities that have been related to central nervous system prophylaxis that included whole-brain irradiation.

5. **Hematologic and immunologic impairment** is usually acute and temporally related to the cancer treatment (e.g., chemotherapy or radiation therapy). In some instances, however, there can be persistent cytopenias as with alkylating agents. Immunologic impairment is a long-term problem for patients with Hodgkin's disease, which may be due to the underlying disease as well as to the treatments that are used. Patients who have undergone splenectomy are also at risk for overwhelming bacterial infections. Complete immunologic reconstitution may take 2 years after marrow ablative therapy requiring stem cell reconstitution.

B. **Second malignancies**

1. **Acute myelogenous leukemia** may occur secondarily to combined-modality treatment (e.g., radiation therapy and chemotherapy in Hodgkin's disease) or prolonged therapy with alkylating agents or nitrosoureas (e.g., for multiple myeloma). In general, this form of treatment-related acute leukemia arises in the setting of myelodysplasia and is refractory to intensive treatment. Treatment with the epipodophyllotoxins also has been associated with the development of acute nonlymphocytic leukemia. This may be the result of a specific gene rearrangement between chromosome 9 and chromosome 11 that creates a new cancer-causing oncogene—ALL-1/AF-9. The peak time of occurrence of secondary acute leukemia in patients with Hodgkin's disease is 5–7 years after treatment, with an actuarial risk of 6–12% by 15 years. Thus a slowly developing anemia in a survivor of Hodgkin's disease should alert the clinician to the possibility of a secondary myelodysplasia or leukemia. Fortunately, secondary leukemias have not been reported in increased frequencies in women treated with standard adjuvant therapy for breast cancer (e.g., cyclophosphamide, methotrexate, and fluorouracil [CMF], though treatments using higher than standard doses of cyclophosphamide (with doxorubicin) have been associated with increased risk for acute nonlymphocytic leukemia.

Table 8-3. Common toxicity criteria used by National Cancer Institute-sponsored clinical trials groups

		0	1	2	3	4
				Grade		
Leukopenia	WBC ($\times 10^3$)	≥ 4.0	3.0–3.9	2.0–2.9	1.0–1.9	< 1.0
	Granulocytes/bands	≥ 2.0	1.5–1.9	1.0–1.4	0.5–0.9	< 0.5
	Lymphocytes	≥ 2.0	1.5–1.9	1.0–1.4	0.5–0.9	< 0.5
Thrombocytopenia	Platelets ($\times 10^3$)	WNL	75.0–normal	50.0–74.9	25.0–49.9	< 25.0
Anemia	Hemoglobin (gm/dl)	WNL	10.0–normal	8.0–10.0	6.5–7.9	< 6.5
Hemorrhage (clinical)		None	Mild, no transfusion	Gross, 1–2 units transfusion/episode	Gross, 3–4 units transfusion/episode	Massive, > 4 units transfusion/episode
*Infection		None	Mild, no active Rx	Moderate, localized infection, requires active Rx	Severe, systemic infection, requires active Rx, specify site	Life-threatening sepsis, specify site
Fever in absence of infection	°C (°F)	None	37.1–38.0 (98.7–100.4)	38.1–40.0 (100.5–104.0)	> 40.0 (> 104.0) for < 24 hr	> 40.0 (104.0) for > 24 hr or fever with hypotension

Fever felt to be caused by drug allergy should be coded as allergy.
Fever due to infection is coded under Infection only.

Genitourinary (GU)	Creatinine	WNL	< 1.5 × N	1.5–3.0 × N	3.1–6.0 × N	> 6.0 × N
	Proteinuria	None or no change	1+ or < 0.3 gm/dl or < 3 gm/liter	2–3+ or 0.3–1.0 gm/dl or 3–10 gm/liter	4+ or > 1.0 gm/dl or > 10 gm/liter	Nephrotic syndrome
	Hematuria	Negative	Micro only	Gross, no clots	Gross with clots	Requires transfusion
	*BUN	< 1.5 × N	1.5–2.5 × N	2.6–5.0 × N	5.1–10.0 × N	> 10.0 × N

Urinary tract infection should be coded under Infection, not GU.
Hematuria resulting from thrombocytopenia should be coded under Hemorrhage, not GU.

Gastrointestinal (GI)	Nausea	None	Able to eat reasonable intake	Intake significantly decreased but can eat	No significant intake	
	Vomiting	None	1 episode in 24 hr	2–5 episodes in 24 hr	6–10 episodes in 24 hr	> 10 episodes in 24 hr or requiring parenteral support
	Diarrhea	None	Increase of 2–3 stools/day over pre-Rx	Increase of 4–6 stools/day, or nocturnal stools, or moderate cramping	Increase of 7–9 stools/day, or incontinence, or severe cramping	Increase of ≥ 10 stools/day or grossly bloody diarrhea, or need for parenteral support

Table 8-3. (continued)

	Grade				
	0	1	2	3	4
Gastrointestinal (GI) (cont.) Stomatitis	None	Painless ulcers, erythema, or mild soreness	Painful erythema, edema, or ulcers, but can eat	Painful erythema, edema, or ulcers, and cannot eat	Requires parenteral or enteral support
Liver Bilirubin	WNL		$< 1.5 \times N$	$1.5–3.0 \times N$	$> 3.0 \times N$
Transaminase (SGOT, SGPT)	WNL	$\leq 2.5 \times N$	$2.6–5.0 \times N$	$5.1–20.0 \times N$	$> 20.0 \times N$
Alkaline phosphatase or 5' nucleotidase	WNL	$\leq 2.5 \times N$	$2.6–5.0 \times N$	$5.1–20.0 \times N$	$> 20.0 \times N$
Liver—clinical	No change from baseline			Precoma	Hepatic coma
Pulmonary	None or no change	Asymptomatic, with abnormality in PFTs	Dyspnea on significant exertion	Dyspnea at normal level of activity	Dyspnea at rest

Viral hepatitis should be coded as infection rather than liver toxicity.

Pneumonia is considered infection and not graded as pulmonary toxicity unless thought to result from pulmonary changes directly induced by treatment.

Cardiac					
Cardiac dysrhythmias	None	Asymptomatic, transient, requiring no therapy	Recurrent or persistent, no therapy required	Requires treatment	Requires monitoring; hypotension; ventricular tachycardia or fibrillation
Cardiac function	Normal	Asymptomatic; decline of resting ejection fraction by < 20% of baseline value	Asymptomatic; decline of resting ejection fraction by > 20% of baseline value	Mild CHF; responsive to therapy	Severe or refractory CHF
Cardiac ischemia	None	Nonspecific T-wave flattening	Asymptomatic, ST and T-wave changes suggesting ischemia	Angina without evidence for infarction	Acute myocardial infarction
Cardiac—pericardial	None	Asymptomatic effusion, no intervention required	Pericarditis (rub, chest pain, ECG changes)	Symptomatic effusion; drainage required	Tamponade; drainage urgently required

Table 8-3. (continued)

		Grade			
		0	1	2	3	4
Blood pressure	Hypertension	None or no change	Asymptomatic, transient increase by > 20 mm Hg (diastolic) or to > 150/100 mm Hg if previously WNL; no treatment required	Recurrent or persistent increase by > 20 mm Hg (diastolic) or to > 150/100 mm Hg if previously WNL; no treatment required	Requires therapy	Hypertensive crisis
	Hypotension	None or no change	Changes requiring no therapy (including transient orthostatic hypotension)	Requires fluid replacement or other therapy but not hospitalization	Requires therapy and hospitalization; resolves within 48 hr of stopping the agent	Requires therapy and hospitalization for > 48 hr after stopping the agent
Skin		None or no change	Scattered macular or papular eruption or erythema that is asymptomatic	Scattered macular or papular eruption or erythema with pruritus or other associated symptoms	Generalized symptomatic macular, papular, or vesicular eruption	Exfoliative dermatitis or ulcerating dermatitis

Allergy	None	Transient rash, drug fever < 38°C (100.4°F)	Urticaria, drug fever ≥ 38°C (100.4°F), mild bronchospasm	Serum sickness, bronchospasm; requires parenteral medication	Anaphylaxis
*Phlebitis, local	None	Arm pain	Thrombophlebitis, leg pain and swelling, with inflammation or phlebitis	Hospitalization or ulceration	Embolus or plastic surgery indicated
Alopecia	No loss	Mild hair loss	Pronounced or total hair loss		
Weight gain or loss	< 5.0%	5.0–9.9%	10.0–19.9%	≥ 20.0%	
Neurologic Sensory					
Neuro-sensory	None or no change	Mild paresthesias, loss of deep tendon reflexes	Mild or moderate objective sensory loss; moderate paresthesias	Severe objective sensory loss or paresthesias that interfere with function	
Neuro-vision	None or no change			Symptomatic subtotal loss of vision	Blindness
Neuro-hearing	None or no change	Asymptomatic, hearing loss on audiometry only	Tinnitus	Hearing loss interfering with function but correctable with hearing aid	Deafness not correctable

Table 8-3. (continued)

		0	1	2	3	4
Motor	Neuro-motor	None or no change	Subjective weakness; no objective findings	Mild objective weakness without significant impairment of function	Objective weakness with impairment of function	Paralysis
	Neuro-constipation	None or no change	Mild	Moderate	Severe	Ileus > 96 hr
Psychologic	Neuro-mood	No change	Mild anxiety or depression	Moderate anxiety or depression	Severe anxiety or depression	Suicidal ideation
Clinical	Neuro-cortical	None	Mild somnolence or agitation	Moderate somnolence or agitation	Severe somnolence or agitation, confusion, disorientation, or hallucinations	Coma, seizures, toxic psychosis

| | Neuro-cerebellar | None | Slight incoordination, dysdiadochokinesis | Intention tremor, dysmetria, slurred speech, nystagmus | Locomotor ataxia | Cerebellar necrosis |
	Neuro-headache	None	Mild	Moderate or severe but transient	Unrelenting and severe	
Metabolic	Hyperglycemia (mg/dl)	< 116	116–160	161–250	251–500	> 500 or ketoacidosis
	Hypoglycemia (mg/dl)	> 64	55–64	40–54	30–39	< 30
	Amylase	WNL	< 1.5 × N	1.5–2.0 × N	2.1–5.0 × N	> 5.1 × N
	Hypercalcemia (mg/dl)	< 10.6	10.6–11.5	11.6–12.5	12.6–13.5	≧ 13.5
	Hypocalcemia (mg/dl)	> 8.4	8.4–7.8	7.7–7.0	6.9–6.1	≦ 6.0
	Hypomagnesemia (mEq/liter)	> 1.4	1.4–1.2	1.1–0.9	0.8–0.6	≦ 0.5
Coagulation	Fibrinogen	WNL	0.99–0.75 × N	0.74–0.50 × N	0.49–0.25 × N	≦ 0.24 × N
	Prothrombin time	WNL	1.01–1.25 × N	1.26–1.50 × N	1.51–2.00 × N	> 2.00 × N
	Partial thromboplastin time	WNL	1.01–1.66 × N	1.67–2.33 × N	2.34–3.00 × N	> 3.00 × N

WNL = within normal limits; N = normal (usually upper limit of normal for laboratory); WBC = white blood cell count; Rx = treatment; BUN = blood urea nitrogen; PFTs = pulmonary function tests; CHF = congestive heart failure.

*Denotes ECOG-specific criteria.

Note: The common toxicity criteria is an example of a systematic scheme for evaluating toxicity due to chemotherapy. This kind of scoring of toxicity helps when assessing the severity of adverse effects for individual patients and for groups of patients undergoing similar or diverse treatments.

2. **Solid tumors** and other malignancies are seen with increased frequency in survivors who have been treated with chemotherapy or radiation therapy. Non-Hodgkin's lymphomas have been reported as a late complication in patients treated for Hodgkin's disease or multiple myeloma. Patients treated with long-term cyclophosphamide are at risk for bladder cancer. Patients who have received mantle radiation therapy for Hodgkin's disease have an increased risk of breast cancer, osteosarcoma, bronchogenic carcinoma, and mesothelioma. In these cases, the second neoplasm is usually in the irradiated field. In general, the risk of solid tumor begins to increase during the second decade of survival after Hodgkin's disease. As a result, young women who have received mantle radiation for Hodgkin's disease should be screened more carefully for breast cancer by starting at an age earlier than what is advised in standard screening recommendations.

C. **Other sequelae**

1. **Endocrine problems** are a result of cancer treatment. Patients receiving radiation therapy to the head and neck region may develop subclinical or clinical hypothyroidism. This is a particular risk in patients receiving mantle radiation therapy for Hodgkin's disease. Biennial assessment of thyroid-stimulating hormone (TSH) should be undertaken in these patients. Thyroid replacement therapy should be given if the TSH level rises, to decrease the risk of thyroid cancer. Short stature may be a result of pituitary radiation and growth hormone deficiency.

2. **Premature menopause** may occur in women who have received certain chemotherapeutic agents (e.g., alkylating agents, procarbazine) or abdominal/pelvic radiation therapy. The risk is age-related, with women older than age 30 at the time of treatment having the greatest risk of treatment-induced amenorrhea and menopause. Early hormone replacement therapy should be considered in such women, if not otherwise contraindicated, to reduce the risk of accelerated osteoporosis and premature heart disease from estrogen deficiency.

3. **Gonadal failure** or dysfunction can lead to infertility in both male and female cancer survivors during their peak reproductive years. Azoospermia is very common, but the condition may improve over time after the completion of therapy. Retroperitoneal dissection in testicular cancer may produce infertility due to retrograde ejaculation. Psychologic counseling should be provided to these patients to help them adjust to these long-term sequelae of therapy. Cryopreservation of sperm prior to treatment should be considered in men. For women, there are limited means available to preserve ova or protect against ovarian failure associated with treatment. Abdomi-

nal radiation in young girls can lead to pregnancy loss due to decreased uterine capacity.
4. **The musculoskeletal system** can be affected by radiation therapy, especially in children and young adults. Radiation may injure the growth plates of long bones and lead to muscle atrophy. Short stature may be a result of direct injury to bone.

Selected Readings

American Joint Committee on Cancer. *Manual for Staging Cancer* (4th ed.). Philadelphia: Lippincott, 1992.

Curtis, R. E., et al. Risk of leukemia after chemotherapy and radiation therapy treatment for breast cancer. *N. Engl. J. Med.* 326:1745, 1992.

Goldhirsch, A., et al. Costs and benefits of adjuvant therapy in breast cancer: a quality adjusted survival analysis. *J. Clin. Oncol.* 7:36, 1989.

Kennealey, G. T., and Mitchell, M. S. Factors That Influence the Therapeutic Response. In F. F. Becker (ed.), *Cancer, A Comprehensive Treatise* (Vol. 5). New York: Plenum Press, 1977.

Loescher, L. J., et al. Surviving adult cancer. Part 1: physiologic effects. *Ann. Intern. Med.* 111:411, 1989.

Oken, M. M., et al. Toxicity and response criteria of the Eastern Cooperative Oncology Group. *Am. J. Clin. Oncol.* 5:649, 1982.

Pedersen-Bjergaard, J., et al. Acute monocytic or myelomonocytic leukemia with balanced chromosome translocations to band 11q23 after therapy with 4-epidoxorubicin and cisplatin or cyclophosphamide for breast cancer. *J. Clin. Oncol.* 10:1444, 1992.

Perry, M. C. (ed.), Toxicity of chemotherapy. *Semin. Oncol.* 19:453, 1992.

Pfeifer, J. D., and Wick, M. R. The Pathologic Evaluation of Neoplastic Diseases. In A. I. Holleb, D. J. Fink, and G. P. Murphy (eds.), *Clinical Oncology*. Atlanta: American Cancer Society, 1991. Pp. 7–24.

Pui, C.-H., et al. Acute myeloid leukemia in children treated with epipodophyllotoxins for acute lymphoblastic leukemia. *N. Engl. J. Med.* 325:1682, 1991.

Smith, M., Rubenstein, L., and Ungerleider, R. Therapy-related acute myeloid leukemia following treatment with epipodophyllotoxins: estimating the risks. *Med. Pediatr. Oncol.* 23:86, 1994.

van Leeuwen, F. E., et al. Second cancer risk following Hodgkin's disease: a 20-year follow-up study. *J. Clin. Oncol.* 12:312, 1994.

Selection of Treatment for the Patient with Cancer

Roland T. Skeel

I. Setting treatment goals

A. Medical perspective. Before a physician decides on a course of treatment for a patient with cancer, the goal of treatment must be clearly defined. If the goal is to cure the patient of cancer, the strategy of therapy is likely to be different from the strategy chosen if the purpose is to prolong life or to relieve symptoms. To set the goal of therapy, the physician must be familiar with the principles and practice of therapy for each of the treatment modalities; well grounded in the ethical principles of the treatment of patients with cancer; knowledgeable about antineoplastic agents; familiar with the particular therapy for the cancer in question; and aware of the patient's individual circumstances, including stage, performance status, social situation, and concurrent illnesses. Armed with this information and with the treatment goals in mind, the physician can plan a course of treatment and make a recommendation to the patient.

Components of the treatment plan include the following.

1. Whether the cancer is to be treated or palliative care is to be given
2. How aggressive the therapy should be
3. Which modalities of therapy will be used and in what sequence
4. How treatment efficacy will be determined
5. Criteria for deciding the duration of therapy

B. Patient perspective. Although most often the medical recommendation is accepted, some patients reject it as inappropriate for them for a variety of reasons. Some ask the physician for another recommendation, and others seek the opinion of a second physician. The physician must clearly present the reasons for the treatment recommendations and why they seem to be the best way to achieve the treatment objective. At the same time, it is important for the physician to allow the patient to share in setting treatment goals, as it is the patient who must undergo the treatment and be willing to abide its consequences. The physician has the obligation to make a treatment recommendation, but the patient always has the right to reject that advice without fear that the physician will be "upset," dislike the patient, or refuse to continue to give him or her care.

II. Choice of cancer treatment modality

A. Surgery. The oldest, most established, and still most effective way to cure most cancers is surgery. Surgery is selected as the treatment if the cancer is limited to one area and if it is anticipated that all cancer cells can be removed without unduly compromising vital structures. If it is believed that the patient can survive the operation and return to a worthwhile life, surgery is recommended. Surgery is not recommended if the risk of surgery is greater than the risk of the cancer, if metastasis always occurs despite complete removal of the primary tumor, or if the patient will be left so debilitated that although cured of cancer he or she feels life is not worthwhile.

Most commonly, surgery is reserved for treatment of the primary neoplasm, although at times it may be used effectively to remove isolated metastases (e.g., in lung, brain, liver) with curative intent. Surgery is also used palliatively, e.g., for decompression of the brain in patients with gliomas or biliary bypass in patients with carcinoma of the pancreas. In nearly all nonhematologic cancers, a surgeon should be consulted to determine the role of surgery in the optimal treatment of the patient. Principles of surgery in cancer management are discussed in Chapter 4.

B. Radiotherapy. Radiotherapy is used for the treatment of local or regional disease when surgery cannot completely remove the cancer or it would unduly disrupt normal structures or functions. In the treatment of some cancers, radiotherapy is as effective as surgery for eradicating the tumor. In this circumstance, factors such as the anticipated side effects of the treatment, the expertise and experience of local oncologists, and the preference of the patient may influence the choice of treatment.

One determinant of the appropriateness of radiotherapy is the inherent sensitivity of the cancer to ionizing radiation. Some kinds of cancer, e.g., the lymphomas and seminomas, are sensitive to radiotherapy. Other kinds, e.g., melanomas and sarcomas, tend to be less sensitive. Such considerations do not preclude the use of radiotherapy, however, and it is helpful to obtain the evaluation of the radiotherapist prior to initiating treatment so that treatment planning can take into consideration the possible contribution of this modality.

Although radiotherapy is frequently used as the primary or curative mode of therapy, it is also well suited to palliative management of problems, e.g., bony metastases, superior vena cava syndrome, and local nodal metastases. The use of radiotherapy in the management of bony metastases and superior vena cava syndrome is discussed in Chapter 30. Principles of radiotherapy in cancer management are discussed in Chapter 5.

C. Chemotherapy. Chemotherapy has as its primary role the treatment of disease that is no longer confined to one site or region and has spread systemically. In the earliest days of chemotherapy, this interpretation directed its use to diseases that regularly presented in a disseminated form, e.g., leukemia, or after disease recurred following primary management with surgery or radiotherapy. It is now understood that widespread systemic micrometastases commonly occur early in cancer. These metastases are associated with certain predictive factors, such as the axillary node metastases of carcinoma of the breast and the large tumor size and poorly differentiated histologic features of sarcomas. Therefore chemotherapy is now applied earlier to treat systemic disease. When this treatment is used for micrometastases, the response of an individual patient cannot be measured. Rather, the effectiveness of therapy must be determined by comparing the survival of high-risk patients who receive therapy with similar (control) patients who do not receive therapy for the micrometastases.

Chemotherapy also has a role in the treatment of localized or regional disease. These specialized uses are discussed in Chapters 36 and 40.

D. Biologic response modifiers. It has long intrigued cancer biologists that cancer does not occur randomly but preferentially selects specific populations: the young, the elderly, the immunosuppressed (certain types of cancer only), and those with a strong family history of cancer. These observations have led cancer biologists to postulate that some kind of biologic control over the emergence of cancer exists, which some people have and others do not, at least at the time the cancer becomes established. One prime candidate for the mechanism of biologic control of cancer has been immunity. That immunity plays some role in controlling the development of cancer has been clearly demonstrated in animal models and a few, though not most, human neoplasms. Other biologic factors including those controlled by oncogenes and tumor suppressor genes, although less well defined at the present, are in all likelihood even more important than immunity in the development of cancer.

In an attempt to exploit and enhance the biologic control that is presumed to exist to some degree in everyone, a variety of agents called *biologic response modifiers* have been used in the treatment of cancer. Two classes of biologic response modifiers, the interferons and lymphokines (of which interleukin-2 is an example), have been intensively studied, and there is evidence of their substantial activity in some types of cancer. This area of intensive research promises to provide an important component of effective cancer therapy. Principles of biologic response modification are discussed in Chapter 3.

E. Combined-modality therapy. Neither surgery, radiotherapy, biotherapy, nor chemotherapy alone is appropriate for the treatment of all cancers. Frequently patients present with cancer in which there is a bulky primary lesion, macroscopically evident regional disease, and presumed microscopic or submicroscopic systemic disease. For this reason, oncologists have turned to a multidisciplinary approach to the treatment of cancer, selecting two or more modalities of therapy for sequential or simultaneous use. This approach requires close cooperation among the surgical oncologist, radiation oncologist, and medical oncologist to provide the patient with the best overall treatment plan. Although combined-modality therapy is not effective or desirable for all kinds or stages of cancers, the regular practice of a multidisciplinary approach provides the best opportunity to exploit the advantages of each mode of treatment.

III. Palliative care. The medical oncologist is often seen as the coordinator of cancer treatment. In this role the cancer is focused on, and the broader perspective of the oncologist as a coordinator of care of the patient—in partnership with the patient—may become obscured. Decisions about what therapy to use and how aggressive to be are critically important to medically sound patient care. Decisions of when to stop active cancer treatment are also vitally important and may be among the most difficult responsibilities for the oncologist. Quality of life is often enhanced in patients responding to chemotherapy and other cancer treatments. It just as surely deteriorates more rapidly when the tumor does not respond to therapy and the patient experiences the toxicity of treatment along with the pain, fatigue, cachexia, and other symptoms from the cancer. For the 50% of patients with cancer who are not cured, the decision to stop antineoplastic therapy is just as important as the selection of chemotherapy regimens earlier in the disease. There comes a time when the best advice a physician can give is for the patient to forgo additional chemotherapy or any other active cancer treatment.

The introduction and rapid acceptance of hospice programs throughout the United States over the past 20 years reflect the need for this kind of care. Hospice programs have effectively addressed the special needs of patients approaching the end of life and have provided the unique skills required to maintain the best possible quality of life as long as possible. Yet too often physicians are reluctant to "give up" and are unable to recognize or to accept when the patient will be helped more by an acknowledgement that active cancer therapy will not improve survival or enhance quality of life.

Oncologists and others caring for patients with cancer who have been trained as acute-care physicians can learn specific techniques to enhance quality of life from those who are expert in palliative care. For example, one might compare the quality of death in hospitalized patients given "maintenance" intravenous hydration versus hospice home care patients offered oral fluids and mouth care to assuage thirst. The former method may result in an overhydrated, edematous patient who dies with an uncomfortable sounding "death rattle" that is disconcerting to family and staff; the latter usually results in a visibly more comfortable patient who is more likely to die with less edema and without as much apparent respiratory distress.

Legitimate questions also can be raised about medical costs toward the end of life that are incurred when physicians give "futile" and "marginal" care. Development of guidelines by physicians and hospitals that define futile care and thoughtful consideration of when the therapy offered patients has marginal value may enable physicians to improve the quality of life for patients and at the same time hold down one component of the rising spiral of health care costs.

Selected Readings

Lundberg, G. O. American health care system management objectives: the aura of inevitability becomes incarnate. *J.A.M.A.* 269:2254, 1993.

Skeel, R. T. Quality of life dimensions that are most important to cancer patients. *Oncology* 7:55, 1993.

Chemotherapeutic and Biologic Agents

Antineoplastic Drugs and Biologic Response Modifiers: Classification, Use, and Toxicity of Clinically Useful Agents

Roland T. Skeel

I. **Classes of drugs.** Chemotherapeutic agents are customarily divided into several classes. For two of the classes, the *alkylating agents* and the *antimetabolites,* the names indicate the mechanism of cytotoxic action of the drugs in their class. For *hormonal agents* the name designates the physiologic type of drug, and for the *natural products* the name reflects the source of the agents. The *biologic response modifiers,* agents that mimic, stimulate, enhance, inhibit, or otherwise alter the host responses to the cancer, are discussed extensively in Chapter 3. Data for individual agents are given in section **III** of this chapter.

Within each class are several types of agents (Table 10-1). As with the criteria for separating into class, the types are also grouped according to the mechanism of action, biochemical structure or derivation, or physiologic action. In some instances these groupings into classes and types are arbitrary, and some drugs seem to fit into either more than one category or none. However, the classification of chemotherapeutic agents in this fashion is helpful in several respects. For example, because the antimetabolites interfere with purine and pyrimidine metabolism and the formation of DNA and RNA, they are all at least cell cycle-specific and in some instances primarily cell cycle phase-specific. The nitrosourea group of alkylating agents, on the other hand, contains drugs that are predominantly or entirely cell cycle-nonspecific. Such knowledge can be helpful in planning therapy for tumors when sufficient kinetic information permits a rational selection of agents and when drugs are selected for use in combination.

The classification scheme also may help to predict cross-resistance between drugs. Tumors that are resistant to one of the nitrogen-mustard types of alkylating agents thus would be likely to be resistant to another of that same type, but not necessarily to one of the other types of alkylating agents, such as the nitrosoureas or the metal salts (cisplatin). The classification system does not help in predicting multidrug resistance, which may have several phenotypes.

A. **Alkylating agents**

1. **General description.** The alkylating agents are a diverse group of chemical compounds capable of forming molecular bonds with nucleic acids, proteins, and many molecules of low molecular weight. The compounds either are electrophiles or generate electrophiles in vivo to produce polarized molecules with positively charged regions. These polarized

Table 10-1. Useful chemotherapeutic agents

Class and type	Agent
Alkylating agents	
Nitrogen mustard	Chlorambucil, cyclophosphamide, ifosfamide, estramustine, mechlorethamine, melphalan
Ethylenimine derivative	Thiotepa (triethylenethiophosphoramide)
Alkyl sulfonate	Busulfan
Nitrosourea	Carmustine, lomustine, semustine,* streptozocin
Triazine	Dacarbazine
Metal salt	Cisplatin, carboplatin
Antimetabolites	
Folic acid analog	Methotrexate
Pyrimidine analog	Azacitidine,* cytarabine, floxuridine, fluorouracil
Purine analog	Mercaptopurine, thioguanine, pentostatin, cladribine, fludarabine
Natural products	
Mitotic inhibitor	Vinblastine, vincristine, vindesine,* vinorelbine
Microtubule polymer stabilizer	Paclitaxel (Taxol), docetaxel*
Podophyllum derivative	Etoposide, teniposide

Antibiotic — Bleomycin, dactinomycin, daunorubicin, doxorubicin (Adriamycin), idarubicin, plicamycin, mitomycin, mitoxantrone, epirubicin*

Enzyme — Asparaginase

Hormones and hormone antagonists

Androgen — Fluoxymesterone and others

Corticosteroid — Prednisone, dexamethasone

Estrogen — Diethylstilbestrol

Progestin — Megestrol acetate, medroxyprogesterone acetate

Estrogen antagonist — Tamoxifen

Androgen antagonist — Flutamide, bicalutamide*

Luteinizing hormone-releasing hormone (LHRH) agonist — Leuprolide, goserelin

Miscellaneous agents

Substituted urea — Hydroxyurea

Methylhydrazine derivative — Procarbazine

Adrenocortical suppressant — Mitotane

Steroid synthesis inhibitor — Aminoglutethimide

Substituted melamine — Altretamine (hexamethylmelamine)

Acridine dye — Amsacrine*

*Investigational agents, not yet approved by the FDA for general use.

molecules then can interact with electron-rich regions of most cellular molecules. The cytotoxic effect of the alkylating agents appears to relate primarily to the interaction between the electrophiles and DNA. This interaction may result in substitution reactions, cross-linking reactions, or strand-breaking reactions. The net effect of the alkylating agent's interaction with DNA is to alter the information coded in the DNA molecule. This alteration results in inhibition or inaccurate replication of DNA with resultant mutation or cell death. One implication of the mutagenic capability of alkylating agents is the possibility that they are teratogenic and carcinogenic. Because they interact with preformed DNA, RNA, and protein, the alkylating agents are not phase-specific, and at least some are cell cycle-nonspecific.

2. **Types of alkylating agents**
   a. **Nitrogen mustards.** This group of compounds produce highly reactive carbonium ions that react with the electron-rich areas of susceptible molecules. They vary in reactivity from mechlorethamine, which is highly unstable in aqueous form, to cyclophosphamide, which must be biochemically activated in the liver.
   b. **Ethylenimine derivatives.** Triethylenethiophosphoramide (thiotepa) is the only compound in this group that has much clinical use. Ethylenimine derivatives are capable of the same kinds of reactions as the nitrogen mustards.
   c. **Alkyl sulfonates.** Busulfan is the only clinically active compound in this group. It appears to interact more with cellular thiol groups than with nucleic acids.
   d. **Triazine.** Dacarbazine, the only agent of this type, was originally thought to be an antimetabolite because of its resemblance to 5-aminoimidazole-4-carboxamide (AIC). Dacarbazine is now known to act as an alkylator after AIC is cleaved from active diazomethane.
   e. **Nitrosoureas.** The nitrosoureas undergo rapid spontaneous activation in aqueous solution to form products capable of alkylation and carbamoylation. They are unique among the alkylating agents with respect to being non-cross-resistant with other alkylating agents, highly lipid-soluble, and having delayed myelosuppressive effects (6–8 weeks).
   f. **Metal salts.** Cisplatin and carboplatin inhibit DNA synthesis probably through the formation of intrastrand cross-links in DNA. They also react with DNA through chelation or through binding to the cell membrane.

B. **Antimetabolites**
   1. **General description.** The antimetabolites are a group of low-molecular-weight compounds that exert

their effect by virtue of their structural or functional similarity to naturally occurring metabolites involved in nucleic acid synthesis. Because they are mistaken by the cell for a normal metabolite, they either inhibit critical enzymes involved in nucleic acid synthesis or become incorporated into the nucleic acid and produce incorrect codes. Both mechanisms result in inhibition of DNA synthesis and ultimate cell death. Because of their primary effect on DNA synthesis, the antimetabolites are most active in cells that are actively growing and are largely cell cycle phase-specific.

2. **Types of antimetabolites**
   a. **Folic acid analogs.** These drugs, of which methotrexate is the only member in wide clinical use, inhibit the enzyme dihydrofolate reductase. This inhibition blocks the production of the reduced N^5-N^{10}-methylenetetrahydrofolate, the coenzyme in the synthesis of thymidylic acid. Other metabolic processes in which there is one carbon unit transfer are also affected but are probably of less importance in the cytotoxic action of methotrexate.
   b. **Pyrimidine analogs.** These compounds inhibit critical enzymes necessary for nucleic acid synthesis and may become incorporated into DNA and RNA (e.g., cytarabine, 5-azacitidine).
   c. **Purine analogs.** The specific site of action for the purine analogs is less well defined than for most pyrimidine analogs, although it is well demonstrated that they interfere with normal purine interconversions and thus with DNA and RNA synthesis. Some of the analogs also are incorporated into the nucleic acids. The adenosine deaminase inhibitor pentostatin increases the intracellular concentration of deoxyadenosine triphosphates in lymphoid cells and inhibits DNA synthesis, probably by blocking ribonucleotide reductase. Among the metabolic alterations is nicotinamide adenine dinucleotide (NAD) depletion, which may result in cell death. Cladribine accumulates in cells as the triphosphate, is incorporated into DNA, and inhibits DNA repair enzymes and RNA synthesis. As with pentostatin, NAD levels are also depleted.

C. **Natural products**
   1. **General description.** The natural products are grouped together not on the basis of activity but because they are derived from natural sources. The clinically useful drugs are (1) plant products, (2) fermentation products of various species of the soil fungus *Streptomyces*, and (3) bacterial products.
   2. **Types of natural products**
      a. **Mitotic inhibitors.** Vincristine, vinblastine, and its semisynthetic derivatives vindesine and vinorelbine are derived from the periwinkle plant (*Catharanthus roseus*), a species of myrtle. They

appear to act primarily through their effect on microtubular protein with a resultant metaphase arrest and inhibition of mitosis.

b. *Podophyllum* derivatives. Etoposide and teniposide, semisynthetic podophyllotoxins derived from the root of the mayapple plant (*Podophyllum peltatum*), form a complex with topoisomerase II, an enzyme that is necessary for the completion of DNA replication. This interaction results in DNA strand breakage and arrest of cells in late S and early G_2 phases of the cell cycle.

c. Antibiotics. The antitumor antibiotics are a group of related antimicrobial compounds produced by *Streptomyces* species in culture. Their cytotoxicity, which limits their antimicrobial usefulness, has proved to be of great value in treating a wide range of cancers. All of the clinically useful antibiotics affect the function and synthesis of nucleic acids.

    (1) Dactinomycin, the anthracyclines (doxorubicin, daunorubicin, and idarubicin), and the anthracenedione mitoxantrone cause topoisomerase II-dependent DNA cleavage and intercalate with the DNA double helix.

    (2) Bleomycins cause DNA-strand scission. The resulting fragmentation is believed to underlie the drug's cytotoxic activity.

    (3) Mitomycin causes cross-links between complementary strands of DNA that impair replication.

    (4) Plicamycin (mithramycin) complexes with Mg^{2+} to DNA and blocks RNA synthesis.

d. Enzymes. Asparaginase, the one example of this type of agent, catalyzes the hydrolysis of asparagine to aspartic acid and ammonia and deprives selected malignant cells of an amino acid essential to their survival.

D. Hormones and hormone antagonists

1. General description. The hormones and hormone antagonists that are clinically active against cancer include steroidal estrogens, progestins, androgens, corticoids and their synthetic derivatives, nonsteroidal synthetic compounds with steroid or steroid-antagonist activity, hypothalamic-pituitary analogs, and thyroid hormones. Each agent has diverse effects. Some effects are mediated directly at the cellular level by the drug binding to specific cytoplasmic receptors or by inhibition or stimulation of the production or action of the hormones. These agents may also act by stimulating or inhibiting natural autocrine and paracrine growth factors (e.g., epidermal growth factor, transforming growth factor-alpha [TGF-α], and TGF-β). The relative role of the various actions of hormones and hormone antagonists is not well understood and probably varies among tumor types. Other effects are mediated through indirect effects on the hypothalamus and its anterior pituitary regulating hormones. The final common pathway in most circumstances appears to lead to the malignant cell, which has retained some sensitivity to direct or indirect hormonal control of its growth. An exception to this mechanism is the effect of corticosteroids on leukemias and lymphomas in which the steroids appear to have direct lytic effects on abnormal lymphoid cells that have high numbers of glucocorticoid receptors.

2. **Types of hormones and hormone antagonists**
   a. **Androgens** may exert their antineoplastic effect by altering pituitary function or directly affecting the neoplastic cell.
   b. **Corticosteroids** cause lysis of lymphoid tumors that are rich in specific cytoplasmic receptors and may have other indirect effects as well.
   c. **Estrogens** suppress testosterone production (through the hypothalamus) in males and alter breast cancer cell response to prolactin.
   d. **Progestins** appear to act directly at the level of the malignant cell receptor to promote differentiation.
   e. **Estrogen antagonists** compete with estrogen for binding on the cytosol estrogen receptor protein in cancer cells and affect the natural growth factors.
   f. **Hypothalamic hormone analogs,** such as the leutenizing hormone (LH)-releasing hormone (LHRH) agonists leuprolide or goserelin can inhibit LH and follicle-stimulating hormone (FSH) (after initial stimulation) and the production of testosterone or estrogen by the gonads.
   g. **Thyroid hormones** inhibit the release of thyroid-stimulating hormone (TSH), thus inhibiting growth of well-differentiated thyroid tumors.

E. **Miscellaneous agents** are listed in Table 10-1. Descriptions of specific agents are found in section **III**, below.

II. **Clinically useful chemotherapeutic and biologic agents.** Section **III** of this chapter contains an alphabetically arranged description of the chemotherapeutic and biologic agents that are recognized to be clinically useful. Each drug is listed by its generic name with other common or trade names included. A brief description is given of the probable mechanism of action, clinical uses, recommended doses and schedules, precautions, and side effects. The role of the biologic agents in the therapy of malignant disease is not as well established as it is for chemotherapy, although it is clear that their indications and use will expand greatly in the near future.

A. **Recommended doses: caution.** Although every effort has been made to ensure that the drug dosages and schedules herein are accurate and in accord with published standards, readers are advised to check the product information sheet included in the package of each

Food and Drug Administration (FDA)-approved drug and to read FDA–NCI (National Cancer Institute) guidelines for drugs not yet approved for general use to verify recommended dosages, contraindications, and precautions and to review potential toxicity.

B. Drug toxicity: frequency designation. The doses are listed using body surface area (square meters) as the base. Adult doses from the literature, which are expressed using a weight base, have been converted by multiplying the milligram per kilogram dose by 37 to give the milligram per square meter dose. Doses using a weight base, which have been taken from the pediatric literature, have been converted using a factor of 25. Because many of the drugs are given in combination with other agents, doses most commonly used in popular combinations may also be indicated. These data should not be used as the sole source of information for any of the drugs but, rather, used as a guide to confirm and compare dose ranges and schedules and to identify potential problems. The designation of the frequency of toxic side effects is indicated as follows (probability of occurrence equals percent of patients).

1. Universal (90–100%)
2. Common (15–90%)
3. Occasional (5–15%)
4. Uncommon (1–5%)
5. Rare (< 1%)

These designations are meant only to be guides, and the likelihood of a side effect in each patient depends on their physical and psychologic status; previous treatment; dose, schedule, and route of drug administration; and other concurrent treatment.

C. Dose modification

  1. Philosophy. The optimal dose and schedule of a drug is one that gives maximum benefit with tolerable toxicity. Most chemotherapeutic agents have a steep dose–response curve; therefore, if no toxicity is seen, as a rule a higher dose should be given to get the best possible therapeutic benefit. If toxicity is great, however, the patient's life may be threatened or the patient may decide that the treatment is worse than the disease and refuse further therapy. How much toxicity the patient and the physician are willing to tolerate depends on the likelihood that more intensive treatment will make a major therapeutic difference (e.g., cure versus no cure) and on the patient's physical and psychologic tolerance for adverse effects.

  2. Guidelines

    a. Nonhematologic toxicity

      (1) Acute effects. Acute drug toxicity that is limited to 1–2 days and is not cumulative is not usually a cause for dose modification unless it is of grade 3–4 (see Table 8-3). Occasionally, repeating a dose that caused intractable nausea and vomiting or a temperature higher than 40°C (104°F) is warranted, but for any other grade 3–4 toxicity, the subsequent doses should be reduced by 25–50%. If the acute drug effects (e.g., severe paresthesias or abnormalities of renal or liver function) last longer than 48 hours, the subsequent doses should be reduced by 35–50%.

A recurrence of the grade 3–4 side effects at the reduced doses would be an indication either to reduce by another 25–50% or to discontinue the drug altogether. Non-dose-related toxicity, e.g., anaphylaxis, is an indication to discontinue the offending drug.

(2) **Chronic effects.** Chronic or cumulative toxicity, e.g., pulmonary function changes with bleomycin or decreased cardiac function with doxorubicin, is nearly always an indication to discontinue the responsible agent. Chronic or cumulative neurotoxicity due to vincristine, cisplatin, or other agents may require no dose change, reduction, or discontinuation dependent on the severity of the resultant neurologic dysfunction.

b. **Hematologic toxicity.** The degree of myelosuppression and attendant risk of infection and bleeding that are acceptable depend on the cancer, the duration of the myelosuppression, the goals of therapy, and the general health of the patient. In addition, one must consider the relative benefit of less aggressive and more aggressive therapy. For example, with acute nonlymphocytic leukemia, remission is unlikely unless sufficient therapy is given to cause profound pancytopenia for at least 1 week. Because there is little benefit with lesser treatment, grade 4 leukopenia and thrombocytopenia are acceptable toxicities in this circumstance. Grade 4 myelosuppression is also acceptable when the goal is cure of a cancer that does not involve the marrow, such as testicular carcinoma. With breast cancer, on the other hand, responses are seen with less aggressive treatment, and prolonged pancytopenia may not be acceptable, particularly if chemotherapy is being used palliatively or in an adjuvant setting in which the proportion of patients expected to benefit from chemotherapy is relatively small and excessive toxicity would pose an unacceptable risk. (Whether higher doses might increase cure is currently under investigation.)

With these caveats in mind, the dose modification schemes shown in Tables 10-2 and 10-3 can serve as a guide to reasonable dose changes for drugs whose major toxicity is myelosuppression. Separate schemes are given for the nitrosoureas

Table 10-2. Dose modifications for myelosuppressive drugs with a nadir[a] at less than 3 weeks

Degree of suppression	ANC (WBC)/μl on day of scheduled treatment[b]		Platelets/μl on day of scheduled treatment	Dose as percentage of immediately preceding cycle
Minimal	≥1800 (≥3500)	and	>100,000	100
Mild	1500–1800 (3000–3500)	or	75,000–100,000	75
Moderate	1000–1500 (2500–3000)	or	50,000–75,000	50
Severe	<1000 (<2500)	or	<50,000	0 (delay 1 week)

[a]If the nadir of the absolute neutrophil count (ANC) is <1000/μl and is associated with fever >38.3°C (101°F) or nadir of platelets is <40,000, decrease dose by 25% in subsequent cycles. If the dose is already to be reduced on the basis of the ANC or platelet count on the day of treatment as per this table, do not reduce further because of the nadir count.

[b]ANC is preferred parameter if available. If counts are rising at the end of a treatment cycle, it is often appropriate to delay 1 week and then treat according to the dose modification scheme shown here.

Table 10-3. Dose modifications for myelosuppressive drugs[a] with a nadir at 3 weeks or later

	ANC (WBC)/μl		Platelets/μl	Dose as percentage of immediately preceding cycle
I. On day of scheduled treatment[b]	> 1800 (> 3500)	and	> 100,000	Dose modified for nadir only
	< 1800 (< 3500)	or	< 100,000	0[c]
II. At last nadir	> 750	and	> 75,000	100
	500–750	or	40,000–75,000	75
	< 500	or	< 40,000	50
III. After 2 weeks' delay	> 1800 (> 3500)	and	> 100,000	Dose modified for nadir only
	1200–1800 (2500–3500)	or	75,000–100,000	75
	< 1200	or	< 75,000	Continue to hold

[a]Nitrosoureas or other agents with prolonged nadir.
[b]Absolute neutrophil count (ANC) is preferred parameter to use.
[c]Withhold treatment and repeat count in 2 weeks. At 2 weeks, treat on basis of lowest dose indicated by nadir (II) or delay (III) section of table.

and for drugs that have less prolonged myelosuppression.

III. Data for clinically useful chemotherapeutic and biologic agents

Note: Although every effort has been made to ensure that the drug dosage and schedules herein are accurate and in accord with published standards, users are advised to check the product information sheet included in the package of each FDA-approved drug and FDA–NCI guidelines for drugs that are not yet approved for general use (see Table 10-1) to verify recommended dosages, contraindications, and precautions.

Agents that have not yet been approved by the FDA are included, either because they have some demonstrated usefulness or are widely used in investigational studies. As their efficacy and toxicity are more firmly established, it is expected that some will be approved by the FDA for general use, whereas others will remain investigational or be dropped from further study.

Aldesleukin

Other names. Interleukin-2 (IL-2), Proleukin.

Mechanism of action. Enhances mitogenesis of T cells, natural killer (NK) cells, and lymphokine-activated killer (LAK) cells; augments cytotoxicity of NK and LAK cells; induces interferon gamma.

Primary indications

1. Renal cell carcinoma.
2. Melanoma.

Usual dosage and schedule. Wide range of doses and routes (IV or SC) have been used. The subcutaneous route has also been used. Examples are given of moderate- and low-intensity regimens. In any of the schedules, therapy may be stopped prematurely for constitutional symptoms, or cardiovascular, renal, hepatic, neurologic, pulmonary, or hematologic toxicity.

1. 600,000 IU/kg (22×10^6 IU/m^2) as a 15-minute IV infusion every 8 hours for up to 14 doses. Repeat once after a 9-day rest period.
2. 18–22×10^6 IU/m^2/24 hours as a continuous IV infusion for 4–5 days, depending on tolerance. Repeat 4–5 day cycle starting day 8 or 15.
3. 18–22×10^6 IU/m^2 as a 15 minute IV infusion daily for 5 days on two successive weeks. Repeat every 3 to 6 weeks as tolerated. In some regimens, it is preceded by 3 days with low-dose cyclophosphamide, 350 mg/m^2 IV push.
4. 30–60×10^6 IU/m^2 IV over 10 minutes three times weekly.

Schedules 1 and 2 require hospitalization. Schedules 3 and 4 can be given in an outpatient setting, but require several hours of observation after treatment.

Special precautions. Patients must be carefully monitored after treatment using any of the dosing regimens. Outpatient regimens require that patients have cardiovascular status observed for up to 5 hours, particularly after the first several doses. With higher doses, capillary leak syndrome resulting in hypotension, pulmonary edema, myocardial infarction, arrhythmias, azotemia, and alterations in mental status may occur. Intensive care, controlled volume replacement, and intubation may be required. The lower doses can be given in an outpatient setting.

Toxicity.   All are dose-dependent.

1. *Myelosuppression.* Uncommon at lower doses, common, but rarely serious at higher doses. Anemia requiring transfusion is common at higher doses. Thrombocytopenia is common at higher doses.
2. *Nausea and vomiting.* Common.
3. *Mucocutaneous effects.* Mucositis is occasional to common. Alopecia is uncommon. Pruritic erythematous rash is common.
4. *Cardiovascular effects*
   a. Arrhythmias are common and dose-related.
   b. Hypotension is dose-related but is occasionally seen at the lower-dose schedules.
   c. Myocardial injury is seen primarily at the higher-dose schedules.
   d. Pulmonary edema from capillary leak syndrome is common with intensive dose regimens.
   e. Weight gain is common from edema, particularly in more intensive dose regimens.
5. *Gastrointestinal effects*
   a. Anorexia—common.
   b. Diarrhea—occasional.
   c. Transient liver function abnormalities, including hyperbilirubinemia, and hypoalbuminemia and elevation of the prothrombin time and partial thromboplastin time—common.
   d. Colonic perforations—rare.
6. *Neuropsychiatric effects*
   a. Mental status changes—common, with dose-related severity.
   b. Dizziness or light-headedness—common.
   c. Blurry vision and other visual disturbances—occasional.
   d. Seizures—uncommon to rare at lower-dose regimens.
7. *Renal function impairment.* Common but reversible. More frequent laboratory abnormalities include creatinine elevation, hypomagnesemia, acidosis, hypocalcemia, hypophosphatemia, hypokalemia, hypouricemia, and hypoalbuminemia.
8. *Fever.* With or without chills—universal and may be severe.
9. *Bacterial infection.* Occasional. Probably related to chemotactic defect induced in granulocytes.
10. *Myalgias and arthralgias.* Occasional to common.
11. *Malaise and fatigue.* Common and dose-related.

Prophylaxis of acute toxicity

1. Acetaminophen 650–1000 mg PO 1 hour prior to therapy and q3h for 2 doses.
2. Cimetidine 800 mg PO prior to therapy and daily for duration of treatment.
3. Antiemetics: ondansetron, metoclopramide, and prochlorperazine may be used. *Do not* use dexamethasone.
4. Meperidine 25–50 mg IV when chills start after first dose. For subsequent doses, meperidine 150 mg PO 1.5 hours before chills are predicated to start, based on the first treatment.
5. Diphenhydramine 50 mg PO q3h for 3 doses may be substituted for meperidine in patients who tolerate the latter drug poorly.

Altretamine

Other names.   Hexamethylmelamine, hexalen, HXM.

Mechanism of action.   Unknown. Although it structurally resembles the known alkaylating agent triethylene-melamine, it has some antimetabolite characteristics.

Primary indication.   Carcinoma of the ovary.

Usual dosage and schedule

1. 200–320 mg/m^2 PO daily in 3 or 4 divided doses for 14 or 21 days every 4 weeks when used as a single agent.
2. 150–200 mg/m^2 PO daily in 3 or 4 divided doses for 2 out of 3 or 4 weeks when used in combination.

Special precautions.   Concurrent altretamine and antidepressants of the monoamine oxidase (MAO) inhibitor class may cause severe orthostatic hypotension. Cimetidine may increase toxicity.

Toxicity

1. *Myelosuppression.* Dose-limiting leukopenia and thrombocytopenia are uncommon. Anemia is common.
2. *Nausea and vomiting.* Usually dose-limiting and associated with anorexia, diarrhea, and abdominal cramps. Tolerance may develop.
3. *Mucocutaneous effects.* Alopecia, skin rash, and pruritus are rare.
4. *Miscellaneous effects*
   a. Peripheral sensory neuropathies—common. May be ameliorated by pyridoxine.
   b. Central nervous system (CNS) effects, including agitation, confusion, hallucinations, depression, and Parkinsonian-like symptoms—less common with recommended intermittent schedule than with continuous treatment.
   c. Decreased renal function—occasional.

Aminoglutethimide

Other names.   Cytadren, Elipten, AG

Mechanism of action.   Inhibits aromatization and cytochrome P-450 hydroxylating enzymes, thereby blocking the conversion of androgens to estrogens and the biosynthesis of all steroid hormones. This drug causes, in effect, a reversible chemical adrenalectomy.

Primary indications.   Breast carcinoma, prostate carcinoma, adrenocortical carcinoma, ectopic Cushing's syndrome.

Usual dosage and schedule.   1000 mg daily in 4 divided doses.

Special precautions.   Hydrocortisone must be given concomitantly (particularly for breast cancer) to prevent adrenal insufficiency. Suggested dose is 100 mg daily in divided doses for 2 weeks, then 40 mg daily in divided doses.

Toxicity

1. *Myelosuppression.* Leukopenia and thrombocytopenia are rare, and if they occur they resolve rapidly when the drug is stopped.
2. *Nausea and vomiting* are occasional and usually mild.
3. *Mucocutaneous effects.* A morbilliform rash is commonly seen during the first week of treatment, but it usually disappears within 1 week.
4. *Hormonal effects*
   a. Adrenal insufficiency—common without replacement hydrocortisone in patients with normal adrenal glands.
   b. Hypothyroidism—uncommon.
   c. Masculinization—possible.
5. *Neurologic effects*
   a. Lethargy is common. Although usually mild and transient, it is occasionally severe.
   b. Vertigo, nystagmus, and ataxia—occasional.
6. *Miscellaneous effects*
   a. Facial flushing—uncommon.
   b. Periorbital edema—uncommon.
   c. Cholestatic jaundice—rare.
   d. Fever—uncommon.

Amsacrine (Investigational)

Other names.   m-AMSA; AMSA.

Mechanism of action.   Binds to DNA through intercalation and external binding. Interaction with topoisomerase II to increase DNA strand breakage.

Primary indications.   Pediatric and adult acute leukemias.

Usual dosage and schedule

1. 120 mg/m^2 IV over 1–2 hours in 500 ml 5% dextrose and water for 3–5 days.
2. 100 mg/m^2 IV over 1–2 hours in 500 ml 5% dextrose and water on days 7, 8, and 9 (in combination regimens).

Special precautions.   Use caution if patient is hypokalemic or was given prior anthracycline, as it may potentiate cardiotoxicity. Solution physically incompatible with sodium chloride solutions. Avoid direct contact with skin.

Toxicity

1. *Myelosuppression.* Universal and dose-limiting.
2. *Nausea and vomiting.* Common.
3. *Mucocutaneous effects.* Mucositis is common and dose-related; occasional skin rash.
4. *Liver.* Common transient liver function abnormalities.
5. *Renal effects.* Rare.
6. *Diarrhea.* Occasional.
7. *Cardiac effects.* Possible. May be affected by prior anthracyclines, e.g., daunorubicin or doxorubicin. Acute arrythmias particularly in association with hypokalemia.
8. *Neurologic effects.* Seizures, neuropathy, headache, dizziness, CNS depression—uncommon.
9. *Phlebitis and local pain.* Common.

Anagrelide (Investigational)

Other names.   Imidazo(2,1-b)quinazolin-2-one, Agrelin.

Mechanism of action.   Mechanism for thrombocytopenia is unknown but may be due to impaired megakaryocyte function. Inhibitor of platelet aggregation. Inhibits cyclic nucleotide phosphodiesterase and the formation of arachidonic acid metabolites from phospholipid stores.

Primary indication.   Uncontrolled thrombocytosis in chronic myeloproliferative disorders, such as essential thrombocythemia, chronic granulocytic leukemia, and polycythemia rubra vera.

Usual dosage and schedule

1. 0.5 mg PO qid (2.0 mg/day). Increase by 0.5 mg/day every 5–7 days if no response. Maximum daily dose is 12 mg. Maximum single dose is 3 mg. Higher doses cause postural hypotension.
2. *Alternate dosing schedules*
   a. Elderly: 0.5 mg PO daily, increase by 0.5 mg daily each week.
   b. Abnormal renal or hepatic function: 0.5 mg PO bid.

Special precautions.   Contraindicated in pregnancy. Use with caution in patients with heart disease. Tachycardia and forceful heartbeat may be exacerbated by caffeine; consumption of caffeine should be avoided for 1 hour before and after anagrelide is taken. Use other drugs that inhibit platelet aggregation (such as nonsteroidal anti-inflamma-tory drugs) with caution.

Toxicity

1. *Myelosuppression.* White cell count—none; anemia—common (36%); thrombocytopenic hemorrhage—uncommon (2%).
2. *Nausea and vomiting.* Nausea—occasional to common (19%); vomiting—uncommon.
3. *Mucocutaneous.* Rash—uncommon (2%); hyperpigmentation—rare; sun sensitivity—possible.
4. *Miscellaneous effects*
   a. Cardiovascular: edema, palpitations, forceful heart beat, and tachycardia—common; congestive heart failure and tachyarrhythmias (including atrial fibrillation and premature atrial beats)—uncommon; angina and cardiomyopathy—rare. Drinking alcoholic beverages may cause flushing. Higher than recommended single doses cause postural hypotension. Cardiovascular effects appear to result from vasodilation, positive inotropy, and decreased renal blood flow.
   b. Neurologic: headaches—common, occasionally severe; dizziness—occasional.
   c. Pulmonary: infiltrates—rare but are cause to stop anagrelide and treat with steroids.
   d. Other gastrointestinal effects: diarrhea, gas, abdominal pain—occasional; pancreatitis—rare. Lactase supplementation eliminates diarrhea (anagrelide formulated with lactose).

Androgens

Other names. Fluoxymesterone (Halotestin), testolactone (Teslac), others.

Mechanism of action. Mechanism of antitumor effects is not clear.

Primary indications

1. Breast carcinoma (in combination with other agents).
2. Anemia of myelodysplastic syndromes.

Usual dosage and schedule

1. *Fluoxymesterone:* 20–40 mg PO daily in 4 divided doses.
2. *Testolactone:* 1000 mg PO daily in 4 divided doses.

Special precautions. Hypercalcemia may occur with initial therapy.

Toxicity

1. *Myelosuppression.* None. Erythropoiesis is stimulated.
2. *Nausea and vomiting.* Mild and dose-related.
3. *Mucocutaneous effects.* Acne.
4. *Miscellaneous effects*
   a. Masculinization—including an increase in facial and

body hair, deepening of voice, acne, baldness, and cli-
toral hypertrophy—is common in females but may be
minimized by dose attenuation.
   b. Intrahepatic biliary stasis with hyperbilirubinemia
is uncommon but may occur at high androgen doses
(17-methyl derivatives only).
   c. Fluid retention may occur, although it is less severe
with androgens than with estrogens—occasional.

Asparaginase

Other names.   L-Asparaginase, Elspar, pegaspargase,
Oncaspar.

Mechanism of action.   Hydrolysis of serum asparagine
occurs, which deprives leukemia cells of the required amino
acid and inhibits protein synthesis. Normal cells are spared
because they generally have the ability to synthesize their
own asparagine. Pegaspargase is a chemically modified formulation of asparaginase in which the L-asparaginase is co-
valently conjugated with monomethoxypolyethylene glycol
(PEG). This modification increases its half-life in the
plasma by a factor of 4 to about 5.7 days and reduces its
recognition by the immune system, which allows the drug
to be used in patients previously hypersensitive to native
L-asparaginase.

Primary indication.   Acute lymphocytic leukemia, primarily for induction therapy.

Usual dosage and schedule.   Both schedules are usually
used in combination with other drugs (see under Special
precautions, item 2, below). The schedules listed are only
two of many acceptable dosing schedules.

1. L-asparaginase: 6000–18,500 IU/m² IV daily for up to 14
   days.
2. Pegaspargase: 2500 IU/m² IM (or IV) once every 14 days,
   in patients who have developed hypersensitivity to native
   forms of asparaginase.

Special precautions

1. Be prepared to treat anaphylaxis at each administration
   of the drug. Epinephrine, antihistamines, corticosteroids,
   and life-support equipment should be readily available.
2. Giving concurrently with or immediately before vincristine may increase vincristine toxicity.
3. The intramuscular route is preferred for pegaspargase,
   because of a lower incidence of hepatotoxicity, coagulopathy, and gastrointestinal and renal disorders compared
   to the intravenous route of administration.

Toxicity

1. *Myelosuppression.* Occasional.
2. *Nausea and vomiting.* Occasional and usually mild.
3. *Mucocutaneous effects.* No toxicity occurs except as a
   sign of hypersensitivity.

4. *Anaphylaxis.* Mild to severe hypersensitivity reactions, including anaphylaxis, occur in 20–30% of patients. Such reaction is less likely to occur during the first few days of treatment. It is particularly common with intermittent schedules or repeat cycles. If the patient develops hypersensitivity to the *Escherichia coli*-derived enzyme (Elspar), *Erwinia*-derived asparaginase may be safely substituted because the two enzyme preparations are not cross-reactive. Note that hypersensitivity may also develop to *Erwinia*-derived asparaginase, and continued preparedness to treat anaphylaxis must be maintained.

   If given IM, asparaginase should be given in an extremity so that a tourniquet can be applied to slow the systemic release of asparaginase should anaphylaxis occur.

   Approximately 30% of patients previously sensitive to L-asparaginase will have a hypersensitivity reaction to pegaspargase, while only 10% of those who were not hypersensitive to the native form will have a hypersensitivity reaction to the PEG-modified drug.

5. *Miscellaneous effects*
   a. Mild fever and malaise are common and occasionally progress to severe chills and malignant hyperthermia.
   b. Hepatotoxicity is common and occasionally severe. Abnormalities observed include elevations of serum glutamic-oxaloacetic transaminase (SGOT), alkaline phosphatase, and bilirubin; depressed levels of hepatic-derived clotting factors and albumin; and hepatocellular fatty metamorphosis.
   c. Renal failure is rare.
   d. Pancreatic endocrine and exocrine dysfunction, often with manifestations of pancreatitis, occasionally occurs. Nonketotic hyperglycemia is uncommon.
   e. CNS effects (depression, somnolence, fatigue, confusion, agitation, hallucinations, or coma) are seen occasionally. They are usually reversible following discontinuation of the drug.

Azacitidine (Investigational)

Other names.   5-Azacitidine, 5 aza-C, ladakamycin.

Mechanism of action.   A pyrimidine analog antimetabolite that causes interference with nucleic acid synthesis and is incorporated into both DNA and RNA, where it acts as a false pyrimidine.

Primary indication.   Acute nonlymphocytic leukemia.

Usual dosage and schedule

1. 100 mg/m² IV push q8h for 5 days *or*
2. 150–200 mg/m² IV daily as continuous infusion for 5 days.

Special precautions. Because of drug instability the dose should be prepared immediately before use and discarded after 8 hours. Infusions should be freshly prepared with Ringer's lactate solution and changed every 8 hours.

Toxicity

1. *Myelosuppression.* Severe in all patients, with the leukocyte nadir occurring at 12–14 days. Occasionally, suppression is prolonged beyond several weeks.
2. *Nausea and vomiting.* Common. Continuous infusion lessens nausea and vomiting.
3. *Mucocutaneous effects.* Stomatitis and rash—occasional.
4. *Miscellaneous effects*
   a. Diarrhea—common.
   b. Neurologic problems with muscle pain, weakness, lethargy, and coma—uncommon.
   c. Hepatotoxicity—rare but may be severe.
   d. Transient fever—occasional.

Bicalutamide (Investigational)

Other name. Casodex.

Mechanism of action. Competitive inhibitor of androgens at the cellular androgen receptor.

Primary indication. Carcinoma of the prostate.

Usual dosage and schedule. 150 mg (1 tablet) daily.

Special precautions. None.

Toxicity

1. *Myelosuppression.* None.
2. *Nausea and vomiting.* Uncommon.
3. *Mucocutaneous effects.* Mild skin rash—occasional.
4. *Miscellaneous effects*
   a. Secondary pharmacologic effects, including breast tenderness, breast swelling, hot flashes, impotence, and loss of libido—common, but reversible following cessation of therapy.
   b. Gastrointestinal effects: diarrhea—uncommon; constipation—occasional.
   c. Elevated liver enzyme levels—uncommon.
   d. Dizziness or vertigo—occasional.

Bleomycin

Other name. Blenoxane.

Mechanism of action. Bleomycin binds to DNA, causes single- and double-strand scission, and inhibits further DNA, RNA, and protein synthesis.

Primary indications

1. Testis, head and neck, penis, cervix, vulva, anus, and skin carcinomas.
2. Hodgkin's and non-Hodgkin's lymphomas.

Usual dosage and schedule

1. 10–20 units/m^2 IV or IM once or twice a week *or*
2. 30 units IV push weekly for 9–12 weeks in combination with other drugs for testis cancer.
3. 60 units in 50 ml of normal saline instilled intrapleurally.

Special precautions

1. In patients with lymphoma, a test dose of 1 or 2 units should be given IM prior to the first dose of bleomycin because of the possibility of anaphylactoid, acute pulmonary, or severe hyperpyretic responses. If no acute reaction occurs within 4 hours, regular dosing may begin.
2. Reduce dose for renal failure.

Serum creatinine	Full dose (%)
2.5–4.0	25
4.0–6.0	20
6.0–10.0	10

3. The cumulative lifetime dose should not exceed 400 units because of the dose-related incidence of severe pulmonary fibrosis. Smaller limits may be appropriate for older patients or those with preexisting pulmonary disease. Frequent evaluation of pulmonary status, including symptoms of cough or dyspnea, rales, infiltrates on chest x-ray film, and pulmonary function studies are recommended to avert serious pulmonary sequelae.
4. Glass containers are recommended for continuous infusion to minimize drug instability.
5. High FiO$_2$ (fraction of inspired oxygen) (such as might be used during surgery) should be avoided as it exacerbates lung injury, sometimes acutely.

Toxicity

1. *Myelosuppression.* Significant depression of counts is uncommon. This factor permits bleomycin to be used in full doses with myelosuppressive drugs.
2. *Nausea and vomiting.* Occasional and self-limiting.
3. *Mucocutaneous effects.* Alopecia, stomatitis, erythema, edema, thickening of nail bed, and hyperpigmentation and desquamation of skin are common.
4. *Pulmonary effects*
   a. Acute anaphylactoid or pulmonary edema–like response—occasional in patients with lymphoma (see Special precautions, above).
   b. Dose-related pneumonitis with cough, dyspnea, rales, and infiltrates, progressing to pulmonary fibrosis.
5. *Fever.* Common. Occasionally severe hyperpyrexia, diaphoresis, dehydration, and hypotension have occurred

and resulted in renal failure and death. Antipyretics help control fever.
6. *Miscellaneous effects*
   a. Lethargy, headache, joint swelling—rare.
   b. IM or SQ injection may cause pain at injection site.

Busulfan

Other name.   Myleran.

Mechanism of action.   Bifunctional alkylating agent. Its effect may be greater on cellular thiol groups than on nucleic acids.

Primary indications

1. *Standard doses:* chronic granulocytic leukemia.
2. *High doses with stem cell rescue:* acute leukemia, lymphoma.

Usual dosage and schedule

1. 3–4 mg/m^2 PO daily for remission induction in adults until the leukocyte count is 50% of the original level, then 1–2 mg/m^2 daily. Busulfan may be given continuously or intermittently for maintenance.
2. High doses with stem cell rescue—consult specific protocols. Not recommended outside research setting. Typical dose is 1 mg/kg PO q6h for 4 consecutive days.

Special precautions.   Obtain complete blood count weekly while patient is on therapy. If leukocyte count falls rapidly to less than 15,000/µl, discontinue therapy until nadir is reached and rising counts indicate a need for further treatment.

Toxicity

1. *Myelosuppression.* Dose-limiting. A fall in the leukocyte count may not begin for 2 weeks after starting therapy, and it is likely to continue for 2 weeks after therapy has been stopped. Recovery of marrow function may be delayed for 3–6 weeks after the drug has been discontinued. High-dose therapy requires stem cell rescue (e.g., bone marrow transplantation).
2. *Nausea and vomiting.* Rare.
3. *Mucocutaneous effects.* Hyperpigmentation occurs occasionally, particularly in skin creases.
4. *Pulmonary effects.* Interstitial pulmonary fibrosis is rare and is an indication to discontinue drug. Corticosteroids may improve symptoms and minimize permanent lung damage.
5. *Metabolic effects.* Adrenal insufficiency syndrome is rare. Hyperuricemia may occur when the leukemia cell count is rapidly reduced. Ovarian suppression and amenorrhea are common.
6. *Miscellaneous effects*
   a. Secondary neoplasia is possible.

b. Fatal hepatovenoocclusive disease with high-dose therapy—occasional.

c. Seizures after high-dose therapy—occasional.

Carboplatin

Other names. Paraplatin, CBDCA.

Mechanism of action. Covalent binding to DNA.

Primary indications. Ovarian, endometrial, and lung cancers, and other cancers in which cisplatin is active.

Usual dosage and schedule

1. 300–400 mg/m^2 IV by infusion over 15–60 minutes or longer, repeated every 4 weeks.
2. *Alternative dosing* uses the area under the curve (AUC): Total dose (mg) = target AUC × (glomerular filtration rate + 25). The target AUC is typically 5–7 depending on previous therapy and concurrent drugs or radiation.
3. Higher doses up to 1600 mg/m^2 divided over several days have been used followed by stem cell rescue (e.g., bone marrow transplantation).

Special precautions. Much less renal toxicity than cisplatin, so there is no need for a vigorous hydration schedule or forced diuresis. Reduce dose to 250 mg/m^2 for creatinine clearance of 41–59 ml/minute, reduce to 200 mg/m^2 for clearance of 16–40 ml/minute.

Toxicity

1. *Myelosuppression.* Anemia, granulocytopenia, and thrombocytopenia are common and dose-limiting. Red blood cell transfusions may be required. Thrombocytopenia may be delayed (days 18–28).
2. *Nausea and vomiting.* Common; but vomiting (65%) is not as frequent or as severe as with cisplatin and can be controlled with combination antiemetic regimens.
3. *Mucocutaneous effects.* Alopecia is uncommon. Mucositis is rare.
4. *Renal tubular abnormalities.* Elevation in serum creatinine or blood urea nitrogen occurs occasionally. More common is electrolyte loss with decreases in serum sodium, potassium, calcium, and magnesium.
5. *Miscellaneous effects*
   a. Liver function abnormalities—common.
   b. Gastrointestinal pain—occasional.
   c. Peripheral neuropathies or central neurotoxicity—uncommon.
   d. Allergic reactions—uncommonly seen with rash, urticaria, pruritus, and rarely bronchospasm and hypotension.
   e. Cardiovascular (cardiac failure, embolism, cerebrovascular accidents)—uncommon.
   f. Hemolytic uremic syndrome—rare.

Carmustine

Other names. BCNU, BiCNU.

Mechanism of action. Alkylation and carbamoylation by carmustine metabolites interfere with the synthesis and function of DNA, RNA, and proteins. Carmustine is lipid-soluble and easily enters the brain.

Primary indications

1. Hodgkin's and non-Hodgkin's lymphomas.
2. Brain tumors.
3. Multiple myeloma.
4. Melanoma.

Usual dosage and schedule

1. 200–240 mg/m^2 IV as a 30- to 45-minute infusion every 6–8 weeks. Dose often is divided and given over 2–3 days. Some recommend limiting the cumulative dose to 1000 mg/m^2 to limit pulmonary and renal toxicity.
2. Higher doses up to 600 mg/m^2 have been used with stem cell rescue (e.g., bone marrow transplantation).

Special precautions. Because of delayed myelosuppression (3–6 weeks), do not administer drug more often than every 6 weeks. Await a return of normal platelet and granulocyte counts before repeating therapy. Amphotericin B may enhance the potential for renal toxicity, bronchospasm, and hypotension.

Toxicity

1. *Myelosuppression.* Delayed and often biphasic, with the nadir at 3–6 weeks, it may be cumulative with successive doses. Recovery may be protracted for several months. High-dose therapy requires stem cell rescue.
2. *Nausea and vomiting.* They begin 2 hours after therapy and last 4–6 hours—common.
3. *Mucocutaneous effects*
   a. Facial flushing and a burning sensation at the IV site may be due to alcohol used to reconstitute the drug—common with rapid injection.
   b. Hyperpigmentation of skin following accidental contact—common.
4. *Miscellaneous effects*
   a. Hepatotoxicity—uncommon but can be severe.
   b. Pulmonary fibrosis—uncommon at low doses, but frequency increases at doses over 1000 mg/m^2.
   c. Secondary neoplasia—possible.
   d. Renal toxicity is uncommon at doses less than 1000 mg/m^2.
   e. With high-dose therapy, encephalopathy, hepatotoxicity, and pulmonary toxicity are common and dose-limiting. Hepatovenoocclusive disease also occurs (occasional).

Chlorambucil

Other name.   Leukeran.

Mechanism of action.   Classic alkylating agent, with primary effect on preformed DNA.

Primary indications
1. Chronic lymphocytic leukemia.
2. Low-grade non-Hodgkin's lymphoma.

Usual dosage and schedule

1. 3–4 mg/m^2 PO daily until a response is seen or cytopenias occur; then, if necessary, maintain with 1–2 mg/m^2 PO daily.
2. 30 mg/m^2 PO once every 2 weeks (with or without prednisone 80 mg/m^2 PO on days 1–5).

Special precautions.   Increased toxicity may occur with prior barbiturate use.

Toxicity

1. *Myelosuppression.* Dose-limiting and may be prolonged.
2. *Nausea and vomiting.* May be seen with higher doses but are uncommon.
3. *Mucocutaneous effects.* Rash—uncommon.
4. *Miscellaneous effects*
   a. Liver function abnormalities—rare.
   b. Secondary neoplasia—possible.
   c. Amenorrhea and azoospermia—common.
   d. Drug fever—uncommon.
   e. Pulmonary fibrosis—rare.
   f. CNS effects including seizure and coma may be seen at very high doses (> 100 mg/m^2).

Cisplatin

Other names.   *cis*-Diamminedichloroplatinum (II), DDP, CDDP, Platinol.

Mechanism of action.   Similar to alkylating agents with respect to binding and cross-linking strands of DNA.

Primary indications.   Usually used in combination with other cytotoxic drugs.

1. Testis, ovary, endometrial, cervical, bladder, head and neck, gastrointestinal, and lung carcinomas.
2. Soft-tissue and bone sarcomas.
3. Non-Hodgkin's lymphoma.

Usual dosage and schedule

1. 40–120 mg/m^2 IV on day 1 as infusion every 3 weeks.
2. 15–20 mg/m^2 IV on days 1–5 as infusion every 3–4 weeks.

Special precautions.   Do not administer if serum creatinine level is more than 1.5 mg/dl. Irreversible renal tubular damage may occur if vigorous diuresis is not maintained, particularly with higher doses (>40 mg/m^2) and with additional concurrent nephrotoxic drugs, such as the aminoglycosides. At higher doses, diuresis with mannitol with or without furosemide plus vigorous hydration are mandatory.

1. An acceptable method for hydration in patients without cardiovascular impairment for cisplatin doses up to 80 mg/m^2 is as follows.
   a. Have patient void, and begin infusion of 5% dextrose in half-normal saline with potassium chloride (KCl) 20 mEq/liter and magnesium sulfate (MgSO$_4$) 1 gm/liter (8 mEq/liter); run at 500 ml/hour for 1.5–2.0 liters.
   b. After 1 hour of infusion, give 12.5 gm of mannitol by IV push.
   c. Immediately thereafter start the cisplatin (mixed in normal saline at 1 mg/ml) and infuse over 1 hour through the sidearm of the IV, while continuing the hydration.
   d. Give additional mannitol (12.5–50.0 gm by IV push) if necessary to maintain urinary output of 250 ml/hour over the duration of the hydration. If patient gets more than 1 liter behind on urinary output or signs or symptoms of congestive heart failure develop, 40 mg of furosemide may be given.
2. For doses more than 80 mg/m^2 a more vigorous hydration is recommended.
   a. Have patient void, and begin infusion of 5% dextrose in half-normal saline with KCl 20 mEq/liter and MgSO$_4$ 1 gm/liter (8 mEq/liter); run at 500 ml/hour for 2.5–3.0 liters.
   b. After 1 hour of infusion, give 25 gm of mannitol by IV push.
   c. Continue hydration.
   d. After 2 hours of hydration, if urinary output is at least 250 ml/hour, start the cisplatin (mixed in normal saline at 1 mg/ml) and infuse over 1–2 hours (1 mg/m^2/minute) through the sidearm of the IV, while continuing the hydration.
   e. Give additional mannitol (12.5–50 gm by IV push) if necessary to maintain urinary output of 250 ml/hour over the duration of the hydration. If patient gets more than 1 liter behind on urinary output or signs or symptoms of congestive heart failure develop, 40 mg of furosemide may be given.
3. For patients with known or suspected cardiovascular impairment (ejection fraction < 45%), a less vigorous rate of hydration may be used, provided the dose of cisplatin is limited (e.g., < 60 mg/m^2). An alternative is to give carboplatin.

Toxicity

1. *Myelosuppression.* Mild to moderate, depending on the dose. Relative lack of myelosuppression allows cisplatin to be used in full doses with more myelosuppressive

drugs. *Anemia* is common and may have a hemolytic component. Anemia often is amenable to erythropoietin therapy.

2. *Nausea and vomiting.* Severe and often intractable vomiting regularly begins within 1 hour of starting cisplatin and lasts 8–12 hours. Prolonged nausea and vomiting occur occasionally. Nausea and vomiting may be minimized by the use of a combination antiemetic regimen, e.g., dexamethasone, ondanseton or metaclopramide, and lorazepam (see Chap. 33).
3. *Mucocutaneous effects.* None.
4. *Renal tubular damage.* Acute reversible and occasionally irreversible nephrotoxicity may occur, particularly if adequate attention is not given to achieving sufficient hydration and diuresis. Nephrotoxic antibiotics increase risk of acute renal failure.
5. *Ototoxicity.* High-tone hearing loss is common, but significant hearing loss in vocal frequencies occurs only occasionally. Tinnitus is uncommon.
6. *Severe electrolyte abnormalities.* These abnormalities, e.g., marked hyponatremia, hypomagnesemia, hypocalcemia, and hypokalemia, may be seen up to several days after treatment.
7. *Anaphylaxis.* May occur after several doses. Responds to epinephrine, antihistamines, and corticosteroids.
8. *Miscellaneous effects*
   a. Peripheral neuropathies—clinically significant signs and symptoms are common at cumulative doses >300 mg/m^2.
   b. Hyperuricemia—uncommon, parallels renal failure.
   c. Autonomic dysfunction with symptomatic postural hypotension—occasional.

Cladribine

Other names.   2-Chlorodeoxyadenosine, Leustatin.

Mechanism of action.   Deoxyadenosine analog with high cellular specificity for lymphoid cells. Resistant to effect of adenosine deaminase. Accumulates in cells as triphosphate, is incorporated into DNA, and inhibits DNA repair enzymes and RNA synthesis. Also results in NAD depletion. Effect is independent of cell division.

Primary indications.   Hairy-cell leukemia, chronic lymphocytic leukemia, and possibly other lymphoid neoplasms.

Usual dosage and schedule.   0.05–0.2 mg/kg (2–8 mg/m^2) IV daily as a continuous 7-day infusion.

Special precautions.   Give allopurinol 300 mg daily as prophylaxis against hyperuricemia.

Toxicity

1. *Myelosuppression.* Moderate granulocyte suppression is common. No other hematologic toxicity has been seen. Serious infection is common.

2. *Nausea and vomiting.* None.
3. *Mucocutaneous effects.* Rash—common.
4. *Other effects.* Fever, possibly due to release of pyrogens from tumor cells, immunosuppression, renal, and neuro-logic effects have been seen.

Corticosteroids

Other names. Prednisone, dexamethasone (Decadron), and others.

Mechanism of action. Unknown but apparently related to the presence of glucocorticoid receptors in tumor cells. Mediated in part by *blc-2* gene and promotion of apoptotic cell death.

Primary indications

1. Carcinoma of the breast.
2. Acute and chronic lymphocytic leukemia.
3. Hodgkin's and non-Hodgkin's lymphomas.
4. Multiple myeloma.
5. Cerebral edema.
6. Nausea and vomiting with chemotherapy.

Usual dosage and schedule

1. *Prednisone*: dose varies with neoplasm and combina-tion. Typical regimen, *except* for acute lymphocytic leu-kemia, is as follows.
    a. 40 mg/m^2 PO days 1–14 every 4 weeks *or*
    b. 100 mg/m^2 PO days 1–5 every 4 weeks.
2. *Prednisone*: for acute lymphocytic leukemia: 40–50 mg/m^2 PO daily for 28 days.
3. *Dexamethasone*: for cerebral edema: 16–32 mg PO daily to start, then reduce to lowest dose at which symptoms remain controlled.

Special precautions. None.

Toxicity

1. *Myelosuppression.* None.
2. *Nausea and vomiting.* None.
3. *Mucocutaneous effects.* Acne; increased risk for oral, rectal, and vaginal thrush. Thinning of skin and striae develop with continuous use.
4. *Suppression of adrenal-pituitary axis.* May lead to ad-renal insufficiency when corticosteroids are withdrawn. This problem is not common with intermittent sched-ules.
5. *Metabolic effects.* Potassium depletion, sodium and fluid retention, diabetes, increased appetite, loss of muscle mass, myopathy, weight gain, osteoporosis, and development of cushingoid features. Their frequency de-pends on dose and duration of therapy.
6. *Miscellaneous effects*
    a. Epigastric pain, extreme hunger, and occasional pep-

tic ulceration with bleeding may occur. Antacids are recommended as prophylaxis.

b. CNS effects, including euphoria, depression, and sleeplessness, are common and may progress to dementia or frank psychosis.

c. Increased susceptibility to infection is common.

d. Subcapsular cataracts in patients are uncommon but have been seen even when used for prophylaxis and treatment of drug-induced emesis.

Cyclophosphamide

Other names. CTX, Cytoxan, Neosar.

Mechanism of action. Metabolism of cyclophosphamide by hepatic microsomal enzymes produces active alkylating metabolites. Cyclophosphamide's primary effect is probably on DNA.

Primary indications

1. Breast, lung, ovary, testis, and bladder carcinomas.
2. Bone and soft-tissue sarcomas.
3. Hodgkin's and non-Hodgkin's lymphomas.
4. Acute and chronic lymphocytic leukemias.
5. Neuroblastoma and Wilms' tumor of childhood.
6. Multiple myeloma.

Usual dosage and schedule

1. 1000–1500 mg/m^2 IV every 3–4 weeks *or*
2. 400 mg/m^2 PO days 1–5 every 3–4 weeks *or*
3. 60–120 mg/m^2 PO daily.
4. High-dose regimens (6–7 gm/m^2 divided over 4 days) are investigational and should only be used with some kind of stem cell rescue (e.g., bone marrow transplantation) and mesna bladder protection.

Special precautions. Give dose in the morning, maintain ample fluid intake, and have patient empty bladder several times daily to diminish the likelihood of cystitis.

Toxicity

1. *Myelosuppression.* Dose-limiting. Platelets are relatively spared. Nadir is reached about 10–14 days after IV dose with recovery by day 21.
2. *Nausea and vomiting.* Frequent with large IV doses; less common after oral doses. Symptoms begin several hours after treatment and are usually over by the next day.
3. *Mucocutaneous effects.* Reversible alopecia is common, usually starting after 2–3 weeks. Skin and nails may become darker. Mucositis is uncommon.
4. *Bladder damage.* Hemorrhagic or nonhemorrhagic cystitis may occur in 5–10% of patients treated. It is usually reversible with discontinuation of the drug, but it may persist and lead to fibrosis or death. Frequency is

diminished by ample fluid intake and morning administration of the drug. Mesna will protect from this effect.
5. *Miscellaneous effects*
   a. Immunosuppression—common.
   b. Amenorrhea and azoospermia—common.
   c. Inhibition of antidiuretic hormone—only of significance with very large doses.
   d. Interstitial pulmonary fibrosis—rare.
   e. Secondary neoplasia—possible.
   f. Acute and potentially fatal cardiotoxicity occurs with high-dose therapy. Abnormalities include pericardial effusion, congestive heart failure, decreased electrocardiographic (ECG) voltage, and fibrin microthrombi in cardiac capillaries with endothelial injury and hemorrhagic necrosis.

Cytarabine

Other names.   Cytosine arabinoside, ara-C, Cytosar-U.

Mechanism of action.   A pyrimidine analog antimetabolite that, when phosphorylated to arabinosyl-cytosinetriphosphate (ara-CTP), is a competitive inhibitor of DNA polymerase.

Primary indication.   Acute nonlymphocytic leukemia.

Usual dosage and schedule

1. *Induction*: 100–200 mg/m^2 IV daily as a continuous infusion for 5–7 days (in combination with other drugs).
2. *Maintenance*: 100 mg/m^2 SQ every 12 hours for 4 or 5 days every 4 weeks (with other drugs).
3. *Intrathecally*: 40–50 mg/m^2 every 4 days in preservative-free buffered isotonic diluent.
4. *High dose*: 2.0–3.0 gm/m^2 IV over 1 hour every 12 hours for up to 12 doses.

Special precautions.   None for standard doses. High dose, give in *1–3-hour infusion*. Longer infusion enhances toxicity.

Toxicity (standard dose only)

1. *Myelosuppression.* Dose-limiting leukopenia and thrombocytopenia occur, with nadir at 7–10 days after treatment has ended and with recovery during the following 2 weeks, depending on the degree of suppression. Megaloblastosis is common.
2. *Nausea and vomiting.* Common, particularly if the drug is given as a push or rapid infusion.
3. *Mucocutaneous effects.* Stomatitis is seen occasionally.
4. *Miscellaneous effects*
   a. Flulike syndrome with fever, arthralgia, and sometimes a rash—occasional.
   b. Transient mild hepatic dysfunction—occasional.

Toxicity (high dose)

1. *Myelosuppression.* Universal.
2. *Nausea and vomiting.* Common.
3. *Mucocutaneous effects.* Occasional to common mucositis.
4. *Neurotoxicity.* Cerebellar toxicity is common, particularly in the elderly, but is usually mild and reversible. However, on occasion it has been severe and permanent or fatal.
5. *Conjunctivitis.* Hydrocortisone 2 drops OU qid for 10 days may ameliorate or prevent keratitis.
6. *Hepatic toxicity with cholestatic jaundice.*
7. *Diarrhea.* Common.

Dacarbazine

Other names.   Imidazole carboxamide, DIC, DTIC-Dome.

Mechanism of action.   Uncertain but probably interacts with preformed macromolecules by alkylation. Inhibits DNA, RNA, and protein synthesis.

Primary indications

1. Melanoma.
2. All soft-tissue sarcomas.
3. Hodgkin's lymphoma.

Usual dosage and schedule

1. 150–250 mg/m^2 IV push or rapid infusion on days 1–5 every 3–4 weeks *or*
2. 400–500 mg/m^2 IV push or rapid infusion on days 1 and 2 every 3–4 weeks.
3. 200 mg/m^2 IV daily as a continuous 96-hour infusion.

Special precautions

1. Administer cautiously to avoid extravasation, as tissue damage may occur.
2. Venous pain along the injection site may be reduced by diluting dacarbazine in 100–200 ml of 5% dextrose in water and infusing over 30 minutes rather than injecting rapidly. Ice application may also reduce pain.

Toxicity

1. *Myelosuppression.* Mild to moderate. This factor allows dacarbazine to be used in full doses with other myelosuppressive drugs.
2. *Nausea and vomiting.* Common and severe but decrease in intensity with each subsequent daily dose. Onset is within 1–3 hours, with duration up to 12 hours.
3. *Mucocutaneous effects*
   a. Moderately severe tissue damage if extravasation occurs.
   b. Alopecia—uncommon.
   c. Erythematous or urticarial rash—uncommon.

4. *Miscellaneous effects*
   a. Flulike syndrome with fever, myalgia, and malaise lasting several days—uncommon.
   b. Hepatic toxicity—uncommon.

Dactinomycin

Other names.   Actinomycin D, act-D, Cosmegen.

Mechanism of action.   Binds to DNA and inhibits DNA-dependent RNA synthesis. Inhibition of topoisomerase II.

Primary indications

1. Gestational trophoblastic neoplasms.
2. Wilms' tumor, rhabdomyosarcoma, and Ewing's sarcoma of childhood.

Usual dosage and schedule

1. *Children*: 0.40–0.45 mg/m^2 (up to a maximum of 0.5 mg) IV daily for 5 days every 3–5 weeks.
2. *Adults*
   a. 0.40–0.45 mg/m^2 IV on days 1–5 every 2–3 weeks.
   b. 0.5 mg IV daily for 5 days every 3–5 weeks.

Special precautions

1. Administer by slow IV push through the sidearm of a running IV infusion, being careful to avoid extravasation, which causes severe soft-tissue damage.
2. If given at or about the time of infection with chickenpox or herpes zoster, a severe generalized disease may occur that sometimes results in death.

Toxicity

1. *Myelosuppression.* May be dose-limiting and severe. It begins within the first week of treatment, but the nadir may not be reached for 21 days.
2. *Nausea and vomiting.* Severe vomiting often occurs during the first few hours after drug administration and lasts up to 24 hours.
3. *Mucocutaneous effects*
   a. Erythema, hyperpigmentation, and desquamation of the skin with potentiation by previous or concurrent radiotherapy are common.
   b. Oropharyngeal mucositis is potentiated by previous or concurrent radiotherapy.
   c. Alopecia is common.
   d. Moderately severe tissue damage occurs with extravasation.
4. *Miscellaneous effects*
   a. Mental depression is rare.
   b. Hepatovenoocclusive disease, worse with higher doses and shorter schedules, e.g., single dose of 2.5 mg versus 5 days at 0.5 mg/day.

Daunorubicin

Other names. Daunomycin, rubidomycin, DNR, Cerubidine; liposomal daunorubicin, DaunoXome.

Mechanism of action. DNA strand breakage mediated by anthracycline effects on topoisomerase II; DNA intercalation; DNA polymerase inhibition.

Primary indications

1. Acute nonlymphocytic leukemia, acute lymphocytic leukemia.
2. Kaposi's sarcoma (liposomal daunorubicin).

Usual dosage and schedule

1. 45–60 mg/m^2 IV push on days 1, 2, and 3 every 2 weeks as induction therapy for 1 or 2 cycles in combination with other drugs.
2. 45 mg/m^2 IV push on days 1 and 2 every 4 weeks as consolidation therapy for 1 or 2 cycles in combination with other drugs.
3. 40 mg/m^2 IV over 30 minutes (liposomal daunorubicin). Repeat every 2 weeks.

Special precautions

1. Administer over several minutes into the sidearm of a running IV infusion, taking precautions to avoid extravasation.
2. Do not give if patient has significantly impaired cardiac function (ejection fraction < 45%), angina pectoris, cardiac arrhythmia, or recent myocardial infarction.
3. Do not exceed cumulative dosage of 550 mg/m^2 (400 mg/m^2 if given previous radiation therapy that has encompassed the heart).
4. Reduce dose if patient has impaired liver or renal function.

Serum bilirubin (mg/dl)		Serum creatinine (mg/dl)	Full dose (%)
1.2–3.0	*or*	—	75
> 3.0		> 3.0	50

Toxicity

1. *Myelosuppression.* Dose-limiting pancytopenia with nadir at 1–2 weeks.
2. *Nausea and vomiting.* Occurs on the day of administration in one-half of patients.
3. *Mucocutaneous effects.* Alopecia is common, but stomatitis is rare. Severe local tissue damage may progress to skin ulceration, and necrosis may occur with subcutaneous extravasation.
4. *Cardiac effects.* Potentially irreversible congestive heart failure may occur owing to cardiomyopathy. The incidence is highly dependent on the lifetime cumulative

dose, which should not exceed 550 mg/m² (400 mg/m² if patient was given previous radiotherapy that encompassed the heart). Congestive heart failure may be predicted by serial measurement of left ventricular function or endomyocardial biopsy. Discontinue drug if there is clinical congestive heart failure or if the ejection fraction falls on the radionuclide angiogram,

a. To less than 45% *or*

b. To less than 50% if the total decrease is 10% or more (e.g., falls from 59% to 49%).

If repeat ejection fraction determination shows return of function, drug may be cautiously restarted, but ejection fraction should be measured before each dose. Transient ECG changes are common and are not usually serious.

5. *Miscellaneous effects*

a. Red urine caused by the drug and its metabolites—common.

b. Chemical phlebitis and phlebothrombosis of veins used for injection—common.

Dibromodulcitol (Investigational)

Other names.   DBD, mitolactol.

Mechanism of action.   A halogenated hexitol, dibromodulcitol acts, at least in part, as an alkylating agent with effects on DNA, RNA, and protein synthesis.

Primary indications

1. Breast and lung carcinomas.
2. Melanoma.
3. Hodgkin's and non-Hodgkin's lymphomas.

Usual dosage and schedule

1. *As a single agent*: 100–130 mg/m² PO daily until mild hematologic suppression develops.
2. *In combination with other drugs*: 130–135 mg/m² PO daily for 10 days every 28 days.

Special precautions.   Use with caution in patients with impaired renal function, as renal excretion is the primary mode of elimination of the drug and its metabolites.

Toxicity

1. *Myelosuppression.* Usually dose-limiting with thrombocytopenia predominating.
2. *Nausea and vomiting.* Uncommon.
3. *Mucocutaneous effects.* Skin pigmentation—uncommon.
4. *Miscellaneous effects*

a. Dyspnea—occasional.

b. Transient liver enzyme elevation—occasional.

c. Somnolence or other neurologic problems—uncommon.

d. Myelodysplasia and acute nonlymphocytic leukemia appear to be increased in incidence.

Docetaxel (Investigational)

Other name. Taxotere.

Mechanism of action. Enhanced formation and stabilization of microtubules. Antineoplastic effect may result from nonfunctional tubules or altered tubulin–microtubule equilibrium. Mitotic arrest is seen and is associated with accumulated polymerized microtubules.

Primary indications. Carcinoma of the breast and non-small-cell lung cancer.

Usual dosage and schedule. 100 mg/m^2 as a 1-hour infusion every 3 weeks.

Special precautions. Severe hypersensitivity reactions with flushing, hypotension, or hypertension with or without dyspnea occur in about 5% of patients (even when premedication is used). The following premedication for each course of docetaxel is required because of the known hypersensitivity reactions.

1. Dexamethasone 20 mg PO or IV 12 and 6 hours prior to receiving docetaxel *and*
2. Diphenhydramine 50 mg IV and cimetidine 300 mg IV 30 minutes prior to receiving docetaxel.

Toxicity

1. *Myelosuppression.* Severe (grade 4) neutropenia is common. Many patients have neutropenic fevers.
2. *Nausea and vomiting.* Common but brief.
3. *Mucocutaneous effects.* Mild mucositis—common; severe mucositis—uncommon; alopecia—common. Maculopapular eruptions that may be associated with desquamation or bullous eruptions from docetaxel occur only occasionally if systemic prophylaxis is used.
4. *Hypersensitivity reactions.* Severe reactions with flushing, hypotension, or hypertension with or without dyspnea and drug fever are uncommon with use of the prophylactic regimen recommended, but may be severe.
5. *Miscellaneous effects*
   a. Fluid retention syndrome—common and cumulative (more commonly after 4 courses); may be helped by prophylactic steroids; may limit continuing therapy.
   b. Neurologic: mild and reversible dysesthesias or paresthesias—common; more severe sensory neuropathies—uncommon.
   c. Hepatic effects: reversible increases in transaminase, alkaline phosphatase, and bilirubin.
   d. Local reactions: reversible peripheral phlebitis.
   e. Mild diarrhea—common; severe diarrhea—rare.
   f. Fatigue, myalgia—common.

Doxorubicin

Other names.   ADR, Adriamycin, Rubex, hydroxyldauno-rubicin.

Mechanism of action.   DNA strand breakage mediated by anthracycline effects on topoisomerase II; DNA intercalation; DNA polymerase inhibition.

Primary indications

1. Breast, bladder, liver, lung, prostate, stomach, and thyroid carcinomas.
2. Bone and soft-tissue sarcomas.
3. Hodgkin's and non-Hodgkin's lymphomas.
4. Acute lymphocytic and acute nonlymphocytic leukemias.
5. Wilms' tumor, neuroblastoma, and rhabdomyosarcoma of childhood.

Usual dosage and schedule

1. 60–75 mg/m^2 IV every 3 weeks.
2. 30 mg/m^2 IV on days 1 and 8 every 4 weeks (in combination with other drugs).
3. 15–20 mg/m^2 IV weekly.
4. 50–60 mg instilled into the bladder weekly for 4 weeks, then every 4 weeks for 6 cycles.

Special precautions

1. Administer over several minutes into the sidearm of a running IV infusion, taking care to avoid extravasation.
2. Do not give if patient has significantly impaired cardiac function (ejection fraction < 45%), angina pectoris, cardiac arrhythmia, or recent myocardial infarction.
3. Do not exceed a lifetime cumulative dose of 550 mg/m^2 (450 mg/m^2 if patient was given prior chest radiotherapy or concomitant cyclophosphamide) unless there are known risk modifiers, such as continuous infusion or weekly dosing, and serial measurements of cardiac ejection fraction show minimal change and adequate function.
4. Reduce or hold dose if patient has impaired liver function.
   a. For serum bilirubin of 1.2–3.0 mg/dl: give one-half the normal dose.
   b. For serum bilirubin of more than 3.0 mg/dl: give one-fourth the normal dose.

Toxicity

1. *Myelosuppression.* Dose-limiting for most patients. Nadir white blood cell (WBC) and platelet counts occur at 10–14 days; recovery by day 21.
2. *Nausea and vomiting.* Mild to moderate in about one-half of patients.
3. *Mucocutaneous effects*
   a. Stomatitis that is dose-dependent.

b. Alopecia beginning 2–5 weeks from start of therapy with recovery following completion of therapy—common.

c. Recall of skin reaction due to prior radiotherapy—common.

d. Severe local tissue damage possibly progressing to skin ulceration and necrosis if subcutaneous extravasation occurs—common.

e. Hyperpigmentation of skin overlying veins used for drug injection in which chemical phlebitis has occurred—common.

4. *Cardiac effects.* Potentially irreversible congestive heart failure may occur owing to cardiomyopathy. The incidence is highly dependent on the lifetime cumulative dose, which should not exceed 550 mg/m^2. This limit is lower (450 mg/m^2) if patient has received prior chest radiotherapy or is taking cyclophosphamide concomitantly. Weekly schedule is less cardiotoxic and higher cumulative doses may be tolerable. Congestive heart failure may be predicted by serial measurement of left ventricular function or endomyocardial biopsy. Discontinue drug if there is clinical congestive heart failure or if the ejection fraction falls on the radionuclide angiogram

a. To less than 45% *or*

b. To less than 50% if the total decrease is 10% or more (e.g., falls from 59% to 49%).

If repeat ejection fraction determination shows return of function, drug may be cautiously restarted, but ejection fraction determination should be done before each dose. Transient ECG changes are common and are not usually serious.

5. *Miscellaneous effects*

a. Red urine caused by drug and its metabolites—common.

b. Chemical phlebitis and phlebosclerosis of veins used for injection, particularly if a vein is used repeatedly—common.

c. Fever, chills, and urticaria—uncommon.

Epirubicin (Investigational)

Other names.   4′Epi-doxorubicin, EPI.

Mechanism of action.   DNA strand breakage, mediated by anthracycline effects on topoisomerase II.

Primary indications.   Breast carcinoma.

Usual dosage and schedule.   70–90 mg/m^2 IV every 3 weeks administered through the sidearm of a freely flowing IV infusion.

Special precautions

1. Take care to avoid extravasation.

2. Do not exceed a lifetime cumulative dose of 1000 mg/m^2

(use a reduced dose for patients with prior chest radio-therapy or prior anthracycline or anthracenedione therapy).

Toxicity

1. *Myelosuppression*. Dose-limiting leukopenia with recovery by day 21.
2. *Nausea and vomiting*. Common.
3. *Mucocutaneous effects*
   a. Stomatitis that is dose-dependent.
   b. Alopecia beginning approximately 10 days after the first treatment with regrowth when cessation of drug treatment occurs—common but not universal (25–50%).
   c. Severe local tissue damage possibly progressing to skin ulceration and necrosis if subcutaneous extravasation occurs—common.
4. *Cardiac effects*
   a. Potentially irreversible congestive heart failure may occur owing to cardiomyopathy. The incidence depends on the lifetime dose, which should not exceed 1000 mg/m^2. This limit is lower if patient has received prior chest radiotherapy or prior anthracycline or anthracenedione therapy. Congestive heart failure may be predicted by serial measurement of left ventricular function or endomyocardial biopsy.
   b. Transient ECG changes are similar in type and frequency to those observed after doxorubicin.
5. *Miscellaneous effects*
   a. Red-orange urine for 24 hours after injection owing to drugs and its metabolites—common.
   b. Diarrhea—occasional.

Erythropoietin

Other names. Epoetin alfa, Epogen.

Mechanism of action. Stimulates red blood cell production.

Primary indications

1. Anemia in patients receiving chemotherapy.
2. Anemia in chronic renal failure.
3. Anemia in zidovudine-treated patients with human immunodeficiency virus (HIV) infection.
4. Myelodysplastic syndrome (uncertain value).

Usual dosage and schedule

1. *Chemotherapy-associated anemia:* 150–300 units/kg (5550–11,000 units/m^2) SQ 3 times a week.
2. *Chronic renal failure:* 50–100 units/kg (1850–3700 units/m^2) IV or SQ 3 times a week as a starting dose. Doses are

increased or decreased by 25 units/kg (925 units/m^2) to achieve a target hematocrit of 30–33%.

3. *Zidovudine-associated anemia:* 100 units/kg (3700 units/m^2) SQ or IV 3 times a week. After 8 weeks, doses may be titrated up or down by 25% to achieve the desired result of decreased transfusion requirement.

Special precautions. Do not use in patients with uncontrolled blood pressure, as a rising hematocrit may result in a further rise in blood pressure.

Toxicity

1. *Myelosuppression.* None.
2. *Nausea and vomiting.* Rare.
3. *Diarrhea.* Occasional.
4. *Miscellaneous effects*—usually mild and short-lived.
   a. Seizures—rarely in patients with chronic renal failure, probably very rare in other patients.
   b. Hypertension—primarily in patients with chronic renal failure.
   c. Edema—occasional.
   d. Potential stimulation of growth of some tumors, particularly myeloid neoplasms.

Estramustine

Other name. Emcyt.

Mechanism of action. A chemical combination of mechlorethamine and estradiol phosphate, estramustine is designed to selectively enter cells with estrogen receptors, and act as an alkylating agent. May promote microtubule disassembly.

Primary indication. Metastatic prostate carcinoma.

Usual dosage and schedule. 300–600 mg/m^2 PO daily in 2–3 divided doses.

Special precautions. Take with meals and antacids to lessen gastrointestinal disturbances.

Toxicity

1. *Myelosuppression.* Occurs only occasionally.
2. *Nausea and vomiting.* Commonly seen soon after starting treatment but usually lessens with continued therapy and antiemetics. If persistent and severe, it may be necessary to discontinue the drug.
3. *Mucocutaneous effects.* Rash with fever is rare.
4. *Miscellaneous effects*
   a. Congestive heart failure—must be watched for in patients with preexisting cardiac disease.
   b. Gynecomastia—occasional.
   c. Vascular (thromboembolism, arterial insufficiency)—uncommon.

Estrogens

Other names. Diethylstilbestrol (DES), chlorotrianisene (TACE), diethylstilbestrol diphosphate (Stilphostrol), and others.

Mechanism of action. Suppression of testosterone production via negative feedback on hypothalamus.

Primary indications. Prostate carcinoma.

Usual dosage and schedule

1. DES, 1–3 mg PO daily.
2. Chlorotrianisene, 12–25 mg PO daily.
3. Diethylstilbestrol diphosphate, 500–1000 mg IV daily for 5–7 days, then 250–500 mg IV 1 or 2 times weekly.

Special precautions

1. Acute fluid retention and pulmonary edema are possible, particularly with high-dose IV therapy.
2. Hypercalcemia may occur with initial therapy.

Toxicity

1. *Myelosuppression.* None.
2. *Nausea and vomiting.* Common at the beginning of therapy but diminish or stop with continued treatment. Severity may be lessened by beginning treatment with doses lower than those recommended.
3. *Mucocutaneous effects.* Darkening of nipples—common.
4. *Miscellaneous effects*
   a. Peripheral edema due to sodium retention is common, but congestive heart failure occurs in fewer than 5% of patients.
   b. Diarrhea is uncommon.
   c. Any patient on estrogens may be at higher risk than normal for thromboemboli. An increase in cardiovascular deaths has been seen in male patients given DES at 5 mg daily for prostate carcinoma.
   d. Increased bone pain, tumor pain, and local disease flare are associated with both good tumor response and tumor progression.
   e. Feminization occurs in male patients.

Etoposide

Other names. Epipodophyllotoxin, VP-16, VP-16–213, VePesid.

Mechanism of action. Interaction with topoisomerase II produces single-strand breaks in DNA. Arrests cells in late S phase or G_2 phase.

Primary indications

1. Small-cell anaplastic and non-small-cell lung carcinoma.
2. Germ cell cancers.
3. Lymphomas.

Usual dosage and schedule

1. 120 mg/m^2 IV on days 1–3 every 3 weeks.
2. 50–100 mg/m^2 IV on days 1–5 every 2–4 weeks.
3. 125–140 mg/m^2 IV on days 1, 3, and 5 every 3–5 weeks.
4. 50 mg/m^2 PO daily for 21 days. Repeat after 1–2 weeks' rest.
5. High-dose therapy (750–2400 mg/m^2) is investigational and should only be used with stem cell rescue (e.g., bone marrow transplantation).

Special precautions

1. Administer as a 30- to 60-minute infusion to avoid severe hypotension. Monitor blood pressure during infusion.
2. Take care to avoid extravasation.
3. Must be diluted in 20–50 volumes (100–250 ml) of isotonic saline before use.
4. Decrease dose by 50% for bilirubin 1.5–3.0 mg/dl; 75% for bilirubin 3.0–5.0 mg/dl; no drug if bilirubin > 5.0 mg/dl.
5. Decrease dose by 25% for creatinine clearance rate < 30 ml/minute.

Toxicity

1. *Myelosuppression.* Dose-limiting leukopenia and less severe thrombocytopenia have a nadir at 16 days with recovery by days 20–22.
2. *Nausea and vomiting.* Usually mild to moderate problems in about one-third of patients receiving standard doses; common with high-dose therapy. Anorexia is common.
3. *Mucocutaneous effects*
   a. Alopecia—common.
   b. Stomatitis—uncommon with standard doses; common with high-dose therapy.
   c. Painful rash may occur with high-dose therapy.
   d. Chemical phlebitis—occasional.
4. *Miscellaneous effects*
   a. Hepatotoxicity—rare.
   b. Diarrhea—uncommon.
   c. Peripheral neurotoxicity—rare.
   d. Allergic reaction—rare.
   e. Hemorrhagic cystitis may occur with high-dose therapy.

Filgrastim

Other names. Granulocyte colony-stimulating factor, G-CSF, Neupogen.

Mechanism of action. Promotes growth and differentiation of myeloid progenitor cells. May improve survival and function of granulocytes.

Primary indications

1. Prophylaxis of granulocytopenia secondary to intensive chemotherapy.

2. Treatment of granulocytopenia secondary to chemotherapy.
3. Granulocytopenia from primary marrow disorders, such as idiopathic neutropenia and aplastic anemia, and myelodysplastic syndrome.
4. Granulocytopenia associated with acquired immunodeficiency syndrome (AIDS) and its therapy.

Usual dosage and schedule

1. *Adjunct to chemotherapy:* commonly 200–400 μg/m^2 (5–10 μg/kg) SQ daily, starting no sooner than 24 hours and no later than 4 days after the last dose of chemotherapy, for 10 to 20 days until the neutrophil count exceeds 10,000/μl after the expected nadir. Because of cost factors, vial size, and comparability of effect with "ballpark" doses, some physicians choose to treat patients weighing less than 75 kg with 300 μg daily and patients weighing more than 75 kg with 480 μg daily.
2. *Other purposes:* 40–500 μg/m^2 SQ, IM, or IV daily. Dose and duration are dependent on the purpose of administration.

Special precautions. Use with caution in disorders of myeloid stem cells, since it may promote growth of leukemic cells.

Toxicity

1. *Myelosuppression.* None (leukocytosis).
2. *Nausea and vomiting.* Rare.
3. *Mucocutaneous effects.* Exacerbation of preexisting dermatologic conditions—occasional; pyoderma gangrenosum—rare.
4. *Miscellaneous effects*—usually mild and short-lived.
   a. Bone pain, musculoskeletal symptoms such as cramps, and back or leg pain—common.
   b. Splenomegaly—with prolonged use.
   c. Exacerbation of preexisting inflammatory or autoimmune disorders—rare.
   d. Mild elevation of lactate dehydrogenase (LDH) and alkaline phosphatase.

Floxuridine

Other name. FUDR.

Mechanism of action. A pyrimidine antimetabolite that, when converted to the active nucleotide, inhibits the enzyme thymidylate synthetase.

Primary indications. Hepatic metastasis of gastrointestinal carcinoma, primary hepatic carcinoma.

Usual dosage and schedule. 4.0–6.0 mg/m^2 as a continuous infusion into the hepatic artery daily for 2 weeks, then off for 2 weeks. Administered via continuous infusion pump.

Special precautions

1. Reduce dose in patients with compromised liver function.
2. Ulcer-like pain or other significant gastrointestinal symptoms are indications to discontinue intraarterial therapy, as hemorrhage or perforation may occur.

Toxicity

1. *Myelosuppression.* Uncommon.
2. *Nausea and vomiting.* Uncommon unless the hepatic artery catheter has become displaced and the stomach and duodenum are being infused.
3. *Mucocutaneous effects*
   a. Stomatitis is an early sign of severe toxicity. It progresses from soreness and erythema to frank ulceration, which may become hemorrhagic in a small number of patients. Esophagitis, proctitis, and diarrhea may also occur.
   b. Partial alopecia is uncommon.
   c. Hyperpigmentation of skin over face, hands, and the vein used for the infusion—occasional.
   d. Maculopapular rash is uncommon.
   e. Sun exposure tends to increase skin reactions.
4. *Miscellaneous effects*
   a. Neurotoxicity, including headache, minor visual disturbances, and cerebellar ataxia—rare.
   b. Increased lacrimation—uncommon.
   c. Abdominal cramps and pain are common if the catheter is displaced and the stomach and duodenum are being infused. Can progress to frank gastritis or duodenal ulcer.
   d. Liver function abnormalities and jaundice—common when given by hepatic arterial infusion. Dose should be reduced during subsequent cycle.
   e. Sclerosing cholangitis when given by hepatic artery infusion—uncommon.

Fludarabine

Other names. FAMP, Fludara.

Mechanism of action. Inhibition of DNA polymerase and ribonucleotide reductase.

Primary indications

1. Chronic lymphocytic leukemia.
2. Macroglobulinemia.
3. Indolent lymphomas.

Usual dosage and schedule. 25 mg/m^2 IV as a 30-minute infusion daily for 5 days. Repeat every 4 weeks.

Special precautions. If there is the potential for tumor lysis syndrome, administer allopurinol and ensure good hydration and close clinical monitoring.

Toxicity

1. *Myelosuppression.* Granulocytopenia and thrombocytopenia are common but appear to become less common in patients who are responding. Infection, particularly pneumonia, is common during early courses; uncommon after sixth course.
2. *Nausea and vomiting.* Common (30%) but not usually severe.
3. *Mucocutaneous effects.* Occasional mucositis, rash, no alopecia.
4. *Neurotoxicity.* Uncommon at usual dosage. Somnolence or fatigue, paresthesias, and twitching of extremities may be seen. Severe neurologic symptoms, including visual disturbances, have been common at higher doses than those recommended.
5. *Miscellaneous effects*
   a. Abnormal liver or renal function—rare.
   b. Allergic pneumonitis—occasional to uncommon.
   c. Edema—occasional.
   d. Diarrhea—occasional.
   e. Tumor lysis syndrome—rare.

Fluorouracil

Other names. 5-FU, Adrucil, 5-fluorouracil.

Mechanism of action. A pyrimidine antimetabolite that, when converted to the active nucleotide, inhibits the enzyme thymidylate synthetase and thereby blocks DNA synthesis.

Primary indications

1. Breast, colorectal, anal, stomach, pancreas, esophagus, liver, head and neck, and bladder carcinomas.
2. Basal and squamous cell carcinomas of skin (topically).

Usual dosage and schedule

1. *Systemic*
   a. 500 mg/m^2 IV on days 1–5 every 4 weeks *or*
   b. 450–600 mg/m^2 IV weekly.
   c. 200–400 mg/m^2 daily as a continuous intravenous infusion.
   d. 1000 mg/m^2 daily for 4 days as a continuous IV infusion every 3–4 weeks.
2. *Intracavitary*: 500–1000 mg for pericardial effusion; 2000–3000 mg for pleural or peritoneal effusions.
3. *Intraarterial* (liver): 800–1200 mg/m^2 as a continuous infusion on days 1–4, followed by 600 mg/m^2 as a continuous infusion on days 5–21.

Special precautions

1. Reduce dose in patients with compromised liver function.
2. For intraarterial infusion, add 5000 units of heparin to 1 liter of 5% dextrose in water together with the daily dose of fluorouracil. The catheter position should be checked

with dye injection every few days to ensure that it has not moved and that the hepatic artery has not thrombosed. Ulcer-like pain or other significant gastrointestinal symptoms are indications to discontinue intraarterial therapy, as hemorrhage or perforation may occur.
3. Precipitation may occur when leucovorin and fluorouracil are mixed in the same bag.

Toxicity

1. *Myelosuppression.* Dose-limiting with a nadir at 10–14 days after the last dose and recovery by 21 days.
2. *Nausea and vomiting.* May occur but are not usually severe.
3. *Mucocutaneous effects*
   a. Stomatitis is an early sign of severe toxicity. It progresses from soreness and erythema to frank ulceration, which becomes hemorrhagic in a small number of patients. Esophagitis, proctitis, and diarrhea may also occur.
   b. Partial alopecia—uncommon.
   c. Hyperpigmentation of skin over face, hands, and the veins used for infusion—occasional.
   d. Maculopapular rash—uncommon.
   e. Sun exposure tends to increase skin reactions.
   f. "Hand-foot syndrome" with painful, erythematous desquamation and fissures of palms and soles—common with continuous infusion, occasional with other schedules or combinations.
4. *Miscellaneous effects*
   a. Neurotoxicity, including headache, minor visual disturbances, and cerebellar ataxia—rare.
   b. Increased lacrimation—uncommon.
   c. Cardiac toxicity, including arrhythmias, angina, ischemia, and sudden death—rare. May be more common with continuous infusion and previous history of coronary artery disease.
   d. Hypertriglyceridemia when given in combination with levamisole.

Flutamide

Other name. Eulexin.

Mechanism of action. Antiandrogen that inhibits binding of dihydrotestosterone at nuclear binding sites.

Primary indication. Carcinoma of the prostate.

Usual dosage and schedule. 250 mg tid daily.

Special precautions. None.

Toxicity

1. *Myelosuppression.* Rare, but occasional WBC fluctuation. Anemia—6%.
2. *Nausea and vomiting.* Occasional.
3. *Mucocutaneous effects.* Rash—uncommon.

4. *Miscellaneous effects*
   a. Gastrointestinal: occasional diarrhea (rarely severe), flatulence, or mild abdominal pains.
   b. Occasional mild elevation of liver enzymes.
   c. Mild breast tenderness and gynecomastia is common in patients who have not had gonadal ablation.
   d. Impotence and loss of libido—common.

Hydroxyurea

Other name.   Hydrea.

Mechanism of action.   Interferes with DNA synthesis, at least in part by inhibiting the enzymatic conversion of ribonucleotides to deoxyribonucleotides.

Primary indications

1. Head and neck carcinomas.
2. Chronic granulocytic leukemia; acute lymphocytic and acute nonlymphocytic leukemia with high blast counts.
3. Essential thrombocythemia.
4. Polycythemia rubra vera.
5. Prevention of retinoic acid syndrome in acute promyelocytic leukemia.

Usual dosage and schedule

1. 800–2000 mg/m² PO as a single or divided daily dose *or*
2. 3200 mg/m² PO as a single dose every third day (not for leukemias).

Special precautions.   The daily dose must be adjusted for blood count trends. Be careful not to change dose too often, because there is a delay in response.

Toxicity

1. *Myelosuppression.* Occurs at doses of more than 1600 mg/m² daily by day 10. Recovery is usually prompt.
2. *Nausea and vomiting.* Common at high doses.
3. *Mucocutaneous effects.* Stomatitis is rare. Maculopapular rash may be seen. Inflammation of mucous membranes caused by radiation may be exaggerated.
4. *Miscellaneous effects*
   a. Temporary renal function impairment or dysuria—uncommon.
   b. CNS disturbances—rare.
   c. Increased red cell mean corpuscular volume (MCV)—common.
   d. May be leukemogenic.

Idarubicin

Other names.   4-Demethoxydaunorubicin, IDA, Idamycin.

Mechanism of action.   DNA strand breakage mediated by anthracycline effects on topoisomerase II or free radicals; DNA intercalation; DNA polymerase inhibition.

Primary indications

1. Acute nonlymphocytic leukemia.
2. Blast crisis of chronic granulocytic leukemia.
3. Acute lymphocytic leukemia.

Usual dosage and schedule.   12–13 mg/m^2 IV daily for 3 days (usually in a combination with cytarabine) during induction; 10–12 mg/m^2 IV daily for 2 days during consolidation.

Special precautions.   Administer over several minutes into the sidearm of a running IV infusion, taking care to avoid extravasation. Cardiac toxicity may be less than that with daunorubicin. Maximum dose not yet established. Cumulative doses > 150 mg/m^2 have been associated with decreased cardiac ejection fraction.

Toxicity

1. *Myelosuppression.* Universal and dose-limiting.
2. *Nausea and vomiting.* Common.
3. *Mucocutaneous effects.* Alopecia—common; mucositis—common but usually not severe.
4. *Hepatic dysfunction.* Common but usually not severe and not clearly due to the idarubicin.
5. *Renal effects.* Common but usually not clinically significant.
6. *Other gastrointestinal effects.* Anorexia—common; diarrhea—occasional to common; bleeding—common in one study.
7. *Cardiac effects.* Uncommon during induction and consolidation (1–5%).
8. *Tissue damage.* If infiltration occurs—probable.
9. *Neurologic effects.* Occasional.

Ifosfamide

Other name.   Ifex.

Mechanism of action.   Metabolic activation by microsomal liver enzymes produces biologically active intermediates that attack nucleophilic sites, particularly on DNA.

Primary indications

1. Testicular and lung cancers.
2. Bone and soft-tissue sarcomas.
3. Lymphoma.

Special precautions.   Must be used with mesna (Mesnex) to prevent hemorrhagic cystitis. Mesna dose is at least 20% of the ifosfamide dose (on a weight basis), administered just prior to (or mixed with) the ifosfamide dose and again at 4 and 8 hours after the ifosfamide to detoxify the urinary metabolites that cause the hemorrhagic cystitis. Higher doses of ifosfamide may require higher doses and longer durations of mesna. Neither mesna nor its only metabolite, mesna disulfide, affect ifosfamide or its antineoplastic metabolites. Mesna disulfide is reduced in the kidney to a free thiol compound, which then reacts chemically with urotoxic metabolites resulting in their detoxification. Vigorous hydration is also required with a minimum of 2 liters of oral or IV hydration daily. Administer as a slow IV infusion over a period of at least 30 minutes.

Usual dosage and schedule

1. 1.2 gm/m^2 IV over 30 minutes or more daily for 5 consecutive days every 3 or 4 weeks, usually with other agents. Mesna 120 mg/m^2 is given just before ifosfamide, then mesna 1200 mg/m^2 as a daily continuous infusion is given until 16 hours after the last dose of ifosfamide.
2. 3.6 gm/m^2 IV daily as a 4-hour infusion for 2 consecutive days, usually with other agents. Mesna is given at a dose of 750 mg/m^2 IV just prior to and at 4 and 8 hours after the start of the ifosfamide.
3. Higher dosage schedules have been used experimentally with up to 14 gm/m^2 being used per course over a 6-day period, with equal or greater doses of mesna.

Toxicity

1. *Myelosuppression.* Dose-limiting. Platelets are relatively spared. Granulocyte nadirs are commonly reached at 10–14 days, and recovery is seen by day 21. Thrombocytopenia may be seen with higher doses.
2. *Nausea and vomiting.* Common without standard antiemetics.
3. *Mucocutaneous effects.* Alopecia—common; mucositis— rarely seen at standard doses; dermatitis—rare.
4. *Hemorrhagic cystitis.* Common and dose-limiting unless a uroprotective agent such as mesna is used. With mesna, the incidence of hemorrhagic cystitis is 5–10%, and gross hematuria is uncommon. Increasing the duration of mesna may alleviate the problem during subsequent cycles.
5. *Miscellaneous effects*
   a. CNS toxicity (somnolence, confusion, depressive psychosis, hallucinations, disorientation, and uncommonly seizures, cranial nerve dysfunction, or coma)— occasional with doses in lower range, more common with larger doses.
   b. Infertility—common in men and women, as with other alkylating agents.
   c. Renal impairment—occasional to common Fanconi syndrome dependent on dose. May be severe acidosis.
   d. Liver dysfunction—uncommon.
   e. Phlebitis—uncommon.
   f. Fever—rare.
   g. Peripheral neuropathy with high-dose therapy—uncommon.

Interferon alpha

Other names. Roferon-A (interferon alfa-2a, recombinant alpha-A interferon), Intron A (interferon alfa-2b, recombinant alpha-2 interferon).

Mechanism of action. Believed to involve direct inhibition of tumor cell growth and modulation of the immune response of the host, including activation of NK cells, modulation of antibody production, and induction of major histocompatibility antigens.

Primary indications

1. Hairy-cell leukemia.
2. Chronic myelogenous leukemia.
3. Non-Hodgkin's lymphoma (low grade), mycosis fungoides.
4. Multiple myeloma.
5. Melanoma.
6. Renal cell carcinoma.
7. Other carcinomas in combination with chemotherapy (e.g., fluorouracil in colon carcinoma).
8. Kaposi's sarcoma.
9. Condyloma acuminatum (intralesional).

Usual dosage and schedule

1. 3–10 million units IM or SQ in various schedules. Daily dosing is often used for several weeks or months, followed by 3 times a week dosing.
2. Investigationally, doses have been higher (up to 50 million units/m^2 per dose), usually IV at doses higher than 10 million units/m^2.

Toxicity

1. *Myelosuppression.* Common but usually mild to moderate and transient, even with continued therapy.
2. *Nausea and vomiting.* Anorexia occurs in about one-half of all patients, nausea in about one-third, and vomiting in 10%.
3. *Mucocutaneous effects.* Rash, dryness, or inflammation of the oropharynx, dry skin or pruritus, and partial alopecia—occasional to common.
4. *Flulike syndrome* with fatigue, fever, chills, myalgias, arthralgias, and headache—common to universal with greater severity at higher doses. Tends to diminish with continuing therapy and acetaminophen.
5. *Neurologic effects*
   a. Peripheral nervous system—occasional paresthesias or numbness.
   b. CNS—uncommon at lower doses, but with higher doses an increased likelihood including headache, somnolence, anxiety, depression, confusion, hallucinations, cerebellar dysfunction, and emotional lability.

6. *General systemic effects.* Fatigue, anorexia, and weight loss—common with chronic administration.
7. *Cardiovascular effects.* Mild hypotension—common but rarely symptomatic.
8. *Infectious effects.* Exacerbation of herpetic eruptions and nonherpetic cold sores—uncommon.
9. *Miscellaneous effects.* Leg cramps, constipation or diarrhea, insomnia, urticaria, hot flashes, coagulation disorders—uncommon.
10. *Metabolic effects and laboratory abnormalities*
    a. Elevated liver enzymes—common.
    b. Mild proteinuria, increase in serum creatinine—occasional.
    c. Hypercalcemia—occasional.
    d. Hypothyroidism and hyperthyroidism with or without antithyroid antibodies.
11. Antibody development (binding and neutralizing) occurs more readily with interferon alfa-2a than with interferon alfa-2b. The significance of this is not clear, though it may be associated with the development of clinical resistance in some patients.

Isotretinoin

Other names.   13-*cis*-retinoic acid, 13-cRA, Accutane.

Mechanism of action.   Binds to cytoplasmic retinoic acid-binding proteins and then is transported to the nucleus where it interacts with nuclear retinoic acid receptors. These then affect expression of the genes that control cell growth and differentiation.

Primary indications

1. Prevention of second primary cancers in patients with surgically or radiotherapeutically cured head and neck cancer.
2. Treatment of carcinomas of the cervix and skin (in combination with interferon alpha).

Usual dosage and schedule

1. *Prevention*
   a. 5.6 mg/m^2 (0.15 mg/kg) PO daily.
   b. 30 mg PO daily.
2. *Treatment:* 40 mg/m^2 (1 mg/kg) PO daily.

Special precautions.   Avoid use in pregnant women because of marked teratogenic potential.

Toxicity

1. *Myelosuppression.* Rare.
2. *Nausea and vomiting.* Occasional and mild.
3. *Mucocutaneous effects.* Universal, particularly at doses at higher end of range. They include redness, dryness, and pruritus of the skin and mucous membranes; possible vesicle formation; peeling of the skin of the palms and soles; cheilitis; and conjunctivitis. There also may

be increased skin photosensitivity (e.g., to sun) and the nails may become brittle. Alopecia is uncommon.
4. *Miscellaneous effects*
   a. Cataracts and corneal ulcerations or opacities—uncommon.
   b. Musculoskeletal: arthralgias, bone pain, muscle aches—occasional to common; skeletal hyperostosis—common at higher doses (80 mg/m^2/day).
   c. Hypertriglyceridemia: mild to moderate elevations—common; marked elevations ($>$ 5 times normal)—uncommon. Hypercholesterolemia occurs to lesser degree.
   d. Neurologic: lethargy, fatigue, headache, and mental depression—uncommon; pseudotumor cerebri—rare.
   e. Gastrointestinal: inflammatory bowel disease—rare.
   f. Hepatotoxicity with increased LDH, SGOT, serum glutamic-pyruvic transaminase (SGPT), gamma-glutamyl transpeptidase (GGTP), alkaline phosphatase—occasional.

Levamisole

Other name. Ergamisol.

Mechanism of action. Restores immune function, but whether this action is related to the mechanism of potentiation of fluorouracil effect in adjuvant therapy of colon cancer is unknown

Primary indications. Dukes' C carcinoma of the colon (with fluorouracil).

Usual dosage and schedule. 50 mg PO q8h for 3 days every 2 weeks for 1 year, beginning with first dose of fluorouracil. (Fluorouracil 450 mg/m^2 IV bolus daily for 5 days, then beginning 28 days later 450 mg/m^2 IV bolus weekly.)

Special precautions. Increased bilirubin may require delay of therapy.

Toxicity

1. *Myelosuppression.* Uncommon.
2. *Nausea and vomiting.* Nausea—common; vomiting—occasionally.
3. *Mucocutaneous effects.* Stomatitis and alopecia are uncommon; rash that may be pruritic—occasional.
4. *Miscellaneous effects*
   a. Dermatitis—occasional.
   b. Fatigue—occasional.
   c. Taste perversion—occasional.
   d. CNS problems (dizziness, somnolence, headache)—uncommon.
   e. Fever and rigors—uncommon.
   f. Musculoskeletal pain—uncommon.
   g. Increased bilirubin and other liver enzymes.
   h. Hypercoagulability leading to venous thrombosis—rare.

    i. Drug interactions with warfarin (increased pro-
thrombin time), phenytoin (increased plasma levels).

    j. Marked elevation of triglyceride levels (with fluoro-
uracil).

Lomustine

Other names.   CCNU, CeeNU.

Mechanism of action.   Alkylation and carbamoylation by
lomustine metabolites interfere with the synthesis and
function of DNA, RNA, and proteins. Lomustine is lipid-
soluble and easily enters the brain.

Primary indications

1. Lung and kidney carcinomas.
2. Hodgkin's and non-Hodgkin's lymphomas.
3. Brain tumors.

Usual dosage and schedule.   100–130 mg/m^2 PO once
every 6–8 weeks (lower dose used for patients with compromised bone marrow function). Some recommend limiting cumulative dose to 1000 mg/m^2 to limit pulmonary and renal
toxicity.

Special precautions.   Because of delayed myelosuppression (3–6 weeks), do not treat more often than every 6
weeks. Await a return of normal platelet and granulocyte
counts before repeating therapy.

Toxicity

1. *Myelosuppression.* Universal and dose-limiting. Leukopenia and thrombocytopenia are delayed 3–6 weeks after therapy begins and may be cumulative with successive doses.
2. *Nausea and vomiting.* Begin 3–6 hours after therapy
and last up to 24 hours.
3. *Mucocutaneous effects.* Stomatitis and alopecia are rare.
4. *Miscellaneous effects*
    a. Confusion, lethargy, and ataxia—rare.
    b. Mild hepatotoxicity—infrequent.
    c. Secondary neoplasia—possible.
    d. Pulmonary fibrosis is uncommon at doses of less than
1000 mg/m^2.
    e. Renal toxicity is uncommon at doses of less than 1000
mg/m^2.

Luteinizing Hormone-Releasing
Hormone Analogs

Other names.   Leuprolide (Lupron, Lupron depot), goserelin (Zoladex depot).

Mechanism of action.   Initial release of FSH and LH
from the anterior pituitary followed by diminution of gonadotropin secretion owing to desensitization of the pituitary to

gonadotropin-releasing hormone (GnRH), and consequent decrease in the respective gonadal hormones. May also have direct effects on cancer cells, at least in cancer of the breast in which GnRH binding sites have been demonstrated.

Primary indications

1. Prostate carcinoma.
2. Breast carcinoma (investigational).

Usual dosage and schedule

1. Leuprolide 1 mg (0.2 ml) as a single daily SQ injection.
2. Leuprolide depot 7.5 mg IM monthly.
3. Goserelin depot 3.6 mg SQ monthly.

Special precautions.   Worsening of symptoms may occur during the first few weeks.

Toxicity

1. *Myelosuppression.* Rare, if at all.
2. *Nausea and vomiting.* Occasional.
3. *Mucocutaneous effects.* Erythema and ecchymosis at the injection site, rash, hair loss, itching—uncommon.
4. *Cardiovascular effects.* Congestive heart failure and thrombotic episodes—uncommon. Peripheral edema—occasional.
5. *Miscellaneous effects*
   a. CNS: dizziness, pain, headache, and paresthesias—uncommon.
   b. Endocrine: hot flashes—common; decreased libido—common; gynecomastia with or without tenderness—uncommon; impotence—uncommon.
   c. Bone pain—"flare," common on initiation of therapy in patients with bony metastasis. Minimized by pretreating with flutamide in men with prostate cancer.
   d. Gastrointestinal: anorexia and constipation—uncommon.

Mechlorethamine

Other names.   Nitrogen mustard, HN2, Mustargen.

Mechanism of action.   Mechlorethamine is a prototype alkylating agent. Its action involves transfer of the alkyl group to amino, carboxyl, hydroxyl, imidazole, phosphate, and sulfhydryl groups within the cell, altering structure and function of DNA (primarily), RNA, and proteins.

Primary indications

1. Hodgkin's lymphoma.
2. Malignant pleural and, less commonly, peritoneal or pericardial effusions.
3. Cutaneous T cell lymphomas (topically).

Usual dosage and schedule

1. 6 mg/m^2 IV on days 1 and 8 every 4 weeks (in MOPP regimen for Hodgkin's disease).

2. 8–16 mg/m² by intracavitary injection.
3. 10 mg in 60 ml of tap water applied to entire body surface (avoid eyes).

Special precautions

1. Administer over several minutes into the sidearm of a running IV infusion, taking care to avoid extravasation.
2. Because mechlorethamine is a potent vesicant, extreme care must be exercised while preparing and administering the drug. Gloves and eye glasses are recommended to protect the preparer. If accidental eye contact should occur, institute copious irrigation with normal saline and follow by prompt ophthalmologic consultation. If accidental skin contact occurs, irrigate the affected part immediately with water for at least 15 minutes and follow by 2.6% sodium thiosulfate solution ($\frac{1}{6}$ M).
3. Mechlorethamine should be used soon after preparation (15–30 minutes) as it decomposes on standing. It *must not* be mixed in the same syringe with any other drug.

Toxicity

1. *Myelosuppression.* Dose-limiting, with the nadir at about 1 week and recovery by 3 weeks.
2. *Nausea and vomiting.* Universal. They usually begin within the first 3 hours and last 4–8 hours.
3. *Mucocutaneous effects.* Severe painful inflammation and necrosis are likely if extravasation occurs. May be ameliorated if 2.6% thiosulfate solution ($\frac{1}{6}$ M) is instilled into the area to neutralize active drug, and ice packs are applied locally for 6–12 hours. Maculopapular rash is uncommon.
4. *Miscellaneous effects*
   a. Phlebitis, thrombosis, or both of the vein used for the injection—common.
   b. Amenorrhea and azoospermia—common.
   c. Hyperuricemia with rapid tumor destruction.
   d. Weakness, sleepiness, and headache—uncommon.
   e. Severe allergic reactions, including anaphylaxis—rare.
   f. Secondary neoplasms—possible.

Melphalan

Other names. Phenylalanine mustard, L-sarcolysin, L-PAM, Alkeran.

Mechanism of action. Alkylating agent with primary effect on DNA. Amino acid-type structure may result in cellular transport that is different from other alkylating agents.

Primary indications

1. Multiple myeloma.
2. Breast and ovarian carcinomas.

Usual dosage and schedule

1. 8 mg/m^2 PO on days 1–4 every 4 weeks *or*
2. 10 mg/m^2 PO on days 1–4 every 6 weeks *or*
3. 3–4 mg/m^2 PO daily for 2–3 weeks, then 1–2 mg/m^2 PO daily for maintenance.
4. High-dose regimens of 140–200 mg/m^2 IV have been used, followed by stem cell rescue (e.g., bone marrow transplantation).
5. 16 mg/m^2 IV every 2 weeks × 4, then every 4 weeks.

Special precaution.   Myelosuppression may be delayed and prolonged to 4–6 weeks. Reduce IV dose by 50% for creatinine > 1.5 × normal.

Toxicity

1. *Myelosuppression.* Dose-limiting; nadir at days 14–21.
2. *Nausea and vomiting.* Uncommon; common with high-dose regimens.
3. *Mucocutaneous effects.* Alopecia, dermatitis, and stomatitis—uncommon; alopecia and mucositis—common with high-dose regimens.
4. *Miscellaneous effects*
   a. Acute nonlymphocytic leukemia—rare but well documented.
   b. Pulmonary fibrosis—rare.
   c. Diarrhea—common with high-dose regimens.

Mercaptopurine

Other names.   6-Mercaptopurine, 6-MP, Purinethol.

Mechanism of action.   A purine antimetabolite that, when converted to the nucleotide, inhibits the formation of nucleotides necessary for DNA and RNA synthesis.

Primary indications.   Acute lymphocytic and juvenile chronic granulocytic leukemias.

Usual dosage and schedule

1. 100 mg/m^2 PO daily if used alone.
2. 50–90 mg/m^2 PO daily if used with methotrexate.

Special precautions

1. Decrease dose by 75% when used concurrently with allopurinol.
2. Increase interval between doses or reduce dose in patients with renal failure.

Toxicity

1. *Myelosuppression.* Common but mild at recommended doses.
2. *Nausea and vomiting.* Uncommon.
3. *Mucocutaneous effects.* Stomatitis may be seen with very large doses. Dry, scaling rash is uncommon.

4. *Miscellaneous effects*
   a. Intrahepatic cholestasis and mild focal centrolobular necrosis with jaundice—uncommon.
   b. Diarrhea—rare.
   c. Hyperuricemia with rapid leukemia cell lysis—common.
   d. Fever—uncommon.

Methotrexate

Other names.   Amethopterin, MTX, Mexate.

Mechanism of action.   Inhibition of dihydrofolate reductase, which results in a block of the reduction of dihydrofolate to tetrahydrofolate. This blockage in turn inhibits the formation of thymidylate and purines, and arrests DNA (predominantly), RNA, and protein synthesis.

Primary indications

1. Breast, head and neck, gastrointestinal, lung, and gestational trophoblastic carcinomas.
2. Osteosarcomas (high-dose methotrexate).
3. Acute lymphocytic leukemia.
4. Meningeal leukemia or carcinomatosis.
5. Non-Hodgkin's lymphoma.

Usual dosage and schedule

1. *Gestational trophoblastic carcinoma:* 15–30 mg PO or IM on days 1–5 every 2 weeks.
2. *Other carcinomas:* 40–80 mg/m^2 IV or PO 2–4 times monthly with a 7- to 14-day interval between doses.
3. *Acute lymphocytic leukemia:* 15–20 mg/m^2 PO or IV weekly (together with mercaptopurine).
4. *Osteogenic sarcoma:* Up to 10 gm/m^2 with leucovorin rescue (high-dose methotrexate). This usage is investigational and should not be applied outside of a research setting.
5. *Intrathecally:* 12 mg/m^2 (not > 20 mg) twice weekly.

Special precautions

1. High-dose methotrexate (> 80 mg/m^2) is experimental and should be administered only by individuals experienced in its use and at institutions where serum methotrexate levels can be readily measured.
2. Intrathecal methotrexate must be mixed in buffered physiologic solution containing no preservative.
3. Avoid aspirin, sulfonamides, tetracycline, phenytoin, and other protein-bound drugs that may displace methotrexate and cause an increase in free drug.
4. Oral anticoagulants, e.g., warfarin, may be potentiated by methotrexate; therefore prothrombin times should be followed carefully.
5. In patients with renal insufficiency it may be necessary to markedly reduce the dose or discontinue methotrexate therapy.

6. Do not give if patient has an effusion, because of "reservoir" effect.

Toxicity

1. *Myelosuppression.* Occurs regularly, with nadir at 6–10 days after a single IV dose. Recovery is rapid.
2. *Nausea and vomiting.* Occasional at standard doses.
3. *Mucocutaneous effects*
   a. Mild stomatitis—common and a sign that a maximum tolerated dose has been reached. Higher doses may result in confluent or hemorrhagic stomal ulcers and bloody diarrhea.
   b. Erythematous rashes, urticaria, and skin pigment changes—uncommon.
   c. Mild alopecia—frequent.
4. *Miscellaneous effects*
   a. Acute hepatocellular injury—uncommon at standard doses.
   b. Hepatic fibrosis—uncommon but seen at low chronic doses.
   c. Pneumonitis—rare.
   d. Polyserositis—rare.
   e. Renal tubular necrosis—rare at standard doses.
   f. Convulsions and a Guillain-Barré-like syndrome following intrathecal therapy—uncommon.

Mitomycin

Other names. Mitomycin C, Mutamycin.

Mechanism of action. Alkylation and cross-linking by mitomycin metabolites interfere with structure and function of DNA.

Primary indications. Bladder (intravesical), esophagus, stomach, anal, and pancreas carcinomas.

Usual dosage and schedule

1. 20 mg/m^2 IV on day 1 every 4–6 weeks *or*
2. 2 mg/m^2 IV on days 1–5 and 8–12 every 4–6 weeks.
3. 10 mg/m^2 IV on day 1 every 8 weeks in combination with fluorouracil and doxorubicin for stomach and pancreatic carcinomas.
4. 30–40 mg instilled into the bladder weekly for 4–8 weeks, then monthly for 6 months.

Special precaution. Administer as slow push or rapid infusion through the sidearm of a rapidly running IV infusion, taking care to avoid extravasation.

Toxicity

1. *Myelosuppression.* Serious, cumulative, and dose-limiting. Nadir is reached usually by 4 weeks but may be delayed. Recovery is often prolonged over many weeks, and occasionally cytopenia never disappears.

2. *Nausea and vomiting.* Common at higher doses, but severity is usually mild to moderate.
3. *Mucocutaneous effects*
   a. Stomatitis and alopecia—common.
   b. Cellulitis at injection site if extravasation occurs—common.
4. *Miscellaneous effects*
   a. Renal toxicity—uncommon.
   b. Pulmonary toxicity—uncommon but may be severe.
   c. Fever—uncommon.
   d. Secondary neoplasia—possible.
   e. Hemolytic-uremic syndrome.

Mitotane

Other names. *o,p'*-DDD, Lysodren.

Mechanism of action. Suppresses adrenal steroid production, modifies peripheral steroid metabolism, and is cytotoxic to adrenal cortical cells.

Primary indication. Adrenocortical carcinoma.

Usual dosage and schedule. Begin with 2–6 gm PO daily in 3 or 4 divided doses and build to a maximum tolerated daily dose that is usually 8–10 gm, although it may range from 2 to 16 gm. Glucocorticoid and mineralocorticoid replacements during mitotane therapy are necessary to prevent hypoadrenalism. Cortisone acetate (25 mg PO in the a.m. and 12.5 mg PO in the p.m.) and fludrocortisone acetate (0.1 mg PO in the a.m.) are recommended.

Special precautions. Patients who experience severe trauma, infection, or shock should be treated with supplemental corticosteroids. Because of the effect of mitotane on peripheral steroid metabolism, larger than usual replacement doses may be necessary.

Toxicity

1. *Myelosuppression.* None.
2. *Nausea and vomiting.* Common and may be dose-limiting.
3. *Mucocutaneous effects.* Skin rash occurs occasionally.
4. *CNS effects.* Lethargy, sedation, vertigo, or dizziness in up to 40% of patients; may be dose-limiting.
5. *Miscellaneous effects.* Albuminuria, hemorrhagic cystitis, hypertension, orthostatic hypotension, and visual disturbances—uncommon.

Mitoxantrone

Other names. Novantrone, dihydroxyanthracenedione, DHAD, DHAQ.

Mechanism of action. DNA strand breakage mediated by anthracenedione effects on topoisomerase II.

Primary indications

1. Acute nonlymphocytic leukemia.
2. Carcinoma of the breast or ovary.
3. Non-Hodgkin's and Hodgkin's lymphoma.

Usual dosage and schedule

1. 12–14 mg/m^2 IV as a 5- to 30-minute infusion once every 3 weeks for solid tumors.
2. 12 mg/m^2 IV as a 5- to 30-minute infusion daily for 3 days for acute nonlymphocytic leukemia.

Special precautions.   Rarely causes extravasation injury if infiltrated. Cardiotoxicity probably less than with doxorubicin; but prior anthracycline, chest irradiation, or underlying cardiac disease increases the risk.

Toxicity

1. *Myelosuppression.* Universal.
2. *Nausea and vomiting.* Common but less frequent and less severe than with doxorubicin.
3. *Mucocutaneous effects.* Alopecia is common, but its frequency and severity is less than with doxorubicin. Mucositis—occasional.
4. *Cardiac toxicity.* Probably less than with doxorubicin; there is no clear maximum dose, though the risk appears to increase at 125 mg/m^2 cumulative dose.
5. *Miscellaneous effects*
   a. Local—erythema and swelling with transient blue discoloration if extravasated, but rarely leads to severe skin damage.
   b. Diarrhea—uncommon.
   c. Green or blue discoloration of urine.
   d. Phlebitis—uncommon.

Octreotide

Other name.   Sandostatin.

Mechanism of action.   Somatostatin analog that inhibits the release of polypeptide hormones, particularly in the pancreas and gut.

Primary indications

1. Carcinoid syndrome.
2. Vasoactive intestinal peptide tumors (VIPomas), and other amine precursor uptake and decarboxylation (APUD) tumors.
3. Chemotherapy-induced diarrhea.
4. Acromegaly.

Usual dosage and schedule.   50 μg SQ twice daily initially, with dose increased up to 450 μg daily in divided doses based on tolerability and response.

Special precautions.   Lower doses indicated if severe renal dysfunction (creatinine > 5.0 mg/dl).

Toxicity

1. *Myelosuppression.* None.
2. *Nausea and vomiting.* Occasional.
3. *Mucocutaneous effects.* Local site reactions—occasional; other effects—rare.
4. *Endocrine effects.* Hypoglycemia or hyperglycemia—uncommon; hypothalamic pituitary dysfunction—rare.
5. *Other gastrointestinal effects,* including diarrhea, loose stools, or bloating—occasional.

Paclitaxel

Other name.   Taxol.

Mechanism of action.   Enhanced formation and stabilization of microtubules. Antineoplastic effect may result from nonfunctional tubules or altered tubulin-microtubule equilibrium. Mitotic arrest is seen and is associated with accumulated polymerized microtubules.

Primary indications

1. Carcinomas of the ovary, breast, lung, head, and neck.
2. Melanoma.

Usual dosage and schedule

1. 135–175 mg/m^2 as a 24-hour infusion every 3–4 weeks.
2. 135–175 mg/m^2 as a 3-hour infusion every 3–4 weeks.

Special precautions.   Anaphylactoid reactions with dyspnea, hypotension (or occasionally hypertension), bronchospasm, urticaria, and erythematous rashes may occur as a result of the paclitaxel itself or the Cremophor vehicle required to make paclitaxel water-soluble. Such reaction is minimized but not totally prevented by pretreatment with antihistamines and corticosteroids and by prolonging the infusion rate (to 24 hours). Paclitaxel must be filtered with a 0.2-micron in-line filter.

Standard pretreatment regimen

1. Dexamethasone 20 mg PO 12 hours and 6 hours prior to treatment.
2. Cimetidine 300 mg IV 30–60 minutes prior to treatment.
3. Diphenhydramine 50 mg IV 30–60 minutes prior to treatment.

Toxicity

1. *Myelosuppression.* Granulocytopenia—universal and dose-limiting; thrombocytopenia—common; anemia—occasional.
2. *Nausea and vomiting.* Common but usually not severe.
3. *Mucocutaneous effects.* Alopecia—universal; mucositis—occasional at recommended doses.
4. *Hypersensitivity reactions.* Dyspnea, hypotension (or occasionally hypertension), bronchospasm, urticaria, and

erythematous rashes—occasionally seen, despite precautions above.
5. *Miscellaneous effects*
   a. Sensory neuropathy—common (30–35%).
   b. Hepatic dysfunction—uncommon.
   c. Diarrhea—occasional and mild.
   d. Myalgias and arthralgias—common (25%).
   e. Seizures—rare.
   f. Abnormal ECG—occasional. If clinically significant bradycardia, stop drug. Restart at slower rate when stable.

Pentostatin

Other names. 2′-Deoxycoformycin, Nipent.

Mechanism of action. Inhibition of adenosine deaminase, increase in deoxyadenosine triphosphates, inhibition of methylation reactions.

Primary indications. Hairy-cell leukemia, chronic lymphocytic leukemia, other lymphoid neoplasms, mycosis fungoides.

Usual dosage and schedule. 2–4 mg/m^2 IV push over 1–2 minutes, after hydration with 1 liter of 5% dextrose with 0.5 N saline or equivalent before pentostatin administration and 500 ml after the drug is given. Repeat every 2 weeks. Higher doses with treatment for 1–3 days may be used in chronic lymphocytic leukemia and other lymphoid neoplasms.

Special precautions. Hydration required to ensure urine output of 2 liters daily on the day pentostatin is administered. Patients often are hospitalized for their first drug administration. Allopurinol 300 mg bid is recommended in patients with a large tumor mass. Sedative and hypnotic drugs should be used with caution or not at all because CNS toxicity may be potentiated. Dose reduction or discontinuation needed for renal impairment (creatinine clearance < 50 ml/minute).

Toxicity
1. *Myelosuppression.* Common but severity variable.
2. *Nausea and vomiting.* Common but usually not severe.
3. *Mucocutaneous effects.* Mucositis—rare; skin rashes—occasional to common.
4. *Miscellaneous effects*
   a. Anorexia—common.
   b. Hepatic dysfunction—occasional.
   c. Diarrhea—uncommon.
   d. Chills and fever—common.
   e. Renal insufficiency—rare at usual doses.
   f. Neuropsychiatric effects. High doses may cause serious neurologic and psychiatric symptoms, including seizures, mental confusion, irritability, and coma.

g. Cough or other respiratory problems—occasional.
h. Infections, probably related both to myelosuppression and lymphocytopenia.

Plicamycin

Other names. Mithramycin, Mithracin.

Mechanism of action. Binds to DNA and inhibits DNA-dependent RNA synthesis.

Primary indications

1. Severe refractory hypercalcemia.
2. Rarely used as antineoplastic agent.

Usual dosage and schedule. 0.6–1.0 mg/m^2 IV for 1–3 days, with doses repeated if necessary and tolerated.

Special precautions

1. Administer as IV infusion over 0.5–3.0 hours to reduce severity of gastrointestinal toxicity.
2. Avoid subcutaneous extravasation.
3. Monitor platelet count, prothrombin time, partial prothrombin time, LDH, SGOT, and blood urea nitrogen (BUN). Discontinue drug if significant abnormality occurs.

Toxicity. High doses, which were used in the past for testicular carcinoma, had severe myelo- and hepatotoxicity.

1. *Myelosuppression.* Dose-related thrombocytopenia—common but usually not severe at doses used for hypercalcemia; leukopenia—not usually significant.
2. *Nausea and vomiting.* Common.
3. *Mucocutaneous effects*
   a. Blushing of the face followed by a coarsening of skin folds, hyperpigmentation, and possible desquamation—occasional with alternate-day therapy.
   b. Stomatitis—common.
   c. Papular skin rash—uncommon.
   d. Alopecia—uncommon.
4. *Hepatic effects.* Coagulopathy due to clotting factor abnormalities and thrombocytopenia occurs occasionally and may be fatal. Prothrombin time, partial thrombin time, SGOT, and LDH must be monitored during therapy.
5. *Miscellaneous effects*
   a. Diarrhea—common.
   b. CNS toxicity manifested by headache, irritability, and lethargy—dose-dependent.
   c. Phlebitis—uncommon.
   d. Renal effects—more than one-half of patients have some abnormality with proteinuria and mild azotemia.
   e. Electrolyte abnormalities (depression of serum calcium, phosphorus, and potassium)—common.

Procarbazine

Other name.   Matulane.

Mechanism of action.   Uncertain but appears to affect preformed DNA, RNA, and protein.

Primary indications.   Hodgkin's and non-Hodgkin's lymphomas.

Usual dosage and schedule.   100 mg/m^2 PO daily for 7–14 days every 4 weeks (in combination with other drugs).

Special precautions.   Many food and drug interactions are possible, although their clinical significance may be low.

Drug or food	Possible result
Ethanol	Disulfiram-like reactions: nausea, vomiting, visual disturbances, headache
Sympathomimetics, tricyclic antidepressants, tyramine-rich foods (cheese, wine, bananas)	Hypertensive crisis, tremors, excitation, angina, cardiac palpitations
CNS depressants	Additive depression

Toxicity

1. *Myelosuppression.* Pancytopenia is dose-limiting. Recovery may be delayed.
2. *Nausea and vomiting.* Frequent during first few days until tolerance develops.
3. *Mucocutaneous effects*
   a. Stomatitis and diarrhea—uncommon.
   b. Alopecia, pruritus, and drug rash—uncommon.
4. *CNS effects.* Paresthesias, neuropathies, headache, dizziness, depression, apprehension, nervousness, insomnia, nightmares, hallucinations, ataxia, confusion, convulsions, and coma have been reported with varying frequency.
5. *Miscellaneous effects*
   a. Secondary neoplasia—possible.
   b. Visual disturbances—rare.
   c. Postural hypotension—rare.
   d. Hypersensitivity reactions—rare.
   e. Teratogenesis—strong potential.

Progestins

Other names.   Medroxyprogesterone acetate (Provera, Depo-Provera), hydroxyprogesterone caproate (Delalutin), megestrol acetate (Megace).

Mechanism of action.   Mechanism of antitumor effects is not clear.

Primary indications.   Endometrial and breast carcinomas.

Usual dosage and schedule

1. Medroxyprogesterone acetate 1000–1500 mg IM weekly or 400–800 mg PO twice weekly.
2. Hydroxyprogesterone caproate 1000–1500 mg IM weekly.
3. Megestrol acetate 80–320 mg PO daily.

Special precautions

1. Acute local hypersensitivity or dyspnea due to oil in IM preparations—uncommon.
2. Hypercalcemia with initial therapy—occasional.

Toxicity

1. *Myelosuppression.* None.
2. *Nausea and vomiting.* Rare.
3. *Mucocutaneous effects.* Mild alopecia or skin rash—uncommon.
4. *Miscellaneous effects*
   a. Mild fluid retention—occasional to common.
   b. Mild liver function abnormalities—occasional; intrahepatic cholestasis may occur.
   c. Menstrual irregularities—common.
   d. Improved appetite, weight gain—common.

Sargramostim

Other names.   Granulocyte-macrophage colony-stimulating factor, GM-CSF, Leukine.

Mechanism of action.   Promotes growth and differentiation of myeloid progenitor cells. May improve survival and function of granulocytes, eosinophils, monocytes, and macrophages. Induces release of secondary cytokines (interleukin-1 and tumor necrosis factor).

Primary indications

1. Acceleration of myeloid recovery and shortening of granulocytopenia secondary to intensive chemotherapy followed by autologous bone marrow transplantation.
2. Granulocytopenia from primary marrow disorders, such as myelodysplastic syndrome or aplastic anemia.
3. Granulocytopenia associated with AIDS and its therapy.

Usual dosage and schedule

1. *Myeloid reconstitution after autologous bone marrow transplantation:* 250 μg/m^2 IV daily as a 2-hour infusion beginning 2–4 hours after the autologous bone marrow infusion and not less than 24 hours after the last dose of chemotherapy or less than 12 hours after the last dose of radiotherapy. Continue for 21 days or until the absolute neutrophil count reaches 20,000/μl.

2. *Bone marrow transplantation failure or engraftment delay:* 250 μg/m² daily for 14 days as 2-hour IV infusion. If no marrow recovery, may be repeated in 7 days at same or higher dose (500 μg/m²). Dose and duration are dependent on the response.
3. *Aplastic anemia, myelodysplastic syndrome, and AIDS:* doses may be much lower (50–100 μg/m² SQ or IM daily).

Special precautions. Flushing, tachycardia, dyspnea, and nausea occur commonly with the first dose of IV therapy; do not infuse for less than 2 hours; longer infusion may help.

Toxicity

1. *Myelosuppression.* None (leukocytosis).
2. *Nausea and vomiting.* Occasional.
3. *Mucocutaneous effects.* Rash—uncommon; exacerbation of preexisting dermatologic conditions—occasional; mild local reactions at injection site—common.
4. *Miscellaneous effects.* Usually mild and short-lived at standard doses, but with increasing dose, may be more severe.
   a. Bone pain, musculoskeletal symptoms such as cramps, and back or leg pain—common.
   b. Pericarditis, fluid retention, and venous thrombosis—dose-related and uncommon at standard doses.
   c. Flulike symptoms (fever, chills, aches, headache)—occasional at standard doses, common at higher doses.

Streptozocin

Other names. Streptozotocin, Zanosar.

Mechanism of action. Inhibition of DNA synthesis, possibly by interference with pyridine nucleotide synthesis. Streptozocin appears to have some specificity for neoplastic pancreatic endocrine cells. Glucose moiety attached to nitrosourea appears to diminish myelotoxicity.

Primary indications

1. Pancreatic islet cell and pancreatic exocrine carcinomas.
2. Carcinoid tumors.

Usual dosage and schedule

1. 1.0–1.5 gm/m² IV weekly for 6 weeks followed by 4 weeks of observation.
2. 500 mg/m² IV on days 1–5 every 6 weeks.

Special precautions

1. A 30- to 60-minute infusion is recommended to reduce local pain and burning around the vein during treatment.
2. Avoid extravasation.
3. Have 50% glucose available to treat sudden hypoglycemia.

Toxicity

1. *Myelosuppression.* Uncommon and mild.
2. *Nausea and vomiting.* Common and severe. May become progressively worse over 5-day course of therapy.
3. *Mucocutaneous effects.* Uncommon.
4. *Nephrotoxicity.* Renal toxicity is common. Although it is not clearly dose-related, it may limit continued drug use in individual patients. Proteinuria, glucosuria, azotemia, and hypophosphatemia, if persistent or severe, are indications to discontinue therapy. Hydration may ameliorate the problem.
5. *Miscellaneous effects*
   a. Hypoglycemia: in patients with insulinoma, hypoglycemia may be severe (although transient) owing to a burst of insulin release.
   b. Hyperglycemia is uncommon in normal or diabetic patients, as normal β cells are usually insensitive to streptozocin's effect.
   c. Transient mild hepatotoxicity—occasional.
   d. Second malignancies—possible.

Suramin (Investigational)

Other names. Antrypol, Bayer 205, Germanin, Moranyl, Naganol, Naphuride NA.

Mechanism of action. Glycosaminoglycan agonist-antagonist that blocks the binding of growth factors to their receptors. Growth factors affected include platelet-derived growth factor, transforming growth factor-beta (TGF-β), and heparin binding growth factor-2 (also known as basic fibroblast growth factor). Inhibition of DNA polymerases and reverse transcriptase and other proteins. Inhibition of glycosaminoglycan metabolism.

Primary indications

1. Adrenocortical carcinoma.
2. Prostate carcinoma that is hormone-refractory.
3. Lymphoma that is refractory to standard agents.

Usual dosage and schedule. 350 mg/m^2 by continuous IV infusion daily for 7 days after an initial test dose of 200 mg over 10 minutes. The plasma level is then measured, the infusion rate adjusted, and the treatment continued until the plasma level reaches 250–300 μg/ml. The infusion is then stopped for 2 months and the treatment cycle repeated.

Special precautions. Measurement of plasma levels is necessary to achieve the narrow concentration that is therapeutic and not prohibitively toxic. Therapy should be stopped when a steady-state drug level of 300 μg/ml is reached. Because of adrenal suppression, patients require hydrocortisone, 25 mg in the morning and 15 mg at bedtime. All patients should also receive vitamin K 10 mg SQ weekly, to reduce the likelihood of coagulopathy. Prothrombin time must be followed closely, and therapy stopped if prothrombin time exceeds 17.5 seconds.

Toxicity

1. *Myelosuppression.* Common but usually not severe.
2. *Nausea and vomiting.* Uncommon.
3. *Mucocutaneous effects.* Transient erythematous rash is common.
4. *Adrenocortical insufficiency.* Common.
5. *Neurotoxicity.* Paresthesias are seen commonly and severe polyradiculopathy occasionally. Motor weakness may be seen following termination of therapy. The degree of toxicity appears to be related to the plasma suramin level, with acute serious reactions uncommon at plasma levels of less than 350 μg/ml.
6. *Miscellaneous effects*
   a. Vortex keratopathy with photophobia, tearing, and blurred vision—common.
   b. Liver function abnormalities—common but reversible.
   c. Coagulopathy—common elevations of the prothrombin time, partial thromboplastin time, and thrombin time, with increased risk of spontaneous bleeding.
   d. Renal effects: proteinuria—common; decrease in creatinine clearance—occasional.
   e. Malaise, fatigue, and lethargy—common after 2–4 months of therapy.

Tamoxifen

Other name. Nolvadex.

Mechanism of action. Tamoxifen is an estrogen agonist-antagonist that binds to cytoplasmic estrogen receptors. This complex is probably transported into the nucleus where it affects nucleic acid function. Also has effects on cellular growth factors, epidermal growth factors, and TGF-α and TGF-β.

Primary indications

1. Breast and endometrial carcinomas.
2. Melanoma, in combination with other drugs.

Usual dosage and schedule

1. 10 mg PO twice daily.
2. 20 mg PO as single daily dose.

Special precautions. Hypercalcemia may be seen during initial therapy. Should not be used as primary cancer preventive agent except under auspices of a controlled clinical trial.

Toxicity

1. *Myelosuppression.* Uncommon and mild.
2. *Nausea and vomiting.* Occur early in the course of ther-

apy in up to 20% of patients, but abate rapidly as therapy is continued.

3. *Mucocutaneous effects.* Skin rash and pruritus vulvae are uncommon. May cause marked decrease in vaginal secretions and result in difficult or painful intercourse.
4. *Miscellaneous effects*
   a. Hot flashes—common.
   b. Vaginal bleeding and menstrual irregularity—uncommon.
   c. Lassitude, headache, leg cramps, and dizziness—uncommon.
   d. Peripheral edema—occasional.
   e. Increased bone pain, tumor pain, and local disease flare (associated both with good tumor response as well as with tumor progression)—occasional.
   f. Diarrhea—occasional.
   g. Slowed progression of osteoporosis.
   h. Reduction in serum cholesterol with favorable changes in lipid profile.
   i. Cataracts and other eye toxicity—rare.
   j. Thromboembolic phenonema—rare.
5. *Carcinogenesis.* Uterine carcinomas—rare (2–4 times the predicted incidence in adjuvant trials).

Teniposide

Other names.   VM-26, Vumon.

Mechanism of action.   Topoisomerase II-mediated double-strand DNA breaks. Causes cells cycle transit delay through S phase and arrest at late S/G_2.

Primary indications

1. Acute lymphocytic leukemia.
2. Neuroblastoma.

Usual dose and schedule

1. 165 mg/m^2 IV over 30–60 minutes twice weekly for 8–9 doses (with cytarabine).
2. 250 mg/m^2 IV over 30–60 minutes weekly for 4–8 weeks (with vincristine and prednisone).

Special precautions

1. Hypersensitivity reactions usually resolve with interruption of the infusion and often can be prevented with diphenhydramine and hydrocortisone pretreatment. Hypotension is alleviated by prolonging the infusion time. It is a possible vesicant.
2. See package insert for IV preparation and administration equipment requirements.

Toxicity

1. *Myelosuppression.* Common and dose-limiting.
2. *Nausea and vomiting.* Common.

3. *Mucocutaneous effects.* Alopecia and mucositis—common.
4. *Miscellaneous effects*
    a. Hepatic and renal dysfunction—rare.
    b. Hypersensitivity reactions with urticaria and flushing—occasional. Anaphylaxis—uncommon.
    c. Hypotension is related to drug infusion rate but should be seen only occasionally at the recommended dose schedules.
    d. Secondary leukemias—uncommon.
    e. Diarrhea—common.
    f. Chemical phlebitis—uncommon.

Thioguanine

Other names. 6-Thioguanine, 6-TG, Tabloid.

Mechanism of action. A purine antimetabolite that, when converted to the active nucleotide, substitutes for the normal guanine nucleotide in DNA synthesis. Thioguanine also inhibits purine synthesis and conversion reactions.

Primary indication. Acute nonlymphocytic leukemia.

Usual dosage and schedule

1. *Induction:* 100 mg/m^2 PO twice daily on days 1–5 (with other drugs).
2. *Maintenance:* 100 mg/m^2 PO twice daily on days 1–5 every 4 weeks (with other drugs).

Special precautions. None (no dose reduction required for concurrent use of allopurinol).

Toxicity

1. *Myelosuppression.* Major dose-limiting toxicity.
2. *Nausea and vomiting.* Occasional but not severe.
3. *Mucocutaneous effects*
    a. Stomatitis and diarrhea, which may necessitate reduction of the dose—uncommon.
    b. Drug rash—rare.
    c. Chemical phlebitis.
4. *Miscellaneous effects.* Hepatotoxicity—rare.

Thiotepa

Other name. Triethylenethiophosphoramide.

Mechanism of action. Alkylating agent similar to mechlorethamine.

Primary indications

1. Superficial papillary carcinoma of urinary bladder.
2. Malignant peritoneal, pleural, or pericardial effusions.
3. Carcinoma of breast and ovary.
4. Neoplastic meningeal infiltrates.

Usual dosage and schedule

1. 12 mg/m^2 IV bolus every 3 weeks in combination with vinblastine and doxorubicin for breast cancer.
2. 30–60 mg in 40–50 ml water instilled into the bladder and retained for 1 hour. Dose is repeated weekly for 3–6 weeks, then every 3 weeks for 5 cycles.
3. 25–30 mg/m^2 in 50–100 ml saline solution as a single intracavitary injection. Dose may be repeated as tolerated by blood counts.
4. 10–15 mg intrathecally.
5. High-dose therapy using 500–1000 mg/m^2 over 3 days has been used followed by stem cell rescue (e.g., bone marrow transplantation).

Special precaution. Dose should be reduced in patients with impaired renal function, as the drug is primarily excreted in the urine.

Toxicity

1. *Myelosuppression.* Dose-limiting. Pancytopenia and sepsis may follow intravesical or intracavitary administration. Nadir counts are reached in 1–2 weeks; recovery by 4 weeks is usual.
2. *Nausea and vomiting.* Uncommon.
3. *Mucocutaneous effects.* Uncommon. Thiotepa is *not* a vesicant. Hyperpigmentation of skin occurs at high doses.
4. *Miscellaneous effects*
   a. Local pain, dizziness, headache, fever—uncommon.
   b. Secondary neoplasms—possible.
   c. Amenorrhea and azoospermia—common.
   d. CNS effects with high-dose therapy.

Topotecan (Investigational)

Other names. None.

Mechanism of action. A semisynthetic camptothecan analog that inhibits topoisomerase I, causing single-strand breaks in DNA.

Primary indications

1. Non-small-cell carcinoma of lung.
2. Ovarian, colorectal, and esophageal carcinomas.

Usual dosage and schedule

1. 1.5–2.0 mg/m^2/day IV as 30-minute infusion on days 1–5 every 3 weeks.
2. 17.5 mg/m^2 IV as 30-minute infusion every 3 weeks.

Special precaution. Prepare in 5% dextrose and water to maintain acidic pH and keep topotecan in its active form.

Toxicity

1. *Myelosuppression.* Universal and dose-limiting.
2. *Nausea and vomiting.* Common, but mild.
3. *Mucocutaneous effects.* Alopecia and skin rash—rare; diarrhea—occasional.
4. *Miscellaneous effects*
   a. Fever and flulike symptoms—common.
   b. Microscopic hematuria—occasional.

Tretinoin (Investigational)

Other names. All-*trans*-retinoic acid, t-RNA, ATRA, Retin-A.

Mechanism of action. Binds to cytoplasmic retinoic acid-binding proteins and then is transported to the nucleus where it interacts with nuclear retinoic acid receptors (RARs). These then affect expression of the genes that control cell growth and differentiation. In acute promyelocytic leukemia, which characteristically has a chromosomal translocation, t(15:17), abnormal mRNA transcripts are seen for RAR-α, the gene for which is on chromosome 17.

Primary indication. Acute promyelocytic leukemia.

Usual dosage and schedule. 45 mg/m² PO daily (divided into 2 doses in the morning and 6 hours later) until complete remission, up to a maximum of 90 days.

Special precautions. Avoid use in pregnant women because of marked teratogenic potential. Retinoic acid syndrome (see below) may require mechanical ventilation and dexamethasone 10 mg every 12 hours at the first signs of fever with respiratory distress until resolution of the acute symptoms (often several days). Continuation of retinoid therapy is controversial.

Toxicity

1. *Myelosuppression.* Rare.
2. *Nausea and vomiting.* Occasional and mild.
3. *Mucocutaneous effects.* Universal, particularly at doses at higher end of range. They include redness, dryness, and pruritus of the skin and mucous membranes; possible vesicle formation; peeling of the skin of the palms and soles; cheilitis; and conjunctivitis. There also may be increased skin photosensitivity (e.g, to sun) and the nails may become brittle. Alopecia is uncommon.
4. *Retinoic acid syndrome.* Leukocytosis, high fever, respiratory distress, diffuse pulmonary infiltrates, pleural or pericardial effusions with the possibility of impaired myocardial contractility, and hypotension—occasional in patients with acute promyelocytic leukemia (15–25%) (see Chap. 23).

5. *Miscellaneous effects*
   a. Cataracts and corneal ulcerations or opacities—uncommon.
   b. Musculoskeletal: arthralgias, bone pain, muscle aches—occasional to common; skeletal hyperostosis—common at higher doses (80 mg/m²/day).
   c. Hypertriglyceridemia: mild to moderate elevations—common; marked elevations (> 5 times normal)—uncommon; hypercholesterolemia occurs to lesser degree.
   d. Neurologic: headache—common; lethargy, fatigue, and mental depression—uncommon; pseudotumor cerebri—rare.
   e. Gastrointestinal: inflammatory bowel disease—rare.
   f. Hepatotoxicity with increased LDH, SGOT, SGPT, GGTP, alkaline phosphatase—occasional.
   g. Hyperhistaminemia with shock—rare.

Trimetrexate (Investigational)

Other name.   TMQ.

Mechanism of action.   Inhibition of dihydrofolate reductase.

Primary indications

1. Head and neck squamous cell cancers.
2. Lung carcinoma.

Usual dosage and schedule.   8 mg/m² IV push daily for 5 days.

Special precautions.   None.

Toxicity

1. *Myelosuppression.* Leukopenia and thrombocytopenia are common.
2. *Nausea and vomiting.* Common but mild to moderate.
3. *Mucocutaneous effects.* Mucositis and skin rash—common (15–25%).
4. *Miscellaneous effects*
   a. Reversible nephrotoxicity—occasional.
   b. Elevated bilirubin—occasional.
   c. Fatigue—occasional.
   d. Diarrhea—uncommon.
   e. Hypersensitivity—uncommon.

Vinblastine

Other names.   VLB, Velban, vincaleukoblastine sulfate.

Mechanism of action.   Mitotic inhibition with reversible metaphase arrest due to action on microtubular and spindle contractile proteins.

Primary indications

1. Testicular, gestational trophoblastic, kidney, and breast carcinomas.
2. Hodgkin's and non-Hodgkin's lymphomas.

Usual dosage and schedule

1. 4–18 mg/m^2 IV weekly.
2. 6 mg/m^2 IV on days 1 and 15 in combination with doxorubicin, bleomycin, and dacarbazine for lymphomas.
3. 4.5 mg/m^2 IV on day 1 every 3 weeks in combination with doxorubicin and thiotepa for breast cancer.

Special precautions.   Administer as a slow push, taking care to avoid extravasation.

Toxicity

1. *Myelosuppression.* Dose-related leukopenia occurs with a nadir at 4–10 days and recovery in 7–10 days. Severe thrombocytopenia is uncommon.
2. *Nausea and vomiting.* Common but not usually severe.
3. *Mucocutaneous effects*
   a. Extravasation may lead to severe inflammation, pain, and tissue damage. Local infiltration with 1–6 ml of hyaluronidase (150 units/ml) may help.
   b. Mild alopecia—common.
   c. Stomatitis—occasionally severe.
4. *Miscellaneous effects*
   a. Neurotoxicity manifested by (1) constipation, adynamic ileus, and abdominal pain if very high doses are used; or (2) paresthesias, peripheral neuropathy, and jaw pain with lower doses. Neurotoxicity is less frequent with vinblastine than with vincristine.
   b. Transient hepatitis—uncommon.
   c. Depression, headache, convulsions, and orthostatic hypotension—rare.

Vincristine

Other names.   VCR, Oncovin.

Mechanism of action.   Mitotic inhibition with reversible metaphase arrest due to drug action on microtubular and spindle contractile proteins.

Primary indications

1. Breast carcinoma.
2. Hodgkin's and non-Hodgkin's lymphomas.
3. Acute lymphocytic leukemia.
4. Wilms' tumor, neuroblastoma, rhabdomyosarcoma, and Ewing's sarcoma of childhood.
5. Multiple myeloma.

Usual dosage and schedule

1. 1–2 mg/m^2 (maximum 2.0–2.4 mg) IV weekly.
2. 0.4 mg/day as a continuous IV infusion on days 1–4.

Special precautions

1. Administer as a slow IV push, taking care to avoid extravasation.
2. Because neurotoxicity is cumulative, neurologic evaluation should be done before each dose and therapy withheld if severe paresthesias, motor weakness, or other severe abnormalities occur. Underlying neurologic problems accentuate vincristine's effect.
3. Reduce dose if liver disease is significant.
4. Stool softeners or high-fiber or bulk diets may avert severe constipation.

Toxicity

1. *Myelosuppression.* Mild and rarely of clinical significance.
2. *Nausea and vomiting.* Not seen unless paralytic ileus occurs.
3. *Mucocutaneous effects.* Severe local inflammation if extravasation occurs. Alopecia is common.
4. *Neurotoxicity.* Dose-dependent and dose-limiting. Mild paresthesias and decreased deep tendon reflexes are to be expected. More extensive peripheral neuropathies, severe constipation, or ileus are indications to reduce or hold therapy. Autonomic dysfunction with orthostatic hypotension or urinary retention may be seen.
5. *Miscellaneous effects*
   a. Uric acid nephropathy due to rapid tumor cell lysis and release of uric acid—always a potential problem when therapy is first given.
   b. Syndrome of inappropriate antidiuretic hormone—rare.
   c. Jaw pain—uncommon.

Vindesine (Investigational)

Other name.   VDS.

Mechanism of action.   Mitotic inhibition with reversible metaphase arrest due to action on microtubule and spindle contractile protein.

Primary indications

1. Lung, breast, and esophageal carcinomas.
2. Hodgkin's and non-Hodgkin's lymphomas.
3. Melanoma.

Usual dosage and schedule.   2–3 mg/m^2 IV bolus (2–3 minutes) weekly for induction, then every 2 weeks.

Special precautions.   Take care to avoid extravasation.

Toxicity

1. *Myelosuppression.* Leukopenia—common but not usually severe.
2. *Nausea and vomiting.* Occasional.
3. *Mucocutaneous effects.* Alopecia—common.

4. *Neurotoxicity.* Dose-dependent and cumulative, consisting in constipation, paralytic ileus, paresthesia, myalgias, and weakness. Severity is intermediate between vincristine and vinblastine.
5. *Miscellaneous effects*
   a. Chills and fever—occasional.
   b. Phlebitis—occasional.
   c. Confusion and lethargy—rare.

Vinorelbine

Other name. Navelbine.

Mechanism of action. Binds to tubulin, depolymerizes microtubules causing mitotic inhibition, similar to other vinca alkaloids. Lower affinity for axonal microtubules associated with lower neurotoxicity.

Primary indications

1. Non-small-cell carcinoma of the lung.
2. Metastatic carcinoma of the breast.

10973/pt1/Miles

Usual dosage and schedule. 30 mg/m^2 IV over 6–10 minutes weekly.

Special precautions. Administer infusion through the sidearm of a freely flowing IV line, taking care to avoid extravasation.

Toxicity

1. *Myelosuppression.* Granulocytopenia—common and dose-limiting with nadir at 7–10 days; thrombocytopenia—uncommon; anemia—occasional to common.
2. *Nausea and vomiting.* Common, but usually mild to moderate.
3. *Mucocutaneous effects.* Alopecia, mild diarrhea, and stomatitis—occasional; severe local inflammation with extravasation.
4. *Miscellaneous effects*
   a. Neurotoxicity: cumulative, but reversible constipation, decreased deep tendon reflexes—occasional; paresthesias—uncommon.
   b. Erythema, pain, and skin discoloration at injection site—common; phlebitis at injection site—occasional.

Selected Readings

Chabner, B. A., and Collins, J. M. *Cancer Chemotherapy. Principles and Practice.* Philadelphia: Lippincott, 1990.

Dorr, R. T., and Van Hoff, D. D. (eds.), *Cancer Chemotherapy Handbook* (2nd ed.). Norwalk, CT: Appleton & Lange, 1994.

Perry, M. C. (ed.), *The Chemotherapy Source Book.* Baltimore: Williams & Wilkins, 1992.

Chemotherapy
of Human Cancer

Carcinomas of the Head and Neck

Ronald C. DeConti

Achievement of a management plan resulting in long-term control or cure for many patients with carcinomas of the head and neck remains an elusive, only partially realized goal for head and neck surgeons, radiation oncologists, and medical oncologists. Important gains in understanding the natural history of these neoplasms have been made, and the individual achievements of irradiation, surgical techniques, and chemotherapy have been stressed. However, only recently these modalities have been combined to form new treatment plans, and increased benefit to the patient that might result from this multidisciplinary effort is now being explored.

This discussion focuses on the squamous cell carcinomas of the lining of the upper aerodigestive tract, which extends from the lip to the esophagus. These tumors account for approximately 5 percent of the new cancer cases seen in the United States each year. Excluded from this discussion are the melanomas, lymphomas, and sarcomas (which also occur in this area), as well as carcinomas of the thyroid, esophagus, and salivary glands. A cross-sectional view of the anatomic regions and the relative frequency of cancer occurring in each area are shown in Figure 11-1. The large number of potential tumor sites and some difficulty in determining the exact site of origin have led to broad use of these larger subdivision terms in an attempt to avoid confusion and to group the related sites. Table 11-1 lists major sites within each of these anatomic subdivisions.

I. **Common and divergent characteristics.** Carcinomas of the head and neck are frequently considered together by students, generalists, and medical oncologists as though they represent a single therapeutic problem. A number of factors promote this concept.

A. **Similarities.** In the United States more than 90% of all lesions are squamous cell carcinomas, occurring predominantly in men (3 : 1). Most patients share common demographic and epidemiologic risk factors. The incidence of head and neck cancer increases with the use of alcohol and tobacco, and with advancing age. Head and neck cancers occur in continuity, one with another, and it is occasionally difficult to determine the precise site of origin in the close confines of the complicated interrelated structures comprising the oral cavity, pharynx, larynx, and sinuses. Furthermore, patterns of spread are similar, with local failure, local recurrence, and regional node failures predominating. For carcinomas originating at most sites, spread below the clavicle is unusual, occurring in only a few patients usually as pulmonary involvement. Bone lesions, usually the result of local extension involving the mandible or floor of the skull, are

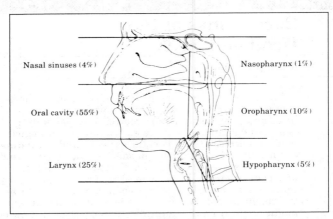

Fig. 11-1. Anatomic divisions of the head and neck. Percentages indicate the relative frequency of carcinoma in these regions.

Table 11-1. Upper aerodigestive tract sites

Region	Area	Site
Oral cavity		Lip
		Buccal mucosa
		Lower alveolar ridge
		Upper alveolar ridge
		Retromolar trigone
		Floor of mouth
		Hard palate
		Oral tongue
Pharynx	Nasopharynx	Posterior wall
		Lateral wall
	Oropharynx	Faucial arch
		Tonsillar fossa and tonsil
		Base of tongue
		Pharyngeal wall
	Hypopharynx	Piriform fossa
		Postcricoid area
		Posterior wall
Larynx	Supraglottis	Ventricular band
		Arytenoid
		Epiglottis
	Glottis	True vocal cords
	Subglottis	Subglottis
Paranasal sinuses		Antrum
		Nasal cavity
		Ethmoid
		Sphenoid
		Frontal

not uncommon, although widespread bone metastases are unusual. A few patients develop hepatic metastases. Inanition, oral ulceration, fistula formation, respiratory difficulty, and aspiration characterize the late course of the disease. Recurrences after primary treatment usually appear within 18 months, and the patients who are not cured are usually dead within 3 years of diagnosis.

B. Differences. For the surgeon or radiation oncologist, the differences among carcinomas at different sites may be more significant than the similarities. Certainly, presenting signs and symptoms differ markedly. For example, patients with an anterior tongue lesion may describe pain, sensation of a mass, and limited motion of the tongue. Hoarseness, dysphagia, or sore throat may predominate in patients with carcinoma of the larynx. More importantly, differences in location influence the frequency of nodal spread and the chances for contralateral node involvement. These factors frequently determine the optimal treatment plan.

II. Primary treatment. A discussion of the specific variations in primary treatment choices for the multitude of sites where head and neck cancers occur is beyond the scope of this chapter. In general, early lesions in most locations are suitable for treatment by surgery or irradiation, and the therapeutic choice usually is made by considering the complications of each treatment, i.e., the deformities of definitive surgery or the complications of irradiation. With increasing failure rates and the likelihood of pathologic, if not clinical, lymph node involvement as tumor bulk increases, clinicians have begun to investigate combined-modality approaches. Radiation can be used electively before operation or postoperatively after a microscopic assessment of regional nodes provides the opportunity for postsurgical pathologic staging. Many studies now report improved local and regional node control after such multimodality approaches. Although substantial progress has been made in improving end results for early-stage lesions at many sites, and in decreasing the morbidity and deformity from the treatment, the outcome for tumors in advanced stages remains poor: For stage III disease, the 3- to 5-year survival rate is 25–60%. For stage IV disease, long-term survival rates of 10–30% are reported.

III. Staging. Any consideration of outcome in relation to treatment relies heavily on detailed pretreatment assessment of the extent of the tumor.

A. TNM classification. A complex site-specific staging system has been devised by the American Joint Committee on Cancer. This system incorporates a TNM classification to identify, clinically and pathologically, the size of the primary tumor (T), the presence and extent of regional node metastases (N), and the presence of distant metastases (M). Table 11-2 outlines the TNM system for carcinoma of the oral cavity. For lesions of the nasopharynx, hypopharynx, and larynx, fixation or anatomic extensions are substituted for tumor size when determining the extent of the primary lesion.

Table 11-2. TNM staging system for carcinomas of the oral cavity

T stage	**Primary tumor**
TX	No available information on primary tumor
T0	No evidence of primary tumor
Tis	Carcinoma in situ
T1	Greatest diameter of tumor $\leq$ 2 cm
T2	Greatest diameter of tumor > 2–4 cm
T3	Greatest diameter of tumor > 4 cm
T4	Invasion to adjacent structures such as antrum, pterygoid muscles, base of tongue, or skin of neck
N stage	**Regional nodal status**
NX	Nodes cannot be assessed
N0	No clinically positive node
N1	Single clinically positive ipsilateral node $\leq$ 3 cm in diameter
N2	Single clinically positive ipsilateral node > 3–6 cm; or multiple clinically positive nodes, none > 6 cm; or bilateral or contralateral nodes, none > 6 cm
N3	Metastasis in a lymph node > 6 cm in greatest dimension
M stage	**Distant metastasis**
MX	Not assessed
M0	No (known) distant metastasis
M1	Distant metastasis present

B. Stages. The stage grouping for head and neck cancers is shown in Table 11-3. Stages I and II are determined by the size of the tumor in the absence of nodal involvement or distant metastases. Stage III comprises both large tumors and tumors of any size with early regional node involvement. Stage IV lesions may be huge with local extension or may be of any size with distant metastatic disease. This stage grouping has been uniformly applied to each tumor site to demonstrate gradations in prognosis.

IV. Chemotherapy

A. Prognostic factors. Whether chemotherapy is considered for the treatment of advanced recurrent head and neck cancer or for preoperative induction treatment, a number of similar, single prognostic variables have now been clearly identified (Table 11-4).

1. Stage of carcinoma. Small lesions with minimal regional node involvement respond better than the massive stage IV tumors. Patients with stage IV disease due to bulky lymph nodes commonly get little benefit from treatment. Response rates are lowest for stage IV disease with pulmonary or visceral metastases. Because patients with head and neck cancers have an increased risk of developing second primary neoplasms, the finding of distant metastases

Table 11-3. Stage grouping for carcinoma of the oral cavity, pharynx, larynx, and paranasal sinuses

Stage	Groups
I	T1, N0, M0
II	T2, N0, M0
III	T3, N0, M0
	T1 *or* T2 *or* T3, N1, M0
IV	T4, N0 *or* N1, M0
	Any T, N2 *or* N3, M0
	Any T, any N, M1

Table 11-4. Factors prognostic for response to chemotherapy

Favorable	Unfavorable
Stage III	Stage IV
No metastasis	Pulmonary metastasis
ECOG performance status 0–1*	ECOG performance status 2–3
No weight loss	Weight loss
Normal immune mechanism	Impaired delayed hypersensitivity
Prior surgery	Prior irradiation
Long disease-free interval	Short disease-free interval
No prior chemotherapy	Prior chemotherapy
Combination chemotherapy	Single-agent chemotherapy
Poorly differentiated tumor	Well-differentiated tumor
Nasopharynx	Other sites

*See Table 8-2.

in the absence of primary site or regional node recurrence suggests this possibility.

2. **State of health.** Both poor ECOG (Eastern Cooperative Oncology Group) performance status (see Table 8-2) and weight loss of more than 5% have been found to adversely affect prognosis. It is still unclear whether aggressive attempts to improve nutrition or restore cellular immunity with hyperalimentation result in gains in the response and survival rates.

3. **Prior treatment.** Many studies have reported the adverse effect of prior radiation therapy on response to chemotherapy. This effect has usually been attributed to an impaired tumor blood supply, a large tumor burden, and poor patient performance status. The failure to respond to irradiation and a rapid relapse after radiation therapy also have been shown to adversely affect response rates.

B. Pretreatment assessment. The extent of evaluation required to determine the suitability of a patient for chemotherapy depends, to a considerable degree, on the intent of therapy and type of program to be employed. The major organ systems affected by the antineoplastic drugs under consideration are bone marrow, lungs, and kidneys. Any pretreatment assessment should consider not only careful evaluation of the size and extent of tumor but also the presence of comorbid disease processes involving these organ systems. A careful history, review of systems, physical assessment, and routine laboratory data may provide clues in these areas.

   1. Bone marrow function. Chronic alcoholism and malnutrition as well as the effect of the tumor on glutition and appetite may contribute to the high incidence of folate deficiency seen in this population. Because of the additive effect of this deficiency and the inhibition of folate metabolism by methotrexate, there is often increased sensitivity to even small doses of methotrexate which is manifested as marked clinical toxicity.

   2. Pulmonary function. Chronic obstructive pulmonary disease is common in this group of patients. Moderate to severe pretreatment reductions in timed forced expiratory volumes may be reduced further with bleomycin. It is recommended that if clinical assessment suggests impaired pulmonary reserve and bleomycin is to be part of the treatment program, pretreatment pulmonary function studies should be performed.

   3. Renal function. Both cisplatin and methotrexate affect renal function. The major cumulative toxicity of cisplatin is renal. Unfortunately, there may be considerable impairment of renal function before the serum creatinine concentration rises; cisplatin doses of 80–120 mg/m^2 require serial determination of creatinine clearance to assess the cumulative effects of the drug on renal function.

   Limited renal excretion of methotrexate prolongs the duration of a high serum concentration, which in turn extends the duration of impaired DNA synthesis for normal as well as neoplastic tissues. Weekly intravenous (IV) methotrexate is usually given to patients with advanced disease after it is established that the serum creatinine level is normal. A careful clinical assessment at the time of each subsequent dose is probably a more reliable indicator of actual and potential methotrexate toxicity than are serial determinations of creatinine in this situation. Most episodes of serious methotrexate toxicity relate to a failure to appreciate intercurrent events that limit excretion of these relatively low doses of the drug. The most common of these toxicities is probably dehydration, which is related to progressive disease, increasingly poor oral intake, nausea and vomiting, or mucositis that may have been caused by prior drug treatment. Third-space reservoirs created by pleural effusions or ascites may lead to delayed clearance, prolonged serum drug levels, and increased toxicity. The addition of any drug that further alters renal clearance of methotrexate may tip the balance toward serious toxicity. Aspirin and other nonsteroidal anti-inflammatory agents, probenecid, sulfonamides, phenytoin, cefoxitin, and gentamicin may decrease methotrexate clearance and increase toxicity. Careful patient assessment at intervals with these considerations in mind helps to avoid these pitfalls.

C. Single-agent responses. Methotrexate, bleomycin, fluorouracil, cisplatin, carboplatin, and doxorubicin (Adriamycin) have been studied extensively as individual agents for head and neck carcinomas, and it is largely from this group that most combinations are derived.

    1. Methotrexate. In efforts to improve its therapeutic index, methotrexate has been investigated for no other solid tumor as extensively as it has been investigated for the management of head and neck cancer.

        a. IV methotrexate in doses of 40–60 mg/m^2 weekly is probably the most widely accepted conventional single-agent treatment for this group of tumors. Treatment with methotrexate results in objective response in 25–50% of patients, 7–10% of which are complete responses. Responses may occur after 1–2 weeks but usually require 4–6 weeks to become evident. Median response durations range from 2 to 6 months. Responders survive significantly longer than nonresponders. Treatment is usually given on an outpatient basis, and drug-related mortality is less than 4%.

        b. Intraarterial infusions of methotrexate, either alone or with systemic leucovorin, have been used in an attempt to improve drug concentrations in tumor tissue and to improve the therapeutic index of treatment. Although these techniques have resulted in marginally superior response rates, the lack of a single predominant blood supply to most tumors, the technical difficulties of the procedure, and the morbidity of problems from clot, embolus, and infection have precluded widespread adoption of this approach; it is not recommended for general use.

        c. Leucovorin rescue has made possible the use of moderate (240–500 mg/m^2) to high (1–3 gm/m^2) doses of methotrexate in attempts to improve response rates. While individual investigators have reported favorable response rates with decreased morbidity using these higher doses of methotrexate, the duration of response is not increased, and two comparative trials have demonstrated no advantage to these treatment approaches compared to weekly IV methotrexate. The need for hydration, urinary alkalinization, careful monitoring of renal clearance, and the high cost of treatment have been important factors in limiting general use of this approach, and it is not recommended outside a research setting.

2. **Bleomycin.** Bleomycin has attracted continued interest for the treatment of head and neck cancers because of its generally mild myelosuppressive effects and the potential for its application in combination with myelosuppressive chemotherapy. Bleomycin 10–30 mg/m^2 is usually given weekly, biweekly, or on a 5-day-per-month schedule by intramuscular (IM) and IV injections. These approaches have the advantage of being convenient for outpatient use. Tumor response rarely occurs at cumulative doses of less than 200 mg/m^2, and response most often requires a total dose of 300 mg/m^2. These doses usually produce significant mucosal toxicity. Response rates range between 15 and 25% and are generally inferior in duration to those achieved with methotrexate. The mucosal toxicity that accompanies the use of bleomycin is generally more frequent and severe than that produced with the use of a weekly methotrexate schedule.

3. **Cisplatin.** Cisplatin 40–60 mg/m^2 IV is given on an every-3-week schedule. Higher doses result in an increased risk of renal toxicity unless special precautions are taken. Doses of 80–120 mg/m^2 may be tolerated if preceded by hydration and accompanied by mannitol administration (with or without furosemide) for diuresis to protect renal function (see Chap. 10). Ondansetron's high degree of control of nausea and vomiting in the first 24 hours after therapy has increased patients' tolerance to cisplatin and has made it considerably easier to administer an intermediate dose of this drug on an outpatient basis. Cisplatin produces objective tumor responses in approximately 25% of patients, many of whom were treated previously with other antineoplastic drugs. Occasionally, dramatic tumor responses occur, although the frequency of complete remission is still low. Its major side effects are severe nausea and vomiting (which may be more of a problem after 24 hours than in the first 24 hours during which ondansetron offers better protection), tinnitus, occasional high-tone deafness, peripheral neuropathy, and most significantly, renal toxicity (with progressive loss in creatinine clearance in some patients).

4. **Carboplatin.** An analog of cisplatin that produces minimal renal toxicity, little peripheral neuropathy, and less emesis, carboplatin has a favorable toxicity profile, which gives it considerable practical utility in head and neck cancer. Doses of 360–400 mg/m^2, usually divided in 3 daily doses and repeated at 4-week intervals, have resulted in response rates ap-

proaching those for cisplatin. Its ease of administration and favorable therapeutic index recommend its use for palliation. Prolonged thrombocytopenia can be dose-limiting.

5. **Other drugs**

   a. Of the remaining agents for which some information is available, **fluorouracil** (5-FU) may be of somewhat greater value for oral cavity lesions than other agents; it has an overall 15% response rate. Use by infusion was popularized by a small phase II study demonstrating a much higher response rate that has not been duplicated. However, most combinations with fluorouracil have used the drug this way. Attempts to improve response rates utilizing leucovorin in conjunction with fluorouracil have not yet demonstrated long-term value.

   b. **Anthracyclines** appear to be of little overall value except in nasopharyngeal cancer. Both doxorubicin and mitoxantrone have led to responses in about 25% of patients.

   c. **Alkylating agents** have had relatively little testing in head and neck cancer, although modest activity was demonstrated for cytoxan. Recent phase II studies showed response rates of 28 and 42% for ifosfamide with mesna as a uroprotector in both bolus and infusion schedules.

   d. Of the taxanes, **paclitaxel** (Taxol) 250 mg/m^2 every 3 weeks with granulocyte colony-stimulating factor (G-CSF) support achieved responses in 40% of advanced head and neck cancers in an ECOG phase II trial. Current investigations are underway to explore lower doses in combination with cisplatin.

   e. Numerous **biologic response modifiers** have been studied, but to date they have not demonstrated any value in routine clinical practice.

D. **Combination-chemotherapy responses.** Multiple attempts have been made to improve single-agent response rates with combination chemotherapy. A number of studies using methotrexate, bleomycin, fluorouracil, cisplatin, and carboplatin in a variety of schedules have been reported.

The ECOG, in a comparison of methotrexate, bleomycin, and cisplatin versus weekly methotrexate, demonstrated a clear-cut response advantage for combination chemotherapy. Forty-eight percent of patients with advanced disease responded to an outpatient program using methotrexate, bleomycin, and cisplatin, compared to 35% using methotrexate alone. Complete remissions were achieved in 16% of patients receiving combination chemotherapy and for 8% treated with methotrexate alone. The median duration of response was the same in both treatment groups, and no survival advantage was demonstrated for the combination treatment. Although neither response rate is exceptional, the careful randomization and stratification procedures used lend weight to the result.

Combinations of cisplatin or carboplatin and fluorouracil or methotrexate demonstrate similar outcomes: improved response rates but no overall gain in survival.

E. **Combined-modality treatment.** Attempts to increase tumor destruction with drugs prior to definitive therapy or together with radiation therapy are not new, although developments in combination chemotherapy reawakened enthusiasm for this approach.

1. **Drugs before irradiation or surgery (neoadjuvant therapy)**

a. **Methotrexate.** In several small, single-institution studies, methotrexate in moderate or high doses with leucovorin rescue was given for several doses or cycles prior to irradiation or surgery. These schedules produced response rates of approximately 75% and avoided the problems of oral mucositis and ulceration reported by the older studies of concomitant chemotherapy with radiotherapy. No data are available to allow comparisons of these rescue programs with weekly methotrexate schedules.

b. **Combination chemotherapy.** A number of combination-drug therapy programs have been developed as initial treatment for advanced local-regional disease. These programs were intended either to reduce tumor bulk and allow more effective radiotherapy or to improve resectability of advanced lesions. In general, the programs use high-dose cisplatin in conjunction with hydration and diuretics (see Chap. 10) combined with either bleomycin or fluorouracil by IV infusion for 3–5 days. Vincristine is frequently included, and methotrexate is usually omitted. These programs produce high response rates (67–94%). Complete clinical disappearance of tumor is achieved in 19–28% of patients, and partial response is achieved in 48–74%. After 1–3 cycles of drug treatment, surgery, irradiation, or both follow. The number of patients with advanced local-regional disease who were made disease-free was higher than expected based on pretreatment staging expectations. Improvement in survival is limited to the patients who achieved complete response.

The achievements and limitations of this plan of therapy are outlined in Table 11-5. In general, neoadjuvant therapy best remains in the context of a clinical investigation.

The most important demonstration of the value of neoadjuvant or induction chemotherapy relates to organ preservation. Trials stimulated by the high response rates achieved by these treatments have shown the ability to preserve the larynx and voice. The best known trial (VA 268) showed that laryngeal

Table 11-5. Achievements of induction or neoadjuvant chemotherapy for patients with head and neck cancers

Major tumor regressions occur in 60–90% of patients with locally advanced disease.

Complete clinical regression occurs in 20–50%.

Response rates increase with the number of cycles given, up to 3.

Pathologic complete regressions are confirmed in 25–60% of patients with clinical complete responses.

Treatment does not adversely affect surgical or radiation therapy complications.

Drug response appears to predict response to irradiation.

Complete responders may achieve local-regional disease control with radiation therapy and avoid surgery.

Quality of life may be improved for some by organ preservation.

Frequency of distant metastasis as cause of treatment failure is reduced.

Complete responders have longer survival.

Overall survival is unchanged.

preservation was possible in 64% of patients who received induction chemotherapy followed by radiation therapy, with survival rates comparable to those for patients treated with laryngectomy and radiation therapy. Survival was not compromised in patients who received chemotherapy. Long-term survival was the same, with evidence of preservation of voice and presumed maintenance of quality of life.

2. **Concurrent chemotherapy and radiotherapy.** Bleomycin, fluorouracil, methotrexate, and cisplatin have been administered synchronously with radiation therapy in attempts to demonstrate synergistic effects. Most uncontrolled studies have suggested improved tumor responses and some gain in survival for patients with unresectable disease. Although randomized trials have found improvement in the initial response or disease-free survival rate, gains in overall survival have been difficult to document. Two studies demonstrated benefit for oral cavity primary lesions with concurrent bleomycin or fluorouracil. Enhanced mucositis has been a common limitation of combined treatment. Cisplatin appears attractive as an agent for concurrent therapy because of its radiosensitizing properties, established activity, and paucity of mucosal toxicity. Weekly dosing of cisplatin during radiotherapy resulted in higher response rates but no overall difference in complete response or survival rate compared with radiotherapy alone. When cisplatin was given as a 100 mg/m^2 bolus every 3 weeks with concurrent ra-

diation therapy in a Radiation Therapy Oncology (RTOG) trial, improvement in the number of complete responders and 4-year survival rates was suggested. As combination chemotherapy has shown itself to be more effective than single-agent therapy, studies are now focusing on combination chemotherapy together with radiation therapy. Because of the more severe local and systemic toxicities that can be associated with these regimens, attempts have been made to modify radiation therapy scheduling to facilitate the administration of combined-modality therapy while avoiding intolerable toxicity. Newer studies are evaluating split-course schedules and rapid alterations of chemotherapy and radiation therapy as well as hyperfractionated radiation. Once again preliminary results suggest improved short-term tumor control, though survival comparisons are difficult to quantitate. This subject continues to be an active and promising area of clinical investigation.

3. **Drugs as posttreatment adjuvants.** Whereas the most recent emphasis in head and neck cancer has been on achieving gains in early tumor control, little attention has been paid to the potential of postoperative or postirradiation therapy adjuvant drug studies. Suggestive phase II data have not been confirmed in larger, randomized phase III comparisons. Reasons for negative results include small sample size, inadequate therapy, poor patient compliance, and statistical analysis based on intention to treat. Posttreatment adjuvant therapy remains investigational.

F. **Selected treatment plans.** Four types of drug treatment programs are displayed in Table 11-6.

1. **Cytoreductive induction treatment**

   a. **Selection of patients.** This treatment is designed to reduce tumor bulk prior to surgery or radiotherapy in patients with advanced-stage disease and no prior therapy. The induction treatment regimen is intended for hospitalized patients following assessment of the extent of their tumor and an evaluation to exclude comorbid disease processes that might unacceptably increase the risks of treatment.

   b. **Administration**

      (1) **Cisplatin + vincristine + bleomycin (COB).** Oral hydration is begun the evening before treatment. On the morning of treatment an IV infusion of 5% dextrose in 0.5 N saline with potassium chloride 20 mEq/liter and magnesium sulfate 1 gm/liter is begun at a rate of 200 ml/hour. One of a number of intensive regimens to alleviate nausea and vomiting should be begun (see Chap. 33). Furosemide 40 mg and mannitol 12.5 gm are given IV after the first liter. Immedi-

ately thereafter, if the patient is voiding freely and adequately, cisplatin 100 mg/m^2 is added to a calibrated solution set and infused IV over a 30-minute period; the second liter of fluid is continued. The volume of subsequent IV fluids for the day and the necessity for additional diuretics are judged by the extent of nausea and vomiting, the urine volume, and evidence of congestive heart failure. On day 2, vincristine 1 mg is given by IV push, and a bleomycin infusion (30 units/day for 4 days) is begun. Bleomycin 15 units is added to each of 2 liters of 5% dextrose in 0.5 N saline with potassium chloride 20 mEq/liter. Two liters are given every 24 hours, and the continuous infusion is maintained for 4 days. On day 5, vincristine 1 mg is given by IV push. If adequate oral intake has not been resumed, additional IV fluids may be given. An infusion pump may be used to help ensure an even rate of flow.

The patient may be discharged after completion of the treatment course, depending on tolerance to the drug and the ability to eat and drink. An interim clinic visit before a second induction course is recommended as a safeguard. A second course of treatment is planned on day 22 but should be administered only after hematologic values and serum creatinine levels are normal and no pulmonary symptoms are reported. If tumor regression is continuing on day 43 after two cycles of treatment, a third cycle may be considered, although the cumulative risks of renal and pulmonary toxicity increase with continued treatment. At this point irradiation, surgery, or both should be considered once again.

(2) **Cisplatin + fluorouracil (CF).** Cisplatin 100 mg/m^2 IV on day 1 is administered with diuresis and antiemetics as described for COB in **1.b.(1)**. Fluorouracil 1000 mg/m^2 is divided between 2 liters of 5% dextrose in 0.5 N saline with potassium chloride 20 mEq/liter to be given every 24 hours. A continuous infusion of fluorouracil is maintained for 5 days, usually with an infusion pump. Follow-up is as described in **1.b.(1)**, although pulmonary toxicity is not a side effect of this program.

2. **Concurrent chemotherapy and radiotherapy.** With this program the dose of cisplatin is reduced to 75 mg/m^2 and fluorouracil infusion duration is limited to 4 days. Treatment is administered with hydration and antiemetics as described in the previous section. Careful attention to fluid and nutritional

Table 11-6. Selected drug treatment programs in head and neck cancer

Intent	Suitability	Scheme
Cytoreductive induction treatment	Advanced stage, no prior treatment	**COB** Cisplatin 100 mg/m² IV on day 1 with induced diuresis *and* Bleomycin 30 units/day as 24-hour infusion on days 2–5 *and* Vincristine 1 mg IV on days 2 and 5 Cycle repeats in 3 weeks
		CF Cisplatin 100 mg/m² IV on day 1 with induced diuresis *and* Fluorouracil 1000 mg/m²/day as 24-hour infusion on days 1–5 Cycle repeats in 3–4 weeks
Concurrent radiotherapy	Advanced stage, no prior treatment	Cisplatin 75 mg/m² IV on day 1 with induced diuresis *and* Fluorouracil 1000 mg/m²/day as 24-hour infusion on days 1–4 Cycle repeats in 4 weeks

		Radiotherapy 30 Gy/15 fractions begun on day 1 Evaluate at week 9: CR or unresectable—repeat third chemotherapy cycle with 30 Gy/15 fractions; PR, stable, and resectable—have surgery with a third cycle of chemotherapy and radiotherapy (30 Gy/15 fractions) 2–6 weeks after operation
Palliation	Any prior treatment	Methotrexate 40 mg/m² IM on days 1 and 15 *and* Bleomycin 10 units IM on days 1, 8, and 15 *and* Cisplatin 50 mg/m² IV day 4 with induced diuresis Cycle repeats in 3 weeks
		Either cisplatin 20 mg/m² IV on days 1–5 *or* Carboplatin 120 mg/m² on days 1–3 *and* Fluorouracil 800 mg/m² on days 1–5 by ambulatory infusion pump Cycle repeats in 3 weeks
Palliation	Prior treatment and contraindications to combination drugs	Methotrexate 40–60 mg/m² IV weekly

CR = complete response; PR = partial response.

support during possible periods of intense mucositis is necessary. In potentially operable patients a decision for surgery is usually made after two courses of chemotherapy and a total of 60 Gy.

3. **Combination chemotherapy for advanced recurrent disease.** The approach to advanced recurrent disease is based on prior treatment and the perceived ability of the patient to tolerate intensive chemotherapy.

   a. **COB or CF.** With advanced recurrent disease, one of two courses of induction treatment with COB or CF (see **IV.F.1** and Table 11-6) may be elected, followed by an intermittent program with lower doses of drug.

   b. An alternative combination-drug treatment using **methotrexate, bleomycin, and cisplatin** administered on an outpatient basis is described in Table 11-6. Methotrexate 40 mg/m^2 and bleomycin 10 units are given IM or IV on day 1. On day 4, cisplatin is given as an IV bolus at 50 mg/m^2. Cisplatin is given approximately 30–60 minutes after starting a 2–3-hour infusion of 2 liters of 5% dextrose in 0.5 N saline with potassium chloride 20 mEq/liter and magnesium sulfate 1 gm/liter. Furosemide 40 mg is given IV at the start of the infusion, and mannitol 12.5 gm is given just before the administration of cisplatin. Less aggressive rates of hydration (500–750 ml/hour) may be necessary in older patients or those with decreased cardiac function to prevent the development of congestive heart failure and pulmonary edema. Antiemetics are given as necessary. On day 8 bleomycin is given at a dose of 10 units, and on day 15 methotrexate and bleomycin are repeated.

   Dosages of methotrexate and cisplatin are reduced 50% for mild or moderate myelosuppression (see Table 10-2). Drugs are withheld if severe myelosuppression occurs. Treatment is resumed as soon as peripheral blood cell counts recover. Methotrexate and bleomycin are withheld if stomatitis is present. Complete blood cell counts, including platelets, should be done on a weekly basis. Serum creatinine levels are measured on day 8 of each cycle to ensure adequate renal function before the next dose of methotrexate is given, and creatinine clearance should be measured if creatinine levels rise 50% or more.

   c. **Ambulatory infusion.** An alternative treatment choice utilizes 3–5 daily doses of cisplatin or carboplatin together with continuous infusion of fluorouracil administered using an ambulatory infusion pump. Either cisplatin 20 mg/m^2 IV daily for 5 days or carboplatin 120 mg/m^2 daily for 3 days as short infusions can be combined with fluorouracil 800 mg/m^2 daily for 5 days as a continuous infusion. Dividing the dosage of cisplatin eliminates the need for aggressive hydration, shortens and simplifies the chemotherapy procedures, and promotes outpatient usage of these regimens.

4. Methotrexate alone for advanced disease

    a. Selection of patients. With a number of reports of increased response rates for drug combinations compared to methotrexate alone, single-agent methotrexate should probably be reserved for selected patients.

        (1) Patients in relapse after induction treatment programs without methotrexate,

        (2) Those who refuse treatment with cisplatin or bleomycin,

        (3) Those whose pulmonary function excludes a bleomycin treatment program, *and*

        (4) Those whose reliability and follow-up opportunities are poor.

    b. Treatment regimens. The usual starting dose of methotrexate is 40 mg/m^2; if advanced age, nutritional status, anemia, borderline renal function, or other factors suggest that the sensitivity of normal tissues to methotrexate might be increased, the initial dose may be reduced to as low as 20 mg/m^2. Blood cell counts are done weekly, and if there is no evidence of mucositis or myelosuppression, the dose is escalated to a maximum of 60 mg/m^2. Most patients tolerate this treatment with minimal nausea and vomiting. A few require antiemetics. Careful attention to oral hygiene (see sec. **V.C.** and Chap. 33) may be helpful for preventing or reducing the severity of mucositis. Candidiasis is common and, if present, should be treated with nystatin (Mycostatin) or another antifungal agent. If mucositis or myelosuppression occurs, treatments are delayed until they clear and blood cell counts are normal.

V. Problems in supportive care

    A. Support systems. The population of patients with head and neck cancer includes many elderly men—often social reprobates, recluses, heavy smokers and drinkers, and occasionally frank derelicts. They are frequently divorced or separated from their families, and many live alone, often in reduced circumstances. Lack of family, friends, resources, and initiative are often impediments to adequate care, especially for those with advanced disease for which close follow-up, regular clinic visits, and adherence to treatment schedules are important. They desperately need a primary caregiver to be in the home or closely allied with the home to promote their well-being and optimal utilization of medical care and to derive advantage from the health care delivery system. Social service, ministerial help, American Cancer Society patient programs (such as I Can Cope), patient support groups, Alcoholics Anonymous, and other social care groups should be enlisted to help the patient cope with illness. Smoking cessation programs may be appropriate for those with early cancers that may be cured.

B. Nutrition. Gradual, progressive weight loss and inanition are common factors in the relentless illness of many patients. Their nutrition is generally inadequate, and repetitive efforts at reinforcing the need for a high-calorie diet, as free of alcohol as possible, must be given. Depending on the location of the tumor and the particular problems with swallowing, efforts need to be extended on a regular basis to ensure adequate patient nutrition. Many patients, or their families, need to be instructed in the use of blended foods, the use of high-protein supplements, or both. Some patients benefit from the use of a pediatric feeding tube when deformities in the anatomy prevent adequate swallowing. In selected patients feeding by a gastrostomy tube may be appropriate, especially early in the clinical course when it may be only a temporary expedient. Most patients benefit from any attempts at oral hyperalimentation. The role of IV hyperalimentation is not clear and needs to be considered early in the management course during the perioperative or radiation therapy period when induction treatment is taking place. Its role for patients with advanced disease is still unclear. Efforts to maintain nutrition must be reinforced at every opportunity with the family, the caregiver, and the patient. Dietary advice or consultation with a dietetic department should be utilized freely.

C. Mouth care. An important problem for some patients with head and neck cancer is mouth care. Many patients have difficulty with secretions. Xerostomia may be produced by radiation therapy and may require treatment with artificial saliva. An additional agent that may be helpful is pilocarpine 5–10 mg PO tid with water. At the opposite extreme, patients with posterior tongue lesions may have edema and swelling that precludes adequate swallowing, and the pooling of secretions and subsequent aspiration become a problem. These patients may benefit from the use of suction to drain their secretions. Cleansing mouthwash (see Chap. 33) may be appropriate, and efforts at dental hygiene need to be maintained. Radiation-induced bone necrosis or fistulas need to be cleaned or debrided and occasionally packed with toothpaste or other material to promote comfort. Dental consultation is helpful in many patients, particularly prior to radiation therapy.

D. Hypothyroidism. Weakness, apathy, listlessness, and weight loss may develop insidiously in patients subjected to thyroid irradiation or resection. Such symptoms may mistakenly be construed as suggesting disease relapse.

E. Hypercalcemia. Hypercalcemia is common in patients with epidermoid carcinoma of the head and neck. As many as 23% of patients with advanced recurrent head and neck cancers may experience hypercalcemia before their death. In general, this phenomenon accompanies late-stage recurrent tumor, often with little evidence of bone involvement. Dehydration, all too common in these patients, may be a precipitating factor; in many patients hypercalcemia is mild and easily controlled with hydration, saline diuresis, or both. Although hydration, saline diuresis, or reduction in tumor bulk (achieved with irradiation, drug therapy, or surgery) frequently reverses this phenomenon, a few patients require pamidronate for adequate treatment (see Chap. 34). If patients have advanced disease without hope of substantial palliation, consideration can also be given to withholding treatment for the hypercalcemia and allowing the patient to die a natural, more comfortable death than might occur if the hypercalcemia were treated and the patient were obliged to die of locally progressive disease.

F. **Aspiration pneumonia.** The anatomic deformities induced by surgery, recurrent tumor, or both make patients with head and neck cancer highly susceptible to aspiration of pooled secretions. Fever, tachycardia, tachypnea, rales, and infiltrates in the lung are usual findings and are often confused with primary bacterial pneumonia. Knowledge of the aspiration or observation of the event may be the only decisive method of proving the diagnosis. Immediate recognition of aspiration should be followed by treatment with steroids, antibiotics, or both.

G. **Granulocytopenia and infection.** There is always an urgent need to identify pulmonary or other infections quickly in the presence of drug-induced granulocytopenia. The mortality due to pneumonia and sepsis is high in this situation. Appropriate cultures are needed in an effort to document infection and help distinguish the problem from aspiration. Fever in a granulocytopenic patient should be treated promptly with broad-spectrum antibiotics without awaiting results of blood or sputum cultures (see Chap. 31). In selected situations the use of G-CSF may reduce the duration of granulocytopenia and ameliorate infections.

VI. **Cancer prevention.** No discussion of treatment of head and neck cancer would be complete without mention of efforts in cancer prevention. Clearly alcohol and tobacco use are synergistic etiologic factors in the development of these neoplasms and all patients should be encouraged in behavior modification and other cessation programs.

Recent evidence suggests that isotretinoin (13-*cis*-retinoic acid) can both clinically improve and histologically mature oral leukoplakia and erythroplakia. Further, the incidence of second head and neck cancers and second primary lung cancers appears to be reduced by this treatment. Although the optimal dose is not yet established, 5.6 mg/m^2 PO daily appears to be a relatively safe and probably effective dosage. This represents a new and challenging area for research.

Selected Readings

Adelstein, D. J., et al. Simultaneous versus sequential combined technique therapy for squamous cell head and neck cancer. *Cancer* 65:1685, 1990.

Al-Kourainy, K., et al. Achievement of superior survival for histologically negative versus histologically positive clinically complete responders to cisplatin combination in patients with locally advanced head and neck cancer. *Cancer* 59:233, 1987.

Al-Sarraf, M., et al. Concurrent radiotherapy and chemotherapy with cisplatin in inoperable squamous cell carcinoma of the head and neck: an RTOG study. *Cancer* 59:259, 1987.

American Joint Committee in Cancer. *Staging Cancer at Head and Neck Sites. Manual for Staging Cancer.* Philadelphia: Lippincott, 1988. P. 27.

The Department of Veterans Affairs Laryngeal Cancer Study Group. Induction chemotherapy plus radiation compared with surgery plus radiation in patients with advanced laryngeal cancer. *N. Engl. J. Med.* 324:1685, 1991.

Merlano, M., et al. Treatment of advanced squamous-cell carcinoma of the head and neck with alternating chemotherapy and radiotherapy. *N. Engl. J. Med.* 327:1115, 1992.

Vogel, S. E., et al. A randomized prospective comparison of methotrexate with a combination of methotrexate, bleomycin and cisplatin in head and neck cancer. *Cancer* 56:432, 1985.

Vokes, E. E., et al. Head and neck cancer. *N. Engl. J. Med.* 328:184, 1993.

Carcinoma of the Lung

Joan H. Schiller

Carcinoma of the lung is responsible for more than 155,000 deaths each year in the United States. This represents one-third of all deaths due to cancer, and more than the number of deaths due to breast, colon, and prostate cancers combined. The incidence of the disease continues to rise, particularly in women and blacks, and thus is likely to present a significant public health problem for years to come.

Lung cancer consists of four major histologic types: adenocarcinoma, squamous cell carcinoma, large-cell carcinoma, and small-cell carcinoma. Because of the unique biologic features of small-cell lung cancer (SCLC), its staging and treatment differ radically from the other three types of lung cancer, which collectively are called non-small-cell lung cancer (NSCLC). Thus these two groups are addressed in two separate sections.

I. **Etiology.** Lung cancer is predominantly a disease of smokers. Eighty percent of lung cancer occurs in active or former smokers, and an additional 5% are estimated to occur as a consequence of passive exposure to tobacco smoke. Tobacco smoke causes an increased incidence of all four histologic types of lung cancer, although adenocarcinoma (particularly the bronchoalveolar variant) is also found in nonsmokers. Other risk factors for lung cancer include exposure to asbestos or radon. Familial factors, such as activity of carcinogen-metabolizing hepatic enzyme systems, e.g., 4-debrisoquine hydroxylase, may also play a role in determining an individual's propensity to develop lung cancer.

II. **Molecular biology.** Numerous genetic changes have been associated with lung tumors. Most common among these include activation or overexpression of the *myc* family of oncogenes in SCLC and NSCLC, and K-*ras* oncogene in NSCLC, particularly adenocarcinoma. Inactivation or deletion of the p53 and retinoblastoma tumor suppressor genes, and a yet-to-be-identified tumor suppressor gene on chromosome 3p, have been found in 50–90% of patients with SCLC. p53 and 3p abnormalities have been associated with 50–70% of NSCLCs. The role of these genetic alterations as prognostic factors and therapeutic targets is under investigation.

III. **Screening.** Screening high-risk patients with chest radiographs or sputum cytology has no impact on mortality, and thus is not recommended.

IV. **Non-small-cell lung cancer.** The prognosis and treatment of NSCLC are dependent primarily on stage of disease at the time of diagnosis. Although histologic differences (adenocarcinoma versus large-cell carcinoma versus squamous cell carcinoma) among the NSCLCs affect their natural history and presentation, these differences are of relatively little importance in determining patient management.

   A. **Staging.** The current TNM staging classification was developed in 1986 by the American Joint Committee on

Cancer and the Union Internationale Contre Cancer (UICC) to reflect the differences in treatment and survival between patients with disease that was locally advanced, but still operable; patients with inoperable, locally advanced disease; and patients with distant metastatic disease. The TNM classification is shown in Table 12-1, and the stage grouping in Table 12-2.

B. **Pretreatment evaluation.** The diagnosis of lung cancer is usually made by bronchial biopsy or percutaneous needle biopsy. Although the disease is usually discovered on chest x-ray films, a computed tomography (CT) scan of the chest is necessary to evaluate the extent of the primary disease, mediastinal extension or lymphadenopathy, and the presence or absence of other parenchymal nodules in patients in whom surgical resection is a consideration. CT of the upper abdomen is performed to look for asymptomatic hepatic or adrenal metastases. Bone scans should be obtained for the patient with bone pain or an elevated alkaline phosphatase level; however, the utility of routine bone scans in the absence of signs or symptoms is controversial. Head CT is not routinely done in the absence of central nervous system (CNS) signs or symptoms. Occasionally thoracoscopy is required. The role of preoperative mediastinoscopy is controversial. Although mediastinoscopy is helpful in determining whether normal-appearing mediastinal nodes on the CT scan contain tumor, the procedure should not be done unless this information will play a role in the management of the patient.

Pulmonary function testing is necessary prior to definitive surgery. Increased postoperative morbidity is associated with a predicted postoperative 1-second forced expiratory volume (FEV_1) < 800–1000 ml; a preoperative maximum voluntary ventilation (MVV) < 35% of predicted; a carbon monoxide diffusing capacity (DLCO) < 60% of predicted; and an arterial oxygen pressure (PO_2) < 60 mm Hg or a carbon dioxide pressure (PCO_2) > 45 mm Hg.

C. **Management**
1. **Stage I disease.** A lobectomy is the treatment of choice for stage I NSCLC, with cure rates of 60–80% reported. Within stage I, patients with T2, N0 disease do not fare as well as those with T1, N0 cancers. In approximately 20% of patients with medical contraindications to surgery but with adequate pulmonary function, high-dose radiotherapy will result in cure. No role of adjuvant chemotherapy for stage I NSCLC has been identified. Patients with a resected stage I NSCLC are at high risk for the development of second lung cancers (approximately 1%/year). Clinical trials are under way to determine the role of isotretinoin (13-*cis*-retinoic acid) in preventing second primary tumors following resection in patients with stage I NSCLC. At the present time, adjuvant isotretinoin should not be considered the standard of therapy.

Table 12-1. TNM definitions for lung cancer

Primary tumor (T)

TX   Tumor proved by the presence of malignant cells in bronchopulmonary secretions but not visualized roentgenographically or bronchoscopically, or any tumor that cannot be assessed.

T0   No evidence of primary tumor.

Tis   Carcinoma in situ.

T1   A tumor ≤ 3.0 cm in greatest dimension, surrounded by lung or visceral pleura, and without evidence of invasion proximal to a lobar bronchus at bronchoscopy.

T2   A tumor > 3.0 cm in greatest dimension, or a tumor of any size that either invades the visceral pleura or has associated atelectasis or obstructive pneumonitis extending to the hilar region. At bronchoscopy, the proximal extent of demonstrable tumor must be within a lobar bronchus or ≥ 2.0 cm distal to the carina. Any associated atelectasis or obstructive pneumonitis must involve less than an entire lung.

T3   A tumor of any size with direct extension into the chest wall (including superior sulcus tumors), diaphragm, or the mediastinal pleura or pericardium without involving the heart, great vessels, trachea, esophagus, or vertebral body, or a tumor in the main bronchus < 2.0 cm from the carina but without involving the carina.

T4   Any tumor of any size with invasion of the mediastinum or involving the heart, great vessels, trachea, esophagus, vertebral body, or carina or the presence of a malignant pleural effusion.

Nodal involvement (N)

N0   No demonstrable metastasis to regional lymph nodes.

N1   Metastasis to lymph nodes in the peribronchial or the ipsilateral hilar region, or both, including direct extension.

N2   Metastasis to ipsilateral mediastinal lymph nodes and subcarinal lymph nodes.

N3   Metastasis to contralateral mediastinal, contralateral hilar, ipsilateral or contralateral scalene or supraclavicular lymph nodes.

Distant metastasis (M)

MX   Cannot be assessed.

M0   No distant metastasis.

M1   Distant metastasis.

Table 12-2. Stage grouping of TNM subsets for lung cancer

Occult carcinoma	TX, N0, M0
Stage 0	Tis, N0, M0
Stage I	T1 or T2, N0, M0
Stage II	T1 or T2, N1, M0
Stage IIIA	T3, N0 or N1, M0
	T1–3, N2, M0
Stage IIIB	Any T, N3, M0
	T4, any N, M0
Stage IV	Any T, any N, M1

2. **Stage II disease.** The treatment for stage II NSCLC is surgical resection. Although the role of neoadjuvant chemotherapy is under investigation (see sec. **C.3.**), it cannot be routinely recommended until the results of randomized clinical trials confirm clinical benefit.

3. **Locally advanced (stage IIIA/IIIB) disease.** Treatment of locally advanced NSCLC is one of the most controversial issues in the management of lung cancer. Treatment options include surgery for less-advanced disease, or radiotherapy, either of which has been given with or without chemotherapy for control of micrometastases. Interpretation of the results of clinical trials involving patients with locally advanced disease has been clouded by a number of issues, including changing diagnostic techniques, different staging systems, and heterogeneous patient populations who may have disease that ranges from "nonbulky" stage IIIA (clinical N1 nodes, with N2 nodes discovered only at the time of surgery or mediastinoscopy), to "bulky" N2 nodes (enlarged adenopathy clearly visible on chest x-ray films, or multiple nodal level involvement), to clearly inoperable stage IIIB disease.

   a. **Nonbulky stage IIIA (and selected stage II).** The primary treatment of stage II disease is surgical resection. Two randomized studies conducted by the Lung Cancer Study Group (LCSG) examined the issue of postoperative adjuvant chemotherapy for stage II and stage IIIA disease. In general, these studies demonstrated an improvement in disease-free survival for patients receiving postoperative chemotherapy, with overall survival bordering on statistical significance. A randomized Intergroup study is currently underway to define further the role of postoperative chemotherapy in patients with resected stage II or IIIA NSCLC; patients are randomized to receive either radiotherapy plus chemotherapy (cisplatin 60 mg/m^2 IV on day 1 and etoposide 120 mg/m^2 IV on days 1–3 every 4 weeks for 4 cycles) or radiotherapy alone. Until these results are available, postoperative adjuvant chemotherapy for this group of patients cannot be routinely recommended.

Postoperative radiotherapy has been shown to reduce local recurrences after resection of stage II or III squamous cell carcinoma of the lung, but does not prolong survival.

b. T3, N0 stage III disease. This subset of stage III disease has a different natural history and treatment strategy compared to stage III N2 disease. Patients with peripheral chest wall invasion should undergo resection of the involved ribs and underlying lung. Chest wall defects are then repaired with chest wall musculature or Marlex mesh and methylmethacrylate. Postoperative radiotherapy is often given. Five-year survival rates as high as 50% have been reported.

c. Pancoast tumors. Pancoast tumors are upper-lobe tumors that adjoin the brachial plexus, and are frequently associated with Horner's syndrome or shoulder and arm pain; the latter is due to rib destruction, involvement of the C-8 or T-1 nerve roots, or both. Treatment consists of a combined-modality approach with radiotherapy and surgery. Five-year survival rates range from 25 to 50%. Combined preoperative chemotherapy and radiotherapy is currently being studied.

d. Bulky stage IIIA (N2) and stage IIIB. The optimal treatment for bulky stage IIIA and stage IIIB disease is also controversial. Current investigational efforts are directed at identifying the optimal combined-modality approach, involving treatments directed at local control of the disease (surgery or radiotherapy) and micrometastatic disease (chemotherapy). Possibilities include radiotherapy only, preoperative chemotherapy, or chemotherapy plus radiotherapy.

(1) Preoperative chemotherapy plus surgery. Several nonrandomized studies in highly selected stage IIIA lung cancer patients suggest that preoperative chemotherapy with and without radiotherapy converts bulky mediastinal disease into a technically resectable tumor, and as a consequence prolongs survival. The Memorial Sloan Kettering Cancer Center has reported response rates of 73% in patients with clinical N2, M0 disease following 2–3 cycles of chemotherapy with cisplatin (120 mg/m^2) on day 1 and vindesine (3 mg/m^2) or vinblastine (5 mg/m^2) on days 1, 8, 15, 22, and 29. The survival rate at 3 years was 34% for all 41 patients, 40% for the 21 who completed the combined treatment (chemotherapy and surgery), and 54% for the 8 patients who had a complete resection. The role of preoperative chemotherapy is being investigated in a randomized Intergroup trial.

A recent randomized trial compared preoperative chemotherapy (mitomycin 6 mg/m^2, ifosfamide 3 gm/m^2 with mesna protection, and cisplatin 50 mg/m^2 each administered once every 3 weeks for 3 courses) followed by surgery, versus surgery without preoperative chemotherapy for patients with stage IIIA disease. (All patients also received postoperative mediastinal radiotherapy after surgery.) Thirty patients in each treatment arm were evaluated; the median survival time was 26 months for patients receiving preoperative chemotherapy plus surgery, compared to 8 months for patients treated with surgery alone. The median disease-free survival period was 20 months in the former group, and 5 months in the latter. Chemotherapy induced responses in 18 (60%) of 30 patients. It should be noted, however, that this patient population did not have bulky disease and included patients with T3, N0–1 disease, and that the prognostic factors were not evenly distributed between groups.

(2) Chemotherapy plus radiation therapy. Radiotherapy as a single agent has been the traditional treatment for patients with bulky stage IIIA or IIIB disease. However, the use of chemotherapy plus radiotherapy continues to remain an area of active investigation. The Cancer and Leukemia Group B (CALGB) conducted a randomized trial of induction chemotherapy plus high-dose radiation, versus radiation alone in patients with favorable prognostic factors who had stage IIIA or IIIB NSCLC. One hundred fifty-five patients were randomized to receive cisplatin (100 mg/m^2 IV on days 1 and 29) and vinblastine (5 mg/m^2 IV on days 1, 8, 15, 22, and 29) followed by radiation therapy on day 50 (60 Gy over a 6-week period), or to radiotherapy alone. The median survival time was significantly longer in the chemotherapy group (13.8 versus 9.7 months).

These results were recently confirmed in a National Cancer Institute (NCI) high-priority study evaluating the role of chemotherapy plus radiotherapy. Four hundred fifty-two patients were randomized to receive standard once-daily fractionation radiotherapy, twice-daily radiotherapy (hyperfractionation), or cisplatin and vinblastine plus radiotherapy. One-year survival rate and median survival time for the standard radiation treatment group were 46% and 11.4 months; for the hyperfractionated radiation therapy group, 51% and 12.3 months; and for chemotherapy plus radiation therapy group, 60% and 13.8 months ($P = 0.03$).

Promising results have also been seen using daily cisplatin (6 mg/m^2) as a radiation sensitizer in conjunction with radiotherapy.

4. Stage IV disease

a. Issues regarding treatment. The role of chemotherapy in the management of patients with metastatic NSCLC is controversial. A recent meta-analysis of randomized controlled trials comparing first-line chemotherapy with supportive care identified a small gain in survival (6 weeks) for patients receiving chemotherapy, with most of the improvement in survival occurring within the first 6 months of treatment. Thus, a discussion must ensue with the patient regarding possible benefits, chance of response, and quality of life with treatment. Since chemotherapy is not curative, goals for treatment should include palliation of symptoms and a modest improvement in survival. Although one study on cost-effectiveness demonstrated a cost benefit for chemotherapy compared to supportive care, studies evaluating quality-of-life issues are clearly needed.

The principal factors predicting response to chemotherapy and survival are performance status and extent of disease. Patients with a poor performance status (Eastern Cooperative Oncology Group (ECOG) performance status of 3–4) and bulky disease are unlikely to respond to treatment, and thus probably should not be treated. Favorable prognostic factors include no weight loss, female sex, normal serum lactic dehydrogenase (LDH) level, and no bone or liver metastases. Since one of the major goals of treatment is palliation of symptoms, it may be reasonable to delay chemotherapy in an asymptomatic patient.

b. First-line chemotherapy. Numerous phase II trials have reported high response rates in metastatic NSCLC. For example, a Canadian trial reported a 62% response rate in 53 patients with stage IIIB or IV NSCLC to cisplatin, vincristine, doxorubicin, and etoposide (CODE) plus antibiotic prophylaxis and supportive corticosteroids. However, no clear advantage to any one chemotherapy regimen has been demonstrated in multiinstitutional randomized trials, which generally report response rates of 15–30%. Cisplatin-based regimens have been the mainstay of treatment, although carboplatin is commonly substituted for cisplatin. One randomized trial comparing cispla-

tin or carboplatin for advanced NSCLC with etoposide reported a slightly higher response rate in
the cisplatin treatment arm, but with increased
toxicity and no improvement in survival. No evidence of a steep dose-response curve for cisplatin
was demonstrated in two randomized trials. Commonly administered chemotherapy regimens are
shown in Table 12-3.

   c. **Second-line chemotherapy.** No second-line
   regimens of value have been identified for metastatic NSCLC. This patient population may be
   appropriate for phase I trials.

   d. **New agents.** New drugs with activity in advanced NSCLC are currently being evaluated;
   their exact role in our chemotherapeutic armamentarium remains undefined. Paclitaxel (Taxol),
   a novel antitubular agent with activity in breast
   and ovarian cancer, resulted in prolonged survival in phase II studies on metastatic NSCLC
   and is currently under investigation in phase
   III randomized trials. Vinorelbine (Navelbine), a
   semisynthetic vinca alkaloid, used alone produced a survival advantage when compared to
   fluorouracil and leucovorin, and when combined
   with cisplatin, it produced a survival advantage
   compared to its use alone or cisplatin plus vindesine. CPT-11, a topoisomerase inhibitor, has
   been reported to have a 32% response rate as a
   single agent, and a 56% response rate in combination with cisplatin.

   Other new chemotherapy agents with possible
   activity in NSCLC, currently being evaluated in
   phase I and II trials, include topotecan, edatrex-
   ate, and gemcitabine.

V. **Small-cell carcinoma.** SCLC differs from NSCLC in a
number of important ways. First, it has a more rapid clini-

**Table 12-3. Common chemotherapy regimens for metastatic
non-small-cell lung cancer**

PE	
Cisplatin	60 mg/m^2 IV on day 1
Etoposide	120 mg/m^2 IV on days 1–3 *or*
	120 mg/m^2 PO bid on days 1–3
	Repeat cycle every 3 weeks
CAP	
Cyclophosphamide	400 mg/m^2 IV on day 1
Doxorubicin (Adriamycin)	40 mg/m^2 IV on day 1
Cisplatin	40 mg/m^2 IV on day 1
	Repeat cycle every 4 weeks
Carbo/VP-16	
Carboplatin	300 mg/m^2 IV on day 1
Etoposide	100 mg/m^2 IV on days 1–3
	Repeat cycle every 3–4 weeks

cal course and natural history, with the rapid development of metastases, symptoms, and death. Untreated, the median survival time for patients with local disease is typically 12–15 weeks, and for those with advanced disease, 6–9 weeks. Second, it exhibits features of neuroendocrine differentiation in many patients (which may be distinguishable histopathologically), and is more often associated with paraneoplastic syndromes. Third, unlike NSCLC, SCLC is exquisitely sensitive to both chemotherapy and radiotherapy, although resistant disease often develops. Because of the rapid development of distant disease and its extreme sensitivity to the cytotoxic effects of chemotherapy, this mode of therapy forms the backbone of treatment for this disease.

A. **Staging.** Because of the propensity of this disease to metastasize so quickly, and the fact that micrometastatic disease is presumed to be present in all patients at the time of diagnosis, this disease is usually classified into either a local or an extensive stage. Local disease is typically defined as disease that can be emcompassed within one radiation port, usually considered limited to the hemithorax and to regional nodes, including mediastinal and ipsilateral supraclavicular nodes. Extensive-stage disease is usually defined as disease that has spread outside those areas.

B. **Pretreatment evaluation.** Common sites of metastases for SCLC include the brain, liver, bone marrow, bone, and CNS. For this reason, a complete staging work-up consists of a complete blood cell count; liver function tests; CT of the brain, chest, and abdomen; a bone scan; and bone marrow aspiration and biopsy. However, this complete staging work-up should not be undertaken unless the patient is a candidate for combined-modality treatment with chest radiation and chemotherapy, the patient is being evaluated for a clinical study, or the information is helpful for prognostic reasons. If the patient is not a candidate for combined-modality treatment or a clinical study, stopping the staging at the first evidence of extensive-stage disease is usually appropriate.

C. **Prognostic factors.** As in NSCLC, the major pretreatment prognostic factors are stage, performance status, and bulky disease. Hepatic metastases also confer a poorer prognosis. If the patient's initial poor performance status is due to the underlying malignancy, these symptoms often disappear quickly with treatment, resulting in a net improvement in quality of life. However, major organ dysfunction from nonmalignant causes often results in an inability of the patient to tolerate chemotherapy.

D. **Therapy.** A number of combination chemotherapeutic regimens are available for SCLC (Table 12-4). However, no clear survival advantage has been demonstrated for any one regimen versus another. With these chemotherapy regimens, overall response rates of 75–90% and complete response rates of 50% for localized disease can

Table 12-4. Chemotherapy regimens for small-cell lung cancer

A. Cisplatin based
  EP

Etoposide	120 mg/m^2 IV on days 1–3 *or*
	120 mg/m^2 PO bid on days 1–3
Cisplatin	60 mg/m^2 IV on day 1

or

Cisplatin	25 mg/m^2 IV on days 1–3
Etoposide	100 mg/m^2 IV on days 1–3
	Repeat cycle every 3 weeks

B. Carboplatin based

Carboplatin	300 mg/m^2 IV on day 1
Etoposide	100 mg/m^2 IV on days 1–3

or

Carboplatin	100 mg/m^2 IV on days 1–3
Etoposide	120 mg/m^2 IV on days 1–3
	Repeat cycle every 4 weeks

C. Adriamycin based
  CAV

Cyclophosphamide	1000 mg/m^2 IV on day 1
Doxorubicin (Adriamycin)	45–50 mg/m^2 IV on day 1
Vincristine	1.4 mg/m^2 IV on day 1 (maximum 2 mg)
	Repeat cycle every 3 weeks

  CAE

Cyclophosphamide	1000 mg/m^2 IV on day 1
Doxorubicin	45 mg/m^2 IV on day 1
Etoposide	50 mg/m^2 IV on days 1–5
	Repeat cycle every 3 weeks

be anticipated. For extensive-stage disease, overall response rates of about 75% with complete response rates of 25% are common. Despite these high response rates, however, the median survival time remains about 14 months for limited-stage disease, and 7–9 months for extensive-stage disease. Only 15–20% of limited-disease patients have long-term survival (> 2 years) with standard therapy, and the long-term survival rate for extensive-disease patients is less than 5%.

   1. Dose intensity. A recent dose intensity meta-analysis of chemotherapy in SCLC, which evaluated doses not requiring bone marrow transplantation support, showed no consistent correlation between dose intensity and outcome. Clinical trials evaluating the role of marrow ablative doses of chemotherapy with subsequent progenitor cell replacement (e.g., autologous bone marrow transplantation) are ongoing.

   Another method for increasing the intensity of chemotherapy is to intensify the schedule. Promising results of weekly intensive chemotherapy with CODE (cisplatin, vincristine, doxorubicin, and etoposide plus prophylactic antibiotics) have been observed (median survival time, 61 weeks; 2-year survival rate, 30%) in extensive-stage SCLC patients.

2. **Alternating therapy and consolidation chemotherapy.** Use of alternating non-cross-resistant chemotherapy regimens has been explored because of the mathematic model created by Goldie and Coldman which predicts improved tumor response when more chemotherapy agents of different mechanisms are used concurrently and early. Despite the mathematic model, randomized trials of alternating chemotherapy regimens versus standard regimens have not consistently yielded significant improvements in survival. The lack of benefit may not represent a failure of the Goldie-Coldman model, but the lack of two totally non-cross-resistant chemotherapy regimens.

A randomized study by the Southeastern Oncology Group found an improvement in median survival time in limited-stage patients who received consolidation cisplatin and etoposide following 6 cycles of cyclophosphamide, doxorubicin (Adriamycin), and vincristine (CAV) compared to patients who received CAV alone (22.8 versus 15.9 months, respectively). Although these results are promising, it is unclear whether they are due to the consolidation chemotherapy or to the introduction of cisplatin and etoposide into a CAV regimen.

Clinical trials involving consolidation with high-dose chemotherapy with bone marrow support are currently ongoing.

3. **Duration of therapy.** Randomized studies have demonstrated that prolonged administration of chemotherapy does not improve survival. The optimal duration of treatment for SCLC is 4–6 months.

4. **Second-line therapy.** No curative regimens for patients with recurrent disease have been identified. Oral etoposide (50 mg/m^2/day for 21 days) resulted in a 45% response rate in 22 patients with recurrent disease, 18 of whom had prior IV etoposide treatment. The median duration of response, however, was only 4 months. Etoposide 37.5 mg/m^2 PO on days 1–14 when combined with ifosfamide 1.2 gm/m^2 IV on days 1–4 and cisplatin 20 mg/m^2 IV on days 1–4 resulted in a 61% response rate in 18 patients with a 25-week median survival time. This was a much more toxic regimen than oral etoposide alone.

5. **New agents.** Promising agents for SCLC include ifosfamide, paclitaxel, the camptothecans CPT-11 and topotecan, and epirubicin. Phase II and III studies with these agents are ongoing.

E. **Chemotherapy plus chest irradiation.** Numerous studies have been done with chemotherapy and thoracic radiotherapy for patients with limited-stage SCLC. Conflicting results have been attributed to differences in chemotherapy regimens and different schedules integrating chemotherapy and thoracic radiation (concurrent, sequential, and "sandwich" approach). Two recent meta-analyses concluded that thoracic radiation does result in a small but significant improvement in survival and major control of the disease in the chest, although no conclusions could be made regarding the optimal sequencing of chemotherapy and thoracic radiation. Preliminary analysis of an Intergroup trial involving concurrent conventional once-daily fractionation (180 cGy/fraction; 5 fractions/week for 5 weeks; total dose = 45 Gy) and cisplatin (60 mg/m^2 day 1) plus etoposide (120 mg/m^2 daily for 3 days) demonstrated a 42% two-year survival rate.

Phase II trials have reported prolonged survival with twice-daily (hyperfractionated) radiotherapy, when given concurrently with cisplatin and etoposide. Results of an Intergroup trial comparing twice-daily (hyperfractionated) radiotherapy with standard radiotherapy are pending and will answer this important question.

F. **Prophylactic cranial irradiation.** Numerous trials have demonstrated that prophylactic brain irradiation (PCI) does not enhance survival. A randomized French study demonstrated that patients with SCLC in complete remission who were randomized to receive PCI (24 Gy/8 fractions/12 days) decreased the risk of brain metastases threefold compared to those who were randomized to the no-PCI group. No effect on survival was seen, and a slight but not significant decrease in mental function was noted in those receiving PCI.

VI. **Palliation**

A. **Radiotherapy.** Palliative radiotherapy is often helpful in controlling the pain of bone metastases or neurologic function in patients with brain metastases. Chest radiotherapy may help control hemoptysis, superior vena cava syndrome, airway obstruction, laryngeal nerve compression, and other local complications.

B. **Pleural effusions.** Common sclerosing agents include tetracycline (no longer available), doxycycline, talc, and bleomycin. A recent review of the literature concluded that doxycycline and minocycline were effective (with success rates of 72 and 86%) and well tolerated, that bleomycin was less effective and substantially more expensive, and that talc, while effective, had the disadvantage of requiring a thoracoscopy and general anesthesia for insufflation.

C. **Brachytherapy.** For patients with bronchial obstruction who have received maximum external beam radiotherapy, the use of high-dose endobronchial irradiation may be of temporary benefit.

D. **Cachexia.** Megesterol acetate 40 mg 4 times daily may improve the appetite of some patients.

E. **Colony-stimulating factors.** Filgrastim (granulocyte colony-stimulating factor, G-CSF) has been shown to decrease the incidence of neutropenic fevers, and decrease the median duration of neutropenia, days of hospitalization, and days of antibiotic treatment in patients with extensive-stage SCLC treated with cyclophosphamide, doxorubicin, and etoposide (CAE) compared to patients who received CAE alone. However, as discussed already, it should be noted that the clinical benefit of maintaining a dose-intense approach in the treatment of SCLC patients has not been established.

Caution must be exercised when using colony-stimulating factors in patients receiving combined-modality treatment with both chemotherapy and thoracic radiation. A randomized study by the Southwestern Oncology Group found patients receiving sargramostim (granulocyte-macrophage colony-stimulating factor, GM-CSF) and chemotherapy with concurrent thoracic irradiation had a significant increase in thrombocytopenia compared to patients receiving concurrent chemotherapy and radiation therapy without growth factor.

Selected Readings

Arriagada, R., et al. Randomized trial on prophylactic cranial irradiation (PCI) for patients (pts) with small cell lung cancer (SCLC) in complete remission (CR). *Proc. Am. Assoc. Clin. Oncol.* 13:334, 1994.

Bonomi, P. D., et al. Combination chemotherapy versus single agents followed by combination chemotherapy in stage IV non-small-cell lung cancer: a study of the Eastern Cooperative Oncology Group. *J. Clin. Oncol.* 7:1602, 1989.

Chang, A., et al. Phase II study of taxol, merbarone, and piroxantrone in stage IV non-small-cell lung cancer: the Eastern Cooperative Oncology Group results. *J. Natl. Cancer Inst.* 85:388, 1993.

Crawford, J., et al. Reduction by granulocyte colony-stimulation factor of fever and neutropenia induced by chemotherapy in patients with small-cell lung cancer. *N. Engl. J. Med.* 325:164, 1991.

Dillman, R. O., et al. A randomized trial of induction chemotherapy plus high-dose radiation versus radiation alone in stage III non-small cell lung cancer. *N. Engl. J. Med.* 323:940, 1990.

Eddy, D. Screening for lung cancer. *Ann. Intern. Med.* 111:232, 1989.

Einhorn, L., et al. Cisplatin plus etoposide consolidation following cyclophosphamide, doxorubicin, and vincristine in limited stage small-cell lung cancer. *J. Clin. Oncol.* 6:451, 1988.

Ettinger, D., et al. Justification for evaluating new anti-cancer drugs in selected untreated patients with a chemotherapy-sensitive advanced cancer: an ECOG randomized study. *Proc. Am. Soc. Clin. Oncol.* 9:224, 1990.

Gandara, D., et al. Evaluation of cisplatin intensity in metastatic non-small-cell lung cancer: a phase III study of the Southwest Oncology Group. *J. Clin. Oncol.* 11:873, 1993.

Giaccone, G., et al. Maintenance chemotherapy in small-cell lung cancer: long-term results of a randomized trial. *J. Clin. Oncol.* 11:1230, 1993.

Grilli, R., Oxman, A., and Julian, J. Chemotherapy for advanced non-small-cell lung cancer: how much benefit is enough? *J. Clin. Oncol.* 11:1866, 1993.

Holmes, E. C., Gail, M., Lung Cancer Study Group. Surgical adjuvant therapy for stage II and III adenocarcinoma and large-cell undifferentiated carcinoma. *J. Clin. Oncol.* 4:710, 1986.

Jaakkimainen, L., et al. Counting the costs of chemotherapy in a National Institute of Canada randomized trial in nonsmall cell lung cancer. *J. Clin. Oncol.* 8:1301, 1990.

Johnson, D., et al. Prolonged administration of oral etoposide in patients with relapsed or refractory small-cell lung cancer: a phase II trial. *J. Clin. Oncol.* 8:1613, 1990.

Johnson, D., et al. Cisplatin (P) and etoposide (E) and concurrent thoracic radiotherapy (TRT) administered once versus twice daily for limited-stage (LS) small cell lung cancer (SCLC): preliminary results of an Intergroup trial. *Proc. Am. Soc. Clin. Oncol.* 13:333, 1994.

Klasa, R., Murray, N., and Coldman, A. Dose-intensity meta-analysis of chemotherapy regimens in small-cell carcinoma of the lung. *J. Clin. Oncol.* 9:499, 1991.

Klastersky, J., et al. A randomized study comparing cisplatin or carboplatin with etoposide in patients with advanced nonsmall-cell lung cancer. European Organization for Research and Treatment of Cancer Protocol 07861. *J. Clin. Oncol.* 8:1556, 1990.

Klastersky, J., et al. A randomized study comparing a high and a standard dose of cisplatin in combination with etoposide in the treatment of advanced non-small-cell lung carcinoma. *J. Clin. Oncol.* 4:1780, 1986.

Lad, T., Rubinstein, L., and Sadeghi, A. The benefit of adjuvant treatment for resected locally advanced nonsmall-cell lung cancer. *J. Clin. Oncol.* 6:9, 1988.

Le Chevalier, T., et al. Randomized study of vinorelbine and cisplatin vs vindesine and cisplatin vs vinorelbine alone in advanced nonsmall-cell lung cancer: results of a European multicenter trial including 12 patients. *J. Clin. Oncol.* 12:360, 1994.

Lilenbaum, R., and Green, R. Novel chemotherapeutic agents in the treatment of non-small cell lung cancer. *J. Clin. Oncol.* 11:1391, 1993.

Lung Cancer Study Group. Effects of post-operative mediastinal radiation on completely resected stage II and stage III epidermoid cancer of the lung. *N. Engl. J. Med.* 315:1377, 1986.

Martini, N., et al. The effects of preoperative chemotherapy on the resectability of non-small cell lung carcinoma with mediastinal lymph node metastases. *Ann. Thorac. Surg.* 45:370, 1988.

Masuda, N., et al. CPT-11 in combination with cisplatin for advanced non-small-cell lung cancer. *J. Clin. Oncol.* 10:1775, 1992.

Murray, N., et al. Brief intensive chemotherapy for metastatic non-small-cell lung cancer: a phase II study of the weekly CODE regimen. *J. Natl. Cancer Inst.* 83:190, 1991.

Murray, N., et al. Intensive weekly chemotherapy for the treatment of extensive stage small cell lung cancer. *J. Clin. Oncol.* 9:1632, 1991.

Neal, C., et al. Pancoast tumor: radiation therapy alone vs preoperative radiation and surgery. *Int. J. Radiat. Oncol. Biol. Phys.* 21:651, 1991.

O'Rourke, M., et al. Survival advantage for patients with stage IV NSCLC treated with single agent Navelbine in a randomized controlled trial. *Proc. Am. Soc. Clin. Oncol.* 12:343, 1993.

Pignon, J.-P., et al. A meta-analysis of thoracic radiotherapy for small-cell lung cancer. *N. Engl. J. Med.* 327:1618, 1992.

Rosell, R., et al. A randomized trial comparing preoperative chemotherapy plus surgery with surgery alone in patients with non-small-cell lung cancer. *N. Engl. J. Med.* 330:153, 1994.

Ruckdeschel, J., et al. A randomized trial of the four most active regimens for metastatic non-small cell lung cancer. *J. Clin. Oncol.* 4:14, 1986.

Sandler, A., et al. A phase II study of daily oral VP-16 plus ifosfamide plus cisplatin (poVIP) for previously treated recurrent small cell lung cancer (SCLC): a Hoosier Oncology Group trial. *Proc. Am. Soc. Clin. Oncol.* 13:327, 1994.

Sause, W., et al. RTOG 8808 ECOG 4588, preliminary analysis of a phase III trial in regionally advanced unresectable non-small cell lung cancer. *Proc. Am. Soc. Clin. Oncol.* 13:325, 1994.

Walker-Renard, P., Vaughan, L., and Sahn, S. Chemical pleurodesis for malignant pleural effusions. *Ann. Intern. Med.* 120:56, 1994.

Warde, P., and Payne, D. Does thoracic irradiation improve survival and local control in limited-stage small-cell carcinoma of the lung? A meta-analysis. *J. Clin. Oncol.* 10:890, 1992.

Weick, J., et al. A randomized trial of five cisplatin-containing treatments in patients with metastatic non-small cell lung cancer: a Southwest Oncology Group study. *J. Clin. Oncol.* 9:1157, 1991.

Wright, C., et al. Superior sulcus long tumors. Results of combined treatment (irradiation and radical resection). *J. Thorac. Cardiovasc. Surg.* 94:69, 1987.

Carcinomas of the Gastrointestinal Tract

John C. Marsh

Cancers of the gastrointestinal (GI) tract (esophagus, stomach, small and large intestines) account for nearly 18 percent of all cancer in the United States and about 17 percent of cancer deaths. Colon cancer is by far the most common of these malignancies, with cancer of the rectum, stomach, esophagus, and small intestine occurring with decreasing frequency. Surgery continues to be the principal curative modality, but irradiation and chemotherapy have increasingly important roles and, in certain adjuvant situations, may improve the cure rate produced by surgery. Chemotherapy alone is not curative. Drugs produce objective remissions in only 15–40 percent of patients. However, there is little question that meaningful palliation and an increase in survival can be achieved in patients who respond to chemotherapy. Controlled clinical trials, often by interinstitutional cooperative groups, have been useful in defining the natural history and therapeutic benefit of various treatment modalities. Participation in such clinical trials should be encouraged.

I. Carcinoma of the esophagus

A. General considerations and aims of therapy

1. **Epidemiology.** Cancer of the esophagus is predominantly of the squamous cell (epidermoid) variety and represents about 1% of the cancers in the United States. Risk factors include heavy tobacco and alcohol use. It is more common in men than women, and blacks than whites. The average patient is in his or her 60s at presentation. In certain parts of China, epidermoid esophageal cancer is the most common kind of cancer, and is thought to be related to dietary habits of the region, and perhaps as a consequence of fungal contamination of pickled vegetables. Other predisposing factors for esophageal cancer include achalasia, a history of lye burns of the esophagus, and prior epidermoid carcinomas of the aerodigestive tract.

   In recent years, the incidence of adenocarcinoma of the esophagus (along with adenocarcinoma of the proximal stomach) has increased greatly. By the mid-1980s, it accounted for about one-third of all esophageal cancer among white men. Adenocarcinoma is predominantly a disease of middle-aged white men, is less clearly associated with alcohol and tobacco use, and is frequently associated with Barrett's esophagus (epithelial metaplasia of the lower esophagus), which is sometimes seen with reflux esophagitis. The rate of increase of adenocarcinomas of the esophagus and gastric cardia during the 1970s and 1980s exceeded that of any other cancer, including lung cancer, non-Hodgkin's lymphoma, and melanoma. This impressive increase is due to entirely unknown causes. Adenocarcinomas of the esophagus tend to involve the lower third of that organ, while the middle third is the most common site for the epidermoid variety. Chemotherapy for the two types of esophageal carcinoma is the same, with little or no difference in response rate in most series.

2. **Clinical manifestations and pretreatment evaluation.** Carcinoma of the esophagus is usually associated with progressive and persistent dysphagia. Pain, hoarseness, weight loss, and chronic cough are unfavorable manifestations that indicate spread to regional structures (e.g., mediastinal nerves), recurrent laryngeal nerve, or fistula formation between the esophagus and the airway. The most common sites of metastases are regional lymph nodes (which may include cervical, supraclavicular, intrathoracic, diaphragmatic, celiac axis, or periaortic), the liver, and the lungs.

   Diagnosis is usually made by barium swallow, endoscopy, and biopsy or lavage cytology. Staging should be based on chest x-ray appearance, computed tomography (CT) scan of the abdomen and chest, and careful physical examination of the cervical and supraclavicular nodes. Endoscopic esophageal ultrasound is still investigational but may be useful in assessing the depth of tumor invasion. The preoperative staging of esophageal cancer is still quite inadequate, due to the inability to evaluate lymph nodes accurately. Bronchoscopy should be done for upper and middle third tumors and a bone scan is useful in patients with bone pain or tenderness. Survival is related to pathologic stage, which can only be defined surgically (Table 13-1).

3. **Treatment and prognosis.** The primary treatment of stage I and II carcinoma of the esophagus is surgical resection. About half of esophageal cancers are operable, and half of these are resectable. Patients with more advanced disease (stage III) are best treated, at least initially, with nonsurgical means, usually a combination of radiation and chemotherapy. In patients who respond to such treatment the carcinoma may subsequently be operable, while patients with metastatic disease to the liver, lung, or bone are best treated with systemic therapy. Palliative feeding procedures, such as with a jejunostomy or gastrostomy tube, may be useful if subsequent surgical resection is not to be done. The overall median survival time is less than a year and the overall 5-year survival rate is about 5%. The prognosis is related to the size of the lesion, the depth of penetration of the esophagus, and nodal involvement. Carcinoembryonic antigen (CEA) may be a useful marker of disease activity in many patients. Current controlled clinical trials are helping to evaluate the

Table 13-1. TNM stages for carcinoma of the esophagus

Primary tumor

Tis	Carcinoma in situ
T1	Invades lamina propria or submucosa
T2	Invades muscularis propria
T3	Invades adventitia
T4	Invades adjacent structures

Regional lymph nodes

N0	No node metastasis
N1	Regional node metastasis

Distant metastasis

M0	None
M1	Present

Stage grouping

0	Tis, N0, M0
I	T1, N0, M0
IIA	T2 or T3, N0, M0
IIB	T1 or T2, N1, M0
III	T3, N1, M0
	T4, any N, M0
IV	Any T, any N, M1

Source: Modified from American Joint Committee on Cancer. In O. H. Beahrs et al. (eds.), *Manual for Staging of Cancer* (4th ed.). Philadelphia: Lippincott, 1992. Pp. 58–59.

relative roles of chemotherapy, radiation, and surgery in all stages of the two predominant histologic types. Participation should be encouraged. Most emphasis has been on preoperative ("neoadjuvant") combined-modality treatment, with few supporting data available for postoperative treatment.

B. **Treatment of advanced (metastatic) disease.** Various agents with modest activity when used alone are available. These include bleomycin, methotrexate, fluorouracil, cisplatin, mitomycin, and doxorubicin. Patients with no prior chemotherapy are more likely to respond than those who have had previous treatment. Single agents are less helpful than combination chemotherapy because of their lower response rates and brief duration of response. Cisplatin-based regimens have been most extensively tested. Among the most active are the following.
   1. **Cisplatin + fluorouracil + interferon alpha**
      a. Cisplatin 100 mg/m^2 IV on day 1 *and*
      b. Fluorouracil 750 mg/m^2 continuous IV infusion on days 1–5 *and*
      c. Interferon alpha 3 × 10^6 units SQ daily on days 1–28.
      Repeat every 28 days. Give cisplatin on every other cycle after the first three cycles.
   A response rate of 53% was reported in a small series, with equal activity in both adenocarcinoma and squamous cell carcinoma.

2. Cisplatin + fluorouracil + doxorubicin
   a. Cisplatin 75 mg/m^2 IV on day 1 *and*
   b. Fluorouracil 600 mg/m^2 IV on days 1 and 8 *and*
   c. Doxorubicin 30 mg/m^2 IV on day 1.
   Repeat every 28 days. This regimen was reported to have a 33% response rate in a small series and to result in a median survival time of 8 months.

3. Second-line therapy may be chosen from the following single agents: methotrexate 40 mg/m^2 IV weekly, mitomycin 20 mg/m^2 IV every 4–6 weeks, or bleomycin 15 mg/m^2 IV twice weekly.

C. Combined-modality therapy for potentially curable patients. Because of the limited success of surgery alone, attempts have been made to combine it with radiation and chemotherapy, or in some instances, omitting surgery altogether. The data are not yet solid enough to allow a definitive choice and controlled clinical trials are critically needed. Neither preoperative nor postoperative radiotherapy has been associated with significant improvement in survival. Postoperative adjuvant therapy with chemotherapy alone, and the combination of chemotherapy and radiation therapy have not yet been shown to be effective. Patients with clinical stage II or III disease are appropriately treated with preoperative radiation, chemotherapy and surgery.

1. Recommended regimen. Some of the best results are those using the following regimen concurrently with radiotherapy.
   a. Vinblastine 1 mg/m^2 IV on days 1–4 and 17–20 of radiotherapy *and*
   b. Cisplatin 20 mg/m^2/day by continuous IV infusion on days 1–5 and 17–21 of radiotherapy *and*
   c. Fluorouracil 300 mg/m^2/day by continuous IV infusion on days 1–21 of radiotherapy.
   Radiation therapy is 3750 cGy in 15 fractions (250 cGy/day). The preoperative regimen is followed by surgery at day 42.
   This program is fairly toxic and should be given largely in the hospital. About 25% of patients treated with this regimen were reported to be tumor-free at surgery. The median survival time was 29 months, and the 5-year survival rate was 34%. A more widely used, less aggressive regimen using fluorouracil and cisplatin intermittently with radiation has been associated with median survival times of 12–18 months and 5-year survival rates of 8–16%.

2. Supportive care. Esophagitis during such a treatment program is nearly universal, and nutritional support frequently will be required, preferably using alimentation by feeding tube. Peripheral alimentation is difficult with the continuous chemotherapy administration. Gastrostomy tubes are to be avoided, because of the usual requirement for a gastric pull-up following resection of the esophageal tumor.

3. Follow-up studies. History and physical examination may be done monthly for a year, then every 3

months for 2 years. Chest x-ray films should be evaluated every 3 months for 2 years and then annually,
with a CT of the abdomen and chest at the end of
combined-modality treatment, then every 6 months
for 2 years, and then annually for a total of 5 years.
Most patients destined to have a recurrence will do
so within that time.

II. Gastric carcinoma

A. General considerations and aims of therapy

1. **Epidemiology.** The incidence of stomach cancer has
   decreased dramatically in the United States since
   the beginning of the century, although it has stabilized in the last 20 years. The leading cause of cancer
   death in 1930, it now ranks twelfth. No improvement
   has been seen, however, in 5-year survival rates,
   which range from 5 to 16%. The only curative modality at present is surgery. The male–female ratio
   is 1.5:1.0. Stomach cancer is still the leading cause
   of cancer death among men in Japan and is also common in China, Finland, Poland, and Chile. A high
   rate of chronic gastritis and intestinal metaplasia of
   the stomach is associated with a high incidence of
   gastric cancer. *Helicobacter pylori* has been implicated in such changes, and in gastric cancer as well
   as in peptic ulcer. While the incidence in the United
   States has fallen, the location of gastric cancers has
   migrated proximally. Cancers in the fundus of the
   stomach have increased from 14% of gastric cancers
   in 1950 to 24% at present.

2. **Clinical manifestations and evaluation.** The
   most common symptoms are weight loss, abdominal
   pain, nausea, vomiting, changes in bowel habits, anorexia, and dysphagia. The diagnosis generally is
   made by endoscopy and biopsy, although barium
   swallow study is frequently helpful. Endoscopic ultrasonography is increasingly used; it is more accurate in gauging the depth of the cancer in the gastric
   wall than it is for determining nodal involvement.
   Metastases are to the liver, pancreas, omentum,
   esophagus, and bile ducts by direct extension and to
   regional and distant lymph nodes, such as those in
   the left supraclavicular area. Pulmonary and bone
   metastases are a late finding. Staging of suspected
   gastric cancer should be based on CT scans of the
   chest, abdomen, and pelvis, and with liver function
   tests. Tumor markers such as CEA, CA 19-9, and CA
   72-4 may be useful for subsequent assessment of the
   response to therapy. Prognosis is reflected by accurate staging (Table 13-2).

3. **Treatment and prognosis.** Most stomach cancers
   are adenocarcinomas. Important prognostic factors
   include tumor grade and gross appearance. Diffusely
   infiltrating lesions are less likely to be cured than
   sharply circumscribed, nonulcerating ones. The presence of regional lymph node involvement or involvement of contiguous organs in the surgical specimen

Table 13-2. TNM stages for carcinoma of the stomach

Primary tumor

Tis	Carcinoma in situ
T1	Invades lamina propria or submucosa
T2	Invades muscularis propria or the subserosa
T3	Penetrates the serosa (visceral peritoneum)
T4	Invades adjacent structures

Regional lymph nodes

N0	No node metastasis
N1	Metastasis in perigastric node(s) within 3 cm of primary tumor
N2	Metastasis in perigastric node(s) beyond 3 cm; or other regional nodes

Distant metastasis

M0	None
M1	Present

Stage grouping

0	Tis, N0, M0
IA	T1, N0, M0
IB	T1, N1, M0
	T2, N0, M0
II	T1, N2, M0
	T2, N1, M0
	T3, N0, M0
IIIA	T2, N2, M0
	T3, N1, M0
	T4, N0, M0
IIIB	T3, N2, M0
	T4, N1, M0
IV	T4, N2, M0
	Any T, any N, M1

Source: Modified from American Joint Committee on Cancer. In O. H. Beahrs et al. (eds.), *Manual for Staging of Cancer* (4th ed.). Philadelphia: Lippincott, 1992. Pp. 64–65.

indicates an increased likelihood of recurrence, as does the presence of dysphagia at the time of diagnosis. Patients with proximal lesions or lesions requiring total, rather than distal subtotal, gastrectomy are also at greater risk.

B. Treatment of advanced (metastatic, locally unresectable, or recurrent) disease

   1. Single agents with activity include epirubicin, mitomycin, doxorubicin, cisplatin, etoposide (VP-16), fluorouracil, hydroxyurea, and the nitrosoureas. Single agents have low response rates (15–35%), brief durations of response, and few complete responses, and have little impact on survival.

   2. Combination of drugs are more widely used than single agents, largely because of higher response rates, more frequent complete responses, and the theoretical potential of longer survival. It must be acknowledged, however, that a controlled trial of fluorouracil alone versus fluorouracil plus doxorubicin (Adriamycin) (FA) versus fluorouracil, doxorubicin, and mitomycin (FAM) failed to show a survival benefit for the combinations, which were more costly and toxic. Response rates, which were measurable in only about half the patients, were higher with the combinations.

Because the effectiveness of "standard" chemotherapy of GI cancer is modest, better treatments, including new drugs, are greatly needed. Before treating patients with standard regimens, consideration should be given to entering the patients into clinical trials. Most new drugs being evaluated for these diseases are available only for patients previously untreated with chemotherapy. One appropriate strategy would be to use an investigational agent or regimen initially, followed by more conventional agents, such as those listed below.

a. ELF. This regimen was designed to be less toxic than the regimen of etoposide, doxorubicin, and cisplatin (EAP), and in the hands of its originators seems to be as effective. Initial experience suggests a response rate of about 50% with an 11-month median survival time.

  (1) Leucovorin 300 mg/m^2 as a 10-minute IV infusion, followed by

  (2) Etoposide 120 mg/m^2 as a 50-minute IV infusion, followed by

  (3) Fluorouracil 500 mg/m^2 as a 10-minute infusion.

  All agents are given on days 1, 2, and 3. The course is repeated in 21–28 days.

b. FAMTX. This regimen compared favorably to FAM in a large European clinical trial and to EAP in the United States. Response rates were 41 and 33% in the two studies, with median survival times of 10.5 and 7.3 months, respectively.

  (1) Hydrate with 1 liter of isotonic sodium bicarbonate (1.4% bicarbonate) prior to methotrexate administration. (Urine pH must be > 7.0.) Infuse 2 liters of an identical solution over 24 hours after methotrexate is given.

  (2) Methotrexate 1.5 gm/m^2 by IV bolus infusion after the hydration and urine alkalinization, day 1.

  (3) Fluorouracil 1.5 gm/m^2 by IV bolus infusion starting 1 hour after the end of the methotrexate infusion.

  (4) Leucovorin 15 mg/m^2 orally starting 24 hours later on day 2, given every 6 hours for 3 days or until the methotrexate level is $< 2 \times 10^{-8}$ M. If the methotrexate level is $\geq 2.5 \times 10^{-6}$ at 24 hours, increase leucovorin dose to 30 mg/m^2 q6h for 96 hours.

  (5) Doxorubicin 30 mg/m^2 IV on day 15 if the white blood cell count (WBC) is > 3000/μl or the absolute neutrophil count (ANC) is $> 1500/\mu l$, and platelet count is $> 70,000/\mu l$. The cycle is repeated every 4 weeks.

Renal function *must* be normal and blood levels of methotrexate should be monitored with this regimen. Doses are modified as shown in Table 13-3.

C. Adjuvant therapy. Despite numerous trials of postoperative chemotherapy following potentially curative gastric resection, its value is uncertain. Until benefit is shown, there is no specific role for adjuvant chemotherapy following surgery.

D. Follow-up studies. Reasonable follow-up studies for patients in remission following surgery consist of history and physical examination every 3 months for 3 years, every 6 months for 2 years, and then annually. Complete blood cell count and liver function tests may be done on the same schedule. Abdominal CT and chest x-ray studies should be done annually. Endoscopy may be done if new symptoms develop.

E. Combined-modality therapy. A large number of patients have locally unresectable or incompletely resectable disease, and it has been known for some time that fluorouracil used in conjunction with radiotherapy adds to the survival of such patients compared with radiotherapy alone, so long as they have no evidence of metastatic disease and have disease that can be encompassed by a treatment port. It is not clear that radiation therapy added to chemotherapy is better, in terms of survival, than chemotherapy alone. However, while the role of radiation therapy in the management of gastric cancer is yet to be defined, the large number of local recurrences seen in this disease suggest a potential value. Thus it seems appropriate to treat such patients at the present time with a combined-modality regimen. While there is no "standard," a reasonable regimen is as follows.

1. Radiotherapy 45 Gy at 180 cGY/day to the tumor (or tumor bed) and nodal chains.
2. Chemotherapy is started on the first or second day of radiotherapy.
   a. Leucovorin 20 mg/m^2 IV bolus on days 1–4.
   b. Fluorouracil 400 mg/m^2 IV bolus on days 1–4, each dose given 1 hour (alternatively immediately) following the leucovorin infusion.
   Repeat chemotherapy at the same daily dose for 3 days on week 5 of radiotherapy.
3. Continuing chemotherapy. After a 4–5-week rest to allow recovery of the WBC to $> 3500/\mu l$ and platelet count to $> 150,000/\mu l$, treat with either
   a. Leucovorin 20 mg/m^2 IV bolus on days 1–5 *and* Fluorouracil 425 mg/m^2 IV bolus on days 1–5, each dose given 1 hour (alternatively immediately) following the leucovorin infusion.
   Repeat for 2–4 cycles.
      or

Table 13-3. Dose modification for FAMTX

	WBC (cells/μl)	Platelets (cells/μl)	Serum creatinine	Action
Day 1 or 15	< 3000	< 70,000		Delay 1 week
After second week of delay	2000–2900	50,000–69,000		50% dose reduction
	< 2000	< 50,000		Discontinue therapy
Nadir	< 1000			25% reduction for fluorouracil and methotrexate
Any day 1			> 50% above baseline	Discontinue therapy

      b. ELF (see sec. **B.2.a**) for at least 2 cycles. Continuation should depend on response and tolerance to the regimen.

The use of preoperative, or "neoadjuvant" chemotherapy is somewhat in vogue at the present time, due to some encouraging responses and apparent conversion of unresectable tumors to resectable ones by the administration of multidrug combinations. Such an approach is still under investigation and is not yet considered standard therapy. Perhaps the most compelling argument is the possibility that early administration of chemotherapy may have a potential benefit on occult metastases.

F. Complications. Hematologic and GI toxicities from the chemotherapy may be accentuated by concurrent radiotherapy. If the complications are sufficiently severe, chemotherapy or radiotherapy, or both, should be withheld until improvement. Consideration is given to treating at reduced doses. Hematopoietic growth factors may be of benefit in preventing severe infections secondary to neutropenia, but their use has not yet resulted in improved survival.

G. Treatment of refractory disease. If the patient's disease recurs or progresses with the recommended regimens, it is reasonable to consider combinations containing drugs not previously administered, or any of the single agents mentioned in sec. **II.B.1.**

III. Cancer of the small intestine

A. General considerations and aims of therapy

    1. Carcinoid tumors. Carcinoid tumors are the most common tumors of the appendix and ileum. They may develop in other parts of the GI tract but much less commonly. The usual histologic criteria of malignancy are not always applicable. Thus, invasion and evidence of distant spread are more useful prognostic features.

In one series, the 60% of patients with intestinal carcinoids that were still confined to the wall of the gut had a 5-year survival rate of 85%, whereas those with tumors invading the serosa or beyond had a 5% survival rate at 5 years. Patients in the latter group were nearly always symptomatic, whereas patients in the former group were not. (Their tumors were discovered at surgery for appendicitis or other causes.) Tumors of the appendix are usually benign by these criteria, whereas those of the ileum are more often invasive. Surgical resection is the definitive therapy.

    2. Carcinoid syndrome. About 10% of patients with carcinoid tumors are afflicted with the carcinoid syndrome, which includes diarrhea, abdominal cramps, malabsorption, and flushing. With tumors of intestinal origin, liver metastases are nearly always present. Serotonin is thought to be responsible for the abdominal symptoms, and its metabolite 5-hydroxyindoleacetic acid (5-HIAA) is excreted in large quantities in the urine and is a useful marker of disease activity. The symptoms may respond to simple anti-diarrheal therapy. The flushing caused by the syndrome has been attributed to bradykinin, formed by the interaction of kallikrein (produced by the tumor) with a plasma protein. If simple symptomatic measures do not suffice, the best treatment is with the synthetic, long-acting somatostatin analog octreotide acetate (Sandostatin). This agent, injected at a dose of 50–150 μg SQ q6–12h, effectively decreases the secretion of serotonin and other gastroentero-pancreatic peptides such as insulin or gastrin. It has been helpful in ameliorating the symptoms of carcinoid tumors, e.g., flushing and diarrhea. There are even modest objective antitumor effects.

3. **Adenocarcinomas.** Adenocarcinomas of the small intestine are so uncommon that there is no large chemotherapy experience to report. Survival of patients with small intestinal cancer is a function of stage (Table 13-4). There is a modest response rate of metastatic disease to FAM and this is a reasonable first choice.

   a. Fluorouracil 600 mg/m² IV on days 1, 8, 29, and 36 *and*

   b. Doxorubicin 30 mg/m² IV on days 1 and 29 *and*

   c. Mitomycin 10 mg/m² IV on day 1.

Table 13-4. TNM stages for carcinoma of the small intestine

Primary tumor

Tis	Carcinoma in situ
T1	Invades lamina propria or submucosa
T2	Invades muscularis propria
T3	Invades through the muscularis propria into the subserosa or into nonperitonealized perimuscular tissue with extension ≤2 cm
T4	Perforates visceral peritoneum or directly invades other organs or structures

Regional lymph nodes

N0	No node metastasis
N1	Regional node metastasis

Distant metastasis

M0	None
M1	Present

Stage grouping

0	Tis, N0, M0
I	T1 or T2, N0, M0
II	T3 or T4, N0, M0
III	Any T, N1, M0
IV	Any T, any N, M1

Source: Modified from American Joint Committee on Cancer. In O. H. Beahrs et al. (eds.), *Manual for Staging of Cancer* (4th ed.). Philadelphia: Lippincott, 1992. P. 70.

B. Treatment of advanced carcinoid tumors

    1. Effective agents. Doxorubicin (Adriamycin), fluorouracil, and streptozotocin have been shown to have some activity in this disease. Responses have also been seen with melphalan, cyclophosphamide, and methotrexate. A major advantage of using streptozotocin in combination is its lack of myelotoxicity. Response rates for combinations of fluorouracil and streptozotocin, or streptozotocin and cyclophosphamide in treating carcinoids of various kinds are 25–35%, with the overall response rate for patients with tumors of intestinal origin 41%. Median durations of response of 7 months may be expected, and patients with a good performance status have the greatest likelihood of response. Tumor response correlates well with reduction of 5-HIAA excretion. Some reports have indicated responses with interferon alpha, including in some patients previously treated with chemotherapy, although the responses are usually transient. When the disease is confined to the liver, it is sometimes possible to achieve good palliation with hepatic artery embolization.

    2. Recommended regimens

        a. Streptozotocin 500 mg/m^2 IV on days 1–5 *and* Fluorouracil 400 mg/m^2 IV on days 1–5.

        Repeat the course every 6 weeks if the disease has responded or is stable.

        b. If the patient does not respond, doxorubicin 60 mg/m^2 IV every 3 weeks can be given with appropriate monitoring of cardiac function and leukocyte count.

        c. Interferon alpha 3 million to 6 million units/ day IM.

C. Precautions. Treatment of carcinoid tumors may precipitate or exacerbate the carcinoid syndrome during the first days of treatment, and the serotonin antagonists cyproheptadine and methysergide should be available.

IV. Cancer of the large intestine

A. General considerations and aims of therapy. Taken together, cancers of the colon and rectum are by far the most frequent malignancies of the GI tract, and they account for the most deaths. Fewer than one-half of patients found to have large-bowel cancers are cured by surgery, although this modality is still the only curative one available. There have been some advances in early diagnosis and in techniques of surgery, but nationwide mortality figures have not really changed appreciably. In some institutions the relative incidence of colon cancer is increasing, whereas the incidence of rectal cancer is decreasing. Local recurrence is much more common for rectal cancer (40–50%). About 50% of large-bowel cancer recurrences are in the liver.

    1. Staging. The most commonly used staging system is that of Dukes or its modifications. This system classifies the tumor in terms of the extent to which it penetrates the bowel wall and involves regional lymph nodes. Dukes A lesions are confined to the mucosa and submucosa and are associated with a 5-year survival rate of more than 80%. B_1 lesions penetrate the muscularis but do not reach the serosa; patient survival rates are 60–80%. B_2 lesions penetrate to the serosa or through it into the pericolic fat; patient survival rates range from 40% to 70%. Dukes C lesions indicate nodal involvement. If the serosa has not been penetrated (in one system of classification) it is called a C_1 lesion, with an associated 35–60% 5-year survival rate; the C_2 lesions are through the serosa, have positive nodes, and are associated with a 15–30% survival rate. Dukes D lesions have distant metastases at the time of initial staging, and there are virtually no 5-year survivors. This pathologic staging method is helpful for selecting patients who are at sufficiently high risk to justify adjuvant therapy, e.g., chemotherapy or irradiation. The TNM system for colorectal cancer is being used increasingly (Table 13-5) but the Dukes classification is still more popular. Staging is most accurately done at

Table 13-5. TNM stages for carcinoma of the colon and rectum

Primary tumor

Tis   Carcinoma in situ and intramucosal (within lamina propria)

T1   Invades through muscularis mucosa into submucosa

T2   Invades muscularis propria

T3   Invades through muscularis propria into subserosa or nonperitonealized pericolic or perirectal tissues

T4   Invades adjacent organs or structures or perforates visceral peritoneum

Regional lymph nodes

N0   No node metastasis

N1   Metastasis in 1–3 regional nodes

N2   Metastasis in $\geq$ 4 regional nodes

N3   Metastasis along course of named vascular trunk or to apical (marked) node

Distant metastasis

M0   None

M1   Present

Stage Grouping

AJCC/UICC		Dukes
0	Tis, N0, M0	—
I	T1 or T2, N0, M0	A
II	T3 or T4, N0, M0	B
III	Any T, N1–3, M0	C
IV	Any T, any N, M1	—

Source: Modified from American Joint Committee on Cancer. In O. H. Beahrs et al. (eds.), *Manual for Staging of Cancer* (4th ed.). Philadelphia: Lippincott, 1992. P. 77.

surgery. Abdominal, chest, and pelvic CT may be helpful for preoperative assessment of extrabowel involvement and for postsurgical follow-up, but the findings may be falsely negative when small peritoneal implants are present. Bone scans are seldom needed except for assessment of bone pain, since bone metastases occur rather late in the course of the disease.

2. **Serum CEA** level may parallel disease activity, although it is not increased in all patients with colon cancer. It is worth measuring preoperatively and, if elevated, postoperatively, as failure of an elevated value to return to normal may signify incomplete removal of the tumor. Likewise, a serial rise in CEA values after an initial fall to normal often indicates recurrence. CEA values may also be an indicator of response during chemotherapy treatment, with a fall signifying improvement and a rise heralding regrowth of tumor. Patients who had a normal serum CEA level preoperatively may still demonstrate an elevated CEA value at the time of recurrence. A rising CEA is an indication for careful staging, with CT, and possibly laparoscopy, since some patients may have isolated, resectable, and thus potentially curable metastases.

B. **Treatment of advanced disease**
   1. **Effective agents and combinations.** For more than 30 years fluorouracil has been the standard agent in the treatment of advanced colorectal disease not amenable to surgical or radiotherapeutic control. Response rates have varied widely, but a generally agreed-on figure is 20%. Several institutions have reported rates of about 40% when fluorouracil was combined with semustine (methyl-CCNU) and, in some instances, vincristine and dacarbazine. However, when these combinations were tested by large cooperative groups, the reported improved response rates did not hold up and survival was not improved. Increased toxicity, particularly myelosuppression, was often observed.

   In recent years, several combinations of other agents with fluorouracil have been reported to have improved response rates and, in some instances, improved survival. They include leucovorin, methotrexate, interferon alpha, and cisplatin. The methotrexate–fluorouracil and leucovorin–fluorouracil combinations have been shown to be superior to fluorouracil alone in controlled trials. Although fluorouracil with a high-dose leucovorin regimen should be superior to a low-dose regimen on the basis of in vitro data, the current clinical data suggest that the low-dose regimen is superior in efficacy, toxicity, and expense; and it is similar in terms of survival. At present, the low-dose regimen is recommended. Moderate-dose methotrexate requiring leucovorin rescue combined with fluorouracil has produced excellent survival in our experience, but only when the fluorouracil and methotrexate are separated by a 24-hour interval (compared to 1 hour). The best of these regimens remains to be determined by controlled studies. Continuous infusion of fluorouracil for varying periods of time also is being evaluated but is not clearly superior to the bolus fluorouracil regimens with modulation. A promising regimen, with good primary activity, and some reasonable activity as a backup or secondary regimen, is the 24-hour weekly infusion of fluorouracil and leucovorin.

2. **Liver metastasis.** If the patient's disease is primarily in the liver, the response rate with IV fluorouracil alone is only about 10%. Intermittent hepatic artery infusion with fluorouracil, which is associated with a response rate of about 50%, should also be considered. Continuous infusion with floxuridine, either by continuous external infusion with permanent catheters or by an implanted or portable pump, has also been used, with response rates averaging 50%. The impact on survival is controversial.

3. **Recommended regimens**
   a. **Fluorouracil + leucovorin.** Leucovorin 20 mg/m^2, IV is followed in 1 hour by fluorouracil 425 mg/m^2 IV. The combination is given daily for 5 days. Courses are repeated at 4 and 8 weeks and at every 5 weeks thereafter.
   b. **Fluorouracil + methotrexate + leucovorin.** Methotrexate 200 mg/m^2 IV is given over 30 minutes after hydration with 1500 ml 5% dextrose in 0.5 N saline. At 24 hours fluorouracil 600 mg/m^2 IV bolus is given followed by leucovorin 10 mg/m^2 to the nearest 5 mg PO q6h × 6. Repeat every 2 weeks.
   c. **Fluorouracil + leucovorin by 24-hour continuous infusion.** Fluorouracil 2600 mg/m^2 and leucovorin 500 mg/m^2 are given concurrently by 24-hour continuous IV infusion weekly. The drugs are administered using two separate infusion pumps to avoid the catheters from being blocked by "stones." The fluorouracil dose is lowered to 2100 mg/m^2 for grade 3 hematologic or GI toxicity.
   d. **Hepatic artery infusion.** The catheter must be carefully positioned by an experienced angiographer through the axillary or femoral artery. A continuous IV heparin infusion of 5000 units/day is given with fluorouracil 800 mg/m^2/day for 4 days, then 600 mg/m^2 for a maximum of 17 days as tolerated. Weekly doses of 600 mg/m^2 IV can then be given to maintain whatever response has occurred, or the hepatic artery infusion can be repeated in the hospital in 4–6 months if the IV therapy does not prevent relapse. The position of the catheter must be checked twice weekly.
   For the implanted pump, the initial dose of

floxuridine is 0.2–0.3 mg/kg/day in heparinized saline given for 2 weeks, alternating with 2 weeks of heparinized saline without floxuridine. Heparin is used in a dose of 200 units/ml. Most patients can tolerate a daily floxuridine dose of 0.15–0.20 mg/kg for repeated cycles of 14 days every 4 weeks.

C. **Adjuvant chemotherapy**

1. **Colon cancer.** For many years surgical adjuvant studies with chemotherapy have shown either marginal benefit or no benefit, and such therapy could not be recommended routinely. The combination of fluorouracil and levamisole has been shown to significantly improve the disease-free as well as the overall survival of patients with node-positive (Dukes C) resectable colon cancer, but not yet those with stage B_2 disease. Although other chemotherapy regimens continue to be reported and appear to be of slight benefit, fluorouracil + levamisole serves as a current standard to which other regimens should be compared. A recently completed clinical trial, yet to be fully analyzed, compared fluorouracil + levamisole to fluorouracil with either high- or low-dose leucovorin (which regimens seem to be more active in advanced disease) or to a regimen with fluorouracil + levamisole + low-dose leucovorin. Although historical data support the use of postoperative radiotherapy for locally advanced colon cancer (Dukes B_3, or C_3 or any T4 lesion), there are as yet no controlled clinical trials that confirm its efficacy. The *recommended regimen* is as follows.

Fluorouracil 450 mg/m^2 IV bolus daily on days 1–5. At day 29, begin 450 mg/m^2 IV weekly × 48 weeks *and*
Levamisole 50 mg PO q8h × 3 days every 2 weeks starting day 1 for 1 year.

Information about the optimum duration of adjuvant therapy (i.e., 6 versus 12 months) should soon be available.

2. **Rectal cancer**

a. **Preoperative irradiation.** Several studies have shown that preoperative irradiation benefits patients with rectal cancer, although there are disadvantages in terms of accuracy of staging, delay before surgery, incomplete knowledge of the extent of tumor for treatment planning, and inappropriate administration of radiation to patients with early (Dukes A or B_1) or advanced (Dukes D) lesions. Accordingly, major attention has been given to trials of postoperative irradiation with and without chemotherapy.

b. **Postoperative irradiation, with and without chemotherapy.** A Gastrointestinal Tumor Study Group (GITSG) trial of Dukes B_2 and C rectal cancer showed that treatment with combined chemotherapy and radiotherapy is significantly better than no treatment after surgical resection in terms of recurrence or survival. Use of either modality alone was inferior to the combined-modality regimen. The chemotherapy used was a combination of semustine (methyl-CCNU) + fluorouracil for 18 months. The same group has observed similar results with a shorter fluorouracil regimen for 6 months, thereby avoiding the use of a drug that is not routinely available and that is associated with a small but significant risk of leukemia. Studies from other groups supported the concept of combined radiation and chemotherapy postoperatively. Variations on chemotherapy including leucovorin with or without levamisole added to fluorouracil are components of studies whose results should be available in the near future. At the present, the following regimen is recommended.

- **(1)** Radiotherapy 4320 cGy in 5 weeks *with* fluorouracil 500 mg/m^2 IV bolus on days 1, 2, and 3 and the last 3 days of radiotherapy, then
- **(2)** Fluorouracil 350 mg/m^2/day IV bolus daily for 5 days, beginning week 11. Repeat every 4 weeks, escalating the dose by 50 mg/m^2 as tolerated to a maximum of 500 mg/m^2 for a total of 6 courses.

D. Follow-up. In the asymptomatic patient, follow-up after treatment includes history and physical examination every 3 months for 3 years, then every 6 months for 2 years. CEA, complete blood cell count, examination of stool for occult blood, and liver function tests are appropriately done at the same intervals. Colonoscopy should be done annually for 3 years, and may then be decreased in frequency to every 3 years if no polyps are found. Annual chest x-ray studies are appropriate. CT of the abdomen, pelvis, or chest should probably not be done routinely except to evaluate symptoms or a rising CEA level, which can indicate recurrent but sometimes resectable disease.

E. Complications of therapy or disease. The complications of chemotherapy are those attributable to the individual drugs. Myelosuppression, nausea, vomiting, and diarrhea are common and may require dose modification and symptomatic treatment. Radiation complications are similar and also include dysuria, tenesmus, and rectal discharge of blood or mucus. Phenazopyridine (Pyridium) is a useful treatment for dysuria, and loperamide (Imodium) or diphenoxylate (Lomotil) is recommended for diarrhea. If toxicity is substantial (grade 3 or 4) during radiotherapy, a delay of at least a week is warranted. During chemotherapy with fluorouracil-based regimens, mild diarrhea (grade 1) may be treated symptomatically. Moderate diarrhea (grade 2 or 3) is an indication for dose reduction by 50%, and severe diarrhea (grade 3 or 4) for a break of a week or longer. Dehydration is a real risk with grade 3 or 4 diarrhea and IV hydration may be necessary. Octreotide 0.05–0.10 mg SQ tid may help to alleviate severe diarrhea. Oral mucositis often can be prevented on subsequent courses without dose reduction by holding ice in the mouth for 20 minutes before and after the IV bolus of fluorouracil. Nausea is usually less of a problem with fluorouracil regimens and usually responds to prochlorperazine or dexamethasone. Hematopoietic growth factors are seldom warranted for the mild neutropenia that is observed with bolus fluorouracil therapy.

F. Treatment of refractory disease. No satisfactory treatment exists for the patient who fails treatment with fluorouracil. Some patients with liver disease failing IV therapy may respond to fluorouracil or floxuridine given as a hepatic artery infusion. The combination cyclophosphamide + methotrexate + vincristine has produced some responses, but response rates are of the order of 10% and are usually brief. The regimen is as follows.

Cyclophosphamide 300 mg/m^2 IV weekly *and*
Vincristine 1.4 mg/m^2 IV weekly (maximum dose 2.0) *and*
Methotrexate 25 mg/m^2 IV weekly.

We also have occasionally seen responses with single-dose mitomycin 15–20 mg/m^2 IV every 6 weeks.

V. Cancer of the anal canal. These cancers, comprising only 1–3% of large-bowel cancers, were historically treated by abdominoperineal resection with an approximately 50% cure rate. They have been seen more commonly in women but, in recent years, have shown an increase in men, particularly homosexuals. The human papilloma virus has been implicated in such patients, and anal warts are sometimes seen as well. Human immunodeficiency virus (HIV)-infected patients also have an increased incidence of anal cancer.

A. Local disease. It has been found that combined-modality treatment with chemotherapy and irradiation is curative in 75–80% of patients and thus allows avoidance of abdominoperineal resection with retention of anal function. The following regimen is recommended.

Radiotherapy 4500 cGy in 25 fractions (5 weeks) *and concurrently*
Fluorouracil 1000 mg/m^2 by continuous IV infusion daily × 4 days (days 1–4 and 29–32) *and*
Mitomycin C 10 mg/m^2 IV on days 1 and 29.

Biopsy again 4 weeks after radiation therapy. If negative, no further treatment is needed. If positive, consider an additional 900 cGy (5 fractions) and 4-day course of fluorouracil 1000 mg/m^2 by continuous IV infusion on days 1–4 and cisplatin 100 mg/m^2 IV on day 2. If biopsy is persistently positive, perform abdominoperineal resection.

B. Metastatic disease. For metastatic disease the following regimen is recommended.
1. Mitomycin 10 mg/m^2 IV every 4 weeks × 2, then every 10 weeks *and*
2. Doxorubicin 30 mg/m^2 IV every 4 weeks × 2, then every 5 weeks *and*
3. Cisplatin 60 mg/m^2 IV, every 4 weeks × 2, then every 5 weeks.

Selected Readings

Ardalan, B., et al. A phase II study of weekly 24-hour infusion with high-dose fluorouracil with leucovorin in colorectal carcinoma. *J. Clin. Oncol.* 9:625, 1991.

Blot, W. J., et al. Rising incidence of adenocarcinoma of the esophagus and gastric cardia. *J.A.M.A.* 265:1287, 1991.

Cullinan, S. A., et al. A comparison of chemotherapeutic regimens in the treatment of advanced pancreatic and gastric carcinoma. *J.A.M.A.* 253:2061, 1985.

Flam, M. S., et al. Definitive combined modality therapy of carcinoma of the anus: a report of 30 cases including results of salvage therapy in patients with residual disease. *Dis. Colon Rectum* 30:495, 1987.

Forastiere, A. A., et al. Preoperative chemoradiation followed by esophagectomy for carcinoma of the esophagus: final report. *J. Clin. Oncol.* 11:1118, 1993.

Gastrointestinal Tumor Study Group (Holyoke, E. D., et al.). Adjuvant chemotherapy and radiotherapy following rectal surgery. *N. Engl. J. Med.* 312:1465, 1985.

Gisselbrecht, C., et al. Fluorouracil, adriamycin and cisplatin combination chemotherapy of advanced esophageal carcinoma. *Cancer* 52:974, 1983.

Kelsen, D., et al. FAMTX versus etoposide, doxorubicin and cisplatin: a random assignment trial in gastric cancer. *J. Clin. Oncol.* 10:541, 1992.

Leichman, L., et al. Cancer of the anal canal: model for preoperative adjuvant combined modality therapy. *Am. J. Med.* 78:211, 1985.

MacDonald, J. S., and Thomas, P. R. M. Therapy for locally advanced gastric cancer. *Adv. Oncol.* 8:17, 1992.

Marsh, J. C. Systemic therapy for gastric cancer. *Adv. Oncol.* 8:23, 1992.

Marsh, J. C., et al. The influence of drug interval on the effect of methotrexate and fluorouracil in the treatment of metastatic colorectal cancer. *J. Clin. Oncol.* 9:371, 1991.

Moertel, C. G., and Hanley, J. A. Combination chemotherapy trials for metastatic carcinoid tumor and the malignant carcinoid syndrome. *Cancer Clin. Trials* 2:327, 1979.

Moertel, C. G., et al. Levamisole and fluorouracil for adjuvant therapy of resected colon carcinoma. *N. Engl. J. Med.* 322:352, 1990.

Nomura, A., et al. *Helicobacter pylori* infection and gastric cancer among Japanese Americans in Hawaii. *N. Engl. J. Med.* 325:1132, 1991.

Poon, M. A., et al. Biochemical modulation of fluorouracil: evidence of significant improvement of survival and quality of life in patients with advanced colorectal carcinoma. *J. Clin. Oncol.* 7:1407, 1989.

Reed, M. I., et al. The practicality of chronic hepatic artery infusion therapy of primary and metastatic hepatic malignancies: ten-year results of 124 patients in a prospective protocol. *Cancer* 47:402, 1981.

Shepard, K., et al. Therapy for metastatic colorectal cancer with hepatic artery infusion chemotherapy using a subcutaneous implanted pump. *J. Clin. Oncol.* 3:161, 1985.

Sirott, M. N., et al. α-Interferon (INF), 5-fluorouracil (FU), and cisplatin (CDDP): an active regimen in advanced adenocarcinoma (ADENOCA) and squamous cell carcinoma (SCC) of the esophagus. *Proc. Am. Soc. Clin. Oncol.* 11:172, 1992.

Stewart, J. R., et al. Improved survival with neoadjuvant therapy and resection for adenocarcinoma of the esophagus. *Ann. Surg.* 218:571, 1993.

Wils, J. A., et al. Sequential high-dose methotrexate and fluorouracil combined with doxorubicin—a step ahead in the treatment of advanced gastric cancer: a trial of the European Organization for Research and Treatment of Cancer Gastrointestinal Tract Cooperative Group. *J. Clin. Oncol.* 9:827, 1991.

Wilke, H., et al. High dose folinic acid/etoposide/5-fluorouracil in advanced gastric cancer—a phase II study in elderly patients or patients with cardiac risk. *Invest. New Drugs* 8:65, 1990.

Willett, C. G., et al. Indications for adjuvant radiotherapy in extrapelvic colonic carcinoma. *Oncology* 3:25, 1989.

Carcinomas of the Pancreas, Liver, Gallbladder, and Bile Ducts

David J. Schifeling

Carcinomas of the pancreas, liver, and biliary passages account for approximately 2 percent of all cancers and 5 percent of all cancer-related deaths in the United States. Virtually all patients with these cancers die. However, recent advances in diagnostic techniques offer hope for early diagnosis and improved survival.

I. Adenocarcinoma of the pancreas

A. **Epidemiology and etiology.** Pancreatic cancer has occurred with increasing incidence over the last several decades and currently is the fifth leading cause of cancer-related death. Risk factors for pancreatic cancer include age, male sex, race (Polynesians, Blacks), and tobacco exposure. It is rare before age 30, and the incidence rises throughout life, with peak occurrence during the seventh decade. Smokers have 1.6–3.9 times the risk of developing pancreatic cancer compared to nonsmokers. Pancreatitis is commonly associated with carcinoma of the pancreas in pathologic specimens. Whether patients with chronic pancreatitis are at greater risk for developing pancreatic cancer is uncertain. Patients with familial pancreatitis appear to have a greater risk. Diabetes mellitus is often discovered just prior to the diagnosis of pancreatic cancer, but patients with diabetes mellitus do not have a greater risk of pancreatic cancer.

B. **Presenting signs and symptoms.** Pain is the most common presenting symptom. It occurs in three-fourths of patients with carcinoma of the head of the pancreas and virtually all patients with carcinoma of the body or tail. Usually the pain is a dull ache in the epigastrium that radiates to the right upper quadrant when the tumor is in the head of the pancreas or to the left upper quadrant when the tumor is in the body or tail. It may be an atypical sharp or intermittent epigastric pain, or it may be located in the lumbar region of the back. As many as one-fifth of patients present with nonspecific symptoms including weight loss, anorexia, nausea, vomiting, and constipation. Seventy percent of patients with carcinoma of the head of the pancreas have jaundice, whereas fewer than 15% of patients with carcinoma of the pancreatic body have jaundice. Physical findings are generally associated with advanced carcinomas and include weight loss, hepatomegaly, and abdominal mass.

C. **Diagnostic evaluation.** Ultrasonography and computed tomography (CT) demonstrate masses in the pancreas or dilatation of the pancreatic duct or the common bile duct. Sensitivity and specificity of CT are approximately 90%. Sensitivity and specificity of ultrasonography are somewhat less. Both tests are limited to detecting relatively large mass lesions of the pancreas and usually miss 1- to 2-cm carcinomas. Endoscopic retrograde cholangiopancreatography (ERCP) demonstrates subtle ductal abnormalities; sensitivity and specificity are in excess of 90%. Endoscopy-directed biopsies of pancreatic ducts have diagnosed tumors less than 1–2 cm in diameter. Percutaneous transhepatic cholangiography may be performed if ERCP is unsuccessful and yields similar information. Percutaneous fine needle aspiration of suspicious abnormalities identified on CT scan can confirm the diagnosis of pancreatic cancer, with 80–90% sensitivity and 100% specificity.

D. Laboratory tests. CA 19-9 is a cell surface glycoprotein associated with pancreatic cancer. Elevated serum levels raise the index of suspicion of pancreatic cancer in patients with a suggestive history. Rising serum levels are a useful early indicator of recurrent disease.

E. Staging and preoperative evaluation

   1. **Staging.** The primary tumor, regional lymph nodes, and potential sites of metastatic disease must be carefully assessed (Table 14-1). CT of the abdomen assesses the primary site, regional lymph nodes, and liver. Chest x-ray screens for metastatic disease in the chest. Routine laboratory studies and physical examination screen for other sites of involvement.

   2. **Preoperative evaluation.** Preoperative evaluation should be performed stepwise from least invasive to most invasive as indicated by the clinical situation. Preoperative evaluation can be stopped when metastatic disease or definite evidence for unresectable local-regional spread is identified. All patients undergo CT. If no hepatic metastasis or major blood vessel involvement is identified, then arteriography should be performed to further assess major blood vessel involvement and tumor blood supply. If no major blood vessel involvement is identified, then laparoscopy should be used to identify small metastases in the liver or peritoneum. Laparoscopy identifies metastatic disease in 40% of patients with pancreatic cancer who have had negative findings on CT and arteriogram. In one series nearly 80% of cancers

Table 14-1. Staging pancreatic cancer

Stage I	T1a (tumor ≤ 2 cm), T1b (tumor > 2 cm, confined to pancreas), or T2 (tumor extends to duodenum, bile duct, or peripancreatic tissue), N0, M0
Stage II	T3 (tumor extends to stomach, spleen, colon, or adjacent large vessels), N0, M0
Stage III	Any T, N1, M0
Stage IV	Any T, N, M1

N1 = any nodal metastases; M1 = any distant metastases.

were resectable when all tests including laparoscopy showed negative results. Whereas after CT and arteriography, only 15–20% of pancreas cancers are found to be resectable at laparotomy.

F. Primary therapy

1. **Surgery.** Three-fourths of patients with pancreatic cancer are operative candidates, but only 15–20% have resectable tumors. Patients without evident metastatic cancer or major blood vessel involvement whose performance status permits operative interventions are candidates for curative surgery. Of the patients whose tumors are resected for cure, 5–10% survive 5 years. Obstructive jaundice and gastric outlet obstruction may be palliated by bypass procedures.

2. **Radiation therapy.** External beam radiation therapy has been used to palliate unresectable carcinomas. It also may be used as a surgical adjuvant in combination with chemotherapy. Great care and expertise must be exercised to plan radiation fields. These fields must encompass known disease without excessive involvement of adjacent normal tissue. If a laparotomy or laparoscopy is performed, surgical clips can be placed to accurately guide treatment.

3. **Combined-modality therapy**
   a. **Resected carcinomas.** On the basis of a randomized study by the Gastrointestinal Tumor Study Group (GITSG), postoperative combined-modality therapy is recommended for patients with resected carcinoma of the pancreas. The GITSG demonstrated that postoperative adjuvant radiotherapy (split course in their study) plus fluorouracil is better than adjuvant radiotherapy alone. On the basis of the demonstrated benefit of prolonged infusion of fluorouracil or fluorouracil modulated by leucovorin in colon and rectal carcinomas, both of these approaches have been safely combined with radiotherapy (40–50 Gy in standard fractionation) in pancreatic cancer. The recommended treatments have the advantage of avoiding split-course radiotherapy. Recommended regimens are as follows.

   (1) Fluorouracil 225 mg/m^2 by continuous IV infusion throughout radiation or 300 mg/m^2 by continuous IV infusion 5 days per week during radiation therapy *or*

   (2) Fluorouracil 425 mg/m^2 by IV push 1 hour following leucovorin 20 mg/m^2 by IV push daily for 4 days during the first week of radiation therapy and for 3 days during the fifth week of radiation therapy *or*

   (3) Fluorouracil 500 mg/m^2 by IV push midway during a 2-hour infusion of leucovorin 500 mg/m^2 weekly for the first 6 weeks of radiation therapy.

At the completion of combined-modality therapy, chemotherapy should be continued for 6 months using weekly IV push fluorouracil or a modulated fluorouracil regimen. Two-year and 5-year survival rates similar to the 43% and 25% rates seen in the combined-modality groups in the GITSG trials may be anticipated, though this has not yet been adequately tested.

b. Localized unresectable carcinoma. A series of randomized trials conducted by the GITSG demonstrated superior survival of patients with localized but unresectable pancreatic cancer when treated with combined-modality therapy compared to patients treated with radiation or chemotherapy alone. These clinical trials also used split-course radiation therapy. As discussed in sec. **F.3.a.,** current clinical trials do not support a specific combined-modality treatment program. However, 60 Gy of radiation should be delivered in a single course of external beam radiation to gross tumor and 40–50 Gy to microscopic cancer. Chemotherapy may be given by any of the regimens noted in sec. **F.3.a.** After completion of combined-modality therapy, chemotherapy should be continued for 6 months using bolus fluorouracil or a modulated fluorouracil regimen. In the GITSG trials the median survival time was 10 months in the combined-modality group compared with 5 months in the radiation-alone group. Specialized modes of administration of the radiation therapy, including intraoperative radiotherapy to boost the dose to the gross tumor or conformational radiation therapy to minimize the dose to surrounding tissues while delivering maximum dose to the tumor, may be considered. Quality-of-life studies have not been reported.

G. Chemotherapy of advanced disease. Patients with pancreatic cancer are often poor candidates for chemotherapy because of severe weight loss, poor performance status, severe pain, lack of measurable or evaluable disease, and the presence of jaundice or hepatic involvement, which may interfere with clearance of therapeutic agents.

1. Single agents. A number of single agents have demonstrated activity (Table 14-2). Most active are fluorouracil and mitomycin, with 20–30% response rates. Many other agents have been evaluated with disappointing activity. Ifosfamide has a response rate of 10–25% in various studies.

2. Combination chemotherapy. Combination chemotherapy has been intensively investigated (Table 14-3). The most commonly used regimens have been fluorouracil + doxorubicin + mitomycin (FAM) and streptozocin + mitomycin + fluorouracil (SMF) with response rates reported between 13 and 43%. A

Table 14-2. Single-agent chemotherapy in pancreatic cancer

Drug	No. of patients	Response rate ± 95% confidence interval (%)
Fluorouracil	251	25 ± 3
Mitomycin	53	21 ± 6
Streptozocin	27	11 ± 6
Semustine (methyl-CCNU)	91	4 ± 2
Doxorubicin	28	7 ± 5
Ifosfamide	113	22

Table 14-3. Combination chemotherapy of carcinoma of exocrine pancreas

Regimens	Dosages
SMF	Streptozocin, 1 gm/m^2 IV on days 1, 8, 29, and 36
	Mitomycin 10 mg/m^2 IV on day 1
	Fluorouracil 600 mg/m^2 IV on days 1, 8, 29, and 36
	Repeat cycle every 8 weeks
FAM	Fluorouracil 600 mg/m^2 IV on days 1, 8, 29, and 36
	Doxorubicin (Adriamycin) 30 mg/m^2 IV on days 1 and 29
	Mitomycin 10 mg/m^2 IV on day 1
	Repeat cycle every 8 weeks

variety of other combination regimens have been investigated, but none has shown advantage over fluorouracil alone.

3. **Current recommendations.** Single-agent therapy with fluorouracil 500 mg/m^2 IV on days 1–5 every 4 weeks or 500–600 mg/m^2 IV weekly is recommended for patients with disseminated pancreatic cancer and an Eastern Cooperative Oncology Group (ECOG) performance status of 0–2, who are not eligible for clinical trials. If the tumor does not respond to the fluorouracil or there is progression following the initial response, the patient could then be treated with mitomycin 20 mg/m^2 IV on day 1 every 4–6 weeks. Because of limited effectiveness of current therapy, participation in clinical trials should be encouraged, particularly with phase II trials of new agents or combinations.

II. **Malignant islet cell carcinomas**

A. **Epidemiology and natural history.** Islet cell neoplasms occur in approximately 1 in 100,000 persons per year. Eighty percent of these tumors secrete one or more hormones excessively: most commonly insulin or gastrin; less commonly glucagon, serotonin, or adrenocorticotropic hormone (ACTH); and rarely vasoactive intestinal peptides (VIP), growth hormone-releasing hormone (GHRH), and somatostatin. Twenty percent are nonfunctional. Islet cell tumors may occur with the multiple endocrine neoplasia (MEN-I) syndrome. In families with this autosomal dominant syndrome, 80% of affected members develop islet cell tumors, most commonly gastrinoma (54%), insulinoma (21%), glucagonoma (3%), or VIPoma (1%). Other endocrine manifestations of MEN-I include parathyroid hyperplasia, pituitary adenomas (often a prolactinoma), and occasionally adrenal or thyroid adenomas. Approximately one-fourth of gastrinomas are associated with MEN-I. Eighty to ninety percent of gastrinomas occur in the head of the pancreas. Insulinomas are common equally in the head, body, and tail. Gastrinomas tend to be multiple small tumors, whereas insulinomas tend to be single tumors and glucagonomas and VIPomas single large tumors. The median age of patients is in the sixth decade. There are no sex or race associations.

Islet cell tumors generally present with symptoms caused by hormone hypersecretion, most commonly fasting hypoglycemia, or the Zollinger-Ellison syndrome followed by others. VIPomas are associated with episodic severe secretory diarrhea with hypokalemia, hypochlorhydria, and metabolic acidosis. Classically, glucagonomas are associated with necrolytic migratory erythema, mild diabetes, severe muscle wasting, and marked hyperaminoaciduria.

Sixty percent of gastrinomas are malignant. Histologic appearance and tumor size do not predict malignancy; only the presence of metastatic disease confirms malignancy. Ninety percent of malignant gastrinomas have liver metastases. Other sites of spread include abdominal nodes, peritoneum, bone, and lung. Median survival from time of diagnosis of metastatic disease is approximately 2.5 years. Only 10% of insulinomas are malignant. They are usually larger than 2.5 cm, whereas benign insulinomas are generally smaller than 2.5 cm. Most glucagonomas and VIPomas are malignant (60–80%).

B. **Treatment of advanced disease**
  1. **Endocrine syndromes.** The first goal of treatment must be to control endocrine syndromes.
     a. **Gastric acid suppression.** The H^+-K^+-ATPase inhibitor omeprazole successfully controls gastric acid secretion in virtually all patients with gastrinoma. The optimal dose must be individualized and periodically reevaluated. Gastric acid secretion in the hour preceding the next dose of omeprazole should be < 10 mEq in patients who have had no previous gastric surgery and < 5 mEq in those who have had an acid-reducing procedure.

The starting dose is 60 mg/day. Doses greater than 80 mg/day should be divided. H_2 blockers are also effective, especially famotidine.

b. Insulin suppression. Diazoxide 3–8 mg/kg/day PO divided in 3 doses (e.g., 50–150 mg PO tid) is the therapy of choice for hypoglycemia associated with insulinoma when dietary measures fail. A diuretic should be given with diazoxide to prevent water retention.

c. Octreotide acetate (Sandostatin). Octreotide acetate is a somatostatin analog that inhibits gut hormone secretion. It is generally useful for carcinoid and VIPoma syndromes and is possibly useful for controlling symptoms in patients with glucagonomas, GHRH tumors, and gastrinomas. In patients with unresectable insulinoma, it can reduce insulin secretion by 50% and return blood glucose levels to normal. However, it must be initiated cautiously with the patient in the hospital, because profound hypoglycemia may occur. The usual starting dose of octreotide is 50 μg SQ bid; thereafter the dose and frequency of injections can be increased to 100 μg tid.

2. Chemotherapy of advanced islet cell tumors. Streptozocin is the most active single agent with a 50% response rate. It is a nonmyelosuppressive nitrosourea with diabetogenic effects in animals. Doxorubicin is also an active agent. The combination of streptozocin and doxorubicin was demonstrated to have a superior response rate (69%), time to tumor progression (20 months), and survival time (2.2 years), than the combination of streptozocin and flurouracil or single-agent chlorozotocin in a recent North Central Cancer Treatment Group (NCCTG) study. This combination is recommended as first-line chemotherapy.

a. Streptozocin 500 mg/m² IV on days 1–5 + doxorubicin 50 mg/m² IV on days 1 and 22. Repeat every 6 weeks.

Renal impairment occurs in approximately 30% of patients receiving a streptozocin-based regimen; approximately one-third of those with renal insufficiency have creatinine levels higher than 2 mg/dl. Nausea and vomiting occur in approximately 60% of patients. Leukopenia occurs in approximately 75%, but only 10% have a white blood cell count of less than 1000/μl. Stomatitis is uncommon. Liver function test abnormalities may also occur. Deaths caused by treatment are rare.

b. Interferon may diminish excess hormone secretion and induce shrinkage of tumors; some trials have reported 50% response rates. This agent can be used after chemotherapy failure.

III. Ampullary carcinomas. In up to 80% of people, the common bile duct and main pancreatic duct empty into a common channel, the ampulla of Vater. Periampullary carcinomas can be classified according to their site of origin. Type I tumors originate in the ampulla of Vater or the duodenal portion of the common bile duct. Type II carcinomas are duodenal tumors involving the ampulla of Vater. Type III are mixed ampullary-periampullary carcinomas, and type IV are pancreatic head carcinomas involving the ampulla. Type IV tumors carry a much worse prognosis and should be distinguished from the ampullary or periampullary carcinomas. Type I–III periampullary and ampullary carcinomas generally can be extirpated surgically. Large tumors require a Whipple resection, whereas local excision may be curative for small tumors. The overall 5-year survival rate is 40–50% for types I–III. The roles of irradiation and chemotherapy are uncertain. Tumors larger than 2 cm in diameter should be treated as adenocarcinoma of the pancreas.

IV. Carcinoma of bile ducts (cholangiocarcinoma)

A. Epidemiology and natural history. The incidence of primary biliary tree carcinoma is approximately 2 per 100,000. Men are affected more commonly than women. Tumors occur most often in late-middle-aged or elderly patients. They are associated with cholelithiasis, ulcerative colitis, obesity, liver flukes, and exposure to thorium oxide (Thorotrast). Patients present with obstructive jaundice, except for the occasional patient with a carcinoma identified at laparotomy for cholelithiasis. Approximately one-half of bile duct tumors are located proximally. Ten percent have multicentric involvement of the bile ducts. Local invasion is common. Liver involvement occurs in nearly one-half of these patients. Surgical cure is uncommon. Bypass procedures or intubation of the biliary tree may offer palliation to patients whose tumors cannot be resected. Radiation therapy may relieve proximal obstruction without intubation or a bypass procedure.

B. Chemotherapy of advanced disease. Few reports are available for this unusual tumor, but its response rate to fluorouracil, alone or in combination with streptozocin, is about 10%. Outside the context of a clinical trial one of the following is recommended.

1. Fluorouracil 500 mg/m^2 IV push on days 1–5 every 4 weeks *or* 500 mg/m^2 IV weekly *or*

2. Fluorouracil 400 mg/m^2 IV on days 1–5 *and* streptozocin 500 mg/m^2 IV on days 1–5. Repeat every 6 weeks.

V. Gallbladder carcinoma

A. Epidemiology and natural history. Carcinomas of the gallbladder are seen predominantly in late-middle-aged or elderly women, with the highest incidence in American Indians and the population of central and eastern Europe and Israel. These areas of high frequency also report a high incidence of cholelithiasis. Patients with "porcelain" or calcified gallbladders on x-ray film have a 12–62% risk of cancer. Carcinoma of the gallbladder most commonly presents with pain, nausea and vomiting, and weight loss. Jaundice occurs in only one-third of patients. Anorexia, abdominal distension, pruritus, and melena occur in some patients. One percent of patients undergoing cholecystectomy are found to have carcinoma of the gallbladder. Overall survival is poor, since less than 5% of patients with resections survive 5 years. However, if the tumor is histologically confined to the mucosa or submucosa, survival rates of 64% at 5 years and 44% at 10 years have been reported. Gallbladder carcinomas may invade locally into the bile ducts, liver, pancreas, stomach, or duodenum. They also may spread to regional lymph nodes and distantly to liver.

B. **Chemotherapy of advanced disease.** Few reports are available for review. Seven (18%) of 40 patients responded to 5-fluorouracil (5-FU). Seven (28%) of 25 patients responded to mitomycin. Four (31%) of 14 patients treated with 5-FU + doxorubicin (Adriamycin) + mitomycin responded. Choices of therapy are as follows.

1. Fluorouracil 500 mg/m^2 IV on days 1–5 every 4 weeks or 500–600 mg/m^2 IV weekly or
2. FAM, a three-drug combination of fluorouracil 600 mg/m^2 IV on days 1, 8, 29, and 36 and doxorubicin 30 mg/m^2 IV on days 1 and 29 and mitomycin 10 mg/m^2 IV on day 1. Repeat every 8 weeks.

Although there may be a slightly improved response rate with FAM, the toxicity is significant and no survival or quality-of-life benefit has been demonstrated.

VI. **Primary carcinoma of the liver**
A. **Epidemiology.** Primary carcinoma of the liver is rare in the United States. There are fewer than 10,000 new patients annually, accounting for less than 2% of all malignancies. However, it is the leading cause of cancer death in parts of Africa and Asia. Ninety percent of primary carcinomas of the liver are hepatocellular carcinomas or hepatoma; the remaining carcinomas include cholangiocarcinomas (about 7%), hepatoblastomas, angiosarcomas, and other sarcomas. Histologic subsets of hepatocellular carcinoma have been recognized. Fibrolamellar carcinomas occur in young patients and are more likely to be resectable and cured. Hepatocellular carcinomas are more common in men than women. The peak occurrence is during the sixth decade, with the highest incidence during the ninth decade.

There appear to be three major factors associated with hepatocellular carcinoma: (1) viral hepatitis B and C; (2) alcohol abuse; and (3) aflatoxin exposure. Seventy-five percent of patients with hepatocellular carcinoma have concomitant cirrhosis, and 4–20% of patients with cirrhosis have hepatocellular carcinoma at autopsy depending on the population studied. Among the patients with hepatocellular carcinoma, 15–80% have hepatitis B surface antigenemia. In China the incidence of hepatocellular carcinoma parallels the incidence of hepatitis B infection. The introduction of an effective hepatitis B vaccine may reduce the risk of hepatocellular carcinoma in these areas. In Africa the increased risk appears to be related to exposure to aflatoxin, which is produced by the fungi *Aspergillus flavus* and *Aspergillus parasiticus* during improper food storage. Three to 27% of patients with long-standing hemochromatosis develop hepatocellular carcinoma. Anabolic steroids also have been associated with hepatocellular carcinoma. These tumors may retain hormone dependence and regress after withdrawal of the steroid.

B. **Presentation.** Patients with primary carcinoma of the liver commonly complain of right upper quadrant pain, abdominal distension, or weight loss. The pain is usually dull or aching but may be acute and radiate to the right shoulder. Fatigue, loss of appetite, and unexplained fever may occur. Patients with underlying cirrhosis may present with hepatic decompensation: new ascites, variceal bleeding, jaundice, or encephalopathy. Rarely, patients present with paraneoplastic syndromes: Erythrocytosis is most common; hypercalcemia, hyperthyroidism, and carcinoid syndrome have been described. Physical findings include nodular hepatomegaly with an arterial bruit and hepatic rub. Extrahepatic spread occurs in approximately 50% of patients during the course of the illness. Twenty percent of patients have lung metastases.

C. **Diagnostic evaluation and screening.** Alpha-fetoprotein levels are elevated in 70% of patients and associated with a poor prognosis. Ultrasonography and CT have a high sensitivity when lesions are larger than 2 cm; however, small lesions are frequently missed. Magnetic resonance imaging is generally equivalent to CT but at a greater cost. Fine needle aspiration with cytology or biopsy usually confirms the diagnosis. Serial alpha-fetoprotein measurements every 3–4 months and liver ultrasound every 4–6 months should be considered in high-risk individuals with hepatitis B antigenemia, or hepatitis C and cirrhosis. Patients with hepatitis C without cirrhosis and patients with hemochromatosis should be considered for less intense screening.

D. **Staging** (Table 14-4). Staging procedures should include a chest x-ray, CT of the abdomen, a complete blood cell count, a blood chemistry profile, and an alpha-fetoprotein measurement. If these do not disclose unresectable cancer or sites of metastatic cancer, then CT of the chest and arteriogram (upper abdominal and hepatic) should be performed to guide surgical intervention and further screening for extrahepatic involvement.

E. **Primary therapy.** At presentation 25% of patients with hepatocellular carcinoma have potentially resectable lesions. At laparotomy, only 10–12% are resected. Operative mortality is 10–30%. Cirrhosis and advanced lesions are the factors limiting resection. Long-term survival is achieved in 15–30% of patients whose tumors are resected. Recurrences appear in liver, regional lymph nodes, lungs, and bone.

F. **Therapy of advanced hepatocellular carcinoma**
   1. **Single agents.** Numerous single agents have been tested in primary hepatocellular carcinoma: Alkyl-

Table 14-4. Staging hepatocellular cancer

Stage I	T1 (solitary tumor ≤ 2 cm, without vascular invasion), N0, M0
Stage II	T2 (solitary tumor ≤ 2 cm with vascular invasion; or multiple tumors in the same lobe which are all ≤ 2 cm and without vascular invasion; or a solitary tumor > 2 cm without vascular invasion), N0, M0
Stage III	T3 (solitary tumor > 2 cm with vascular invasion; or multiple tumors in the same lobe which are all ≤ 2 cm with vascular invasion; or multiple tumors any of which are > 2 cm in the same lobe with or without vascular invasion), N1 (regional nodes involved), M0
Stage IVA	T4 (multiple tumors involving more than one lobe or a major branch of the portal or hepatic veins), N0, M0
Stage IVB	Any T, any N, M1

ating agents, antimetabolites, plant alkaloids, and cisplatin have been ineffective. Doxorubicin 60 mg/m^2 IV every 21 days is recommended. This regimen results in a partial response rate of about 16%.

2. **Combination chemotherapy and other modes of treatment.** Combination chemotherapy has not had better success than single agents. Hepatic artery infusion has been studied, and appears to have an increased response rate compared to IV chemotherapy. To date, no survival advantage has been proved for intraarterial therapy. Similarly chemoembolization has been employed, with high response rates but uncertain survival advantage. Immunotherapy has not shown promise in hepatocellular carcinoma. Irradiation has had a limited role in treating liver tumors because of hepatic intolerance to radiation.

Selected Readings

Andrews, W. B., and Smith, F. P. Chemotherapy for cholangiocarcinoma and gallbladder cancer. *Sci. Pract. Surg.* 8:453, 1987.

Evans, D. B., et al. Preoperative chemoradiation and pancreaticoduodenectomy for adenocarcinoma of the pancreas. *Arch. Surg.* 127:1335, 1992.

Gastrointestinal Tumor Study Group. Further evidence of effective adjuvant combined radiation and chemotherapy following curative resection of pancreatic cancer. *Cancer* 59: 2006, 1987.

Kalser, M. H., and Ellenberg, S. S. Pancreatic cancer: adjuvant combined radiation and chemotherapy following curative resection. *Arch. Surg.* 120:899, 1985.

McMahon, B. J., and London, T. Workshop on screening for hepatocellular carcinoma. *J. Natl. Cancer Inst.* 83:916, 1991.

Moertel, C. G., et al. Early evaluation of combined fluorouracil and leucovorin as a radiation enhancer for locally unresectable, residual, or recurrent gastrointestinal carcinoma. *J. Clin. Oncol.* 12:21, 1994.

Moertel, C. G., Hahn, R. G., and O'Connell, M. S. Therapy of locally unresectable pancreatic carcinoma: a randomized comparison of high dose (6000 rads) radiation alone, moderate dose radiation (4000 rads + 5-fluorouracil), and high dose radiation + 5-fluorouracil: Gastrointestinal Tumor Study Group. *Cancer* 48:1705, 1981.

Moertel, C. G., et al. Streptozocin-doxorubicin, streptozocin-fluorouracil, or chlorozotocin in the treatment of advanced islet-cell carcinoma. *N. Engl. J. Med.* 326:519, 1992.

Schifeling, D. J., et al. Radiation therapy and 5-fluorouracil modulated by leucovorin for adenocarcinoma of the pancreas. *Int. J. Pancreatol.* 12:239, 1992.

Shutze, W. P., Sack, J., and Aldrete, J. S. Long-term follow-up of 24 patients undergoing radical resection for ampullary carcinoma, 1953 to 1988. *Cancer* 66:1717, 1990.

Tsukuma, H., et al. Risk factors for hepatocellular carcinoma among patients with chronic liver disease. *N. Engl. J. Med.* 328:1797, 1993.

Warshaw, A. L., and Castillo, C. F. Pancreatic carcinoma. *N. Engl. J. Med.* 326:455, 1992.

Warshaw, A. L., et al. Preoperative staging and assessment of resectability of pancreatic cancer. *Arch. Surg.* 125:230, 1990.

Wynick, D., and Bloom, S. R. Clinical review 23: the use of the long-acting somatostatin analog octreotide in the treatment of gut neuroendocrine tumors. *J. Clin. Endocrinol. Metab.* 73:1, 1991.

Carcinoma of the Breast

Roland T. Skeel

I. Natural history, evaluation, and modes of treatment

A. Epidemiology and etiology. Carcinoma of the breast gave way to carcinoma of the lung as the most common cause of cancer deaths among women in the United States in 1986. Nonetheless, in 1994 more than 182,000 new cases of breast cancer were diagnosed, and there were approximately 46,000 deaths. The incidence of breast cancer varies widely among different populations. Women in western Europe and the United States have a higher incidence than women in most other parts of the world, possibly in part because of the high intake of animal protein and fat. Although discrete causes of breast cancer are not known, many factors increase a woman's risk for developing the disease. Among the strongest of the risk factors is family history, particularly if more than one family member has developed breast cancer at an early age. Genetic linkage analysis has shown a germ-line mutation in a gene (*BRCA-1*) localized to chromosome 17. Although this mutation accounts for < 5% of all breast cancers, carriers may face an 85% lifetime risk of breast cancer. Other factors that increase the risk are early menarche, late age at first birth, and prior benign breast disease (particularly if there is a high degree of benign epithelial atypia). Prior or present use of birth control pills appears to play little or no role in the risk for developing breast cancer. Although breast cancer may occur among men, such cases represent fewer than 1% of all breast cancers and is uncommonly seen in most hospitals.

B. Detection, diagnosis, and pretreatment evaluation

   1. Screening. Because more lives can be saved if breast cancer is diagnosed at an early stage, many programs have been designed to detect small, early cancers. Monthly breast self-examination for all women after puberty and yearly breast examinations by a physician or other trained professional after age 30 are recommended. Mammography, when done on a regular basis, can reduce mortality due to breast cancer by 30% in women ≥ 50 years old. The benefit for women age 40–50 (or > 65) is less certain. It is recommended at age 40 as a baseline, once every 1–2 years (depending on risk factors) between the ages of 40 and 50, and yearly after age 50. Although each method can be of some help in detecting early lesions that can be successfully removed before metastasis has occurred, mammography is capable of detecting the smallest and therefore the most curable lesions. Thus despite the high cost of screening mammography ($75–$140 in many areas of the United States), it is highly recommended that the above guidelines be followed. As an incentive to patients to follow these recommendations, physicians may inform patients that lesions amenable to tumorectomy (followed by irradiation) are more likely to be found, avoiding the necessity for mastectomy.

2. **Presenting signs and symptoms.** Although increasing numbers of nonpalpable cancers are being found by mammography, breast cancer is still most often discovered by a woman herself as an isolated, painless lump in the breast. If the mass has gone unnoticed or ignored for a time, there may be fixation to the skin or underlying chest wall, ulceration, pain, or inflammation. Some early lesions present with discharge or bleeding from the nipple. At times the primary lesion is not discovered, and the woman presents with symptoms of metastatic disease, e.g., pleural effusion, nodal disease, or bony metastases. About one-half of all lesions are in the upper outer quadrant of the breast (where most of the glandular tissue of the breast is). About 20% are central masses, and 10% are in each of the other quadrants. One-half of all women with breast cancer have axillary node metastasis unless the primary tumor has been detected by screening mammography or other screening method.

3. **Staging.** Carcinoma of the breast is staged according to the size and characteristics of the primary tumor (T), the involvement of regional lymph nodes (N), and the presence of metastatic disease (M). An abridged version of the commonly used TNM classification of breast cancer is shown in Table 15-1, and the stage grouping is outlined in Table 15-2. Although preliminary staging is commonly done prior to surgery, definitive staging that can be used for prognostic and further treatment planning purposes usually must await postsurgical pathologic evaluation when the primary tumor size and the histologic involvement of the lymph nodes are established. It is important to note that in 30% of patients with palpable breast masses, but without clinical evidence of axillary lymph node involvement, the histologic evaluation reveals cancer; and in a somewhat smaller number, nodes that clinically appear positive contain no cancer when examined histologically.

4. **Diagnostic evaluation**
   a. **Prior to biopsy** the woman should have a careful **history,** during which attention should be paid to *risk factors,* and a **physical examination,** with a focus not only on the involved breast but also on the opposite breast, all regional lymph node areas, the lungs, bone, and liver. This examination should be followed by bilateral mammography to help assess the extent of involvement and to look for additional ipsilateral or contralateral disease.
   b. **Excisional biopsy** of the primary lesion is performed, and the specimen is given intact (not in

Table 15-1. Abridged TNM classification of breast cancer

Stage	Description
Primary tumor (T)	
Tis	Carcinoma in situ: intraductal carcinoma, lobular carcinoma in situ, or Paget's disease of the nipple with no tumor
T1	Tumor $\leq$ 2 cm
T1a	$\leq$ 0.5 cm
T1b	> 0.5 to $\leq$ 1.0 cm
T1c	> 1.0 to $\leq$ 2.0 cm
T2	Tumor > 2.0 to $\leq$ 5 cm
T3	Tumor > 5 cm
T4	Any size with extension to chest wall or skin. Chest wall includes ribs, intercostal muscles, and serratus anterior muscle, but not pectoral muscles
T4a	Extension to chest wall
T4b	Edema, skin ulceration, or satellite skin nodules confined to same breast
T4c	Both (T4a and T4b) criteria
T4d	Inflammatory carcinoma
Nodal involvement (N)—pathologic	
pN0	No regional lymph node metastasis
pN1	Metastasis to movable ipsilateral axillary nodes
pN1a	Only micrometastasis ($\leq$ 0.2 cm) (prognosis of patients with pN1a similar to that of patients with pN0)
pN1b	Macrometastasis (> 0.2 cm)
i	To 1–3 nodes, any > 0.2 cm, all < 2.0 cm
ii	To 4 or more nodes, any > 0.2 cm, all < 2.0 cm
iii	Extension of tumor (< 2.0 cm) beyond capsule of node
iv	Any metastatic focus $\geq$ 2.0 cm
pN2	Fixed metastasis to ipsilateral axillary nodes
pN3	Metastasis to ipsilateral internal mammary nodes
Distant metastasis (M)	
M0	None known
M1	Metastases present, including to ipsilateral supraclavicular lymph nodes

Table 15-2. Stage grouping of breast cancer

Stage	T	N	M
0	Tis	N0	M0
I	T1	N0	M0
IIA	T0, T1	N1	M0
	T2	N0	M0
IIB	T2	N1	M0
	T3	N0	M0
IIIA	T0–2	N2	M0
	T3	N1, N2	M0
IIIB	T4	Any N	M0
	Any T	N3	M0
IV	Any T	Any N	M1

Note: Patients are staged in the highest group possible for their composite TNM. For example, a patient with T1a, N2, M0 would be a stage IIIA because of the N2 status.

formalin) to the pathologist, who can divide the specimen for histologic examination, hormone receptor assays, flow cytometric measurements of ploidy and the percent of cells in the S phase, or other tests.

  c. After confirmation of the histology, the patient is evaluated for possible metastatic disease.

    (1) Mandatory studies include a chest x-ray film, complete blood count, blood chemistry profile, and estrogen and progesterone receptor assays on the primary breast carcinoma and grossly cancerous nodal tissues.

    (2) Other studies, including radionuclide scan of the bones, skeletal survey (usually obtained only if the radionuclide scan is positive), and computed tomography (CT) scan of the liver (abdomen) are optional unless the history, physical examination, or blood studies suggest a poor prognosis or point to specific organ involvement. A carcinoembryonic antigen (CEA) assay is also often performed. Additional studies that may impart clinically useful prognostic information include evaluation of the ploidy of the malignant cells, their DNA synthesis rate (percent in S phase), and the content of other markers such as cathepsin D and the c-*erbB-2 (HER-2)* oncogene and its protein product.

5. Histology. About 75–80% of all breast cancers are infiltrating ductal carcinomas, and 10% are infiltrating lobular carcinomas; these two types have similar biologic behavior. The remainder of the histologic types of invasive breast carcinoma may have

a somewhat better prognosis but are usually managed more according to the stage than to the histologic type.

C. Approach to therapy

1. **Surgery** has been and remains the most frequently
utilized mode of primary therapy for most women
with carcinoma of the breast. The role of surgery in
the primary management of carcinoma of the breast
has been evolving with a trend to lesser surgery, e.g.,
wide local excision, together with axillary dissection.
This step is then followed by radiotherapy to control
the microscopic cancer remaining in the breast.

   For most women this therapy yields therapeutic
results just as good as mastectomy without the need
for amputating the breast and its attendant physical
deformity and psychological trauma. These therapeutic changes notwithstanding, the operation that
is still most commonly performed is some version
of the modified radical mastectomy in which the
breast, pectoralis fascia (with or without the pectoralis minor muscle), and lymph nodes are removed.
There are wide geographic variations in the use of
breast-conserving surgery throughout the United
States. For most women operations more extensive
than the modified radical mastectomy are probably
of no benefit, and lesser operations, unless combined
with radiotherapy, are insufficient in terms of providing important prognostic information regarding
the status of the axillary lymph nodes and controlling the local disease (40% of women treated with excisional biopsy alone have recurrence in the ipsilateral breast).

   For patients who have had mastectomy, reconstruction is being done with increasing frequency. It
may be done at the time of mastectomy or delayed
for a period (usually 1–2 years). Options include insertion of a silicone or saline implant or transposi-
tion of a rectus muscle flap. Neither procedure has
resulted in worsening of the prognosis from the
breast cancer or a significant increase in the difficulty in detecting local recurrences.

2. **Radiotherapy**'s role in the management of carcinoma of the breast has been expanded since the early
1970s. Radiotherapy is now commonly used in conjunction with excisional biopsy of varying degree as
part of the primary therapy. In this circumstance the
radiotherapy is commonly delivered using external
beam therapy to the entire breast and a boost of therapy to the tumor bed with either external beam therapy or implantation of radioactive substances. Radiotherapy may also be given after mastectomy in
women who have a high likelihood of local recurrence, and it is highly effective in preventing the
reappearance of disease in the treated fields. Local
recurrences and distant metastases also are frequently treated successfully with radiotherapy. This

mode of treatment is particularly critical to the management of painful bony lesions or sites of impending pathologic fracture.

3. **Chemotherapy and endocrine therapy** are used for the treatment of early disease to reduce the likelihood of recurrence as well as for the treatment of advanced disease with distant metastasis. *Endocrine therapy* may consist in surgical, chemotherapeutic, or radiotherapeutic ablation or inhibition of the ovaries, adrenal glands, or anterior pituitary gland; or it may consist in additive therapy with estrogens, progestins, androgens, antiestrogens, or luteinizing hormone-releasing hormone (LHRH) agonists. Endocrine therapy is generally ineffective (as sole therapy) for the treatment of metastatic disease in those patients with low levels of estrogen and progesterone receptors (ERs and PRs) in their cancer and increasingly effective as the level of receptors rises. The best responses can be expected in women in whom the ER level is high and PRs are present. Chemotherapy is apparently equally effective regardless of the level of hormone receptors in the cancer cell.

4. **Multimodal therapy** has had more impact on carcinoma of the breast than on any other common cancer affecting adults.

   a. **Postoperative chemotherapy or hormonal therapy** (including ovarian ablation in premenopausal women) for women with a high risk of recurrence owing to positive axillary nodes (i.e., nodes containing cancer) has varying effects, depending on the menopausal status of the woman and the hormone receptor status of the tumor. Most node-positive patients benefit from adjuvant therapy, with a decrease in the annual rates of recurrence by 25–30% and of death by 15–30%.

   Studies have shown that many women with negative nodes also benefit from adjuvant chemotherapy or hormonal (tamoxifen) therapy. While the percent decrease in mortality is similar to that for node-positive women, the lower baseline mortality for node-negative women results in less absolute benefit per 100 women treated. Current clinical trials use tumor size, hormone receptor status, DNA synthesis rate (percent of cells in S phase), and other factors to aid in determining the patients, among those with negative nodes, who are most likely to relapse and thus most likely to benefit from adjuvant therapy.

   b. **Radiotherapy** to the breast and nodal areas following excisional biopsy or quadrantectomy of the breast cancer is as effective a treatment as mastectomy in terms of local recurrence and survival. For most patients it is not only equivalent but preferable treatment because of the preservation of the breast.

    c. Consultation with a surgeon, radiotherapist, and medical oncologist is critical once the diagnosis of carcinoma is highly suspected or histologically confirmed. It is important to have all of these oncology specialists see the patient *before any decisions regarding therapy are made,* so the primary physician and the patient can have opinions from several perspectives about optimal management.

        It is critical to have the patient (and her family if she desires) share in the therapy decisions after she has heard the options, the relative advantages and disadvantages of each option, *and the recommendations* of the consultants. The patient should be given an opportunity to hear why the recommended treatment is thought by the physicians to be best and to decide whether that is acceptable to her.

D. Prognosis. There is a broad spectrum in the biologic behavior of breast carcinoma from the aggressive, rapidly fatal, inflammatory carcinoma to the relatively indolent disease with late-appearing metastasis and survival of 10–15 years. The likelihood of relapse and survival are influenced by the stage of the disease and the hormone receptor status at diagnosis, pathologic characteristics of the tumor, measures of proliferative activity of the cancer cell, oncogene expression or amplification (c-*erbB-2*, c-*myc*), and age and general health of the patient.

    1. Stage. Axillary node involvement and the size of the primary tumor are determinants of the likelihood of survival.

        a. Nodes. In one large National Surgical Adjuvant Breast Project study, 65% of all patients who had a radical mastectomy survived 5 years and 45% survived 10 years. If no axillary nodes were positive, the 5-year survival rate was nearly 80% and the 10-year survival rate 65%. If any axillary nodes were positive, the 5-year survival rate was less than 50% and the 10-year survival rate 25%. If four or more nodes were positive, the 5-year survival rate was 30% and the 10-year survival rate less than 15%. Since that time (1975), there appears to be some improvement with 5-year survival rates of 85% for stage I, 66% for stage II, 41% for stage III, and 10% for stage IV breast cancer.

        b. Primary tumor. Patients with large primary tumors do not do as well as patients with small tumors, irrespective of the nodal status, although those patients with a large primary tumor are more likely to have node involvement. Tumors that are fixed to the skin or to the chest wall do worse than those that are not. Patients with inflammatory carcinomas have a particularly poor prognosis with a median survival time of less than 2 years and a 5-year survival rate of less than 10% in some series. Aggressive initial chemotherapy may improve the outlook for some patients.

2. **Estrogen and progesterone receptors.** Patients without estrogen or progesterone receptors (or with very low levels) are twice as likely to relapse during the first 2 years after diagnosis as those who are receptor-positive. This observation is true for both premenopausal and postmenopausal patients within each major node group (0, 1–3, ≥4).

3. **Other prognostic factors** are emerging as independent prognostic factors, particularly for node-negative cancers, and include the ploidy of the breast cancer cells (diploid better than aneuploid) and the percent of cells in DNA synthesis (low percent S better than high percent). Additional tumor markers that may have predictive value include cathepsin D, c-*erbB-2* and c-*myc* oncogene amplification, and p53 suppressor gene expression.

II. Chemotherapy and endocrine therapy

A. **General considerations and aims of therapy.** Carcinoma of the breast is responsive to many cytotoxic chemotherapeutic agents, hormonal agents, and other endocrine manipulations.

1. **Endocrine therapy** is presumed to be effective because the breast cancer tissue retains some of the endocrine sensitivity of the normal breast tissue. In the premenopausal woman, if the breast cancer growth is supported by estrogen production from the ovary, antiestrogen therapy, removal of endogenous estrogen by oophorectomy, or suppression of estrogen production using an LHRH agonist logically results in regression of the cancer, at least those tumor cells that are dependent on the estrogen. (The dependent cells seem to be those that have the ERs.) Other mechanisms of action of the antiestrogen, tamoxifen, include inhibition of the epithelial growth factor, transforming growth factor-alpha (TGF-α), and stimulation of the epithelial inhibitory factor TGF-β.

2. **Chemotherapy.** As with other cancers, the basis for the effectiveness of cytotoxic drugs in the treatment of carcinoma of the breast is not well understood. It is clear, however, that combinations of drugs are considerably more effective than single agents (although how many is enough is not as clear), and nearly all treatment programs use the drugs in various combinations. In addition to their cytotoxic effects, chemotherapeutic agents may induce menopause in premenopausal women, thus affecting estrogen production as well as killing cells directly.

3. **Aims of therapy** differ depending on the stage of disease being treated.

a. **For early disease** the aim is to eradicate micrometastases in order to render the patient free of disease and prevent recurrence of the disease. If eradication of cancer cells cannot be achieved, long-term suppression is desirable. Coincident with this aim is the goal of avoiding unnecessarily excessive drug-induced toxicity, both short and long term. Of particular theoretical concern is the possibility of second cancers arising many years after the completion of chemotherapy. Thus a goal of investigational studies has been to try to determine the minimum therapy that is effective for preventing the maximum number of recurrences in any given clinical situation.

If micrometastases cannot be eradicated, long-term suppression is also a reasonable goal of therapy. This may in fact be what is accomplished by tamoxifen and the reason why chronic therapy is needed.

b. **For advanced disease** the aim is usually to temporarily reduce the tumor burden and the resultant disability in order to alleviate the patient's symptoms, improve performance, and prolong meaningful survival. Whereas long-term toxicity is not usually of great import, short-term toxicity is a major area of concern for both physician and patient, as the aim of therapy is to improve how the patient feels (quality of life) as well as to prolong the time of her remaining life.

B. **Effective agents** for treating carcinoma of the breast can be found among the alkylating agents, antimetabolites, natural products (antibiotics, vinca alkaloids, and paclitaxel), hormones, and hormone antagonists.

1. **Among the cytotoxic drugs,** the most commonly used agents include doxorubicin (Adriamycin), cyclophosphamide, methotrexate, fluorouracil, paclitaxel, thiotepa, mitoxantrone, and vincristine. Each of these agents has response rates of 20–40% when used as a single agent. Because combinations are so much more effective (60–80% responses) than single agents, these drugs are rarely used alone.

2. **Among the hormones and antihormones,** the most commonly used agents are tamoxifen, various progestins (e.g., megestrol acetate), aminoglutethimide, fluoxymesterone, the LHRH agonists (leuprolide and goserelin), and prednisone. The first five may be used alone, in combination with cytotoxic drugs or sequentially with cytotoxic drugs; prednisone is nearly always used together with cytotoxic agents.

C. **Treatment of early disease.** As indicated already, standard treatment of early disease depends on primary tumor size, nodal status, menopausal status of the woman, hormone receptor status of the tumor, and other tumor characteristics. Because there is not yet optimal therapy for any subset of women with breast cancer, the women and their physicians should be encouraged to participate in a clinical trial. If none is available or the woman declines, Table 15-3 can be used as a guide for

**Table 15-3. Prognostic factors for assessing risk
of recurrence of breast cancer**

Parameter	Value
Lymph node involvement	Risk increased with presence of metastasis and numbers of nodes involved
Tumor size	Risk increases with tumor size independent of nodal status
Estrogen and progesterone receptors	Positive receptors confer better prognosis
Age	Complex factor. Women age 45–49 have best prognosis, with increasing likelihood of deaths from their breast cancer in older and younger age groups
Morphology	Higher nuclear and histologic grade tumors have worse prognosis
DNA content and proliferative capacity	Tumors that are diploid and have low S-phase fraction do better than those that are aneuploid or have a high S-phase fraction (by flow cytometry)
Oncogene expression	c-erbB-2 and c-myc amplification have possible association with earlier relapse and shorter survival

assessing risk. Table 15-4 may be used as a guide to select the type of therapy, depending on menopausal state,
age, and other risk factors.

1. **Cytotoxic therapy** is recommended for premenopausal women with positive nodes, irrespective of
   hormone receptor status. It should also be used in
   high-risk premenopausal patients with negative
   nodes and high-risk postmenopausal women with
   negative hormone receptors. We are less inclined to
   use cytotoxic therapy in the adjuvant treatment of
   women over age 70. We use CAF more commonly in
   women with a higher risk of recurrence, and CMF
   more in those with lesser risks (e.g., node-negative).
   There may be a slight advantage to CAF in terms of
   overall survival, but the difference, if present, is
   small (10%). The *recommended regimens* are as follows.
   a. **CAF**

   Cyclophosphamide 100 mg/m^2 PO daily on days
   1–14 (given as a single daily dose) *and*
   Doxorubicin 30 mg/m^2 IV push on days 1 and 8,
   through the side arm of a free-flowing IV infusion of normal saline *and*

Table 15-4. Adjuvant therapy of breast cancer

	Premenopausal women[a]	Postmenopausal women	
		≤ 70 years	> 70 years
Node-positive			
ER/PR-positive[c]	CT → ± TAM	TAM ± CT	TAM
ER/PR-negative[c]	CT	CT → ± TAM	TAM
Node-negative			
ER/PR-positive			
≤ 2 cm	Low risk[b]	TAM	TAM
	None		
	High risk[b]		
	CT → ± TAM		
> 2 cm	CT → ± TAM	TAM ± CT	TAM
ER/PR-negative	CT	CT → ± TAM	TAM

CT = CAF, CMF, or CMFP for six cycles; TAM = tamoxifen for at least 5 years, alone or after completion of chemotherapy; ER/PR = estrogen receptor/progesterone receptor.
[a]Ovarian ablation may be equally or more effective in premenopausal women than chemotherapy, though direct comparisons are not available.
[b]Based on factors such as proliferative capacity (% S phase) as in Table 15-3.
[c]ER/PR-negative is used to designate that both receptors are negative. ER/PR-positive is used to designate that either receptor (or both) is positive.

Fluorouracil 500 mg/m² IV push on days 1 and 8. Repeat every 28 days for 6 cycles.

b. CMF

Cyclophosphamide 100 mg/m² PO on days 1–14 *and*
Methotrexate 40 mg/m² IV on days 1 and 8 *and*
Fluorouracil 600 mg/m² IV on days 1 and 8.
Repeat cycle every 28 days for 6 cycles.

c. Dose modifications are outlined in Table 15-5.
2. **Tamoxifen** 10 mg PO bid (or 20 mg once daily) is recommended in hormone receptor-positive postmenopausal women with positive nodes. It should be continued for at least 2 years and perhaps for life, so long as the woman remains disease-free. It is probably also beneficial in hormone receptor-positive premenopausal and postmenopausal women with negative nodes and may be of greater benefit than chemotherapy or no therapy in all women over age 70. It may also benefit other groups of women following cytotoxic chemotherapy, though this benefit is less clear, except for women between ages 50 and 69 in whom the benefit is established. It does appear to present low risk in the adjuvant setting and our current recommendations generally include tamoxifen where it is indicated as an option in Table 15-4.

Table 15-5. Dose modification for chemotherapy of breast carcinoma

Dysfunction		Percent of full dose	
Hematologic toxicity ANC (WBC)/μl on day of scheduled treatment		**Platelets/μl on** day of scheduled treatment	**Dose as** **percentage of** **immediately** **preceding** **cycle**
≥ 1800 (≥ 3500)	and	> 100,000	100
1500–1800 (3000–3500)	or	75,000–100,000	75
1000–1500 (2500–3000)	or	50,000–75,000	50
< 1000 (< 2500)	or	< 50,000	0 (delay 1 week)

Note: Absolute neutrophil count (ANC) is the preferred parameter if available. If counts are rising at the end of a treatment cycle, it is often appropriate to delay 1 or even 2 weeks and then treat according to the dose modification scheme shown here. If the ANC is < 1000/μl and is associated with fever > 38.3°C (101°F) or the nadir platelet count is < 40,000, decrease dose by 25% in subsequent cycles. If the nadir WBC count is >3500/μl and the platelet count is >125,000/μl, increase the dose by 25%.

Renal dysfunction (serum creatinine, mg/dl)	M	T	Others
<1.5	100	100	100
1.5–2.0	50	75	100
2.0–3.5	0	50	100
>3.5	0*	0*	0*

Hepatic dysfunction (serum bilirubin, mg/dl)	A, VLB, VCR	C, M, F, T
<1.5	100	100
1.5–3.0	50	100
3.1–5.0	25	100
>5.0	0*	0*

Hemorrhagic cystitis	Discontinue cyclophosphamide and substitute melphalan 4 mg/m² PO on days 1–5 of each cycle
Gastrointestinal toxicity	For debilitating vomiting or diarrhea, reduce doses of C, M, F, and A by 25% for one cycle. For severe mucositis (ulcerations that inhibit eating), reduce subsequent F, M, and A by 50%. Reescalate if possible
Cardiotoxicity	Discontinue doxorubicin

Table 15-5. (continued)

Dysfunction	Percent of full dose
Hypercorticism	If side effects such as hypertension, severe insomnia, psychosis, or uncontrolled diabetes occur, reduce or stop prednisone
Neurotoxicity	Reduce vincristine or vinblastine dose by 50% for moderate paresthesias or severe constipation. Discontinue for severe paresthesias, decreased strength, difficulty walking, cranial nerve palsies, etc.

A = doxorubicin (Adriamycin); C = cyclophosphamide; F = fluoroura-cil; M = methotrexate; T = thiotepa; VCR = vincristine; VLB = vin-blastine.
*Safe guidelines cannot be given, and expert evaluation is required be-fore therapy is applied.

3. **Response to therapy.** It is impossible to determine if individual patients have responded to treatment for micrometastatic disease unless they relapse, as there are no parameters to measure. The effectiveness of such treatment must therefore depend on population studies. Because breast cancer may have a long natural history, and the disease may recur after 5–10 years, it is critical to defer final conclusions regarding any study until at least 5 years and preferably 10 years have passed. It is possible to make some observations, however, regarding the benefits of this kind of multimodal therapy.

   a. **In node-positive premenopausal and post-menopausal women,** both disease-free survival and absolute survival are longer in women treated with various cytotoxic regimens or ovarian ablation (premenopausal only) than in those who receive no therapy after mastectomy.

   b. **In node-positive postmenopausal women,** the disease-free and absolute survival benefit to tamoxifen in receptor-positive women is also clear. Chemotherapy plus tamoxifen may also be better in this group.

   It is apparent that there is a minimal effective dose and duration of drugs that are required for therapy of micrometastases to be effective. If women are arbitrarily given less therapy than they can tolerate, their likelihood of remaining disease-free seems to be less than in women who are given full doses of the drugs. This observation has led to the recommendation that if postoperative chemotherapy is to be given, doses should be as high as the patient can tolerate and should be continued for the entire planned period (usually 6 months).

 c. In all node-negative women, the benefit of therapy is less certain. It does appear that the disease-free survival and survival are improved in women who are treated but because the likelihood of recurrence is lower in most of the node-negative women, the absolute survival benefit is less and must be weighed against the toxicity of any proposed therapy.

D. Treatment of advanced disease is undergoing continuing evolution with the aim of improving the quality and duration of remissions and survivals. In patients with bony metastasis or cerebral metastasis radiotherapy usually has an important role to play in their management, and a radiotherapist should participate in planning the patients' treatment. Regardless of the role of radiotherapy, however, chemotherapy or endocrine therapy is generally indicated in patients who have advanced disease.

 1. Endocrine therapy is indicated in women who have a positive test for estrogen or progesterone receptors in their tumor tissue. It is not generally recommended as the sole therapy for women who have low receptor levels or have previously been shown to be unresponsive to hormonal manipulation. It is also not appropriate therapy for women with brain metastasis, lymphangitic pulmonary metastasis, or other dire visceral disease such as extensive liver metastasis in which a slow response could jeopardize survival.

  a. Premenopausal women. Oophorectomy is the treatment of choice. If the woman is a poor surgical risk, the LHRH analogs goserelin and leuprolide are reasonable alternatives with or without tamoxifen.

  b. Postmenopausal women. Tamoxifen 10 mg PO twice daily or 20 mg PO once daily is the treatment of choice.

  c. Secondary endocrine therapy may be indicated in women who have had a good response to the primary endocrine manipulation and then relapsed. Choices for therapy in this circumstance include the following.

   (1) Tamoxifen 10 mg PO twice daily or 20 mg PO once daily for premenopausal women who fail after responding to oophorectomy.

   (2) Megestrol acetate 40 mg PO qid.

   (3) Aminoglutethimide 250 mg PO qid + hydrocortisone 100 mg PO in divided doses daily for the first 2 weeks, then 40 mg PO in divided doses daily. Fludrocortisone 0.05 to 0.1 mg PO may be given daily or every other day if there is evidence of salt wasting. (Aminoglutethimide is not approved by the Food and Drug Administration for the treatment of breast cancer.)

(4) Fluoxymesterone 10 mg PO bid.

2. **Cytotoxic chemotherapy,** rather than endocrine therapy, is commonly used as the first treatment for advanced disease, particularly in premenopausal patients, because the responses are more rapid and the rate of response is greater when drugs are used in combination than when endocrine therapy is used alone. For patients over age 65, however, initiation of hormone therapy may be justified, with cytotoxic therapy being reserved for patients who have failed on tamoxifen.

a. **Primary therapy** is used as the first nonendocrine therapy for patients with advanced disease. Although several regimens have been shown to be effective, two are recommended. The first is for patients in whom doxorubicin (Adriamycin) is not contraindicated, and the second is for patients with recent myocardial infarction or congestive heart failure in whom the risk of any further myocardial compromise by doxorubicin would be too great.

(1) CAF

Cyclophosphamide 100 mg/m^2 PO on days 1–14 *and*

Doxorubicin 30 mg/m^2 IV on days 1 and 8 *and*

Fluorouracil 500 mg/m^2 IV on days 1 and 8. Repeat the cycle every 4 weeks.

When the cumulative doxorubicin dose reaches 550 mg/m^2, substitute methotrexate 40 mg/m^2.

(2) CMFP

Cyclophosphamide 100 mg/m^2 PO on days 1–14 *and*

Methotrexate 40 mg/m^2 IV on days 1 and 8 *and*

Fluorouracil 600 mg/m^2 IV on days 1 and 8 *and*

Prednisone 40 mg/m^2 PO on days 1–14, during the first 3 cycles only.

Repeat the cycle every 4 weeks.

b. **Secondary therapy** depends on what treatment the patient has had previously. If the patient relapses while on CMF or CMFP treatment, or within 6 months after finishing CMF treatment for micrometastatic disease, it is not likely that these drugs used in combination can be helpful in achieving a second remission. Because doxorubicin is among the most effective agents against breast carcinoma, it should be used in any combination in this situation. An effective combination (VATH) is as follows.

Vinblastine 4.5 mg/m² IV on day 1 *and*

Doxorubicin 45 mg/m² IV on day 1 (maximum cumulative dose 550 mg/m²) *and*

Thiotepa 12 mg/m² IV on day 1 *and*

Fluoxymesterone (Halotestin) 20 mg PO daily.

Repeat cycle every 3 weeks if blood counts permit.

Other agents with activity include paclitaxel, mitomycin, mitoxantrone, and the investigational agents dibromodulcitol, epirubicin, and vindesine. Paclitaxel appears to be a particularly active agent in previously treated breast cancer. It is likely that it will become a component of some initial combination programs both for advanced disease and as adjuvant therapy.

3. **Dose modifications** are outlined in Table 15-5.
4. **Response to therapy**
   a. **Endocrine therapy.** Of patients who are ER-negative, fewer than 10% have a response to either additive or ablative endocrine therapy. Among ER-positive patients, about 60% have a partial, or better, response to either additive or ablative endocrine therapy. Responses to endocrine therapy tend to last somewhat longer than responses to cytotoxic chemotherapy, frequently lasting 12–24 months.
   b. **Cytotoxic chemotherapy** produces responses in 60–80% of patients regardless of their ER status. The responses to therapy at times are durable, but the median duration in most studies is less than 1 year.
E. **Dose-intensive therapy, with or without bone marrow transplantation or other progenitor cell replacement.** As discussed in Chapter 2, the role of dose-intensive therapy and autologous bone marrow transplantation for carcinoma of the breast remains very controversial. The complete remission rates following intensive combination chemotherapy are in the range of 50%, compared to 5–10% following standard therapy. Unfortunately, most of these complete remissions are not durable, with about 20% of patients alive and free of disease at 6–7 years, although the overall survival rate seems to be in the range of 40–50%, which is better than the 20% five-year survival rate that would be expected with standard therapy. Phase II studies that demonstrate comparable activity of high-dose regimens given with filgrastim (G-CSF), but without progenitor cell replacement, may extend the number of patients who can be treated with high-dose therapy. Nonetheless, pending completion of a randomized trial of high-dose therapy with bone marrow transplantation versus standard therapy in metastatic disease, this controversy will probably not be laid to rest in the medical literature. There is no clearly best dose-intensive regimen, although the CPB, CEP, and DICEP regimens (see Chap.

2) have the longest follow-up times and are comparable in outcomes. Several randomized trials are currently evaluating the use of dose-intensive therapy in the adjuvant setting and there is no place for this outside the context of a well-controlled clinical trial.

F. **Complications of therapy.** Acute toxicities are primarily hematologic and gastrointestinal. Subacute toxicities include alopecia, hemorrhagic cystitis, hypertension, edema, and psychoneurologic abnormalities. Chronic or long-term toxicities may be cardiac or neoplastic. Dose modifications for the more common problems are given in Table 15-5. These guidelines are designed to be helpful in selecting a course of therapy that will be effective with the least risk of life-threatening toxicity. Because of individual differences, toxicities that are worse than expected may occur, and the responsible physician must always be alert for special circumstances that dictate further attenuation of the drug doses. The drug data listed in Chapter 10 should be consulted for the individual precautions and toxicities of each drug.

Adjuvant tamoxifen therapy also has consequences that must be watched for. These include a twofold to fourfold increase in endometrial cancer and an increase in thromboembolic disease. Hot flashes are common, but can be helped in some women using a clonidine patch (Catapress TTS-1). There are also beneficial effects of tamoxifen on lipid profiles, the rate of osteoporosis, and possibly the rate of myocardial infarction.

Selected Readings

American Joint Committee on Cancer. In Beahrs, O. H., et al. (eds.), *Manual for Staging Cancer* (4th ed.). Philadelphia: Lippincott, 1992.

Benner, S. E., Clark, G. M., and McGuire, W. L. Review: steroid receptors, cellular kinetics, and lymph node status as prognostic factors in breast cancer. *Am. J. Med. Sci.* 296:59, 1988.

Bonanonna, G., and Valagussa, P. Adjuvant systemic therapy for resectable breast cancer. *J. Clin. Oncol.* 3:259, 1985.

Buzdar, A. U., et al. Bioequivalence of 20-mg once-daily tamoxifen relative to 10-mg twice-daily tamoxifen regimens for breast cancer. *J. Clin. Oncol.* 12:50, 1994.

Carpenter, J. T., et al. Five year results of a randomized comparison of cyclophosphamide, doxorubicin (Adriamycin) and fluorouracil (CAF) vs cyclophosphamide, methotrexate, and fluorouracil (CMF) for node positive breast cancer: a Southeastern Cancer Study Group study. *Proc. Am. Soc. Clin. Oncol.* 13:66, 1994.

Clark, G. M., and McGuire, W. L. Prediction of relapse or survival in patients with node-negative breast cancer by DNA flow cytometry. *N. Engl. J. Med.* 320:627, 1990.

Claus, E. B., Risch, N., and Thompson, W. D. Autosomal dominant inheritance of early-onset breast cancer: implications for risk prediction. *Cancer* 73:643, 1994.

Early Breast Cancer Trialists Collaborative Group. Effects of adjuvant tamoxifen and of cytotoxic therapy on mortality in early breast cancer. *N. Engl. J. Med.* 319:1681, 1988.

Early Breast Cancer Trialists' Collaborative Group. I. Systemic treatment of early breast cancer by hormonal, cytotoxic, or immune therapy: 133 randomised trials involving 31,000 recurrences and 24,000 deaths among 75,000 women. *Lancet* 339:1, 1992.

Early Breast Cancer Trialists' Collaborative Group: II. Systemic treatment of early breast cancer by hormonal, cytotoxic, or immune therapy: 133 randomised trials involving 31,000 recurrences and 24,000 deaths among 75,000 women. *Lancet* 339:71, 1992.

Eddy, D. M. High-dose chemotherapy with autologous bone marrow transplantation for the treatment of metastatic breast cancer. *J. Clin. Oncol.* 10:657, 1992.

Fisher, B., et al. Ten year follow-up results of patients with carcinoma of the breast in a cooperative clinical trial evaluating surgical adjuvant chemotherapy. *Surg. Gynecol. Obstet.* 140:528, 1975.

Fisher, B., et al. Relative worth of estrogen or progesterone receptor and pathologic characteristics of differentiation as indicators of prognosis in node-negative breast cancer. *J. Clin. Oncol.* 6:1076, 1988.

Fisher, B., et al. A randomized clinical trial evaluating sequential methotrexate and fluorouracil in the treatment of node-negative breast cancer who have estrogen negative tumor. *N. Engl. J. Med.* 320:473, 1989.

Fisher, B., et al. A randomized trial evaluating tamoxifen in the treatment of patients with node-negative breast cancer who have estrogen-receptor positive tumors. *N. Engl. J. Med.* 320:479, 1989.

Fisher, B., et al. Eight-year results of a randomized clinical trial comparing total mastectomy and lumpectomy with or without irradiation in the treatment of breast cancer. *N. Engl. J. Med.* 320:822, 1989.

Fisher, B., et al. Endometrial cancer in tamoxifen-treated breast cancer patients: findings from the National Surgical Adjuvant Breast and Bowel Project (NSABP) B-14. *J. Natl. Cancer Inst.* 86:527, 1994.

Fowble, B. L., et al. Ten year results of conservative surgery and irradiation for stage I and II breast cancer. *Int. J. Radiat. Oncol. Biol. Phys.* 21:269, 1991.

Gail, M. H., et al. Projecting individualized probabilities of developing breast cancer for white females who are being examined annually. *J. Natl. Cancer Inst.* 81:1879, 1989.

Gasparini, G., et al. Tumor microvessel density, p53 expression, tumor size, and peritumoral lymphatic vessel invasion are relevant prognostic markers in node-negative breast carcinoma. *J. Clin. Oncol.* 12:454, 1994.

Goldberg, R. M., et al. Transdermal clonidine for ameliorating tamoxifen-induced hot flashes. *J. Clin. Oncol.* 12:155, 1994.

Hryniuk, W., and Bush, H. The importance of dose intensity in chemotherapy of metastatic breast cancer. *J. Clin. Oncol.* 2:1281, 1984.

Ingle, J. N., et al. Randomized trial of bilateral oophorectomy versus tamoxifen in premenopausal women with metastatic breast cancer. *J. Clin. Oncol.* 4:178, 1986.

LiVolsi, V. A., et al. Fibrocystic disease in oral contraceptive users. *N. Engl. J. Med.* 299:381, 1978.

Love, R. R. Tamoxifen therapy in breast cancer: biology, efficacy, and side effects. *J. Clin. Oncol.* 7:803, 1989.

Mansour, E. G., et al. Efficacy of adjuvant chemotherapy in high-risk node-negative breast cancer: an intergroup study. *N. Engl. J. Med.* 320:485, 1989.

McGuire, W. L., et al. How to use prognostic factors in axillary node-negative breast cancer patients. *J. Natl. Cancer Inst.* 82:1006, 1990.

National Institutes of Health Consensus Development Conference statement: adjuvant chemotherapy for breast cancer. *J.A.M.A.* 254:3461, 1985.

Nattinger, A. B., et al. Geographic variation in the use of breast-conserving treatment for breast cancer. *N. Engl. J. Med.* 326:1102, 1992.

Peters, W. P., et al. High-dose chemotherapy and autologous bone marrow support as consolidation after standard-dose adjuvant therapy for high-risk primary breast cancer. *J. Clin. Oncol.* 11:1132, 1993.

Pickle, L. W. Estimating the long-term probability of developing breast cancer. *J. Natl. Cancer Inst.* 81:1854, 1990.

Pritchard, K. I., et al. CMF added to tamoxifen as adjuvant therapy in postmenopausal women with node-positive estrogen and/or progesterone positive breast cancer: negative results from a randomized clinical trial. *Proc. Am. Soc. Clin. Oncol.* 13:65, 1994.

Rivkin, S. E., et al. Adjuvant CMFVP vs tamoxifen vs concurrent CMFVP and tamoxifen for postmenopausal, node-positive, and estrogen receptor-positive breast cancer patients: a Southwest Oncology Group study. *J. Clin. Oncol.* 12:2078, 1994.

Rosen, P. P., et al. Pathological prognostic factors in stage I (T1 N0 M0) and stage II (T1 N1 M0) breast carcinoma: a study of 644 patients with median follow-up of 18 years. *J. Clin. Oncol.* 7:1239, 1989.

Rosen, P. P., et al. Factors influencing prognosis in node-negative breast carcinoma: analysis of 767 T1N0M0/T2N0M0 patients with long-term follow-up. *J. Clin. Oncol.* 11:2090, 1993.

Rutqvist, L. E., and Mattsson, A. Cardiac and thromboembolic morbidity among postmenopausal women with early-stage breast cancer in a randomized trial of adjuvant tamoxifen. *J. Natl. Cancer Inst.* 85:1398, 1993.

Sawka, C. A., et al. Role and mechanism of action of tamoxifen in premenopausal women with metastatic breast carcinoma. *Cancer Res.* 46:3152, 1986.

Sigurdsson, H., et al. Indicators of prognosis in node-negative breast cancer. *N. Engl. J. Med.* 322:1045, 1990.

Slamon, D. J., et al. Studies of HER-2/neu proto-oncogene in human breast and ovarian cancer. *Science* 244:707, 1989.

Smalley, R. V., et al. A comparison of CAF and CMFVP in patients with metastatic breast cancer. *Cancer* 40:625, 1977.

Taylor, S. G., et al. Combination chemotherapy compared to tamoxifen as initial therapy for stage IV breast cancer in elderly women. *Ann. Intern. Med.* 104:455, 1986.

Tormey, D. C., et al. A randomized trial of five and three drug chemotherapy and chemoimmunotherapy in women with operable node positive breast cancer. *J. Clin. Oncol.* 1:138, 1983.

Veronesi, U., et al. Comparing radical mastectomy with quadrantectomy, axillary dissection, and radiotherapy in patients with small cancers of the breast. *N. Engl. J. Med.* 305:6, 1981.

Gynecologic Cancer

C. O. Granai and Walter H. Gajewski

I. Carcinoma of the cervix. Cervical cancer is the most common female malignancy worldwide but ranks only eighth in the United States. The 70% reduction in cervical cancer deaths in the United States in the last 30 years is the result of effective screening by Papanicolaou's smear ("Pap" smear), which identifies disease while it is preinvasive. Nevertheless, there will be 13,500 new cases and 4400 deaths from cervical cancer in the United States this year. Cervical cancer correlates with sexual intercourse at an early age, multiple sex partners, high parity, human papilloma virus (HPV) infection (particularly types 16 and 18), human immunodeficiency virus (HIV) infection, and cigarette smoking. The established relationship with sexual and social behavior permits squamous cancer of the cervix to be categorized as a sexually-socially transmitted disease, and thus is theoretically preventable.

A. Pathology and patterns of spread

1. Histology. Over 90% of cervical cancers are of the squamous cell histologic type. The other 10% are various adenocarcinomas. Squamous cancer arises from the exocervix, while adenocarcinoma is from the columnar epithelium of the endocervix. Less common cervical malignancies also occur, each having unique biologic behaviors. For example, adenosquamous and adenoid cystic carcinomas are aggressive tumors and thus have a relatively poor prognosis. Adenoid basal and verrucous cancers behave in the opposite fashion. More virulent yet is the infrequent small-cell cancer of neuroendocrine origin which sometimes presents with confusing paraendocrine symptoms. Lymphomas, embryomas, embryonal rhabdomyosarcomas, leiomyosarcomas, malignant mixed müllerian tumors, melanomas, carcinoids, and primary sarcomas also develop on the cervix. Finally, not all neoplasms on the cervix are primary from that site. Metastasis to the cervix can arise from the uterus, breast, colon, and kidney. Discussed here are the management principles pertaining to squamous cancer only.

2. The continuum of neoplasia. Cervical neoplasia is a disease "continuum" spanning from mild dysplasia (cervical intraepithelial neoplasia type I [CIN I]) to invasive cancer. Often preinvasive neoplasia will spontaneously stabilize or resolve, but rapid, unpredictable progression to malignancy also can occur.

Management of preinvasive neoplasia is not discussed here. The next step beyond the highest degree of preinvasive neoplasia is "microinvasion." Expert opinions differ on what parameters best define this lesion. Fundamental to all concepts of microinvasion, however, is localized, readily resectable disease without or with a low risk of metastases. The Society of Gynecologic Oncologists defines microinvasion as a malignancy with a depth of invasion 3 mm or less, without vascular/lymphatic space invasion (VSI), and without multiple foci. In contrast, the International Federation of Gynecology and Obstetrics (FIGO) stage IA2 allows for deeper penetration (≤ 5 mm). This more liberal definition of microinvasion has been associated with a small risk of nodal metastasis.

Unlike squamous neoplasia where there is a clearcut histologic demarcation (the basement membrane) beyond which the "invasion" becomes obvious, there are no equivalent histologic boundaries within the cervical stroma by which to delineate degrees of glandular ("adeno") neoplasia. This makes diagnostic distinctions between preinvasion, microinvasion, and true invasion more precarious with glandular histologies.

3. **Spread pattern.** Expanding through the cervical stroma, the squamous cancer extends onto the vagina and uterus and laterally into the paracervical and parametrial soft tissues, ultimately to involve the pelvic sidewall and obstruct the ureters. Direct extension into the bladder or rectum is uncommon. While invading the stroma, the cancer can enter lymphatic vessel spaces, with consequent spread to the obturator and iliac lymph nodes, and ascension to the aortic and supraclavicular groups. Hematogenous dissemination is found in 10% of patients. Distant sites of metastases include the lungs, mediastinum, bone, and liver.

B. **Diagnosis and staging**

1. **Clinical manifestations.** Because of effective screening, many diagnoses of cervical cancer are made prior to the onset of symptoms. However, intermenstrual bleeding, postcoital bleeding ("classic" but uncommon), postmenopausal bleeding, and vaginal discharge can result from friable, ulcerated, often necrotic cervical epithelium. Pelvic, lumbosacral, gluteal, and back pains are worrisome symptoms for advanced disease (e.g., nodal metastasis). Hematuria or rectal bleeding rarely occur, but if so suggest organ involvement.

2. **Diagnosis.** The actual diagnosis of cervical cancer can be proved only by biopsy, not by Pap smear. Though the correlation between Pap smear (cytology) and biopsy (histology) results is good (60–85%), cytology per se is insufficient for diagnosing any degree of cervical neoplasia, let alone malignancy. Practically, an abnormal Pap smear should be considered a "red flag," warning of possible neoplasia, thus demanding further investigation (e.g., colposcopy and biopsy).

3. **Staging** (Table 16-1). In contrast to ovarian and en-

Table 16-1. FIGO staging classification of cervical carcinoma

	Description
Stage 0	Carcinoma in situ, intraepithelial carcinoma.
Stage I	Carcinoma strictly confined to the cervix (extension to the corpus should be disregarded).
IA	Preclinical carcinoma of the cervix, diagnosed only by microscopy.
A1	Minimal microscopically evident stromal invasion.
A2	Lesion detected microscopically that can be measured. The upper limit of the measurement should not show a depth of invasion of > 5 mm taken from the base of the epithelium, either surface or glandular, from which it originates, and a second dimension, the horizontal spread, must not exceed 7 mm. Larger lesions should be staged as IB.
IB	Lesions of greater dimension than stage IA but confined to the cervix (extension to the corpus should be disregarded).
Stage II	The lesion extends beyond the limits of the cervix but has not extended to the pelvic wall. Involves the vagina but not as far as the lower third.
IIA	The lesion extends to the upper two-thirds of the vagina. No obvious parametrial involvement.
IIB	The lesion extends to the parametrium but does not reach the pelvic side wall.
Stage III	The lesion extends to the lower third of vagina. On rectal examination, there is no tumor-free space between the cervix and the pelvic side wall. The lesion reaches the pelvic side wall. There is hydronephrosis or a nonfunctioning kidney known not to be due to other causes.
IIIA	The lesion extends to the lower third of the vagina. No extension to the pelvic side wall.
IIIB	The lesion extends to the pelvic side wall. Presence of hydronephrosis or nonfunctioning kidney.
Stage IV	The lesion has extended beyond the true pelvis or has clinically involved the mucosa of the bladder or rectum. A bullous edema does not permit a carcinoma to be staged as IV.
IVA	The lesion extends to the bladder or rectum.
IVB	There are distant metastases.

dometrial cancers, which are staged surgically, cervical cancer is staged clinically. As such, the most important determinant of stage is the clinical examination, with particular emphasis on the pelvic and rectal examination. Chest x-ray studies and evaluation of the ureters using computed tomography (CT) are also done. In clinically early disease, cystoscopy and proctoscopy are neither helpful nor cost-effective.

C. Treatment

1. Early clinical disease

a. **Stage IA1** can be treated by either cone biopsy, simple total hysterectomy, or at times, modified radical hysterectomy. Theoretically the same option exists for stage IA2 disease, but the recurrence rate is higher after cone biopsy compared to radical surgery. The extra risk inherent in pursuing a "minimalist" treatment strategy (i.e., cone biopsy) must be assumed by the well-informed patient, who often has a strong desire to preserve fertility.

b. For **stages IB–IIA** either a radical hysterectomy with pelvic lymphadenectomy or radical radiation therapy (whole pelvis plus brachytherapy) can be used. Both approaches produce comparable 5-year survival rates. Surgery, however, offers certain advantages: less long-term morbidity, ovarian conservation, better posttreatment sexual function, and surgical-pathologic staging permitting risk stratification.

c. **Risk stratification.** Nodal metastasis significantly worsens prognosis. With stage IB cervical cancer, factors correlating with pelvic node involvement are lesion size, tumor grade, VSI, parametrial extension, and depth of stromal invasion. High-risk patients identified by surgical staging are candidates for adjuvant treatment, preferably on protocol, because of the yet unproved survival benefit of adjuvant radiotherapy or chemotherapy.

d. **Special cases.** The optimal therapy for the bulky cervical cancer is controversial. Neoadjuvant (upfront) chemotherapy followed by either radical surgery or radiation is being used as an alternative approach to brachytherapy radiation in managing the bulky cervical cancer.

   Other special cases of cervical cancer include cervical cancer/neoplasia occurring during pregnancy, carcinoma of the cervical stump after supracervical hysterectomy, the unexpected finding of cancer after "benign hysterectomy," cervical cancer and a coexisting pelvic mass or pelvic inflammatory disease, cervical cancer and ureteral obstruction, and cervical cancer and acquired immunodeficiency syndrome (AIDS). Each of these complex situations needs appropriate, often unique, interventions (or no intervention) in the context of the actual tumor biology, anatomic circumstances, and the specific patient.

2. **Advanced disease**
   a. **Stage IIB–IVA cervical cancers,** by default, have been managed by radical radiation therapy. The modest 5-year survival rates reported vary with stage and institution but generally range from 20 to 50%. With stage IVA, barring evidence of distant or unresectable disease, cure is also occasionally possible using ultraradical surgery (i.e., primary pelvic exenteration).
   b. **Stage IVB is incurable.** Accordingly treatment is individualized and palliative.
   c. **Chemotherapy in advanced disease,** using either single agents or combinations, can produce short-term responses. Cisplatin, carboplatin, bleomycin, vincristine, mitomycin, ifosfamide, fluorouracil, etoposide, methotrexate, and combinations such as BOMP (bleomycin 20–30 units/m^2 IV on days 1–4 plus vincristine 0.5 mg/m^2 IV on days 2–4 plus mitomycin 10 mg/m^2 IV on day 1 plus cisplatin 50 mg/m^2 IV on day 1 every 3 weeks) have been used. At present, the relative toxicity of combination regimens seems unjustified since cisplatin alone prolongs survival equivalently. With recurrent squamous cancer, cisplatin produces a 20–30% response rate, 10% being complete. Surprisingly, no clear dose-response relation has been demonstrated, so cisplatin 50 mg/m^2 IV every 4 weeks is currently recommended.
   d. **New approaches to advanced disease.** Use of neoadjuvant chemotherapy in certain clinical situations seems logical, but the results of limited studies using neoadjuvant platinum, BOMP, fluorouracil and cisplatin (cisplatin 50 mg/m^2 IV on day 1 plus fluorouracil 1000 mg/m^2/day as a continuous IV infusion on days 1–5 every 3 weeks), and others are mixed as to benefit. Chemotherapy is being prospectively tested as a radiation sensitizer. Several small series suggested that better local control and survival are achieved using radiation concurrent with hydroxyurea, fluorouracil, cisplatin, or combinations of these agents.

3. **Recurrent cervical cancer.** The recurrence rate for all cervical cancer is 35%. In contrast, only 10–20% of patients with stage IB have a recurrence. This rate increases to 45–60%, however, if lymph nodes contain metastasis. Recurrences generally develop within 2–3 years of primary treatment, and most with recurrence die from disease. Recurrent cervical cancer must be treated within the constraints presented by the site of the recurrence and

by the type of treatment originally rendered (i.e., surgery and/or radiation). Sites of recurrence are categorized as local/central (resectable, thus potentially curable), regional (in the pelvis but unresectable, extending to the sidewall, or to lymph nodes, thus rarely curable), and distant.

A true central recurrence following primary surgery can be managed with radiation (possibly with sensitizing chemotherapy). Salvage rates as high as 25–50% are reported. A curative alternative for central recurrence, particularly in previously radiated patients, is the select use of ultraradical surgery. Employed under ideal clinical circumstances, pelvic exenteration offers a 30–60% five-year survival rate, if complete, negative margin resection proves possible. However, because of the high surgical complication rate and the risk for major long-term physical and psychologic morbidities, exenterative surgery is indicated only with the intent of cure.

D. Survival. The overall 5-year survival rate for cervical cancer is only 50%. Stage is the most significant predictor. The survival rate for stage IA is 98%; stage IB–IIA, 75–85%; stage IIB, 55%; stage III, 10–50%; and stage IVB, essentially none. Discouragingly, despite improvements in radiotherapy technology and better delineation of disease, survival rates have not improved in 30 years.

II. Endometrial cancer. Endometrial cancer is the most common gynecologic pelvic malignancy in developed nations. Because endometrial cancer usually presents as postmenopausal bleeding, any amount of postmenopausal bleeding is suspect. Epidemiologic risk factors for endometrial cancer include obesity, nulliparity, diet, advancing age, and unopposed estrogen use. The use of oral contraception and, surprisingly, smoking are negatively correlated. The diagnosis is established by simple, cost-effective, endometrial biopsy performed in the office. The physical examination and Pap smear are not usually contributory to diagnosis.

A. Pathology and patterns of spread

    1. Histology. The dominant histologic type of endometrial cancer is endometrioid. Together with the other less common adenocarcinomas of the endometrium (adenosquamous, papillary serous, and clear cell cancers), they constitute 90% of uterine cancer. Differentiating between the adenocarcinoma subtypes is important as each has its own biologic behavior and outcome. For example, the patterns of spread and the 90% five-year survival rate for early-stage endometrioid cancer differ greatly from those of papillary serous and clear cell carcinomas which have 40 and 44% survival rates, respectively.

    2. Patterns of spread. Endometrioid carcinoma first invades the myometrium and then the vascular/lymphatic space. Metastases to the pelvic lymph nodes, and then to the periaortic lymph nodes, follow. The vagina is another common site of lymphatic spread. Thus, metastases in the vagina usually represent only the "visible tip of the iceberg," rather than an innocuous, truly isolated lesion. The presence of simultaneous, but occult lymphatic metastasis accounts for the high failure rate of treatment focused only on the obvious vaginal site. In another means of dissemination, malignant cells can exfoliate from the endometrial primary tumor and implant throughout the peritoneal cavity. Hematogenous metastases to the lungs, liver, bone, and brain are usually late-occurring events. Concomitant endometrioid cancer found in both the endometrium and ovaries is surprisingly frequent. Distinguishing whether the simultaneous involvement of organs represents metastasis, one site to the other, or two separate stage I primary tumors has therapeutic relevance.

B. Pretreatment evaluation

1. **Diagnostic tests.** In "clinically early" endometrial cancer, few preoperative tests are fruitful. Still, chest x-ray and CT studies are generally obtained to look for advanced disease. CA-125 levels are occasionally elevated in endometrial neoplasms and, if so, are useful in monitoring treatment response. Cystoscopy, sigmoidoscopy, and pelvic ultrasound invariably show negative results, and hence should be avoided unless symptoms indicate otherwise. Magnetic resonance imaging (MRI) shows promise for determining the extent and depth of myometrial invasion but is expensive and rarely alters current treatment.

2. **Staging.** FIGO staging of endometrial cancer is surgical (Table 16-2). Stage according to disease distribution is further subcategorized by tumor grade. Because most endometrial cancers are heralded by abnormal bleeding, diagnosing the problem while in a low stage is facilitated; consequently, 75% are stage I and 15% stage II at the time of diagnosis.

3. **Risk stratification.** Risk factors in stage I endometrial cancer are tumor grade (G1, G2, G3), depth of myometrial invasion, VSI, age, hormonal receptor status, tumor histology, DNA ploidy, and S-phase fraction. In a major Gynecologic Oncology Group (GOG) study of stage I endometrioid cancer, there was only a 3% risk of pelvic nodal involvement for G1 lesions, compared to 18% with G3 lesions. Without myometrial invasion, the risk of nodal metastases was 1%. This risk increased to 25% with myometrial penetration to the outer third. Among patients with cancer showing no VSI, 7% had pelvic nodal metastases, compared to 27% if there was VSI. Finding malignant cells on cytology of abdominal and pelvic washings is another independent predictor of risk. In recognition of this fact, FIGO has changed the stage for patients with malignant cytology to stage IIIA.

   Following surgery, the combined power of all the pathologically confirmed prognostic factors is used

Table 16-2. FIGO staging for carcinoma of the corpus uteri

Stage IA G123	Tumor limited to endometrium
Stage IB G123	Invasion to less than one-half the myometrium
Stage IC G123	Invasion to more than one-half the myometrium
Stage IIA G123	Endocervical glandular involvement only
Stage IIB G123	Cervical stromal invasion
Stage IIIA G123	Tumor invades serosa and/or adnexa, and/or positive peritoneal cytology
Stage IIIB G123	Vaginal metastases
Stage IIIC G123	Metastases to pelvic and/or periaortic lymph nodes
Stage IVA G123	Tumor invasion of bladder and/or bowel mucosa
Stage IVB	Distant metastases including intraabdominal and/or inguinal lymph nodes

for risk stratification, thus determining the need for adjuvant treatment.

C. Management

1. **Surgery.** Traditionally, endometrial cancer was treated with radiation followed by hysterectomy. The same survival is achieved when surgery, rather than radiation, is the initial and primary intervention. Moreover, by not giving up-front radiation, the true scope of pathology is not obscured by radiation-induced changes. Overall, performing surgery first is a more informative and cost-effective strategy.

   Surgery for endometrial cancer consists of exploratory laparotomy, cytologic washings, extrafascial total hysterectomy, bilateral salpingo-oophorectomy, intraoperative assessment of myometrial invasion and disease distribution, and lymph node sampling and other staging if indicated. Specific adjustments in the operation are made according to patient age, histology, tumor grade, and intraoperative findings.

2. **For the rare patient** deemed "absolutely inoperable" for medical reasons, radiation (external beam and intracavitary implants) as sole treatment becomes an alternative. The cure rate achieved by radiation alone, even with early-stage disease, is inferior to that of hysterectomy, and hormonal therapy, as a medical alternative to surgery, is rarely of sustained benefit.

3. **Postoperative management**

   a. **Adjuvant treatment.** Based on the surgical pathology, patients with a poor prognosis can be identified. Pelvic radiation is still the most common type of adjuvant treatment given patients considered at high risk for local recurrence. At Women and Infants Hospital/Brown University, adjuvant treatment protocols for stage I endometrioid cancer currently employ postoperative whole pelvic radiation if there is deep myometrial invasion, VSI, G3 lesions, or extension to the endocervix stroma—assuming in each patient that the lymph nodes are negative for cancer. On the other hand, if the lymph nodes have metastasis, extrauterine disease is present, or abdominal/pelvic washings contain malignant cells, then the potential rationale of adjuvant radiation is less obvious. Therefore, we view such patients as better candidates for advanced-disease treatment.

b. Advanced-disease treatment

    (1) Radiotherapy. Effective treatment for advanced endometrial cancer remains elusive. Lacking other options, pelvic radiation therapy is often tried, even with high-risk or high-stage regional disease. The generally poor outcome is understandable, since treating a simultaneously bulky and diffuse malignant process with necessarily constrained, nontumoricidal radiation doses is bound to fail.

    (2) Systemic therapy. Hormonal therapy, though logical and once highly touted, has proved largely ineffective in controlled studies. Occasionally, however, meaningful responses to high-dose progestins do occur, particularly with late-recurring grade 1 tumors, at sites outside the radiated field. Similarly, there are individual responses to systemic chemotherapy but larger studies have yet to identify a routine role, if any, for potentially toxic current drugs, especially administered to asymptomatic patients. At present, despite a lack of compelling response data, cyclophosphamide, doxorubicin, cisplatin, etoposide, and combinations of these agents may be given for their short-term benefit. Paclitaxel and other agents are also being studied.

        (a) Doxorubicin (Adriamycin) 60 mg/m^2 IV *plus*

        Cisplatin 50 mg/m^2 IV every 3 weeks.

        (b) CAP. Cyclophosphamide 500 mg/m^2 IV *plus*

        Doxorubicin 50 mg/m^2 IV *plus*

        Cisplatin 50 mg/m^2 IV every 3 weeks.

c. Recurrent disease. In select patients with a presumably limited recurrence of endometrial cancer, surgical restaging can be helpful in the final decision-making process. When possible, complete resection of the recurrent tumor (e.g., upper vaginectomy) seems to enhance subsequent salvage therapy. In general, however, for advanced or recurrent endometrial cancer, surgery and radiation are of limited, local-control value, and systemic therapies are briefly palliative. But since individual good responses can occur, thoughtful chemotherapy, surgery, and radiation, especially in the protocol setting, is justified for the informed patient wishing to try.

4. **Special cases.** A variety of less common uterine neoplasms also can occur. These need to be managed according to their own unique biology, which differs from that of the "endometrioid" histology.

   a. **Papillary serous carcinoma (PSC)** of the endometrium behaves biologically like the histologically identical PSC of the ovary. In an ovarian-like fashion, the endometrial PSC spreads and recurs diffusely on peritoneal serosal surfaces throughout the entire abdomen. Disappointingly, even the use of postsurgery ovarian cancer–like cisplatin-based combination chemotherapy has had little impact. Nevertheless, systemic adjuvant therapy seems called for, given the biologic behavior of PSC.

   b. **Other uterine malignancies.** About 5% of uterine malignancies are sarcomas, which can emanate from the myometrium or the endometrial stroma. The mixed müllerian mesodermal tumor (MMMT), formally called *carcinosarcoma*, is the most common type, followed by leiomyosarcoma.

      In general, the primary treatment for MMMT and leiomyosarcomas is surgery: total abdominal hysterectomy and bilateral salpingo-oophorectomy and staging, followed by consideration of adjuvant treatment. Both lesions recur locally/regionally and distantly; thus adjuvant pelvic radiation may reduce local recurrence but has no overall survival benefit. Doxorubicin as adjuvant chemotherapy proved unsuccessful. Currently, combinations are receiving the greatest interest.

      (1) Ifosfamide 1.2–1.5 gm/m^2 IV days 1–4 with mesna protection *plus*

      (2) Cisplatin 20 mg/m^2/day IV for 4 days every 3 weeks for 8 cycles.

      Limit the ifosfamide dose to 1.2 gm/m^2 if the patient was previously treated with radiation therapy.

      Other neoplasms (e.g., endometrial stromal tumors) occasionally will develop in the uterine connective tissues as well. Most often, advanced or recurrent connective tissue tumors are of higher grade or are unresectable, and thus must be treated systemically. Depending on hormonal receptor status and the type of histology, dramatic responses to hormonal ablation with high-dose progesterone such as **megestrol acetate (Megace) 260–1000 mg PO daily** can occur. Others sometimes respond to chemotherapy, including etoposide, doxorubicin combinations, ifosfamide, or cisplatin. Unfortunately, the majority of high-grade sarcomas, not cured surgically, do not have prolonged responses to systemic treatment.

c. **Preserving fertility.** Infrequently, a young woman desirous of fertility will develop a well-differentiated endometrioid adenocarcinoma of the endometrium. Barring evidence of advanced disease or an MRI suggesting myometrial invasion, extremely informed patients can consider, as primary management, intensive hormonal therapy using high-dose progesterone (e.g., megestrol acetate 260–1000 mg PO daily × 3 months) instead of hysterectomy. The anticipated response to medical management is amenorrhea. A thorough dilation and curettage with or without hysteroscopy follows the limited trial of hormones (or sooner if the clinical behavior does not conform to expectations). If the cancer is "resolved," reproductive assistance with ovulation stimulation can be done in hopes of completing fertility desires before a need for hysterectomy develops. Generally, however, the odds for achieving a successful pregnancy under these circumstances are considered poor.

III. Fallopian tube cancer. Despite their direct physical and anatomic relation with the uterus, the rare tubal cancer is biologically and behaviorally more analogous to serous epithelial ovarian cancer. As a practical matter then, fallopian tube cancer is staged and managed in a fashion similar to ovarian and not uterine malignancy. The diagnosis of a tubal cancer is usually fortuitous, or comes about retrospectively, after surgery is performed to address some other process. Preoperative symptoms are sometimes present, the classic being a profuse, intermittent, watery, vaginal discharge. Pelvic pain and an abnormal Pap smear suggesting adenocarcinoma that are not otherwise explained by routine testings such as colposcopy, endocervical curettage (ECC), and dilation and curettage can also lead to the diagnosis of fallopian tube cancer.

Treatment is primarily surgical, but radiotherapy and chemotherapy, as in ovarian cancer, have also been used successfully.

IV. Ovarian cancer. Ovarian cancer is the leading killer among female pelvic malignancies in the United States. In 1994 there were 24,000 new cases and 13,600 deaths. Contrary to the common perception, ovarian cancer is a heterologous group of biologically diverse neoplasms, often sharing only their anatomic site, the ovary, in common. Thus, broad generalizations about ovarian cancer are difficult but are best made by subcategorizing them into three groups based on their embryologic origin.

A. Histologic types

1. **Germ cell ovarian cancers.** These malignancies typically occur in young women and are curable. They often present as an asymptomatic pelvic mass and in the past, were usually lethal (e.g., immature teratomas, endodermal sinus tumors, dysgermino-

mas), even though they are confined to the ovary. Today's therapeutic breakthrough is curative chemotherapy which, as an added benefit, does not compromise future fertility. Following surgery, which is done to remove the involved ovary, establish the diagnosis, and stage the disease, the same agents effective against male germ cell tumors (see Chap. 17) also work well against their less common female counterparts.

2. **Stromal tumors.** Stromal tumors of the ovary are rare anachronistic neoplasms occurring at any age but are "stereotyped" by their occasional sex hormone production. The uncommon but often discussed childhood granulosa cell tumor causing precocious puberty is a classic example. After surgical resection, the typical patient with a stromal tumor is observed without further intervention. This management strategy is chosen in part because most stromal tumors are benign or low grade (or of inscrutable malignant potential), and hence are resolved by simple removal. Recurrences can occur, sometimes many years later. If so, or with advanced or unresectable disease, chemotherapy (e.g., BEP, see Chap. 17) can be beneficial, even if not curative.

3. **Epithelial ovarian cancer.** Seventy percent of ovarian malignancies belong to the "epithelial" subgroup (e.g., serous, mucinous, endometrioid, clear cell). In contrast to germ cell tumors, epithelial ovarian cancer (EOC) generally occurs after menopause, is advanced at the time of diagnosis, and is rarely curable. The remainder of this chapter deals with the diagnosis and management of this common variety of ovarian cancer.

B. **Diagnosis and screening**

1. **Early diagnosis.** Diagnosing EOC at an early stage is a difficult, almost fortuitous occurrence because patients usually lack specific symptoms and findings. Little actual merit has come from attempts to screen healthy asymptomatic women for EOCs by using tumor markers with or without ultrasound. CA-125, alone or together with other tumor markers (e.g., CA-125 plus LASA, plus NB70K), lacks sufficient sensitivity and specificity for general screening. By its nature, the normal ovary has a dynamic "everyday" cyst-forming physiology. By comparison, the chance of developing an EOC—an estimated lifetime risk of 1 in 70 (1.4%) American women—is very rare. Most impressively, today's ultrasound technology can detect even the tiniest ovarian cysts. In terms of early cancer diagnosis, the question then becomes, "Which small 'lesion' identified by ultrasound merits surgical intervention?" Consequently, routine screening programs for EOC are inappropriate as a current standard of care.

In contrast, however, two classes of serum tumor markers, monoclonal antibodies (e.g., CA-125 with

EOCs) and peptide markers (e.g., alpha-fetoprotein with endodermal sinus tumors, müllerian inhibiting factor and inhibin with granulosa cell tumors), have proved useful in monitoring the treatment of, not the screening for, ovarian cancer. Additionally, tumor markers evaluated prior to surgery can help differentiate between benign and malignant pelvic masses (i.e., a complex ovarian mass plus an elevated CA-125 level in postmenopausal women correlates with EOC).

2. **Risk stratification for "screening."** As mentioned, screening is not recommended for the general population. However, women deemed at high risk for EOC are still being advised to undergo extra surveillance and, at the extreme, prophylactic oophorectomy. Accepting for the moment the underlying premise of cancer prevention benefit, because the criteria defining "high risk" are not yet specific or proved, that designation can be subjectively extrapolated to encompass too many women.

Epidemiologically, low parity with a history of infertility correlates with an increased risk of EOC. In contrast, high parity, tubal ligation, and oral contraceptive use negatively correlate with risk of EOC, with oral contraceptive use reducing the relative risk up to 50%. Ironically, in this era which clamors for cancer prevention, the use of safe, low-dose birth control pills stands out as a real, but often ignored option that would be immediately advantageous.

More objective risk criteria, such as loss of DNA tumor suppressor genes on chromosomes 13q and 17p, have been associated with the development of some EOCs. Similarly, genetic abnormalities on chromosome 2 and *BRCA 1* suggest a linkage of certain breast, colon, uterus, and ovary cancers. Hopefully, based on this type of cellular research, reliable molecular markers will soon become available, making categorization into high- and low-risk groups impartial and meaningful.

Meanwhile, under present limitations, risk stratification for EOC relies largely on the family history. Fortunately, lacking multiple first-degree relatives with EOC, or repetitive generations (maternal or paternal) affected by the cancer, there is little (e.g., 5–7% lifetime risk) increase in risk. However, a validated strong family history suggests an autosomal dominant inheritance (with incomplete penetrance) whereby females may have a 50% chance of developing EOC. In this very rare high-risk situation, prophylactic oophorectomy is being advocated, and may have benefit. However, even after oophorectomy, serous carcinoma of the peritoneum, a disease similar to EOC, can still occur.

3. **The role of surgery.** After a minimal work-up and assessment of tumor markers, the key diagnostic and staging step in the evaluation of a pelvic/

abdominal mass with or without ascites (i.e., poten-EOC) is surgery. Indeed, surgery becomes the primary intervention, almost without regard for patient age, clinically presumed diagnosis, or stage of disease. Preoperative diagnostic tests, such as needle biopsies and paracenteses, are generally meddlesome, risk disseminating disease, and do not alter the ultimate need for surgery.

C. Management

    1. Early disease and surgical staging (Table 16-3). At laparotomy, the ovarian mass is resected intact if possible (i.e., without rupture) and diagnosis is established based on frozen-section evaluation. During surgery, 20% of EOCs will *appear* visually or grossly

Table 16-3. FIGO surgical staging for ovarian carcinoma

	Definition
Stage I	Growth limited to the ovaries.
IA	Growth limited to one ovary; no ascites. No tumor on the external surface; capsule intact.
IB	Growth limited to both ovaries; no ascites. No tumor on the external surfaces; capsule intact.
IC	Tumor either stage IA or IB but with tumor on surfaces of one or both ovaries; or with capsule ruptured; or with ascites containing malignant cells or with positive peritoneal washings.
Stage II	Growth involving one or both ovaries with pelvic extension.
IIA	Extension and/or metastases to the uterus and/or tubes.
IIB	Extension to other pelvic tissues.
IIC	Tumor either stage IIA or IIB, but with tumor on surface of one or both ovaries; or with capsule(s) ruptured; or with ascites containing malignant cells or with positive peritoneal washings.
Stage III	Tumor involving one or both ovaries with peritoneal implants outside the pelvis and/or positive retroperitoneal or inguinal nodes. Superficial liver metastasis equals stage III. Tumor is limited to the true pelvis but with histologically proved malignant extension to the small bowel or omentum.
IIIA	Tumor grossly limited to the true pelvis with negative nodes but with histologically confirmed microscopic seeding of abdominal peritoneal surfaces.
IIIB	Tumor of one or both ovaries with histologically confirmed implants of abdominal peritoneal surfaces, none exceeding 2 cm in diameter. Nodes are negative.
IIIC	Abdominal implants > 2 cm in diameter and/or positive retroperitoneal or inguinal nodes.
Stage IV	Growth involving one or both ovaries, with distant metastases. If pleural effusion is present, there must be positive cytology to classify a tumor stage IV. Parenchymal liver metastasis equals stage IV.

confined to the ovary (i.e., stage I), but 30–50% of patients will have extraovarian microscopic disease—thus the stage of disease is more advanced. Surgical staging then permits postoperative treatment to be realistically directed at the true EOC distribution.

2. **Advanced disease**
    a. **Intraabdominal metastasis.** Unfortunately, at initial laparotomy, 80% of women with EOC have blatantly advanced disease, visible throughout the abdominal cavity.
    b. **Debulking.** The finding of advanced EOC often portrays a seemingly insurmountable picture of "unresectable" peritoneal and bulky pelvic and abdominal tumor. Fortunately, with the proper surgical approach, maximal tumor resection is possible in 80% of patients. While the surgical risks of debulking are real and substantial, they seem justified by the improved survival experienced by patients whose tumor was optimally debulked relative to those in whom cytoreduction was suboptimal or not carried out. Therefore, if technically feasible, as is usual in experienced hands, optimal debulking remains the recommended surgical intervention for advanced EOCs.
3. **Postsurgery chemotherapy.** The need for postsurgery chemotherapy is determined in the context of histology, grade, stage, amount of residual tumor, and other prognostic factors like DNA ploidy and proliferative index. Except for those with "borderline" histology, generally treated with bilateral salpingo-oophorectomy alone, or for the occasional patient with stage I low-grade EOC, most patients potentially benefit from postoperative therapy.
    a. In early-stage, high-grade EOC, **adjuvant chemotherapy** has proved to prolong disease-free survival and possibly survival itself. Various adjuvants have been used, among them intraperitoneal phosphorus 32 (^{32}P) and systemic treatment with melphalan and platinum-based chemotherapy. For the occasional patient with high-grade stage I EOC, judicious adjuvant platinum-based therapy for 4 cycles is a current recommendation.
        (1) Carboplatin 350–400 mg/m^2 (or calculated with area under the curve (AUC) of 6–7) *plus* Cyclophosphamide 500–600 mg/m^2.

        An older alternative follows. It has no apparent advantage compared to the less toxic carboplatin regimen.
        (2) Cisplatin 75 mg/m^2 IV *plus* Cyclophosphamide 600 mg/m^2 IV.

        Along with the physical examination, CA-125 levels are monitored, though under these circumstances, both the physical findings and CA-125 levels are generally normal from the outset. The best adjuvant regimen has yet to be defined and might include additional agents such as paclitaxel.

b. Patients with more advanced disease have traditionally been treated with the cisplatin-cyclophosphamide regimen (just described) after debulking surgery, but the carboplatin regimen appears to be equivalent in effectiveness. Overall, the response rate (complete response plus partial response) is 70–80%, of which 50% are complete clinical responses and 30% complete pathologic responses. Because of its more favorable toxicity profile, carboplatin is being substituted for the parent compound in most nonpaclitaxel (Taxol) EOC regimens. Standard frontline treatment is currently as follows.

Carboplatin 350–400 mg/m^2 IV (or calculated by formula with AUC of 6–7) in combination with Cyclophosphamide 500 mg/m^2 IV.

This regimen is administered every 4 weeks for 6–8 cycles. The dose intensity of the carboplatin is increased to 600 mg/m^2 as toxicity permits. Only occasionally needed, filgrastim (G-CSF) may be used to support the bone marrow, thus maintaining dose intensity.

Patients are carefully monitored to determine treatment efficacy. Prior to receiving each cycle, they undergo physical examination, including pelvic examination, CA-125 determination, and less frequently, other studies. If any parameter suggests treatment failure (i.e., progression of disease), the regimen is immediately curtailed and strategic options that remain are presented to the patient. Patients opting for second-line treatment, on or off protocols, do so realistically and with a great concern for maintaining the best possible quality of life under difficult circumstances.

Clinical trials are now comparing the paclitaxel class of drugs to standard therapy. Preliminary evidence strongly suggests that paclitaxel-cisplatin combinations will produce a modestly higher response rate and survival.

Paclitaxel 135 mg/m^2 IV with or without Cisplatin 75 mg/m^2 IV.

4. Second-look laparotomy. At the end of primary treatment, if there is a complete clinical response, a normal CA-125 level, and a normal-appearing CT scan, selected patients are offered a "second-look laparotomy." This is appropriate only in a protocol setting, where the information gained from surgery is used to determine further protocol treatment. In spite of a preoperative impression of no evidence of disease, approximately one-third of second-look laparotomies reveal gross disease. Though controversial, under such circumstances, if optimal secondary debulking is technically feasible without undue morbidity, the effort seems prudent. Of the remaining second-look laparotomies, one-third will reveal microscopic residual disease, and one-third will be negative (i.e., all of the restaging biopsy and cytology studies are normal).

5. **Intraperitoneal chemotherapy.** Intraperitoneal (IP) chemotherapy has no role in the standard management of bulky EOC. An exception to this, where IP chemotherapy may still have value, is after a second-look laparotomy, where at most only microscopic disease was found. In the setting of exceedingly minimal disease, the limited but very high-dose drug intensity IP chemotherapy delivers to the peritoneal surfaces at risk for EOC is theoretically advantageous compared to IV administration. Samples of regimens include the following.

1. ^{32}P, or
2. Cisplatin 100 mg/m^2 IP every 3 weeks × 6, or
3. Cisplatin 200 mg/m^2 IP plus
   Etoposide (VP-16) 350 mg/m^2 in 2 liters of normal saline every 3 weeks × 6.

Thiosulfate should be utilized during high-dose IP cisplatin to protect against nephrotoxicity. Thiosulfate 4 gm/m^2 IV bolus over 30 minutes at the start of IP therapy and then 2 gm/m^2/hour continuous IV infusion for a total of 6 hours has been employed.

Access to the peritoneal cavity is gained prior to each IP infusion using a Veries needle under local anesthesia and with fluoroscopic confirmation of proper needle location and free peritoneal cavity dispension of contrast dye prior to installation of the drugs. If IP chemotherapy is to be considered for a seemingly ideal patient, informed entry into a proper protocol remains important.

D. **Follow-up.** Unfortunately, even the patients with negative findings at second-look laparotomies (i.e., the best-responding patients) eventually develop recurrent disease. Current treatment has greatly improved survival and quality of life, but patients are not, in the strictest sense, cured. Time to recurrence can range greatly, from a few months to more than 15 years. Nevertheless, it seems that if patients are followed long enough, recurrences develop. It may be that a recurrence many years later is actually a new or second malignant process (e.g., de novo peritoneal disease) and not a treatment failure.

E. **Recurrent/persistent disease.** Various second-line chemotherapies have yielded modest responses and some relative improvement in survival. Platinum-based agents can be retried if the interval from complete response to recurrence was at least 6 months. Paclitaxel (Taxol) 135 mg/m^2 IV can be given if it was not used upfront. Other agents with reported activity include the following.

1. Altretamine (hexamethylmelamine) 260 mg/m^2/day PO on days 1–14 in a 28-day cycle.
2. Ifosfamide 1.2–1.5 gm/m^2 IV on days 1–5 every 3 weeks.

   A common side effect of ifosfamide is hemorrhagic cystitis. Mesna is administered as a uroprotectant. It is given as a bolus 120 mg/m^2 on day 1 prior to ifosfamide, then as a continuous infusion at 1.5 gm/m^2/24 hours on days 1–6.
3. Tamoxifen 20 mg PO bid.

Responses with second-line treatment range from 20 to 40%. Most are short but occasionally can exceed 1–2 years, justifying the concept of second-line chemotherapy for the informed patient who still wishes to try.

V. **Gestational trophoblastic neoplasm.** Gestational trophoblastic disease encompasses a spectrum of neoplasms arising from fetal chorionic tissue. These tumors range from benign hydatidiform mole, to invasive or metastatic molar tissue, to malignant choriocarcinoma. All histologic classifications of this disease exhibit proliferation of cytotrophoblast and syncytiotrophoblast secreting human chorionic gonadotropin (β-hCG), which is a sensitive and specific tumor marker for gestational trophoblastic neoplasm (GTN). Historically, metastatic gestational choriocarcinoma was the first solid tumor to be cured with systemic chemotherapy. Indeed, today most GTNs can be cured with systemic chemotherapy, even in the presence of widespread metastases.

A. **Hydatidiform mole.** By far the most common form of GTN is the hydatidiform mole. Cytogenetic techniques have established two distinct molar syndromes: complete moles and partial moles. The complete moles arise from a paternal diploid genotype (46XX) and constitute 95% of GTNs overall. In contrast, partial moles are associated with triploidy incorporating an extra haploid paternal chromosome (69XXX). All hydatidiform moles have the potential for developing malignant sequelae. Indeed, malignant transformation occurs in 20% of complete moles but only 4–6% overall develop metastatis. Only 10% of partial moles have malignant sequelae and these usually take the form of nonmetastatic, postmolar GTN.

1. **Initial management.** The evaluation and primary management of both complete and partial hydatidiform moles are similar: surgical evacuation of the uterus and then close monitoring of postevacuation β-hCG levels until proof of cure or malignant sequelae occur. Often the diagnosis of hydatidiform mole is only established retrospectively, following what was presumed to be an otherwise unremarkable spontaneous or elective abortion. If, however, the actual diagnosis is made prior to evacuating the uterus (typically by antenatal ultrasound), a physi-

cal examination, complete blood cell count, chest x-ray, and baseline β-hCG measurement should be done preoperatively. Liver and thyroid function tests should be considered. It is important to note that hydatidiform moles cause and present with a variety of severe medical syndromes, classic among them is early-gestational-age preeclampsia. Occasionally ultrasound will identify a concomitant viable fetus with or without large ovarian theca-lutein cysts. Uncommonly, metastatic disease will be found, requiring a more extensive work-up and staging (to be discussed). Considering the complex array of problems associated with hydatidiform moles, if the diagnosis is known preoperatively, clinical management is best rendered by physicians with extensive knowledge and experience with GTN.

2. **Monitoring.** Following evacuation of a molar pregnancy, serum β-hCG levels are monitored weekly until three consecutive measurements are normal, and then titers are followed monthly for 6 months. Resolution of the β-hCG to a normal value typically occurs by 12 weeks. Throughout the entire observation period, patients are recommended to practice effective birth control to prevent pregnancy and its attendant β-hCG elevation, which confuses the situation.

3. **Malignant transformation.** Malignant transformation of a hydatidiform mole expresses itself as a prolonged plateau, or even a rise, in the β-hCG titer during the follow-up period. Under these circumstances, prompt referral to an oncologist is recommended to expedite further evaluation and treatment. Such patients are staged and managed in the manner described in the next section. The risk for a specific hydatidiform mole undergoing malignant transformation may be predicted by a number of factors (e.g., β-hCG titer, age). At some centers, patients deemed at high risk for developing malignant sequelae are recommended to receive single-agent prophylactic chemotherapy to reduce the transformation risk. But because the accuracy of prognostic factors is less than absolute, and the transformation rate of hydatidiform mole overall is only 15%, most experts do not recommend or use prophylactic chemotherapy, even for high-risk patients. Instead, all patients are observed, and treatment is reserved until such time actual malignant transformation is documented.

B. **Malignant GTN.** The FIGO staging system for GTN, and that of the American College of Obstetricians and Gynecologists (ACOG), are shown in Tables 16-4 and 16-5. The latter means of classification has greater clinical utility, as it facilitates treatment selection as well as classification. Prognostic factors including age, β-hCG titer, number and sites of metastases, antecedent pregnancy, interval between antecedent pregnancy and start of chemo-

Table 16-4. FIGO staging for gestational trophoblastic neoplasia

Stage	Characteristics
I	Strictly confined to uterine corpus
II	Extends outside the uterus, but limited to genital structures
III	Extends to the lungs, with or without genital tract involvement
IV	All other metastatic sites

Source: Modified from F. Pettersson et al. *Annual Report on the Results of Treatment of Gynecologic Cancer* (Vol. 19). Stockholm: International Federation of Gynecology and Obstetrics, 1985.

Table 16-5. Modified ACOG classification of gestational trophoblastic neoplasm (GTN)

I. Nonmalignant GTN
      Hydatidiform mole
         Complete
         Incomplete
II. Malignant GTN
    A. Nonmetastatic GTN: no evidence of disease outside of uterus, not assigned to prognostic category
    B. Metastatic GTN: any metastases
        1. Good-prognosis metastatic GTN
            Short duration (<4 months)
            Low β-hCG level (<40,000 mIU/ml serum β-hCG)
            No metastases to brain or liver
            No antecedent term pregnancy
            No prior chemotherapy
        2. Poor-prognosis metastatic GTN: any high risk factor
            Long duration (>4 months since last pregnancy)
            High pretreatment β-hCG level (>40,000 mIU/ml serum β-hCG)
            Brain or liver metastases
            Antecedent term pregnancy
            Prior chemotherapy

therapy, and prior chemotherapy are considered as part of the ACOG classification system for malignant GTN.

Unlike patients with hydatidiform moles, everyone with malignant GTN is ultimately treated with chemotherapy. Before treatment is initiated, however, they undergo a more extensive metastatic survey. For example, chest x-ray studies and CT of the chest, abdomen, brain, and pelvis are usually done. Usually, however, in the setting of normal-appearing chest x-ray films (and normal vaginal findings), metastases are rarely identified by any of the other more sophisticated tests. As such, clinicians experienced in GTN management often exercise cost-effective selectivity in the actual pretreatment evaluation of patients with malignant GTN.

The key treatment monitor for malignant GTN, as with all GTNs, is the serum β-hCG level. As a matter of further surveillance, the complete blood cell count, along with renal and liver functions, are also followed starting from their pretreatment baseline. As a further safeguard, a pretreatment ultrasound to exclude the possibility of an intrauterine pregnancy should be considered. Once the patient's malignant GTN data base is collected, permitting ACOG classification, those unlikely to be cured using single-agent chemotherapy can be identified. Such high-risk patients are then treated with aggressive combination chemotherapy.

1. **Treatment of malignant nonmetastatic GTN.** Malignant GTN is divided into two subsets according to the presence or absence of metastatic disease. For the nonmetastatic group, most centers report almost 100% cure rates using single-agent treatment with either methotrexate or dactinomycin.

   a. Methotrexate 0.4 mg/kg IM for 5 days with cycles repeated every 14 days has been standard, *but*
   b. Methotrexate 40 mg/m² IM weekly has emerged as the preferred alternative because of its simplicity and relative lack of toxicity.

   Alternative schedules for methotrexate with folinic acid rescue have been used, but with no obvious therapeutic advantage and possibly with greater toxicity.

   Whichever primary treatment regimen is selected for nonmetastatic GTN, additional controversy exists regarding the number of cycles of therapy required for disease resolution. In the United States nonmetastatic GTN has been treated using repeated doses, given at short intervals, until one or two negative β-hCG titers are achieved. This tact is in recognition of the subpopulation of trophoblastic cells that can theoretically persist even when the β-hCG titer is zero.

   Fortunately, few patients with malignant nonmetastatic GTN fail primary therapy. The majority of those who fail methotrexate, however, can still be salvaged using single-agent dactinomycin. Dactinomycin is given IV in doses of 9–13 μg/kg/day for 5 days recycled at 14-day intervals or a single IV bolus 40 μg/kg (1.5 mg/m²) administered every 2 weeks. As mentioned, dactinomycin can also be used as an alternative to methotrexate as initial therapy of nonmetastatic disease. Patients prefer the latter, however, particularly since it does not cause alopecia.

   For patients not desiring further fertility, hysterectomy is an alternative approach to the use of extended chemotherapy alone. The advantage is that performing hysterectomy concomitant with chemotherapy reduces the total number of chemotherapy cycles needed to produce remission. However, given the high effectiveness of chemotherapy in treating GTN, and the uncertainty of most young patients regarding their future fertility, the hysterectomy option is rarely taken.

2. **Treatment of malignant metastatic GTN.** As defined by the ACOG criteria, patients with malignant metastatic GTN are further separated into low- and high-risk groups. This distinction is of major clinical relevance.

   a. **Low-risk (good-prognosis) metastatic GTN.** This is treated in the identical fashion to nonmetastatic GTN discussed already. Approximately two-thirds of low-risk patients will have complete remission after single-agent therapy. Similar to their nonmetastatic peers, nearly all low-risk patients with metastases who develop disease resistant to initial therapy are subsequently cured with either an alternate single-agent, or combination chemotherapy.

   b. **High-risk (poor-prognosis) metastatic GTN.** Not all patients with metastatic high-risk GTN survive. Most American centers treat patients with high-risk metastatic GTN using multiagent chemotherapy. The overall success rate in high-risk disease ranges between 63 and 80% for multiagent chemotherapy using methotrexate- and dactinomycin-based combinations. The two most commonly used combination regimens are outlined in Table 16-6. MAC chemotherapy has been the combination regimen most often reported in American centers. MAC frequently produces significant toxic side effects, particularly when cycled at intervals of less than 21 days. Because of MAC's severe toxicity, this regimen has fallen out of favor in deference to less-toxic therapy. The alternative, increasingly preferred regimen is EMA-CO (see Table 16-6) given on an outpatient basis. This combination is attractive because its primary complete response rate appears to be slightly better than that from MAC therapy.

3. **Special situations**

   a. **Central nervous system metastases.** Patients with metastases to the central nervous system (CNS) have a greater risk for failure of primary therapy than do patients with disease limited to the lungs or vagina. Radiation therapy is often administered to patients with CNS metastasis in conjunction with their primary multiagent chemotherapy. Delivered in 10 equal fractions, 3000 cGy has been safely administered with concurrent MAC chemotherapy. Survival rates are approximate 70–89% for patients treated with primary brain metastasis; however, the survival rate falls to 30% for those who receive salvage treatment for brain metastasis. Patients with

Table 16-6. Multiagent chemotherapy for high-risk metastatic gestational trophoblastic disease (GTD)

MAC

Days 1–5	Methotrexate	0.3 mg/kg (11.1 mg/m^2)	IM IV
	Dactinomycin	8–10 µg/kg (0.30–0.37 mg/m^2)	IV
	Cyclophosphamide	250 mg	

Cycles repeated every 14–21 days

EMA-CO

Course A

Day 1	Dactinomycin	500 µg	IV bolus
	Etoposide	100 mg/m^2	IV infusion over 30 minutes
	Methotrexate[a]	100 mg/m^2	IV bolus
		200 mg/m^2	IV infusion over 12 hours
Day 2	Dactinomycin	500 µg	IV bolus
	Etoposide	100 mg/m^2	IV infusion over 30 minutes
	Folinic acid	15 mg	IM/PO q6h × 4 doses; begin 12 hours after methotrexate infusion is completed

Course B

Day 8[b]	Vincristine	1.0 mg/m^2	IV bolus
	Cyclophosphamide	600 mg/m^2	IV infusion
Day 15	Recycle course A		

[a]In patients with CNS metastases, increase methotrexate to 1 gm/m^2 as 24-hour IV infusion. Increase folinic acid to 15 mg IM/PO q8h × 9 doses beginning 12 hours after methotrexate infusion is completed.

[b]Patients with CNS metastases or with high-risk World Health Organization (WHO) prognostic index scores receive 12.5 mg of methotrexate by intrathecal injection.

Source: Modified from E. S. Newlands et al. Developments in chemotherapy for medium- and high-risk patients with gestation trophoblastic tumors (1979–1984). *Br. J. Obstet. Gynaecol.* 93:63, 1986.

CNS metastasis are at risk for neurologic decompensation caused by cerebral edema and acute hemorrhage. Therefore, dexamethasone is frequently used throughout their course of whole-brain radiation to minimize cerebral edema. Surgical extirpation is generally reserved for patients who demonstrate neurologic decompensation or those who require salvage therapy for recurrent CNS disease.

b. **Metastases to the liver.** Liver metastases occur in 2–8% of patients presenting for primary therapy of metastatic GTN. Survival rates of 40–50%

are reported for patients with primary involvement of the liver. Since these metastases tend to be highly vascular and death is frequently caused by intraabdominal hemorrhage, whole-liver radiation to 2000 cGy in conjunction with combination chemotherapy is recommended.

c. **Drug-resistant disease.** Patients with high-risk metastatic GTN who have not responded to primary chemotherapy have a very poor prognosis. Surgical excision of drug-resistant foci of disease should be considered in patients with limited systemic metastases and has been curative when all else has failed. β-hCG imaging techniques are available to identify small sites of drug-resistant disease. Regimens including cisplatin or etoposide (VP-16) and cisplatin in patients who did not respond to EMA-CO can be effective. Other experimental drugs can be considered as a last resort. Total parenteral nutrition (TPN) and other systemic supports can be essential. In short, no therapeutic approach or support should be ignored on behalf of these compelling patients since they are young and salvage for cure is occasionally still possible.

4. **Posttreatment follow-up.** Most women with malignant gestational trophoblastic disease can be cured using chemotherapy alone, thus preserving the potential for future childbearing. During the first year after completion of therapy, pregnancy is deferred so that β-hCG surveillance is not disrupted by an intercurrent pregnancy. Several series of women treated with simple chemotherapy for non-metastatic or low-risk metastatic GTN have shown normal reproductive capacity after treatment.

VI. **Vulvar cancer.** Vulvar cancer is relatively uncommon, accounting for only 4–5% of gynecologic malignancies. Squamous histology comprises 85% of vulvar malignancies, but cancer of other cell types including melanoma, Bartholin gland adenocarcinoma, Paget's disease, and sarcoma can occur as well. Because vulvar squamous cancers anatomically involve external skin and are slow-growing, early diagnosis is possible and generally leads to high cure rates. Cancers of the other cell types can be more insidious and have variable prognoses.

A. **Pathology.** Squamous cancers of the vulva typically occur in older, often elderly, women and may be preceded by or associated with vulvar intraepithelial neoplasia (VIN). The risk factors correlating with disease include lower socioeconomic status, smoking, history of lower genital tract malignancies (particularly squamous neoplasia of the cervix), and immune-compromised states. Biologically, squamous cancers tend to be indolent, spread initially by direct extension to adjacent organs (e.g., to the vulva, vagina, urethra, anus), and at some point send tumor emboli to regional lymph nodes (inguinal and femoral nodes) and then to distant nodes. Hematogenous spread to the lungs and distant organs is usually a late finding.

B. **Diagnosis and work-up.** Diagnosing vulvar cancer, based simply on gross appearance, is generally not possible. To the contrary, clinical impression is notoriously incorrect, both overestimating and underestimating the degree of neoplasia present. Therefore, a biopsy of abnormal vulvar lesions is needed for definitive diagnosis. After malignancy is diagnosed, establishing the lesion size and location, as well as the regional lymph node status by clinical examination, is important. Further workup includes a thorough examination (e.g., colposcopy) of the cervix and vagina looking for concomitant neoplasia, CT of the pelvis and abdomen to evaluate disease and nodes, and a chest x-ray.

C. **Treatment**

1. **Surgery.** Due to the biologic behavior and anatomic site, vulvar cancer is often ideal for surgical cure. Indeed, radiation is a poorly tolerated alternative in that anatomic area, leading to high morbidity with skin breakdown, infection, and pain. Currently the extent of surgical resection (i.e., the radicalness of the vulvectomy) required to achieve cure is in the midst of reconsideration, but a trend toward less extensive, but still radical surgery seems to be emerging. In addition to radical vulvectomy, inguinal lymphadenectomy is also part of the surgical management for vulvar cancer. Here too, the radicalness of the inguinal dissection is being reconsidered. Consideration is given to superficial or superficial and deep node dissection, and whether ipsilateral or bilateral dissection is needed, based on lesion size, depth of invasion, and clinical status of the groin nodes.

2. **Staging, risk stratification, and management principles.** Staging for vulvar cancer has been changed from clinical to surgical (Table 16-7). Based on surgical-pathologic findings (e.g., depth of invasion, nodal status), coupled with clinical prognostic factors (e.g., lesion size, location), risk stratification is possible and helps with further treatment planning. Most commonly after surgery, the lesion is found to be completely resected and the lymph nodes are negative. The good-prognosis patients are generally observed and do well. In contrast, if groin nodes are positive, the prognosis is worse. In this circumstance, adjuvant radiation to the inguinal region as well as to the whole pelvis is usually recommended. In this poor-prognosis situation, the use of radiation has increased survival relative to that of the former strategy (ultraradical surgery) including pelvic lymph node dissection.

3. **Candidates for chemotherapy.** Patients with distant metastasis and those with locally advanced disease who would otherwise require exenterative-type,

Table 16-7. FIGO staging for vulvar carcinoma

Stage 0	
Tis	Carcinoma in situ, intraepithelial carcinoma
Stage I	
T1, N0, M0	Tumor confined to the vulva and/or perineum, ≤ 2 cm in greatest dimension; nodes are not palpable
Stage II	
T2, N0, M0	Tumor confined to the vulva and/or perineum, > 2 cm in greatest dimension; nodes are not palpable
Stage III	
T3, N0, M0	Tumor of any size with
T1–3, N1, M0	(1) adjacent spread to the lower urethra and/or the vagina, or the anus, *and/or* (2) unilateral regional lymph node metastasis
Stage IVA	
T1–3, N2, M0	Tumor invades upper urethra, bladder mucosa, rectal mucosa, and/or pelvic bone, and/or bilateral regional node metastasis
T4, any N, M0	
Stage IVB	
Any T, any N, M1	Any distant metastasis including pelvic lymph nodes

Rules for clinical staging

T (primary tumor)	
Tis	Preinvasive carcinoma (carcinoma in situ)
T1	Tumor confined to the vulva and/or perineum, ≤ 2 cm in greatest dimension
T2	Tumor confined to the vulva and/or perineum, > 2 cm in greatest dimension
T3	Tumor of any size with adjacent spread to the urethra and/or vagina and/or to the anus
T4	Tumor of any size infiltrating the bladder mucosa and/or the rectal mucosa including the upper part of the urethral mucosa and/or fixed to the bone
N (regional lymph nodes)	
N0	No nodes palpable
N1	Unilateral regional lymph node metastasis
N2	Bilateral regional lymph node metastasis
M (distant metastasis)	
M0	No clinical metastasis
M1	Distant metastasis

ultraradical surgery for complete resection are candidates for chemotherapy. The latter group can receive as an alternative neoadjuvant chemotherapy with or without radiation given preoperatively followed by a less radical resection.

Experience with cytotoxic drugs in managing vulvar malignancy is largely restricted to treating squamous cell tumors. As would be expected, most agents effective against squamous neoplasms occurring at other sites also have an effect on the vulva. Cisplatin, bleomycin, fluorouracil, methotrexate, mitomycin, and doxorubicin have some reported activity, albeit brief. Various combinations of these agents have been used, particularly as neoadjuvant treatment or given in conjunction with radiation therapy.

  a. Cisplatin 50 mg/m²/day IV on day 1 *and* Fluorouracil 1000 mg/m² on days 1–4, continuous IV infusion every 3 weeks.
  b. Mitomycin 10 mg/m² IV day 1 *and* Fluorouracil 1000 mg/m²/day continuous IV infusion on days 1–4.

Cycles may be repeated in 3 or 4 weeks, depending on recovery of the blood cell counts and whether or not subsequent surgery is planned. When used together with radiation therapy, these regimens have been reported to shrink locally advanced lesions, making them amenable to a lesser surgical resection.

D. Summary. At this time, it is impossible to determine the optimal combination, or even the role of, chemotherapy in the treatment of vulvar cancer. Studies are ongoing. Fortunately, most patients with vulvar cancers are cured surgically. Moreover, there is an optimistic trend toward more limited, less-disfiguring surgical management, at times creatively combined with chemotherapy with or without radiation.

For their essential assistance in the preparation of this chapter, the authors acknowledge Hector Tarraza, M.D., Amanda S. Goldstein, R.N., B.S.N., O.C.N., and Cheryl Merolla, R.N., B.S.N., O.C.N.

Selected Readings

Carcinoma of the Cervix

Alberts, D. S., Garcia, D., and Mason-Liddil, N. Cisplatin in advanced cancer of the cervix: an update. *Semin. Oncol.* 18(suppl. 3):11, 1991.

Ambros, R. A., and Kurman, R. J. Current concepts in the relationship of human papilloma virus infection to the pathogenesis and classification of precancerous lesions of the uterine cervix. *Semin. Diagn. Pathol.* 7:158, 1990.

Dottino, P. R., et al. Induction chemotherapy followed by radical surgery in cervical cancer. *Gynecol. Oncol.* 40:7, 1991.

Killackey, M. A., Boardman, L., and Carroll, D. S. Adjuvant chemotherapy and radiation in patients with poor prognostic stage Ib/IIa cervical cancer. *Gynecol. Oncol.* 49:377, 1993.

Park, R. C., and Thigpen, J. T. Chemotherapy in advanced and recurrent cervical cancer: a review. *Cancer* 71:1446, 1993.

van Nagell, J. R., et al. Surgical Therapy for Cervical Cancer. In D. M. Gershenson, A. H. DeCherney, and S. L. Curry (eds.), *Operative Gynecology*. Philadelphia: Saunders, 1993. P. 271.

Endometrial Carcinoma

Burk, T. W., and Morris, M. Surgery for Malignant Tumors of the Uterine Corpus. In D. M. Gershenson, A. H. DeCherney, and S. L. Curry (eds.), *Operative Gynecology*. Philadelphia: Saunders, 1993. Pp. 371–393.

Carcangiu, M. L., and Chambers, J. T. Uterine papillary serous carcinoma: a study on 108 cases with emphasis on the prognostic significance of associated endometrioid carcinoma, absence of invasion, and concomitant ovarian carcinoma. *Gynecol. Oncol.* 47:298, 1992.

Creasman, W. T., et al. Surgical pathologic spread patterns of endometrial cancer: A Gynecologic Oncology Group Study. *Cancer* 60:2035, 1987.

Davies, J. L., et al. A review of the risk factors for endometrial carcinoma. *Obstet. Gynecol. Surv.* 36:107, 1981.

Gurney, H., Murphy, D., and Crowther, D. The management of primary fallopian tube carcinoma. *Br. J. Obstet. Gynaecol.* 97:822, 1990.

Lesko, S. M., et al. Cigarette Smoking and the Risk of Endometrial Cancer. *N. Engl. J. Med.* 313:593, 1985.

Morris, P. J., and Malt, R. A. (eds.), *Oxford Textbook of Surgery* (Vol. 12). Oxford: Oxford Medical, 1994. Pp. 1438–1443.

Morrow, C. P., et al. Relationship between surgical-pathological risk factors and outcome in clinical stage I and II carcinoma of the endometrium: a GOG study. *Gynecol. Oncol.* 40:55, 1991.

Muntz, H. G., et al. Primary adenocarcinoma of the fallopian tube. *Eur. J. Gynaecol. Oncol.* 10:239, 1989.

Silverberg, S. G., et al. Carcinosarcoma (malignant mixed mesodermal tumor) of the uterus. A Gynecologic Oncology Group pathologic study of 203 cases. *Int. J. Gynecol. Pathol.* 9:1, 1990.

Thigpen, J. T., et al. A randomized comparison of doxorubicin alone versus doxorubicin plus cyclophosphamide in the management of advanced or recurrent endometrial carcinoma: a Gynecologic Oncology Group study. *J. Clin. Oncol.* 12:1408, 1994.

Carcinoma of the Ovary

Advanced Ovarian Trialists Group. Chemotherapy in advanced ovarian cancer: an overview of randomized clinical trials. *Br. Med. J.* 303:884, 1991.

Arbuck, S. G. Paclitaxel: what schedule? What dose? *J. Clin. Oncol.* 12:233, 1994.

Baker, T. R., Piver, M. S., and Hempling, R. E. Long term survival by cytoreductive surgery to less than 1 cm, induction weekly cisplatin and monthly cisplatin, doxorubicin, and cyclophosphamide therapy in advanced ovarian adenocarcinoma. *Cancer* 74:656, 1994.

Friedman, J. B., and Weiss, N. S. Second thoughts about second look laparotomy in advanced ovarian cancer. *N. Engl. J. Med.* 322:1079, 1990.

Gallion, H. H., et al. Molecular genetic changes in human epithelial ovarian malignancies. *Gynecol. Oncol.* 47:137, 1992.

Granai, C. O., Gajewski, W. H., and Arena, B. Ovarian cancer: issues and management. *Cancer* 7:1, 1994.

Kirmani, S., et al. *Intraperitoneal Cisplatin/Etoposide (IP/CDDP/VP-16) for Consolidation of Pathologic Complete Response (PCR) in Ovarian Carcinoma. Proc. Am. Soc. Clin. Oncol.* 9:167, 1990.

National Conference on Gynecologic Cancers. Orlando, FL, April, 1992. *Cancer* 71:4, 1993.

NIH Consensus Conference. Ovarian cancer screening, treatment and follow-up. *J.A.M.A.* 273:491, 1995.

Rossing, M. A., et al. Ovarian tumors in a cohort of infertile women. *N. Engl. J. Med.* 331:771, 1994.

Swenerton, K., et al. Cisplatin-cyclophosphamide versus carboplatin-cyclophosphamide in advanced ovarian cancer. *J. Clin. Oncol.* 10:718, 1992.

Thigpen, J. T., et al. Phase II trial of paclitaxel in patients with progressive ovarian cancer after platinum-based chemotherapy. A Gynecologic Oncology Group study. *J. Clin. Oncol.* 12:1748, 1994.

Young, R. C., et al. Adjuvant therapy in stage I and stage II epithelial ovarian cancer: results of two prospective randomized trials. *N. Engl. J. Med.* 322:1021, 1990.

Gestational Trophoblastic Neoplasms

Bolis, G., et al. EMA/CO regimen in high-risk gestational trophoblastic tumor (GTT). *Gynecol. Oncol.* 31:439, 1988.

Holmseley, H. D., et al. Weekly intramuscular methotrexate for nonmetastatic gestational trophoblastic disease. *Obstet. Gynecol.* 72:413, 1988.

Mutch, D. G., et al. Recurrent gestational trophoblastic disease: experience of the Southeastern Regional Trophoblastic Disease Center. *Cancer* 66:978, 1990.

Theodore, C., et al. Treatment of high-risk gestational trophoblastic disease with chemotherapy combinations containing cisplatin and etoposide. *Cancer* 64:1824, 1989.

Willemse, P. H., et al. Chemotherapy of resistant gestational trophoblastic neoplasia treated successfully with cisplatin, etoposide, and bleomycin. *Obstet. Gynecol.* 71:438, 1988.

Carcinoma of the Vulva

Berek, J. S., et al. Concurrent cisplatin and 5-fluorouracil chemotherapy. *Gynecol. Oncol.* 42:197, 1991.

Figge, D. C., Tamimi, H. K., and Greer, B. E. Lymphatic spread in carcinoma of the vulva. *Am. J. Obstet. Gynecol.* 152:387, 1985.

Hacker, N. F., et al. Management of regional lymph nodes and their prognostic influence in vulvar cancer. *Obstet. Gynecol.* 61:408, 1983.

Homesley, H. D., et al. Radiation therapy versus pelvic node resection for carcinoma of the vulva with positive groin nodes. *Obstet. Gynecol.* 68:733, 1986.

Homesley, H. D., et al. Assessment of current International Federation of Gynecology and Obstetrics staging of vulvar carcinoma relative to prognostic factors for survival (a Gynecologic Oncology Group study). *Am. J. Obstet. Gynecol.* 164:997, 1991.

Levin, W., et al. The use of concomitant chemotherapy and radiotherapy prior to surgery in advanced stage carcinoma of the vulva. *Gynecol. Oncol.* 25:20, 1986.

Podratz, K. C., et al. Carcinoma of the vulva: analysis of treatment and survival. *Obstet. Gynecol.* 61:63, 1983.

Thomas, G., et al. Concurrent radiation and chemotherapy in vulvar carcinoma. *Gynecol. Oncol.* 34:263, 1989.

Urologic and Male Genital Malignancies

Scott B. Saxman and Craig R. Nichols

Malignancies that arise from the urinary and male genital tract are highly diverse in their biologic behavior. They span a spectrum that includes one of the most chemotherapeutically curable of cancers (testicular germ cell tumors [GCTs]) and one of the most resistant (renal cell carcinoma [RCC]). The therapeutic approach to these tumors is also diverse and should be multidisciplinary, since chemotherapy, surgery, and radiation therapy all have important roles.

I. **Carcinoma of the kidney**
   A. **Background.** RCC, which is an adenocarcinoma that arises from the parenchyma of the kidney, accounts for 85% of primary renal neoplasms. Transitional cell carcinomas (TCCs) arise from the cells lining the collecting system. Their behavior and response to therapy are similar to those seen arising in the bladder (see sec. **II**). Other rare malignancies of the kidney include oncocytomas (well-differentiated adenocarcinomas), undifferentiated carcinomas, and sarcomas. Wilms' tumor (nephroblastoma) is a cancer that is seen predominantly in childhood and is not covered here. The term *hypernephroma* is a misnomer and should no longer be used.
   B. **Staging.** Staging for RCC should include a computed tomography (CT) scan of the chest and abdomen, bone scan, and usually arteriography and/or venography if nephrectomy is being considered. The TNM staging system is as follows.

Stage I	Tumor 2.5 cm or smaller confined to the kidney (T1, N0, M0)
Stage II	Tumor larger than 2.5 cm confined to the kidney (T2, N0, M0)
Stage III	Tumor extending into major veins, adrenal gland, or perinephric tissues but not beyond Gerota's fascia *or* metastasis to single node smaller than 2 cm (T3, N0, M0 or T1–3, N1, M0)
Stage IV	Tumor invading beyond Gerota's fascia *or* multiple lymph node metastasis *or* distant metastatic disease (T4, any N, M0; any T, N2–3, M0; or any T, any N, M1)

   C. **General therapeutic approach.** The treatment of choice for RCC is radical nephrectomy including removal of the perinephric fat and regional lymph nodes. Partial nephrectomy is an option in patients with bilateral RCC or a solitary kidney to prevent the need for dialysis or kidney transplantation. Rarely, patients with solitary metastatic lesions can be cured by surgical removal of the metastasis at the time of nephrectomy. RCC is relatively radioresistant; thus, adjuvant radiation therapy does not improve survival. Radiation therapy can be useful for palliation of painful metastasis. Although it is reasonable to consider patients with inoperable metastatic disease for treatment with biologic agents or chemotherapy, in most patients these systemic therapies are of minimal benefit.

D. Treatment regimens

1. **Biologic response modifiers**

   a. **Interleukin (IL)-2** mediates its antitumor effects through activation of the patient's immune system. IL-2 alone or in combination with lymphokine-activated killer (LAK) cells or interferon results in tumor regression in 15% of patients treated. Although some of these responses have been complete and long-lasting, it is not yet known whether this represents a therapeutic advance, since patients in the reported studies were carefully selected. There is a wide dosage range in various protocols. Some generally accepted treatment regimens and schedules are shown in Table 17-1. Although the greatest experience has been with the high-dose bolus regimen, it is not recommended for most patients because of its greater toxicity. Outpatient bolus therapy is probably equally efficacious and has less morbidity.

   b. **Interferon** produces regressions in 15% of treated patients. The optimal treatment regimen or duration of treatment is not known. Most commonly used is an intermediate-dose regimen of 5–10 $\times$ 10^6 IU/m^2 given SQ 3–5 times a week. The average response duration is 6–10 months. Response correlates with prior nephrectomy, good performance status, long disease-free interval, and lung-predominant disease.

   c. **Combination therapy** in which IL-2 is combined with either interferon or cyclophosphamide has been used (see Table 17-1). While the advantage of these combinations over single-agent therapy is not established, they are based on solid theoretical considerations and can be administered safely to patients with an Eastern Cooperative Oncology Group (ECOG) performance status of 0–1.

2. **Cytotoxic chemotherapy.** The most commonly used regimen is vinblastine 5–6 mg/m^2 given intravenously (IV) weekly, which produces responses in 10% of patients. The major dose-limiting toxicity is hematologic, and therapy should be delayed for a white blood cell count less than 3000/μl or a platelet count less than 100,000/μl. Chemotherapy does not prolong survival in these patients, and therefore the minimal potential palliative benefit should be carefully weighed against the added toxicity.

3. **Hormonal therapy.** Hormonal therapy (medroxy-

Table 17-1. IL-2–based regimens for renal cell carcinoma

Regimen	Treatment plan*
High-dose bolus IL-2 (inpatient therapy; may require intensive care unit support)	**IL-2:** 22×10^6 IU/m^2 IV bolus over 15 minutes every 8 hours for 14 doses. Repeat once after a 9-day rest period. Repeat the cycle every 10 weeks if stable or responding disease.
Continuous infusion IL-2 (inpatient therapy; requires close monitoring; less likely to require intensive care support)	**IL-2:** 18×10^6 IU/m^2 CIV per day, for 4–5 days, depending on tolerance. Repeat starting day 15. Repeat entire cycle starting on day 43.
Outpatient bolus IL-2	**IL-2:** 30–60×10^6 IU/m^2 IV bolus over 10 minutes 3 times weekly.

CIV = continuous IV infusion over 24 hours.
*Daily premedication and additional symptomatic medication are required on all regimens.** Examples of medication for symptom control include ondansetron 30 mg IV on each day of the IL-2; acetaminophen 650 mg PO pretreatment and q4h PRN; cimetidine 800 mg PO daily; diphenoxylate with atropine (Lomotil), one tablet up to 6 times daily for diarrhea; hydroxyzine 25–50 mg q4–6h for itching. In any of the schedules, therapy may be stopped prematurely for constitutional symptoms, or cardiovascular, renal, hepatic, neurologic, pulmonary, or hematologic toxicity.

progesterone acetate or tamoxifen) has historically been the mainstay of treatment, initially used because of preclinical data suggesting activity. More recent studies do not support any beneficial effect of these agents. At best these agents produce responses in fewer than 5% of patients and therefore cannot be recommended.

E. **Complications of therapy.** Complications of IL-2, particularly with higher doses, include fever, agitation, and a capillary leak syndrome that results in increased interstitial water in the lungs and respiratory insufficiency. This situation usually requires management in an intensive care unit. Interferon can cause nausea, anorexia, fatigue, myalgia, headache, and fever. Complications of cytotoxic therapy include nausea, mucositis, myalgias, and myelosuppression. Hormonal therapy is usually free from side effects other than fluid retention.

F. **Recommendations.** The majority of patients with metastatic RCC should be managed expectantly with the aggressive use of narcotics and radiation therapy for pain control or be placed in clinical trials. Well-informed patients with excellent performance status and cardiac and pulmonary function can be considered for treatment with one of the IL-2 or interferon regimens. More enthusiasm for the use of these agents will have to await the results of phase III trials.

II. Bladder cancer

A. General considerations and staging.

Cancer arising in the bladder is usually TCC, although occasionally squamous cell carcinomas or adenocarcinoma can be seen. TCC falls into two major groups—superficial and invasive. The biology and natural history of these two groups are quite different. When planning treatment for bladder cancer, one must take into account the stage of the tumor (0–IV), histologic grade (1–3), and the location of the tumor within the bladder (related to surgical considerations of partial versus total cystectomy).

The standard evaluation of a patient with invasive bladder cancer should include a CT scan of the abdomen and pelvis, chest x-ray study, complete blood cell count, and serum chemistry profile. The TNM staging system can be summarized as follows.

Tis	Carcinoma in situ
Ta	Noninvasive papillary carcinoma
T1	Tumor invading subepithelial connective tissue
T2	Tumor invading superficial muscle
T3	Tumor invading deep muscle or perivesical fat
T4	Local invasion including prostate, uterus, vagina, or pelvic/abdominal wall

Stage 0	Tis/Ta	N0	M0
Stage I	T1	N0	M0
Stage II	T2	N0	M0
Stage III	T3	N0	M0
Stage IV	T4	Any N	Any M

B. General approach to therapy

1. **Superficial-stage, low-grade tumors.** Patients with stage 0 or I tumors are usually treated with transurethral resection (TUR) and fulguration, with a local control rate higher than 80%. However, TUR does not reduce the risk of recurrence at other sites in the bladder. This risk may be reduced by administration of intravesical therapy. Diffuse carcinoma in situ may also be treated with intravesical therapy.

2. **Deep-stage, high-grade tumors.** Patients with larger stage II lesions or with stage III disease are usually managed with partial or radical cystectomy (depending on the size and location of the tumor). Several trials have investigated the role of preoperative radiation therapy and/or chemotherapy with inconclusive results. The role of neoadjuvant therapy remains controversial and should not be considered standard care.

3. **Advanced and metastatic tumors.** Patients with locally advanced disease or local recurrences can be considered for radiation therapy. Patients with metastatic disease are candidates for systemic chemotherapy. There is evidence that chemotherapy can prolong survival, and that combinations are superior to single agents.

C. **Treatment regimens and evaluation of response**
1. **Intravesical chemotherapy**
   a. **Method of administration and follow-up.** Intravesical therapy is usually administered in a volume of 40–60 ml through a Foley catheter. The catheter is then clamped and the agent retained for 2 hours. This procedure delivers a high local concentration to the tumor area while usually avoiding systemic effects. Patients with superficial bladder cancers require lifelong surveillance with periodic cystoscopy (initially every 3 months, then every 6 months, then annually) because even with intravesical therapy an increased risk of new primary tumors persists. Patients being treated for diffuse carcinoma in situ should have biopsy confirmation of the return of normal mucosa after the installation therapy has been completed. These patients also require lifelong cystoscopic surveillance.
   b. **Selection of patients for intravesical therapy.** Only patients with superficial or small, minimally invasive tumors (T1) should be treated. The grade of the tumor is also a significant predictor of progression. Patients with grade 3 lesions should be considered for more aggressive treatment than intravesical therapy. Possible objectives for intravesical therapy are as follows.
      (1) **Prevention of relapse** in patients with Ta grades 2–3, and stage I lesions treated with TUR.
      (2) **Prevention of occurrence of new bladder tumors.** Patients with two or more previously resected bladder tumors should be treated in an effort to prevent development of new de novo malignancies.
      (3) **Carcinoma in situ** may involve the bladder diffusely and thus not be amenable to TUR. A course of installation therapy is usually given, followed by repeat biopsies. Persistence of carcinoma in situ is an indication for radical cystectomy.
   c. **Specific intravesical therapeutic regimens**
      (1) Bacillus Calmette-Guérin (BCG) 120 mg weekly for 6–8 weeks *or*
      (2) Thiotepa 30–60 mg weekly for 4–6 weeks *or*
      (3) Mitomycin 20–40 mg weekly for 6–8 weeks *or*
      (4) Doxorubicin 50–60 mg weekly for 6–8 weeks.

    d. Selection of therapy. Although few controlled studies have been done, it appears that thiotepa, mitomycin, and doxorubicin are equally effective. Two separate studies have shown BCG to be superior to thiotepa and doxorubicin in preventing recurrence. Thus, BCG should be considered the agent of choice for intravesical therapy.

    e. Response to therapy. Approximately 40–70% of patients with existing or residual tumor following TUR respond to therapy. Whether adjuvant intravesical therapy prevents progression to invasive or metastatic bladder cancer or improves survival will require further study.

    f. Complications of therapy. All of the agents mentioned can cause symptoms of bladder irritation (pain, urgency, hematuria) and allergic reactions. Thiotepa is systemically absorbed and can occasionally cause myelosuppression. This is rare with mitomycin and doxorubicin. Patients receiving thiotepa should have their blood cell counts monitored closely. Mitomycin can cause dermatitis in the perineal area and hands. BCG is occasionally associated with systemic symptoms including fever, chills, malaise, arthralgias, and skin rash.

2. Adjuvant chemotherapy. Chemotherapy has been studied both preoperatively and postoperatively in patients with deeply invasive tumors or positive lymph nodes. To date, no randomized trial has demonstrated a clear-cut benefit. While this question is still under study, neoadjuvant or adjuvant chemotherapy is not generally considered standard in this patient population.

3. Systemic chemotherapy for advanced disease

    a. Active drugs against bladder cancer. These include cisplatin, doxorubicin, vinblastine, fluorouracil, cyclophosphamide, carboplatin, mitoxantrone, and methotrexate. Of these, cisplatin is probably the most active as a single agent. The combination of methotrexate, vinblastine, doxorubicin, and cisplatin (MVAC) is the most commonly used. A randomized trial showed MVAC to have a survival advantage over single-agent cisplatin.

    b. Specific regimens (Table 17-2). Combination chemotherapy that includes three or four agents should be considered standard first-line therapy. Single agents can be used for patients with congestive heart failure, renal dysfunction, or poor bone marrow reserve who are unable to tolerate more aggressive treatment.

    c. Response to therapy. MVAC may be expected to produce a complete response in 15% and a partial response in 35% of patients treated, for an overall response rate of approximately 50%. The median

Table 17-2. Combination chemotherapy and active single agents for cancer of the bladder

Regimen or single agent	Doses and schedules
MVAC	Methotrexate 30 mg/m^2 IV on day 1. Vinblastine 3 mg/m^2 IV on day 2. Doxorubicin 30 mg/m^2 IV on day 2. Cisplatin 70 mg/m^2 IV on day 2 (with vigorous diuresis). Repeat methotrexate and vinblastine on days 15 and 22 if WBC count > 2000/μl and platelet count > 50,000/μl. Cycles should be repeated every 28 days.
CMV	Vinblastine 4 mg/m^2 IV on days 1 and 8. Methotrexate 30 mg/m^2 IV on days 1 and 8. Cisplatin 100 mg/m^2 IV on day 1 (given 12 hours after methotrexate). Repeat cycle every 21 days.
Cisplatin	40–60 mg/m^2 IV every 3 weeks.
Doxorubicin	60 mg/m^2 IV every 3 weeks.
Cyclophosphamide	1 gm/m^2 IV every 3 weeks.
Fluorouracil	500 mg/m^2 IV weekly.

survival time is about 13 months. The toxicity of this regimen is substantial and must be weighed against the expected benefit when selecting therapy. Drug delivery can be enhanced by the coadministration of granulocyte colony-stimulating factor (G-CSF). However, there is no evidence that this improves survival. Response to any chemotherapy is monitored by periodic measurement of tumor masses with the expectation that most patients who respond will do so within the first 1–2 cycles of treatment. Patients who relapse after or progress during MVAC will occasionally respond to a second-line regimen. This should be done for palliative reasons only, since any survival benefit is minimal. Such patients should be considered for clinical trials.

d. **Complications of systemic therapy.** The major dose-limiting toxicity of MVAC is myelosuppression, which often precludes the administration of chemotherapy on days 15 and 22. Cisplatin can cause renal damage, but this can usually be prevented by vigorous hydration and saline diuresis. Mucositis, nausea and vomiting, and malaise are also commonly seen.

e. **Follow-up.** Patients can be followed every few months for symptomatic progression. Serial x-ray studies or bone scans are costly and are of minimal value.

III. Prostatic cancer

A. Background. Carcinoma of the prostate is the most common cancer in the United States, with the exception of nonmelanoma skin cancers. Largely because of aggressive "screening" using prostatic specific antigen (PSA), the incidence of new cases increased 50% between 1980 and 1990, so that by 1994 approximately 200,000 new cases were diagnosed annually. Whether the earlier diagnosis and aggressive surgical or radiotherapeutic management of these patients will change the natural history of prostate cancer and decrease the mortality of this disease of older men is presently indeterminant.

B. Staging. Staging is usually done using a combination of clinical and pathologic indicators. Pathologic staging is necessary for completely accurate staging of low-stage disease, but often is not needed once the disease has become metastatic to the bones or visceral organs. Accurate determination of extension beyond the prostate capsule and into lymph nodes requires pathologic evaluation in most circumstances. The modified Whitmore-Jewett or American Urologic Association (AUA) staging system is the one most commonly used in the United States.

A1	Well-differentiated tumor in a few prostatic chips found incidentally at transurethral prostatectomy (TURP)
A2	Poorly differentiated tumor or multiple prostatic chips found incidentally at TURP
B	Palpable nodule with no extension outside the prostate
C	Local extension beyond the prostate
D1	Metastatic disease to pelvic or abdominal lymph nodes
D2	Metastatic disease to bones or visceral organs

In the TNM system, stages I, II, III, and IV correspond fairly closely to stages A, B, C, and D in the AUA system. The TNM system has the potential to provide more detail about tumor extent and spread, but has not been adopted widely for this tumor. Additional prognostic information can be obtained by evaluating the differentiation of the tumor using the Gleason Grading System and the degree of elevation of the PSA.

Staging for prostate cancer should include abdominal and pelvic CT scans, chest x-ray films, bone scans, liver function tests (LFTs), and serum PSA and acid phosphatase measurements.

C. General considerations and goals of therapy. Selection of therapy for prostate cancer is complex and based on the extent of the disease as well as the age and general medical condition of the patient. Although many biases exist, there are no good randomized studies comparing treatment modalities in patients with organ-confined disease.

With the possible exception of very young patients ($<$ age 60), stage A1 prostate cancer should be followed without further therapy since survival is equal to that in age-matched controls. For other patients with organ-confined disease (stages A2, B), radical prostatectomy and high-dose radiation therapy are treatment options that probably have equal effectiveness. Observation alone may also be reasonable for patients with low-grade, organ-confined tumors. The choice between these three options must take into account the patient's performance status and the toxicities of each modality, which include anesthesia, blood loss, and incontinence for surgery versus tenesmus, rectal bleeding, and diarrhea for radiation. Stage C tumors are usually treated with radiation therapy, although it is unclear whether this therapy prolongs survival. Very elderly patients or patients who have poor general health can be observed without therapy since the natural history is usually slow with progression over years rather than months. Patients with metastatic disease (stages D1, D2) are usually treated initially with hormonal therapy with or without radiation therapy to severely affected vertebral bodies or long bones. Asymptomatic patients with metastasis can have treatment delayed until symptoms develop, with no decrease in likelihood of benefit from therapy.

D. Treatment of symptomatic metastatic disease

1. **Hormonal therapy.** Hormonal therapy results in a subjective response in nearly 75% of patients treated, lasting an average of 18 months. Most of these patients also have objective evidence of response, measured either radiographically or by a falling PSA level. In general, there is little evidence to suggest that one hormonal manipulation is superior to any other, so the choice can be based on patient preference, existing medical conditions, and cost. No good predictive markers for response currently exist in clinical practice.

   a. **Orchiectomy** is often the treatment of choice because it is relatively inexpensive and obviates the need for injections or daily medications. This procedure can be done on an outpatient basis in all but the sickest of patients with minimal morbidity.

   b. **Estrogens** are effective but less frequently used because of concern about potential cardiotoxicity and thrombophlebitis. Historically 3–5 mg/day of diethylstilbestrol (DES) has been given; however, 1 mg/day produces fewer side effects without shortening survival. Painful gynecomastia can be prevented by superficial radiation (5 Gy) to the breast tissue before the start of therapy.

   c. **Luteinizing hormone (LH)–releasing hormone (LHRH) analogs** are synthetic peptides administered by parenteral injection that occupy the receptors for LHRH in the pituitary gland. Initially the release of LH is increased, causing a rise in the serum testosterone level. The continuous administration of therapeutic (super physiologic) doses of the LHRH analog blocks the physiologic pulsatile LH release from the pituitary, causing a fall in the serum testosterone to castrate levels. These agents can be administered either by SQ injection daily, or monthly in a depot form. Current agents include the following.

(1) Leuprolide 1.0 mg SQ daily

(2) Leuprolide depot 7.5 mg IM monthly

(3) Goserelin depot 3.6 mg SQ monthly

Advantages of these agents are that they avoid the trauma of orchiectomy as well as the side effects of DES. Disadvantages include the potential for rapid worsening during the initial few weeks due to a paradoxical transient increase in testosterone production. This flare can usually be avoided by the concurrent use of antiandrogens. Other disadvantages include the potential for poor patient compliance, and the extremely high cost—over $500 a month.

d. LHRH analogs and antiandrogens (total androgen blockade) have been used in combination. Synthetic antiandrogens (e.g., flutamide) act by competing with testosterone at the level of the cellular receptor. Some randomized studies suggest a marginal advantage in survival when flutamide (250 mg tid) is added to LHRH analogs. However, this is controversial and clinical trials are ongoing. This must be weighed against its side effects (mostly diarrhea) as well as its price. Flutamide adds approximately $300 per month to the cost of therapy.

e. Second-line hormonal therapies that have been tried include orchiectomy (if not used as initial therapy), adrenalectomy, hypophysectomy, antiandrogens, progestins, and adrenal suppressants. The response rates to these therapies are low (< 15%) and of brief duration. Patients who were initially treated with combined-modality therapy will occasionally respond to withdrawal of the flutamide. This should be considered before proceeding to more toxic therapies.

2. Cytotoxic chemotherapy. Patients who relapse from or fail to respond to hormonal therapies can be considered for cytotoxic chemotherapy. In general however, chemotherapy trials have been disappointing, with most agents having response rates lower than 10%. The most commonly used drugs are shown below. Except for the combination of estramustine and vinblastine, they are used as single agents.

a. Doxorubicin 60 mg/m^2 IV every 3 weeks

b. Cyclophosphamide 1 gm/m^2 every 3 weeks

c. Fluorouracil 500 mg/m^2 IV weekly

d. Methotrexate 40 mg/m^2 IV weekly

e. Cisplatin 40 mg/m^2 IV every 3 weeks

f. Estramustine 600 mg/m^2 PO days 1–42 *and* Vinblastine 4 mg/m^2 IV weekly for 6 weeks.

Courses of estramustine and vinblastine are repeated every 8 weeks

Suramin is an investigational agent that has been shown to be active in hormone-refractory patients. Its role in the treatment of prostate cancer has yet to be determined.

Patients who have received extensive radiation therapy should have their initial chemotherapy dose reduced by 20%. Patients who progress with hormonal therapy can still have severe symptomatic worsening if testosterone levels rise. Therefore, patients who have not undergone orchiectomy should continue with estrogen or LHRH therapy.

There is no evidence that chemotherapy improves survival in these patients, and no drug combination is clearly better than single agents. Most of the time these patients are best managed with narcotic analgesics and the prudent use of radiation therapy.

3. **Evaluation of response.** Evaluating the response is often difficult since many patients do not have measurable disease. However, the serum PSA or alkaline phosphatase level is often elevated and can be serially measured as a marker for response. Bone scans are difficult to interpret since "hot spots" can reflect either the presence of disease or healing of bone in response to tumor regression.

4. **Complications of therapy.** All hormonal therapies can cause sexual dysfunction including impotence and decreased libido. Orchiectomy can rarely be complicated by local infection or hematoma. LHRH analogs can cause an initial flare of the disease and are frequently associated with "hot flashes." Flutamide can cause diarrhea and hepatic dysfunction. Estrogens are associated with thromboembolic disease, fluid retention, and cardiac disease. Chemotherapy side effects include nausea and vomiting, mucositis, marrow suppression, and alopecia.

E. **Follow-up.** Patients treated with radical prostatectomy can be followed with PSA measurements every 4 months. Patients with a rising PSA, evidence of local recurrence, and no evidence of metastatic disease can be considered for radiation to the prostatic bed. Otherwise there is no role for serial PSA measurements (except as a marker for response to hormonal therapy noted in sec. **III.D.3**) or bone scans since patients are treated only for symptomatic progression.

IV. **Testicular cancer (germ cell tumors)**

A. **Overview.** Although primary neoplasms of the testis can arise from Leydig or Sertoli cells, less than 95% of testicular cancers are of spermatogenic or germ cell origin. GCTs are rare, accounting for 1% of all malignancies in males. However, they are important malignancies because they represent the most common solid tumor in young males and because of their high degree of curability. With the advent of cisplatin-based chemotherapy, accurate tumor markers, and aggressive surgical approaches, overall cure rates for patients with disseminated disease approach 80%, and patients with early-stage disease are cured nearly 100% of the time. GCTs are also one of the few solid tumors for which salvage chemotherapy can be curative.

B. Histology. GCTs are categorized as either seminoma or a variety of other histologies (embryonal cell carcinoma, choriocarcinoma, yolk sac tumor) that are collectively referred to as nonseminomatous GCTs. Pure seminoma accounts for 40% of patients with GCTs. Although mild elevations of the beta subunit of human chorionic gonadotropin (HCG) may be seen, pure seminoma is never associated with an elevation of alpha-fetoprotein (AFP). Nonseminomatous GCT can cause elevations of either the HCG or AFP or both.

C. Staging. Pretreatment staging should include serum tumor markers (AFP, HCG) and CT of the abdomen and chest. Other radiographic procedures should be undertaken only if symptoms or physical examination dictate.

Stage I   Tumor confined to the testis with or without involvement of the spermatic cord or epididymis

Stage II   Tumor with metastasis limited to retroperitoneal lymph nodes

Stage III   Tumor spread beyond retroperitoneal lymph nodes

D. Treatment strategies and management of specific situations. The therapeutic approach to the patient with testicular cancer depends on the histology of the tumor and the clinical or pathologic stage of the disease.

   1. Seminoma. Most patients with seminoma present with early-stage disease and nearly always are cured with radiation therapy. Patients with stage I disease are treated with 2500 cGy given to abdominal nodes in daily fractions over 3–4 weeks. Patients with lymph node involvement on lymphangiogram or CT scans receive a slightly higher dose of 3000–3500 cGy. The contralateral testis should be shielded to maintain fertility. Radiation to the mediastinum is contraindicated and can compromise salvage chemotherapy. Residual radiographic abnormalities are most often scar tissue or necrosis and do not need to be surgically resected. Patients with bulky retroperitoneal disease larger than 5 cm or stage III disease should be treated with chemotherapy (sec. **IV.D.2.**).

   2. Nonseminoma

      a. Stage I disease. Historically these patients have been pathologically staged and treated with a retroperitoneal lymph node dissection (RPLND). Patients with pathologically confirmed stage I disease do not need any further therapy since less than 10% will ever show relapse. In approximately 25% of patients, clinical stage I disease will be found to be stage II pathologically and treatment for these patients is discussed in the following section. The major complication of RPLND is retrograde ejaculation with subsequent infertility, although this is rare with the currently used nerve-sparing procedure. The other option for selected patients is surveillance without RPLND. These patients should be chosen carefully, and should not have any poor prognostic features for extratesticular involvement: microscopic evidence of lymphatic or vascular invasion, invasion of the tunica albuginea or epididymis, or embryonal cell carcinoma. Since 30% of these patients eventually experience relapse, they must be followed closely with monthly measurements of serum markers and chest x-ray studies for the first year and every other month the year after that. Abdominal CT scans should also be performed every 2 months the first year and every 4 months thereafter. If patients are selected and followed appropriately, overall survival is the same as for patients undergoing RPLND.

b. Stage II disease. Patients with lymph nodes larger than 3 cm should be treated primarily with chemotherapy. If the lymph nodes measure less than 3 cm, a RPLND should be performed. Patients with pathologically confirmed and completely resected stage II disease have a relapse rate of approximately 30%. These patients either can be treated with 2 cycles of adjuvant chemotherapy after RPLND or can be closely followed and treated with standard chemotherapy if they show relapse. Patients who choose observation should receive monthly chest x-ray and serum marker evaluations and be treated immediately if the disease recurs. Patients with stage II disease who have elevated markers after RPLND or whose disease is not completely resected should be treated the same as patients with stage III disease.

c. Stage III disease. Approximately 30% of patients will present with stage III disease. The most common site of involvement is the lungs, but liver, bone, and brain can also be involved with metastatic disease. These patients are further categorized as good risk or poor risk based on the number, size, and sites of metastatic involvement. Poor-risk patients according to the Indiana Classification System include those with

(1) Advanced chest disease (mediastinal mass > 50% of the intrathoracic diameter or > 10 pulmonary metastases per lung or multiple pulmonary metastases > 3 cm), or

(2) Palpable abdominal mass plus pulmonary metastases, or

(3) Hepatic, osseous, or central nervous system (CNS) metastasis.

d. Recommended therapy. All patients with stage II or III disease who require chemotherapy should receive cisplatin-based BEP chemotherapy, as follows.

Cisplatin 20 mg/m² IV over 30 minutes on days 1–5, *and*
Etoposide 100 mg/m² IV on days 1–5, *and*
Bleomycin 30 units IV push weekly on days 1, 8, and 15.

Repeat every 21 days regardless of blood cell counts for 2 (adjuvant therapy), 3 (good-risk patients), or 4 (poor-risk patients) cycles.

If the patient has fever associated with granulocytopenia, we would give the next cycle at the same doses followed by daily SQ injections of G-CSF. Other chemotherapy regimens such as VIP (etoposide, ifosfamide, cisplatin) have not improved outcome and are more toxic.

  e. **Surgery for residual disease.** Patients who have a complete response with chemotherapy should be followed and do not require any further treatment. Patients whose marker levels normalize but who have not achieved a radiographic complete response should undergo complete surgical resection of residual disease. If the resected material reveals only teratoma, necrosis, or fibrosis, then no further therapy is necessary and the patient should be followed. If there is carcinoma in the resected specimen, the patient should receive 2 more cycles of BEP chemotherapy.
  f. **Follow-up.** The majority of patients who experience relapse do so within the first 2 years, although late relapses do occur. In general, patients should be followed with monthly physical examination, chest x-ray studies, and serum marker measurements during the first year and every 2 months the second year. Patients should then be followed approximately every 4 months for the third year, twice the fourth year, and yearly thereafter. Since tumors can arise in the contralateral testis, patients should be taught to do testicular self-examination.
E. **Salvage chemotherapy**
  1. **Standard-dose therapy.** Patients who respond to first-line chemotherapy and then relapse are still curable with salvage regimens such as **VIP.**

Vinblastine 0.11 mg/kg (4.1 mg/m²) IV push on days 1 and 2, *and*
Ifosfamide 1.2 gm/m² IV over 30 minutes on days 1–5, *and*
Cisplatin 20 mg/m² IV over 30 minutes on days 1–5.

Repeat every 21 days for 4 cycles. Any radiographic abnormalities that persist after salvage chemotherapy should be surgically resected.
  2. **High-dose chemotherapy with autologous bone marrow transplantation (ABMT).** High-dose che-

motherapy with carboplatin and etoposide with or without ifosfamide followed by ABMT should be considered for patients who have a relapse after salvage chemotherapy or who progress during first-line chemotherapy. Overall approximately 15% of these patients are long-term survivors. The role of ABMT as first-line salvage therapy is currently being evaluated and should be considered experimental.

F. Prognosis. With these strategies, the overall cure rate for patients with stage I disease is more than 98%; stage II disease, more than 95%; and stage III disease, more than 80%.

G. Complications of therapy. Since the majority of patients are cured, the short- and long-term toxicities are of considerable importance. The short-term toxicities of the described chemotherapy regimens include nausea and vomiting, myelosuppression, renal toxicity, and hemorrhagic cystitis. The major long-term morbidities include infertility, pulmonary fibrosis, and a small but definite risk of secondary leukemia.

H. Mediastinal and other midline germ cell tumors. GCTs can arise in several midline structures including the retroperitoneum, mediastinum, and pineal gland. All patients with GCTs at these sites should have a testicular ultrasound examination to exclude an occult primary tumor. Mediastinal nonseminomatous GCTs are associated with Klinefelter's syndrome and with rare hematologic malignancies (particularly acute megakaryocytic leukemia). Small mediastinal seminomas can be treated with radiation therapy alone. Widespread tumors or nonseminomatous tumors should be treated with 4 cycles of BEP chemotherapy. Salvage chemotherapy (including ABMT) in patients with nonseminomatous mediastinal GCT is ineffective.

V. Cancer of the penis

A. General considerations. Penile cancer is rare in North America, but is a significant health problem in many Third World countries. These tumors are nearly always squamous cell in origin and are associated with the presence of a foreskin and poor hygiene. Typically these tumors present as a nonhealing ulcer or mass on the foreskin or glans. The most common treatment is wide surgical excision or penectomy depending on the size and location of the lesion. Prophylactic inguinal lymph node dissection is indicated in certain subgroups of patients. Radiation therapy can also provide local control, although 15–20% of patients will require surgical salvage.

B. Chemotherapy for systemic disease. Active single agents include bleomycin, cisplatin, and methotrexate, with response rates of 20–50%. Combination chemotherapy results in high response rates, but whether survival is improved over that with single agents is unknown. A reasonable regimen is cisplatin 100 mg/m^2 on day 1 with fluorouracil 1000 mg/m^2/day given by continuous infusion on days 1–4. Cycles can be repeated every 21 days.

Selected Readings

Kidney

Provet, J., et al. Partial nephrectomy for renal cell carcinoma: indications, results and implications. *J. Urol.* 145:472, 1991.

Quesada, J. R. Role of interferons in the therapy of metastatic renal cell carcinoma. *Urology* 34:80, 1989.

Rosenberg, S. A., et al. Combination therapy with interleukin-2 and alpha-interferon for the treatment of patients with advanced cancer. *J. Clin. Oncol.* 7:1863, 1989.

Wirth, M. P. Immunotherapy for metastatic renal cell carcinoma. *Urol. Clin. North Am.* 20:283, 1993.

Bladder

Gospodarowicz, M. K., and Warde, P. The role of radiation therapy in the management of transitional cell carcinoma of the bladder. *Hematol. Oncol. Clin. North Am.* 6:147, 1992.

Lamm, D. L., et al. A randomized trial of intravesical doxorubicin and immunotherapy with bacille Calmette-Guerin for transitional-cell carcinoma of the bladder. *N. Engl. J. Med.* 325:1205, 1991.

Loehrer, P. J., et al. A randomized comparison of cisplatin alone or in combination with methotrexate, vinblastine, and doxorubicin in patients with metastatic urothelial carcinoma: a cooperative group study. *J. Clin. Oncol.* 10:1066, 1992.

Lum, B. L., and Torti, F. M. Adjuvant intravesicular pharmacotherapy for superficial bladder cancer. *J. Natl. Cancer Inst.* 83:682, 1991.

Presti, J. C., et al. Molecular genetic alterations in superficial and locally advanced human bladder cancer. *Cancer Res.* 51:5405, 1991.

Raghavan, D., et al. Biology and management of bladder cancer. *N. Engl. J. Med.* 322:1129, 1990.

Smith, J. A., et al. A randomized prospective trial of preoperative irradiation plus radical cystectomy versus surgery alone for transitional cell carcinoma of the bladder: a Southwest Oncology Group study. *J. Urol.* 139:266A, 1988.

Prostate

Chodak, G. W., Thisted, R. A., and Gerber G. S. Results of conservative management of clinically localized prostate cancer. *N. Engl. J. Med.* 330:242, 1994.

Crawford, E. D., et al. A controlled trial of leuprolide with and without flutamide in prostatic carcinoma. *N. Engl. J. Med.* 321:419, 1989.

Eisenberger, M. A., et al. Suramin, an active drug for prostate cancer. Interim observations in a phase I trial. *J. Natl. Cancer Inst.* 85:594, 1993.

Garnick, M. B. Prostate cancer: screening, diagnosis and management. *Ann. Intern. Med.* 118:804, 1993.

Gittes, R. F. Carcinoma of the prostate. *N. Engl. J. Med.* 324:236, 1991.

Hudes, G. R., et al. Phase II study of estramustine and vinblastine, two microtubule inhibitors, in hormone-refractory prostate cancer. *J. Clin. Oncol.* 10:1754, 1992.

Oesterling, J. E. Prostate specific antigen. A critical assessment of the most useful tumor marker for adenocarcinoma of the prostate. *J. Urol.* 145:907, 1991.

Pienta, K. J., and Esper, P. S. Risk factors for prostate cancer. *Ann. Intern. Med.* 118:793, 1993.

Tannock, I. F. Is there evidence that chemotherapy is of benefit to patients with carcinoma of the prostate? *J. Clin. Oncol.* 3:1013, 1985.

Testis

Bosl, G. J., Geller, N. L., and Bajorin, D. Identification and management of poor risk patients with germ cell tumors: the Memorial Sloan-Kettering Cancer Center experience. *Semin. Oncol.* 15:339, 1989.

Broun, E. R., et al. Long-term outcome of patients with relapsed and refractory germ cell tumors treated with high-dose chemotherapy and autologous bone marrow rescue. *Ann. Intern. Med.* 117:124, 1992.

Einhorn, L. H. Treatment of testicular cancer: a new and improved model. *J. Clin. Oncol.* 8:1777, 1990.

Einhorn, L. H., et al. Evaluation of optimal duration of chemotherapy in favorable-prognosis disseminated germ cell tumors: a Southeastern Cancer Study group protocol. *J. Clin. Oncol.* 7:387, 1989.

Nichols, C. R., et al. Secondary leukemia associated with a conventional dose of etoposide: review of serial germ cell tumor protocols. *J. Natl. Cancer Inst.* 85:36, 1993.

Nichols, C. R., et al. Randomized study of cisplatin dose intensity in poor-risk germ cell tumors: a Southeastern Cancer Study group and Southwest Oncology Group protocol. *J. Clin. Oncol.* 9:1163, 1991.

Nichols, C. R., et al. Primary mediastinal nonseminomatous germ cell tumors. A modern single institution experience. *Cancer* 65:1641, 1990.

Saxman, S. Salvage therapy in recurrent testicular cancer. *Semin. Oncol.* 19:143, 1992.

Williams, S. D., et al. Treatment of disseminated germ cell tumors with cisplatin, bleomycin and either vinblastine or etoposide. *N. Engl. J. Med.* 316:1435, 1987.

Williams, S. D., et al. Immediate adjuvant chemotherapy versus observation with treatment of relapse in pathological stage II testicular cancer. *N. Engl. J. Med.* 317:1433, 1987.

Penis

Abi-Aad, A. S., and deKemion, J. B. Controversies in ilioinguinal lymphadenectomy for cancer of the penis. *Urol. Clin. North Am.* 19:319, 1992.

Burgers, J. K., Badalament, R. A., and Drago, J. R. Penile cancer: clinical presentation, diagnosis, and staging. *Urol. Clin. North Am.* 19:247, 1992.

Thyroid and Adrenal Carcinomas

Samir N. Khleif

Endocrine cancers account for 1.5 percent of all cancers diagnosed and 0.4 percent of cancer deaths. Thyroid cancer is the most common endocrine malignancy, accounting for 90 percent of endocrine cancers and 60–70 percent of the deaths from this group of diseases. Although the role of cytotoxic chemotherapy is limited in endocrine cancer, it is beneficial in selected patients. Pancreatic islet cell carcinomas and other pancreatic malignancies are discussed in Chapter 14. Here thyroid and adrenal carcinomas are discussed. The pathology, presentation, and biologic behavior of thyroid and adrenal carcinomas are important determinants of therapy, and they are briefly considered.

I. Thyroid carcinoma

A. Background

1. **Incidence.** About 14,000 new cases of thyroid carcinoma are diagnosed each year, and according to the American Cancer Society there will be an estimated 1120 deaths due to this cancer in 1995. The incidence of thyroid carcinoma is 5.9/100,000 women and 2.2/100,000 men. The prevalence in autopsied subjects is 5–15/100,000. Thyroid carcinoma usually affects persons between the ages of 25 and 65 years.

2. **Etiology and prevention.** In most instances, the cause of thyroid carcinoma is unknown, although experimentally prolonged stimulation by thyroid-stimulating hormone (TSH) may lead to the development of thyroid carcinoma. Some cases appear to be related to a dose-dependent phenomenon involving radiation to the neck during childhood. Thyroid malignancy has been observed 20–25 years after the exposure in atomic bomb survivors and in children treated with radiation therapy for benign conditions of the head and neck. The frequency increases exponentially with doses up to 12 Gy and then decreases, so that with doses over 20 Gy the risk of developing malignancy becomes relatively low. Some cases of thyroid carcinoma (usually medullary carcinoma) are familial, as seen in the multiple endocrine neoplasia (MEN) syndromes, particularly MEN-IIa or MEN-IIb. Although ionizing radiation for benign conditions of the head and neck is no longer being used, thyroid carcinomas related to this usage are still being seen. In cases of accidental nuclear exposure, it is thought that the use of potassium iodide to block the thyroid uptake of radioactive iodine (RAI) in children is helpful in reducing the incidence of subsequent thyroid cancer. This measure was used in eastern Europe following the Chernobyl accident.

3. **Histologic types.** The most common histologic types of thyroid carcinoma are as follows.

    a. Well-differentiated adenocarcinoma, which included papillary carcinoma (40–50%), follicular carcinoma (25%), and mixed papillary-follicular adenocarcinoma (20%). Well-differentiated adenocarcinomas are derived from thyroglobulin-producing follicular cells.

    b. Anaplastic or undifferentiated carcinoma (15–20%).

    c. Medullary carcinoma (1–5%). Medullary carcinomas are derived from thyroid parafollicular or C cells. These cells produce both immunoreactive calcitonin and carcinoembryonic antigen (CEA).

    d. Hürthle cell carcinoma (2–5%), which used to be considered a variant of follicular carcinoma. Recently, it was shown to be a separate pathological entity.

    e. Thyroid lymphoma (5%).

4. Prognosis

    a. Cell types. Patients with papillary or mixed papillary-follicular histology (which have similar biologic and prognostic behaviors) have an excellent prognosis, with less than 15% mortality at 20 years. Patients with pure follicular carcinoma do not do as well as those with papillary elements, at least in part because there is a tendency for the follicular carcinoma to spread via the bloodstream, whereas the papillary carcinoma spreads more by lymphatic channels. About 50% of medullary carcinomas are familial, as part of three clinical syndromes (MEN-IIa, MEN-IIb, and familial non-MEN medullary thyroid carcinoma). Regional lymph node and distant metastases are common in patients with medullary carcinomas and occur in early stages of the disease. The 10-year survival rate following surgical resection is 40–60%. Patients with anaplastic thyroid carcinoma have an abysmal prognosis, with a median survival time of 4 months, although occasional patients may be cured with combined radiotherapy and chemotherapy.

    b. Other factors. In addition to the cell type, the prognosis of thyroid carcinoma is shown to be worse if the following factors are present.

        (1) A large tumor size, especially more than 4 cm.

        (2) Patient age more than 40 years.

        (3) Distant metastases. Well-differentiated carcinoma tends to metastasize to the lung or bone. Patients with bone metastases have survival rates at 5, 10, and 15 years of 53, 38, and 30%, respectively.

        (4) Abnormal DNA content in tumor cells in the papillary type; the more pronounced the aneuploidy, the more aggressively the cancer behaves.

(5) Male sex. This difference may be related to the fact that men tend to be older at the time of diagnosis and are more likely to have a worse histologic type.

In contrast to most other cancers, limited regional lymph node metastasis of well-differentiated thyroid carcinomas does not influence survival substantially, and radiation-induced thyroid carcinoma is not associated with a worse prognosis.

B. Diagnosis and staging. Any solitary nonfunctioning thyroid nodule (cold nodule) should be considered a possible malignant tumor until proved otherwise, especially in patients younger than 25 years and men older than 60 years. The overall incidence of cancer in a "cold" nodule is 25%. Although toxic goiters are less likely to contain carcinoma, a hyperfunctioning thyroid nodule does not automatically confer benignity. As most thyroid tumors spread primarily by local extension and regional nodal metastasis, assessment of the extent of disease is concentrated on the neck. Presurgical studies include inspection and palpation, indirect laryngoscopy, radionuclide scanning, esophagram, computed tomography (CT) scan of the neck, and needle aspiration cytology. The accuracy of needle aspiration biopsy ranges between 50 and 97%, depending on the pathologist and the institution. Whereas the best method for the diagnosis of well-differentiated thyroid and medullary carcinoma is surgical resection, large-needle biopsy is the method of choice for diagnosing thyroid lymphoma and anaplastic carcinoma. Chest radiography should be performed before surgery to rule out pulmonary metastasis. If there is any clinical or laboratory suggestion of bone metastases, a radionuclide bone scan should be performed. Patients with thyroid carcinoma are typically euthyroid. Thyroid carcinoma rarely destroys thyroid function to the point of frank hypothyroidism. However elevated TSH levels with increased antimicrosomal antibodies may be seen with Hashimoto's thyroiditis, which may coexist in 20% of patients with papillary thyroid carcinoma.

C. Treatment. The therapeutic approach to patients with thyroid carcinoma depends considerably on the histologic type.

1. Well-differentiated thyroid carcinoma. The management approach to the patient with well-differentiated thyroid carcinoma is illustrated in Table 18-1.

a. Surgery is the only definitive therapy. Although the surgical approach may differ among surgeons and institutions, many surgeons prefer a bilateral near-total thyroidectomy, taking into consideration that with well-differentiated thyroid carcinoma the incidence of the disease in the contralateral lobe is 20–87%. Limited lymph node involvement does not substantially influence the survival rate, but it is associated with an increase

Table 18-1. Guidelines for the treatment of well-differentiated thyroid carcinoma

Patient age	Extent of the disease (cm)	Treatment
≤ 45 years	< 2	Lobectomy or NTT + HS
	≥ 2	NTT + HS
	Metastasis	NTT + HS + RAI
> 45 years	< 2	NTT + HS
	≥ 2	NTT + HS + RAI
	Metastasis	NTT + HS + RAI

NTT = near-total thyroidectomy; HS = thyroid-stimulating hormone suppression; RAI = radioactive iodine.

in local recurrence. Total thyroidectomy with modified neck dissection is often preferred for those who have cervical lymph node involvement. Mortality after thyroidectomy in well-differentiated thyroid carcinoma approaches 0%. Complications include permanent recurrent laryngeal nerve damage in 2% of patients and permanent hypoparathyroidism in 1–2%.

   b. **TSH suppression** is an essential component in the treatment of all of these tumors (see Table 18-1), because there is good evidence that well-differentiated thyroid cancer cells are usually responsive to TSH. TSH suppresses the growth of malignant as well as normal thyroid tissue, and therefore the recurrence rate is reduced; in a few patients metastatic lesions are diminished markedly. This hormonal suppression can be achieved by the administration of exogenous thyroid hormone. Usually 200–250 μg of levothyroxine (T_4) daily is necessary to obliterate the pituitary response to thyrotropin-releasing hormone (TRH), although the dose should be individualized to a maximum tolerable level. Side effects and dose-limiting factors include symptoms of thyrotoxicosis, angina, and cardiac arrhythmia. Other alternatives include liothyronine (T_3) and desiccated thyroid preparations.

   c. **Radiotherapy** depends to a large degree on the clinical practice of the institution. Treatment with RAI (^{131}I) is usually recommended for patients with well-differentiated thyroid carcinoma and known postoperative residual disease, patients with distant metastases, or patients with locally invasive lesions. It is also recommended in patients older than 45 years and those with large lesions (see Table 18-1). When ablation of a thyroid remnant is carried out postoperatively, it is usually done 4–6 weeks after thyroidectomy. Although the effect of RAI on survival is not well determined, it is clear that the use of RAI and T_4

markedly decreases the recurrence rate. Effective use of RAI treatment requires the following.

  (1) Tumor cells that are capable of receiving and concentrating iodide (i.e., well-differentiated papillary or follicular carcinoma) *and*
  (2) Appropriate patient preparation by withholding thyroid hormone administration for 2–4 weeks to provide the iodine-concentrating cells with the highest endogenous TSH stimulation.

Triiodothyronine (T_3) is cleared from the body much more rapidly than levothyroxine. The shorter period of withdrawal minimizes the period of hypothyroidism. Accordingly, patients are switched from suppression therapy with levothyroxine to a corresponding dose of T_3 for 2–4 weeks to allow metabolic disposal of the levothyroxine. This is followed by 2 weeks of T_3 withdrawal. Effective doses of thyroid ablation usually are 50–150 mCi, depending on the size and extent of the disease. Isolation of the patients is required by federal regulations until the total-body radiation activity decreases below 30 mCi. Postablation TSH follow-up should identify individuals who do not respond to the therapy. Ideally serum levels should exceed 30 μm/ml. Potential side effects expected after radioiodine therapy include temporary bone marrow depression, nausea, sialoadenitis with possible permanent cessation of salivary flow (radiation mumps), skin reaction over the tissue concentrating the radioiodine, pulmonary fibrosis, and a small risk of later development of acute leukemia (2%). Once ablation is successful, patients are placed on suppressive therapy. Patients with lung metastases treated with RAI have a 20-year survival rate of 54%. In contrast, patients with bony involvement have a 10-year survival rate of 0%. Scintigraphy should be performed 4–6 weeks after therapy to detect any residual carcinoma. Most well-differentiated thyroid carcinomas grow very slowly. The rate of recurrence is 0.5–1.6% per year. Therefore, lifelong annual serum thyroglobulin assays are recommended. Scintigraphy is suggested if the thyroglobulin is found to be elevated (>23 ng/ml). The role of external radiation therapy in well-differentiated thyroid carcinoma is limited. It is considered for tumors that concentrate little or no iodine.

2. **Medullary thyroid carcinoma.** With familial medullary carcinoma, the disease is almost always bilateral. Regional lymph node involvement is common in early stages. Therefore, total thyroidectomy and central lymph node dissection are required. The overall 10-year survival rate following surgical resection is 40–60%. Postoperative annual evaluation is recom-

mended by measuring levels of calcitonin and CEA, both of which are secreted by the medullary thyroid carcinoma cells, as a follow-up for residual disease or recurrence. Suppressive therapy is of no benefit because medullary cells do not have TSH receptors. RAI and cytotoxic chemotherapy are of little utility. Cisplatin, streptozocin, carmustine, methotrexate, and fluorouracil have shown little if any benefit. However, some studies have shown chemotherapy to produce occasional responses of metastatic disease (see sec. **I.C.4.**). Local radiation therapy is useful in some patients as palliative therapy.

3. **Anaplastic thyroid carcinoma.** Most anaplastic tumors are unresectable at the time of presentation. Combination chemotherapy or chemotherapy plus irradiation have shown encouraging results for local control, and some partial and complete remissions have been seen.

4. **Chemotherapy**

   a. **Single-agent chemotherapy.** The most widely applied cytotoxic agents are doxorubicin (Adriamycin), bleomycin, cisplatin, and etoposide. Each of these medications has demonstrated some activity against anaplastic and medullary thyroid carcinomas. Improved survival may be achieved in those patients responding to sequential exposure to these agents. Doxorubicin has proved to be the best single chemotherapeutic agent with the highest response rate. Doxorubicin at 60–75 mg/m^2 IV every 3 weeks has resulted in objective responses in 20–45% (median, 34%) of patients with advanced refractory metastatic thyroid carcinoma. The response rate is probably highest for the medullary type and lowest for undifferentiated thyroid carcinoma. A high single dose of doxorubicin, which should be increased in patients with no response, appears to be essential for a therapeutic effect. Because of its lower cardiotoxicity, 4-epidoxorubicin (epirubicin—still investigational), although almost as effective as doxorubicin, may be given at higher doses and over longer periods and is therefore preferred by some investigators.

   b. **Combination chemotherapy** usually includes doxorubicin. Cisplatin 40 mg/m^2 IV + doxorubicin 60 mg/m^2 IV given every 3 weeks yielded a higher rate and quality of response than did doxorubicin alone. These results included complete remission in 12% of patients, several of whom survived more than 2 years. Toxicity was no worse with the combination therapy. Other combination chemotherapy used includes doxorubicin + bleomycin + vincristine + melphalan with a response rate of 36%. Doxorubicin + bleomycin + vincristine, another combination, showed an improved 64% response rate. Doxorubicin 10 mg/m^2

IV has been used in combination with external radiotherapy 90 minutes prior to the first radiation treatment and weekly thereafter. In this combination, the radiotherapy was given at a dose of 1.6 Gy per treatment twice a day for 3 consecutive days weekly for 6 weeks. Patients with undifferentiated thyroid carcinoma who are treated in this fashion showed an improvement in the median survival compared to historical control subjects. In general, the highest response is observed in patients with pulmonary metastasis. If anaplastic thyroid carcinoma responds to chemotherapy, a prolongation of the median survival time from 3–5 months to 15–20 months can be achieved.

5. **Lymphoma** is more thoroughly addressed in Chapter 26. The discussion here briefly highlights its significance concerning thyroid malignancies. By definition, lymphoma of the thyroid is the one that at the time of diagnosis is confined to the gland or to the gland and regional lymph nodes. The major histologic type is non-Hodgkin's lymphoma. Autoimmune thyroiditis is a predisposing factor. Lymphoma of the thyroid usually presents with rapid enlargement of the gland within a few weeks and is bilateral in 25% of patients. If the tumor is confined to the thyroid, surgical excision alone yields a 5-year survival rate of 70–90%. However, once the lymphoma extends beyond the thyroid gland, surgical therapy does not improve survival, and irradiation and chemotherapy are indicated.

II. Adrenal carcinoma
A. Adrenocortical carcinoma

1. **Incidence and etiology.** Adrenocortical carcinoma is a rare tumor, with fewer than 200 new cases occurring yearly in the United States. It accounts for 0.05–0.20% of all cancers and 0.2% of cancer deaths. It has a prevalence of 2/1,000,000 worldwide. The peak incidence of adrenocortical carcinoma occurs during the fourth and fifth decades of life. The incidence in women in most reports is about 2.5 times higher than that in men, who tend to be older at diagnosis. Women have a tendency to develop a functional carcinoma, whereas males usually develop a nonfunctional malignancy. There is no family predilection, and no etiologic factors have been established.

2. **Clinical picture.** Adrenal carcinoma may present in several modes.
   a. A palpable **abdominal mass** or an abdominal mass detected incidentally by abdominal imaging for some other purpose. Approximately 50% of patients have a palpable abdominal mass at the time of diagnosis.
   b. A **functioning tumor** with or without endocrine signs and symptoms of Cushing's syndrome, virilization, or feminization. More than 60% of pa-

tients present with functioning tumor, depending on the age and sex of the patient. Such manifestations are due to an increase in the production of a wide variety of steroid hormones. Ten percent of adrenocortical carcinomas are associated with virilization and 12% with feminization. Adrenal carcinoma is the cause of 10% of all cases of Cushing's syndrome.

  c. **Other frequent presenting symptoms** include upper abdominal pain, weight loss, anorexia, and malaise. Usually these symptoms are associated with advanced disease.

3. **Pathology and diagnosis.** Most malignant adrenal masses represent carcinomatous metastatic lesions, primarily from the lung and breast. Whether the coincidental finding of an adrenal mass requires complete screening of the patient for a hidden primary adrenal tumor depends on the clinical situation. There may be some difficulty distinguishing adenoma from carcinoma. Criteria for differentiating benign from malignant primary adrenal tumors (Table 18-2) were suggested by Page, DeLellis, and Hough of the Armed Forces Institute of Pathology. Adrenocortical carcinoma can further be divided into two categories according to the pathologic patterns of cellular arrangement and the cellular pleomorphism.

  a. Well-differentiated adrenocortical carcinoma, which occurs more commonly in women and usually presents with a functioning tumor, *and*

  b. Anaplastic carcinoma, which is more common in men and is often associated with a lack of hormone production.

4. **Staging and prognosis.** Most patients (70%) present with stage III or IV disease. Adrenocortical carcinoma is a highly malignant cancer with an overall 5-year mortality of 75–90%, depending on the stage and morphology of the disease. The most commonly used staging system (derived from the TNM classification system) for adrenocortical carcinoma is as follows.

Stage	Size (cm)	Node or local invasion	Metastasis
I	< 5	−	−
II	> 5	−	−
III	Any	+	−
IV	Any	Both	−
		±	+

Metastases of adrenocortical carcinoma most commonly occur in the lung (71%), lymph nodes (68%), liver (42%), and bone (26%). The median survival time of patients with well-differentiated carcinoma is 40 months, whereas patients with anaplastic carcinoma have a more dismal median survival time of 5 months. The median survival time of patients with

Table 18-2. Diagnosis of malignancy in adrenocortical neoplasms

Reliability	Clinical criteria	Pathologic criteria
Diagnostic of malignancy	Weight loss, feminization, nodal or distant metastases	Tumor weight > 100 gm, tumor necrosis, fibrous bands, vascular invasion, mitoses
Consistent with malignancy	Virilism, Cushing's syndrome/virilism, no hormone production	Nuclear pleomorphism
Suggestive of malignancy	Elevated urinary 17-ketosteroid levels	Capsular invasion
Unreliable	Hypercortisolism, hyperaldosteronism	Tumor giant cells, cytoplasmic size variations, ratio between compact and clear cells

Source: Adapted from D. L. Page, R. A. DeLellis, and A. J. Hough. Tumors of the Adrenal. In: W. H. Hartmann, L. H. Sobin (eds.), *Atlas of Tumor Pathology.* Washington, D.C.: Armed Forces Institute of Pathology, 1986.

stages I, II, or III disease is 24–28 months, and for stage IV disease, 12 months.

5. **Treatment.** Because of the extremely low incidence of this disease, very few medical centers have sufficient experience treating it and an effort should be made to refer these patients to centers that have clinical trials pertaining to this disease. This caveat notwithstanding, several guidelines regarding its treatment can be given.

   a. **Surgery.** In up to one-half of patients, adrenocortical carcinomas can be resected, although incompletely in some patients; however, the remainder of patients have either local invasion that is too extensive or metastases to other sites in the abdomen, liver, lung, or other locations. Of the patients whose tumors are resected for cure, 40% remain disease-free. The remainder die, usually with extensive metastatic disease, within an average of less than 1 year. Patients who undergo complete resection should initially be followed on a monthly basis (with measurements of steroid levels if they have a functioning tumor) to detect recurrence. Serial magnetic resonance imaging (MRI) may also be used to evaluate for recurrence.

   b. **Radiotherapy.** This provides symptomatic relief from pain due to local or metastatic disease, especially bony metastases. It has also been used to prevent local recurrence following surgical resection (40–55 Gy over 4 weeks), but the benefit is uncertain and there is no proof that it improves survival.

   c. **Chemotherapy.** Indications include recurrent, metastatic, and nonresectable adrenocortical carcinoma. Agents used are the following.

      (1) **Adrenocortical suppressants**

         (a) **Mitotane** (o,p-DDD, Lysodren). An unconventional chemotherapy and a close chemical relative of the insecticide DDT, mitotane has been used to treat adrenocortical carcinoma since 1960. It inhibits corticosteroid biosynthesis and destroys adrenocortical cells secreting cortisol. The cytotoxic effect of mitotane has been considered transient and inconsistent. Included in its effects is the destruction of the adrenocortical cells. The part that is most affected by this action is the zona reticularis and the least is the zona glomerulosa. Forty percent of the medication is absorbed from the gastrointestinal tract. The drug is highly lipid-soluble and subsequently is concentrated in both normal and malignant adrenocortical cells. Reports of its plasma half-life range from 18 to 159 days.

    (i) **Dosage and administration.** Treatment with mitotane is started at 2–6 gm/day PO in 3 divided doses, then gradually increased monthly by 1 gm/day until 9–10 gm/day is reached or until the maximum tolerated dose is achieved with no side effects. Blood levels of o,p-DDD should be maintained at more than 14 μg/ml to demonstrate a therapeutic response. Levels of more than 20 μg/ml have a higher incidence of toxicity.

    (ii) **Response and follow-up.** Objective tumor regression usually occurs within 6 weeks after the initiation of therapy and is seen in 70% of patients as a decrease in excessive hormone production. However, the reduction in hormone production is not regularly accompanied by an objective tumor response. In about 30–40% of patients, the tumor size is reduced significantly but complete remission is unlikely. The median duration of response is 10.5 months. If no clinical benefit is demonstrated at the maximum tolerated dose after 3 months, the case may be considered a clinical failure. Postoperative adjuvant therapy with mitotane has resulted in no improvement in survival. The combination of mitotane and radiation therapy has not conferred any additional benefit over mitotane alone.

    (iii) **Side effects.** Nausea and vomiting occur in 80% of patients. Severe neurotoxicity, which may occur during long-term treatment, presents as somnolence, depression, ataxia, and weakness in 60% of patients. Reversible diffuse electroencephalographic (EEG) changes may also occur. Adrenal insufficiency occurs in 50% of patients (without replacement), and dermatitis develops in 20% of patients. As the maximal dosage is often limited by the severity of, and the patient's tolerance to, the side effects, the total dose may range widely from patient to patient.

(iv) Glucocorticoid replacement. During mitotane treatment, it is necessary to prevent hypoadrenalism. Replacement can be achieved by administering cortisone acetate 25 mg PO in the morning and 12.5 mg PO in the evening plus fludrocortisone acetate 0.1 mg PO in the morning. Plasma cortisol rather than 17-hydroxycorticosterol should be used to monitor adrenal function during mitotane use. If severe trauma or shock develops, mitotane should be discontinued immediately and larger doses of corticosteroids (e.g., hydrocortisone 100 mg tid) should be administered.

(v) Nonresponders to mitotane. These patients can be treated with other adrenocortical suppressants, including metyrapone (75 mg PO q4h) or aminoglutethimide (250 mg PO q6h initially, with a stepwise increase in dosage to a total of 2 gm/day or until limiting side effects that resemble those of mitotane appear). The latter drug inhibits conversion of cholesterol to pregnenolone. Metyrapone can induce hypertension and hypokalemic alkalosis. Neither of these medications have antitumor effects, but they are effective in relieving the signs and symptoms of excessive hormonal secretion. Another medication that can be used is ketoconazole 200–600 mg/day. It is a potent adrenal inhibitor that produces clinical alleviation of the signs and symptoms within 4–6 weeks. In addition, it may cause regression of pulmonary and hepatic metastases though the mechanism is not clear. Other drugs that might be of benefit in controlling symptoms include those that block the action of steroids in their target tissues, e.g., antimineralocorticoid and antiandrogenic agents

and more recently antiglucocorti-
coid agents, e.g., mifepristone (RU
486). None of these medications
has an effect on tumor regression.

(2) **Cytotoxic chemotherapy.** This therapy is
usually used in patients who show no response to mitotane. Because of the small
number of patients who require such therapy, the experience with this treatment is
limited despite many clinical trials. No cytotoxic drug has shown definite effectiveness in the treatment of adrenocortical
carcinoma, although doxorubicin, cisplatin,
and suramin have been reported to produce
partial responses in patients with metastatic disease. Few combination chemotherapy
regimens have been effective. Cyclophosphamide 600 mg/m^2 IV + doxorubicin 40 mg/m^2
IV + cisplatin 50 mg/m^2 IV given in cycles
every 3 weeks led to partial remission in 2 of
11 patients with adrenocortical carcinoma.
The only combination that induced complete
remission is cisplatin 40 mg/m^2 IV + etoposide 100 mg/m^2 IV + bleomycin 30 units IV
given every 4 weeks. Three of 4 patients responded, 1 with complete remission. Severe
side effects occurred in patients in both of
these studies.

Chemotherapy can also be given in combination with mitotane. Cisplatin 75–100
mg/m^2 was combined with mitotane 4 gm PO
daily. This resulted in a 30% objective response that lasted for 7.9 months. The survival duration in this study was 11.8 months.
Other combinations of natural product chemotherapy with mitotane are being tested;
this may be pharmacologically advantageous, because mitotane has been shown to
be a multidrug resistance (MDR) blocking
agent.

d. **Arterial embolization.** Another modality used
for palliation of adrenocortical carcinoma is arterial embolization. It is used to decrease the
bulk of the tumor, suppress tumor function, and
relieve pain. Embolic agents used include polyvi-
nyl alcohol foam and surgical gelatin.

B. **Pheochromocytoma**

1. **Description and diagnosis.** Pheochromocytoma is
a tumor that arises from chromaffin cells mainly in
the adrenal medulla (90% of cases), as well as other
places (e.g., the urinary bladder, heart, and organ of
Zuckerkandl). It is an uncommon tumor, with an estimated 800 cases diagnosed in the United States
every year. It is found in up to 0.3% of autopsied subjects and is responsible for fewer than 0.1–0.5% of all
cases of hypertension. Pheochromocytoma can be he-

reditary, as part of the MEN syndrome (MEN-IIa, MEN-IIb), or familial with no other manifestation of the MEN syndrome, and when part of the syndrome it is never malignant. The risk of developing a contralateral tumor in hereditary pheochromocytoma is more than 50%. The incidence of malignant pheochromocytoma ranges between 5 and 45%. Although it may be difficult to differentiate between benign and malignant pheochromocytoma on the basis of pathologic criteria, cells in malignant pheochromocytomas are usually larger and have more mitoses with greater polyploidy than do those in benign pheochromocytoma. The only definite proof of malignancy is the presence of tumor in secondary sites where chromaffin tissue is not normally present. The diagnosis of pheochromocytoma depends on a thorough history and physical examination, increased catecholamine levels in the plasma and the urine (including epinephrine, norepinephrine, dopamine, total metanephrines, and vanillylmandelic acid), an abnormal result on the clonidine suppression test, cross-sectional imaging such as with CT or MRI, and ^{131}I-metaiodobenzylguanidine (MIBG) scintigraphy. The overall 5-year survival rate for malignant pheochromocytoma is 36–44%. Although pheochromocytoma is a rare tumor, early detection and treatment are crucial, owing to its high morbidity and potential mortality.

2. **Treatment**

   a. **Surgery.** Surgery is the only definitive therapy for pheochromocytoma. It is done for localized and regional unilateral or bilateral disease. Surgery requires careful preoperative preparation to achieve control of the blood pressure, blood volume, and heart rate. Phenoxybenzamine, an alpha-adrenergic blocker, is started 1–2 weeks prior to surgery in a dose of 10–20 mg PO 3–4 times a day. Some patients require the addition of beta blockers, e.g., propranolol 80–120 mg/day, which are indicated for persistent supraventricular tachycardia or the presence of angina. To prevent hypertensive crisis secondary to unopposed vasoconstriction, the beta blocker should never be given prior to the alpha antagonist. Other alpha-adrenergic blockers are used for the same purpose, including prazocin, which is a selective alpha-1 antagonist that has also been used successfully for preoperative preparation of pheochromocytoma. Intraoperatively, blood pressure can be controlled by titration with nitroprusside. Postoperatively, blood pressure is best controlled with diuretics.

   Catecholamine levels should be measured 1 week following surgery to confirm total removal of the tumor. Operative mortality should be less than 2–3%. Patients whose localized disease is fully resected should have normal life expectancy. Close postoperative follow-up is mandatory because of the possibility of postoperative residual tumor, and because 10% of patients have metastasis and another 10% have multiple primary tumors at the time of diagnosis.

The follow-up should include a history and physical examination and catecholamine measurements every 3 months for a year, then every 6 months for another year, followed by a similar evaluation yearly for life. Redevelopment of any sign or symptom suggesting pheochromocytoma or a rising trend in catecholamine levels requires imaging, including ^{131}I MIBG scintigraphy. Some groups recommend that ^{131}I MIBG scintigraphy be done yearly regardless of the catecholamine levels or the clinical picture. The recurrence rate of pheochromocytoma postoperatively is 5% per year. Contralateral adrenalectomy of a normal gland is generally not recommended in patients with a high incidence of bilateral disease (e.g., MEN-II), despite the high risk for subsequent involvement. In patients with metastatic disease, there is no evidence to support improved survival after local debulking.

b. **Chemotherapy and radiation therapy.** These are reserved for locally invasive, metastatic, and inoperable lesions. Response to both of these treatments is evaluated by regression of tumor size and a decrease in the catecholamine levels. Owing to the small number of patients with pheochromocytoma, limited data are available regarding the effect of chemotherapy. Because of the functional and biologic similarities between pheochromocytoma and neuroblastoma, the combination of cyclophosphamide and dacarbazine, which induces an 80% response in neuroblastoma, was used in two series to treat pheochromocytoma. The chemotherapy regimen consisted of cyclophosphamide 750 mg/m^2 IV plus vincristine 1.4 mg/m^2 IV on day 1 and dacarbazine 600 mg/m^2 IV on days 1 and 2; it was repeated in 21- to 28-day cycles. Analysis of 23 patients showed objective tumor size regression in 61% of patients, and the urinary catecholamine levels decreased in 74% of patients. The median response time averaged 28 months. Improvement of blood pressure control and performance status occurred with minimal toxicity. Because streptozocin has yielded favorable results in the treatment of neuroendocrine tumor in the gastrointestinal tract, it was used as a single agent in a patient with malignant pheochromocytoma. Streptozocin showed promising results, with a 73% reduction in urinary vanillylmandelic acid level and significant tumor size regression.

c. **Radiation therapy.** MIBG is actively taken up and concentrated by pheochromocytoma cells with high sensitivity and specificity. Consequently, a high dose of ^{131}I MIBG is used to treat pheochromocytoma. This treatment has shown some evidence of response in terms of tumor size regression and decreased catecholamine levels. The uptake of MIBG by pheochromocytoma requires the presence of an active neuronal pump mechanism, which limits the use of this agent to patients with pheochromocytoma who have the ability to concentrate ^{131}I MIBG in the cells. Therefore, initial screening of the ability of the pheochromocytoma to concentrate small doses of ^{131}I MIBG is necessary to determine the probable efficacy of the treatment.

d. **Supportive pharmacologic therapy.** Alpha blockers should be used to prevent severe hypertension-related morbidity and mortality, especially in untreated patients or those receiving chemotherapy. Another pharmacologic agent that can be used is α-methyl-L-tyrosine (metyrosine), which inhibits tyrosine hydroxylase, a rate-limiting step in catecholamine biosynthesis. Metyrosine allows the use of lower doses of alpha blockers, and has been shown to be effective in catecholamine-induced cardiomyopathy. Other medications include beta blockers which are used to control arrhythmias; angiotensin-converting enzyme (ACE) inhibitors; and calcium channel blockers, which are also used for hypertension control.

Selected Readings

Thyroid Carcinoma

Ahuja, S., and Ernst, H. Chemotherapy of thyroid carcinoma. *J. Endocrinol. Invest.* 10:303, 1987.

Bierwaltes, W. H., et al. An analysis of "ablation of thyroid remnants" with I-131 in 511 patients from 1947–1984 experience at University of Michigan. *J. Nucl. Med.* 25:1287, 1984.

Blahd, W. H. Management of thyroid cancer. *Compr. Ther.* 19(5):197, 1993.

Cady, B., and Rossi, R. An expanded view of risk group definition in differentiated thyroid carcinoma. *Surgery* 104:945, 1988.

Colson, Y. L., et al. Medullary thyroid carcinoma. *Am. J. Otolaryngol.* 14(20):73, 1993.

Doria, R., et al. Thyroid lymphoma. *Cancer* 73:200, 1993.

Hay, I. D., and Klee, G. G. Thyroid cancer diagnosis and management. *Clin. Lab. Med.* 13:725, 1993.

Hoskin, P. J., and Harmer, C. Chemotherapy for thyroid cancer. *Radiother. Oncol.* 10:187, 1987.

Liung, S. F., et al. Efficacy of low dose iodine-131 ablation of post-operative thyroid remnants: a study of 69 cases. *Br. J. Radiol.* 65:905, 1992.

Schlumberger, M., et al. Long-term results of treatment of 283 patients with lung and bone metastases from differentiated thyroid carcinoma. *J. Clin. Endocrinol. Metab.* 63:960, 1986.

Shiamoka, K., et al. A randomized trial of doxorubicin versus doxorubicin plus cisplatin with advanced thyroid carcinoma. *Cancer* 56:2155, 1985.

Adrenocortical Carcinoma

Bukowski, R. M., et al. Phase II trial of mitotane and cisplatin in patients with adrenal carcinoma: a Southwest Oncology Group study. *J. Clin. Oncol.* 11:161, 1993.

Carpenter, P. C. Mitotane failure in adrenocortical cancer: where next? *Cancer* 71:2900, 1993.

Dunnick, R. N. Adrenal carcinoma. *Radiol. Clin. North Am.* 31:99, 1994.

Haak, H. R., et al. Optimal treatment of adrenocortical carcinoma with mitotane: results in a consecutive series of 96 patients. *Br. J. Cancer* 69:947, 1994.

Haq, M. M., et al. Cytotoxic chemotherapy in adrenal cortical carcinoma. *Cancer Treat. Rep.* 64:909, 1980.

Luton, J. P., et al. Clinical features of adrenocortical carcinoma, prognostic factors, and the effect of mitotane therapy. *N. Engl. J. Med.* 322:1195, 1990.

Medeiros, J. L., and Weiss, L. M. New development in the pathologic diagnosis of the adrenal cortical neoplasm. *Am. J. Clin. Pathol.* 97:73, 1992.

Page, D. L., DeLellis, R. A., and Hough, A. J. Tumors of the Adrenal. In W. H. Hartmann, L. H. Sobin (eds.), *Atlas of Tumor Pathology.* Washington, D.C.: Armed Forces Institute of Pathology, 1986.

Pommier, R. F., and Brennan, M. F. An eleven year experience with adrenocortical carcinoma. *Surgery* 112:963, 1992.

Wooten, M. D., et al. Adrenal cortical carcinoma. Epidemiology and treatment with mitotane and review of the literature. *Cancer* 72:3145, 1993.

Pheochromocytoma

Averbuch, S. D., et al. Neoplasm of the Neuroendocrine System. In J. F. Holand et al. (eds.), *Cancer Medicine* (3rd ed.). Philadelphia: Lea & Febiger, 1993. Pp. 1153–1180.

Bravo, E. L., et al. Pheochromocytoma. *Endocrinol. Metab. Clin. North Am.* 20:329, 1993.

Feldmann, J. M. Treatment of metastatic pheochromocytoma with streptozotocin. *Arch. Intern. Med.* 143:1799, 1983.

Keiser, H. R., et al. Treatment of malignant pheochromocytoma with combination chemotherapy. *Hypertension* 7:I18, 1985.

Manger, M., et al. Pheochromocytoma: current diagnosis and management. *Cleve. Clin. J. Med.* 60:365, 1993.

Sclumberger, M., et al. Malignant pheochromocytoma: clinical, biologic, histologic and therapeutic data in a series of 20 patients with distant metastasis. *J. Endocrinol. Invest.* 15:631, 1992.

Shapro, B., et al. Malignant pheochromocytoma: effective treatment with a combination of cyclophosphamide, vincristine, and dacarbazine. *Ann. Intern. Med.* 109:267, 1988.

Melanomas and Other Skin Malignancies

Larry Nathanson

I. Melanoma
A. Introduction
1. Natural history

a. Origin and occurrence. The normal precursor cell of malignant melanoma is the melanocyte. During embryologic development these cells differentiate in the neural crest and migrate to the skin and eye. In adults they are responsible for the formation of skin pigment. About 10% of melanomas occur in some extradermal site, primarily in the eye, mucous membrane, anus, or external genitalia. The incidence of the disease has tripled since the early 1970s, with a current lifetime risk in the general population of about 0.7%. This striking increase in incidence, the largest of any cancer in the United States, is presumably due to increased exposure to actinic radiation, particularly in the ultraviolet B spectrum. Melanoma is equally prevalent in men and women, and its peak age of incidence is during the sixth decade. Early recognition and early diagnosis of this disease result in prompt and curative surgical management.

b. Precursor lesions and familial melanoma. Congenital and dysplastic nevi may be precursor lesions for melanoma. Although the dysplastic nevi may be sporadic or familial, they constitute markers of increased risk for melanoma. Attention should be paid to careful follow-up of patients and families with dysplastic nevi whether or not there is a history of melanoma. Early excision of suspect lesions may result in prevention of disease that might otherwise prove fatal.

c. Types of primary lesions. There are four major types of cutaneous melanoma. In order of increasing aggressiveness, they are lentigo maligna melanoma, superficial spreading melanoma, nodular melanoma, and palmar-plantar-mucosal melanoma. These lesions vary in size from the larger lentigos ($\geq$ 5 cm) to the smaller, palpable nodular melanoma. When the lesions become actively malignant, they share a characteristic history of recent growth in association with one or more of these signs or symptoms: change in pigmentation, ulceration, itching, or bleeding. On examination, they share a tendency to have absent hair follicles, irregular margins, and variegated coloring in hues of blue, red, or white. These signs help distinguish them from benign nevi.

Persons who have fair complexion, intermittent intense sun exposure in childhood, more than 40 benign nevi, dysplastic nevi, family history of melanoma, or other risk factors should be counseled in prevention, including use of sunscreens and protective clothing.

d. **Metastasis.** At initial presentation, up to 25% of patients have disease that has clinically spread beyond the local lesion. In about one-half of these patients, the disease has spread no further than regional nodes. In the other half, there is evidence of distant metastasis. Of the patients who do not have metastatic melanoma at presentation, about one-sixth subsequently develop metastasis. Of these patients, one-fifth experience metastases in soft tissues alone (lymph nodes, skin, subcutaneous tissue). In the other four-fifths, metastases appear in other tissues and organs (particularly liver, lung, brain, or bone) alone or together with soft-tissue disease. Forty-five percent of patients with melanoma that is not cured develop central nervous system (CNS) metastases during the course of the disease.

e. **Ocular melanoma,** the most common malignancy of the eye in adults, is one type of melanoma that deserves special mention. Although enucleation was the standard therapy for primary ocular melanoma, studies are now under way to evaluate use of local radiotherapy with or without sight-preserving surgery. When metastatic (usually to the liver), the same therapy as described for cutaneous melanoma is employed. It is said by some that metastatic ocular melanoma is less chemosensitive than that of cutaneous origin. Further discussion of this type of melanoma is beyond the scope of this chapter.

2. **Staging.** Melanomas are staged based on the thickness of the primary tumor and the extent of spread (Table 19-1). Clinical staging is often difficult because of the poor resolution of diagnostic radiologic studies. All patients should have a complete history and physical examination. Particular attention should be paid to examination of the regional lymph nodes and of all cutaneous and assessable mucous membrane areas. A chemistry profile may give clues to bony or hepatic metastasis. A chest x-ray study is relatively inexpensive and should be done to ensure that there are no apparent pulmonary metastases. In addition, in patients at high risk for advanced disease (e.g., tumor thickness > 3.0 mm), radionuclide scans, sonograms, computed tomography (CT), and magnetic resonance imaging (MRI) of the head and body may be helpful staging procedures, but are only cost-effective when signs, symptoms, or screening blood tests demonstrate an abnormality. MRI utilizing optimal technology has been demonstrated to be

Table 19-1. Staging and prognosis in malignant melanoma

Stage	TNM	Site	Approximate 5-year survival rate
		Primary tumor thickness (mm)	
I	pT1	< 0.75	97
	pT2	0.75–1.50	90
II	pT3a	1.5–3.0	80
	pT3b	3.0–4.0	70
	pT4a	> 4.0	40
	pT4b	Local (satellite) metastases (< 2 cm from primary)	48
		Regional metastases	
III	N1	Lymph nodes ≤ 3 cm	40
	N2a	Lymph node > 3 cm	15
	N2b	In transit metastases*	30
	N2c	Both N2a and N2b	15
		Distant metastases	
IV	M1a	Skin, subcutaneous, lymph node	10
	M1b	Visceral	5

*Cutaneous or subcutaneous lesions > 2 cm from the primary tumor.

a more specific and sensitive test for CNS metastasis than is CT. Gallium scanning and lymphangiography are occasionally useful.

3. **Surgical treatment and prognosis.** Standard treatment for melanoma is initial excisional biopsy and wide excision (1–2-cm tumor-free margin) of the primary lesion. Routine prophylactic regional lymph node dissection has not proved to increase survival. Retrospective data, however, strongly suggest benefit following lymph node dissection in the patient with a primary lesion thickness of 1.5–4.0 mm. Visual identification of a "sentinel" node by use of lymphoscintograph and patent blue-V or isosulfan blue dye on biopsied frozen section has been used to predict which lymph node drains the cutaneous site of a primary melanoma. This procedure may determine whether node dissection is necessary, and which nodes to dissect when there may be multiple possible draining node groups. The prognosis of an excised primary lesion varies inversely according to the thickness of the lesion (see Table 19-1). The prognosis is also better in women and for primary cutaneous lesions of the extremities (compared with trunk, head, or neck). Survival decreases sharply as the extent of disease increases. Surgery is occasionally indicated in the patient with metastatic disease,

especially with an asymptomatic solitary lesion of the brain, lung, or elsewhere.

B. Chemotherapeutic interventions

  1. Systemic therapy

   a. Patient selection. When patients with metastatic melanomas are considered for chemotherapy, favorable clinical factors predicting the likelihood of chemotherapeutic response must be kept in mind. These factors include the following.

   (1) Good performance status (Eastern Cooperative Oncology Group [ECOG] 0–2)

   (2) Soft-tissue disease or a relatively small number of visceral sites (pulmonary metastases are most sensitive)

   (3) Youth (< 65 years old)

   (4) No prior chemotherapy

   (5) Normal hemogram and normal hepatic and renal function

   (6) Absence of CNS metastases

   b. Single-agent chemotherapy. A number of single agents have been found to have antitumor activity against melanoma. The response rates to these agents vary widely as reported by various authors. It must be emphasized that despite these reports, metastatic melanoma remains one of the neoplasms most refractory to chemotherapy, and asymptomatic patients achieve a few months' gain in survival at best.

   (1) Dacarbazine (DTIC), the standard single agent for treatment of this disease, is usually given at a dose of 200 mg/m^2 IV on days 1–5 every 3 weeks or 750 mg/m^2 IV on day 1 every 6 weeks. The response rate is 20–25%.

   (2) Nitrosoureas have each been used for melanoma and probably have similar efficacy.

    (a) Carmustine (BCNU) 150 mg/m^2 IV every 6 weeks *or*

    (b) Lomustine (CCNU) 100–130 mg/m^2 PO every 3–6 weeks.

    These regimens are the most commonly used, and each has a response rate of 15–20%.

   (3) Platinum-containing drugs. Cisplatin 100 mg/m^2 IV every 3 weeks or carboplatin 400 mg/m^2 every 3 weeks appear to have similar efficacy. The dose may be cautiously escalated for optimal response.

   (4) Paclitaxel (Taxol), dactinomycin, ifosfamide (+ mesna), alkylating agents, vinca alkaloids, and procarbazine have response rates of 10–15%.

   (5) Very high-dose chemotherapy with either carmustine or melphalan with or without **autologous bone marrow transplantation** is now being evaluated; initial studies have not been promising.

Table 19-2. Combination chemotherapy for malignant melanoma

Regimen	Dosage
PDB-T *or* PDB-M	Cisplatin (Platinol) 30 mg/m² IV on days 1–3 and 22–24
	Dacarbazine (DTIC) 220 mg/m² IV on days 1–3 and 22–24
	Carmustine (BCNU) 150 mg/m² IV on day 1 Repeat cycle every 6 weeks *plus*
	Tamoxifen 10 mg bid PO continuously *or* megestrol acetate 40 mg qid PO continuously Repeat cycle every 6 weeks
VDP	Vinblastine 5 mg/m² IV on days 1 and 2
	Dacarbazine 150 mg/m² IV on days 1–5
	Cisplatin 75 mg/m² IV on day 5 Repeat cycle every 3 weeks
DTIC-Act-D	Dacarbazine (DTIC) 750 mg/m² IV on day 1
	Dactinomycin (actinomycin D) 1 mg/m² IV on day 1 Repeat cycle every 4 weeks

    c. Multiple-agent chemotherapy. A number of chemotherapeutic combinations have been used for melanoma. Some of the regimens with data from significant numbers of patients are listed in Table 19-2. Although definitive studies have not been completed, the substitution of carboplatin for cisplatin in the above-mentioned combinations may give just as good results while avoiding the nephrotoxicity and neurotoxicity associated with that drug.

      (1) PDB-T. The first combination listed employs cisplatin, dacarbazine, carmustine, and tamoxifen. This drug combination is associated with a 55% objective response rate and a median survival time of 10 months (more in responding patients). A similar regimen utilizing megestrol (Megace) instead of the tamoxifen plus the same chemotherapy has been reported, with a 56% objective response rate and 12.5-month median duration of survival.

      (2) DTIC-Act-D. Dactinomycin and dacarbazine are given together in large single-pulse doses approximately every 3–4 weeks. This combination was reported by the Southwest Oncology Group to have a response rate of approximately 30–40%, but the median survival time is only 8–10 months.

      (3) Vinblastine, dacarbazine, and cisplatin. This combination has achieved a 35–45% objective response rate in patients with advanced disease. The median survival time is similar to that for regimens previously mentioned.

One of the major problems with these programs has been the high incidence of relapse in the CNS, a metastatic site that tends to respond poorly to chemotherapy. Any of the regimens in Table 19-2 should be considered if the patient has a good performance status and can be expected to tolerate an intensive chemotherapy regimen.

2. Regional chemotherapy

a. Infusion and perfusion.
Arteriovenous isolation with perfusion chemotherapy has long been used in patients with regional melanoma, particularly that confined to the lower extremities. A variety of drugs have been employed and include the alkylating agents (especially nitrogen mustard and melphalan) and more recently dacarbazine and carmustine. The perfusate is heated (usually to 40°C) in most studies (see also the discussion in sec. **I.D.**). This therapy should only be done by those who have specific training and experience in the technique.

Intraarterial infusion has been carried out with the previously mentioned drugs, as well as with doxorubicin or cisplatin. This treatment is technically much easier than perfusion. It may represent the optimal treatment for patients with regional extremity disease, especially when used with external tourniquet control, or dominant hepatic metastasis.

b. Intracavitary chemotherapy.
Intracavitary thiotepa, doxycycline, or bleomycin may be of benefit in reducing the rate of progression of malignant pleural or peritoneal effusions. Colloidal gold (^{98}Au) or chromic phosphate (^{32}P) is occasionally helpful for this complication. Each of these drugs should be administered through an indwelling chest tube, as described in Chapter 36.

3. Hormones.
The use of hormones for treating melanoma has been suggested by the discovery that some melanoma tumor cells contain cortisol-binding protein receptors.

a. Megestrol
may have antitumor effects in melanoma as demonstrated in a randomized study where adjuvant megestrol alone increased survival in patients with stage II or III melanoma compared to nontreated control subjects.

b.
The use of **tamoxifen** with chemotherapy is an example of possible clinical synergy, and may represent the ability of this drug to abrogate the multidrug resistance phenotype.

4. Retinoids.
These agents inhibit pigment formation and slow tumor growth in a variety of experimental melanomas. This technique is experimental in humans.

5. **Radiopotentiating agents.** These may have a place in the treatment of melanoma. For example, the use of cisplatin may potentiate the antitumor effects of radiation. Hyperthermia either alone or as a radiopotentiator has been shown to have anti-tumor effects on superficial lesions of metastatic melanomas.

6. **Antipigmentary chemotherapy.** Antipigmentary chemotherapy, particularly with drugs that are tyrosinase inhibitors or that may inhibit cysteine incorporation into nucleic acid polymerases, has anti-tumor effects on experimental melanomas. These drugs include alpha-methyl-L-tyrosine (metyrosine, Demser), 6-hydroxydopa, pimozide, and 4-hydroxy-anisole. Their efficacy has not yet been demonstrated in any clinical study.

C. **Biologic response modifiers (BRMs).** BRMs have been used to treat gross or microscopic metastatic disease as initial therapy, together with chemotherapy either simultaneously or in a planned sequence, or following chemotherapy failure. Whether it is better to use chemotherapy or BRM therapy first probably depends on the stage of the disease. Combination chemotherapy regimens have a higher response rate than does interferon alone in metastatic disease. Conversely, chemotherapy has no demonstrable effectiveness as an adjuvant after surgery in high-risk patients, but there are indications that BRM therapy may delay recurrences. The toxicity of higher-dose regimens of interleukin (IL)-2 makes it undesirable as the initial standard therapy.

1. **Recombinant interferon alpha (IFN-α)** gives a 5–15% objective response. Interferon is used alone and in combination with chemotherapy. Doses of IFN-α range from 3×10^6 to 10×10^6 IU SQ, with dose frequency ranging from 3 times weekly to daily. There are conflicting data on the question of additive or synergistic effects of IFN-α and chemotherapy.

2. **Interleukin (IL)-2,** a potent lymphokine, has been used with or without lymphokine-activated killer (LAK) cells for melanoma. This treatment is toxic and requires special facilities for its use in the more commonly used high-dose regimens. The development of continuous infusion schedules and low-dose bolus schedules for IL-2 diminishes toxicity. Substitution of tumor-infiltrating lymphocytes (TILs) for LAK cells may have more potent tumor lytic activity.

   Response rates in these treatments vary from 20 to 50%. The use of IL-2 plus IFN-α may be more effective and less toxic than use of either agent alone. Combinations of cisplatin, vinblastine, and dacarbazine (CVD) chemotherapy with IL-2 and IFN-α (interferon alfa-2a starting on the first day of IL-2) treatment have been reported to be more effective than the use of CVD alone if CVD is given immediately prior to IL-2 + IFN-α.

D. **Adjuvant therapy.** A variety of chemotherapy and BRM therapy programs have been used in patients with high-risk primary melanoma (lesion thickness > 1.5 mm) or patients with node metastasis. The efficacy of adjuvant chemotherapy in this setting is controversial. A prospective randomized adjuvant study of 107 hyperthermic chemotherapy perfusions found a statistically significant superior survival rate in patients with primary melanoma, stages I, II, or III, in an extremity.

A large recent (ECOG) prospective randomized study of IFN-α (interferon alfa-2b) 20 × 10^6 IU/m^2 IV 5 days a week for 4 weeks, then 10 × 10^6 IU/m^2/day SQ 3 times a week for 48 weeks, showed a statistically significant increase in disease-free survival time in treated (41 months) than in control (19 months) patients. Ninety-one percent of these patients had pathologic stage III (regional node–positive) disease and only 9% had T4 primary cutaneous melanoma only, thickness > 4.0 mm. There was no difference in survival at 41-month median follow-up time. Another (World Health Organization) study utilizing IFN-α 3 × 10^6 IU/m^2 seems to confirm these findings.

E. **Other regional therapy**
1. **Brain metastases.** Melanoma of the CNS has been a particularly difficult problem and is a relatively common occurrence. The standard approach is radiotherapy to the whole brain in one of several dosage schedules accompanied initially by corticosteroids. The use of high-dose fractions (400–800 cGy) may be somewhat superior to conventional radiotherapy but does not increase survival. Some patients may respond for long periods to CNS radiotherapy, particularly if no other visceral site is involved. A new nitrosourea, fotemustine (100 mg/m^2 IV), used in Europe produced a significant objective response rate in patients with CNS metastases.
2. **Intralesional immunotherapy.** Intralesional immunotherapy, particularly with bacillus Calmette-Guérin (BCG), lymphokines, or interferon, according to a number of reports controlled both injected and uninjected regional intradermal metastases (satellitosis). Although this treatment is not applicable to patients who have distant disease or bulky regional disease, in patients with early recurrence it may produce long disease-free survival periods. Occasional cases of systemic BCG infection occurring with this treatment are usually easy to control with antituberculous chemotherapy.
3. **Radiotherapy.** This may be helpful in controlling circumscribed and symptomatic extra-CNS lesions such as painful bony metastases.

II. **Nonmelanoma skin cancer**
A. **Etiology and epidemiology.** Nonmelanoma skin cancer is the most common malignancy in the United

States, with an estimated number of new cases in excess of 700,000 annually in the United States.

The most common types of skin cancer are basal cell carcinoma (BCC) (or epithelioma) and squamous cell carcinoma (SCC). This summary excludes other types of skin tumor such as mycosis fungoides, tumors of the skin appendages, and Kaposi's sarcoma (see Chap. 29). BCC and SCC are more common in men than in women. Like melanoma, SCC is increasing in incidence in the United States. The most frequent etiologic factor is exposure to actinic radiation. Accordingly, individuals with fair skin and light hair and eyes tend to have a high incidence of the diseases. In addition, it is more common on the lower extremities in the female, and on the ear in the male. Individuals with chronic sun exposure are at particular risk for this disease. Whites have a greater incidence than Asians, who in turn have a greater incidence than blacks. BCC is more common than SCC in whites, and SCC is more common than BCC in blacks. Multiple primary skin cancers can be seen in affected individuals. Other etiologic factors include exposure to x-rays, chronic scarring (especially from burns), chronic inflammatory states, and exposure to arsenic.

B. Actinic keratosis

   1. Natural history. Actinic keratoses (e.g., solar keratosis) are lesions found in the exposed areas of the skin. They are assumed to be precancerous, since SCCs may arise from them. In the patient predisposed to the development of such lesions, use of sun protective creams (e.g., p-aminobenzoic acid) and clothing may be an important preventive medical practice.

   2. Topical chemotherapy. Fluorouracil is used as a 1% solution or cream on the face and up to a 5% concentration on the arms. It is applied twice daily for 2–4 weeks by the patient rubbing it in with the fingertips. Care must be taken around the eyes, but the periorbital skin may be treated. Fluorouracil must be applied smoothly with avoidance of accumulated ointment in the nasolabial folds. After application, the hands must be washed. Erythema begins 3–7 days after treatment. The reaction progresses from erythema to scaling, erosion, and tenderness, at which time the application should be stopped. The reaction subsides rapidly, and lesions on the face heal within 2–6 weeks (a somewhat longer period for those on the arms). Repeated courses of fluorouracil may be used. An overly brisk reaction may be treated locally with topical steroids. Because topical steroids protect against the inflammatory effect of fluorouracil but do not diminish its antitumor effect, it seems likely that fluorouracil exerts its effects by a cytotoxic mechanism, rather than by a nonspecific inflammatory sloughing of superficial skin layers. Sloughing, however, may be in part from a local delayed hypersensitivity reaction.

C. Basal cell carcinoma

1. **Natural history.** The most common type of BCC is the noduloulcerative or "rodent ulcer" form. It presents as a well-defined nodule that has rolled, pearly or translucent borders traversed by telangiectases and a central concave area that is often ulcerated. Histologic subtypes of this tumor, including solid, keratotic, cystic, and adenoid varieties exist. Pigmented types, which may resemble malignant melanoma (pigmented basal cell epithelioma), are important because of this differential diagnosis. These lesions have a low metastatic potential, and 85% of them are present on the skin of the head and neck. In patients with neglected disease (0.1–0.2% of total patients) metastases may occur. Such metastases occur an average of 11 years after the primary lesion was first noted. Lymph nodes, lung, and bone may be involved in decreasing order of likelihood.

2. **Topical treatment.** Superficial surgery, electrodesiccation, chemosurgery, or radiation therapy (especially with electron beam) may be used on these lesions. The cure rate should be above 95% regardless of the technique employed. Chemosurgery employs the use of zinc chloride fixative paste (Mohs' technique).

   The use of fluorouracil in a topical solution or ointment, as described in sec. **II.B.2**, is usually reserved for patients with multiple or widespread lesions because of the efficacy of the nonchemotherapeutic techniques for treating localized disease. Deeply invasive tumors are not appropriately treated with fluorouracil because the drug penetrates only a few millimeters into the skin.

D. Squamous cell carcinoma

1. **Natural history.** SCC may occur at any site on the skin, as well as on mucous membranes, particularly on the lips, vulva, penis, and anus. The area from which SCC arises rarely appears normal but usually has the changes associated with actinic keratosis. The latter process may be considered an in situ state of SCC. A rough, scaly surface with thickening of the skin and often well-circumscribed macular changes are frequently present. A reddish, brownish, or grayish cast to the skin may also be present. Crusting, thickening, or ulceration strongly suggest malignant change. An indurated border is suggestive of malignancy.

   The primary lesion histopathologically is in the epidermis, with cells penetrating the dermis. Keratinization and epidermal pearl formation are often present. The degree of cellular differentiation, atypicality of cells, and depth of penetration of the tumor are prognostic factors.

   About 0.2% of patients develop metastatic tumors, and 90% of these metastases are to the lymph nodes only. Only one-half of patients with lymph node metastases and 60% of patients with distant metastases die within 5 years.

The exceptional lesions that arise in normal-appearing skin or in other preexisting lesions (scars of thermal, chemical, or radiation injury) tend to be more aggressive than those that arise in actinically damaged skin. Surgery by a variety of means is the conventional treatment of SCC, as it is for BCC. The choices include curettage and desiccation after biopsy. Radiation therapy, cryotherapy, and chemosurgery have also been used, and all produce cure rates in excess of 94%. Treatment of locally recurrent tumors is less satisfactory, and the importance of patients receiving prompt and adequate treatment early in the disease must be emphasized. As for BCC, the use of Mohs' chemosurgery with zinc chloride fixative paste may be highly effective in SCC.

2. **Topical chemotherapy.** Superficial SCCs may be effectively treated with 5% topical fluorouracil with relatively little toxicity and an essentially 100% cure rate. However, it is important with more invasive lesions to avoid the possibility that fluorouracil may fail to control microscopic islands of invasive SCC and, therefore, may delay appropriate therapy. When treatment of more invasive or noduloulcerative SCC is contemplated, 20% fluorouracil under occlusive dressings may be employed if standard therapy is refused or contraindicated. As a rule, treatment for at least 3 weeks is required, although at times, it is necessary to treat for up to 12 weeks.

E. **Multifocal tumors.** In patients who have widespread multifocal superficial tumors, as in xeroderma pigmentosum, chronic arsenic exposure, Bowen's disease (multiple intraepidermal squamous carcinomas), extensive or long-term extensive radiation dermatitis, or long-term extensive actinic changes, the use of surgical techniques may be impossible. In these patients, applications of dinitrochlorobenzene, purified protein derivative of tuberculin, streptokinase-streptodornase, or other agents may be clinically useful. These medications are applied in a topical fashion to large areas of the skin in increasing concentrations. They can produce selective lytic effects on malignant epidermal cells even when the cells are present in microscopic foci that otherwise would not be readily detectable. The allergic contact dermatitis that results from the application of these immunoadjuvants appears to destroy most microscopic BCC. Whether these allergic reactions are directly responsible for tumor lysis, or whether they simply result from an attraction of sensitized "killer" lymphocytes to the areas where microscopic deposits of epidermoid neoplastic epidermal cells are present, is not yet known. The fact that neoplastic epidermal cells are selectively killed has an important clinical implication. Scarring rarely develops from this type of treatment because normal epidermal cells remain viable and are not replaced by proliferating fibroblasts.

Selected Readings

Balch, C. M., et al. Efficacy of 2 cm surgical margins for intermediate-thickness melanomas (1–4 mm). Results of a multi-institutional randomized surgical trial. *Ann. Surg.* 218:262, 1993.

Carey, R. W., et al. Treatment of metastatic malignant melanoma with vinblastine, dacarbazine, and cisplatin: a report from the Cancer and Leukemia Group B. *Cancer Treat. Rep.* 70:329, 1986.

Clark, W. H., et al. Model predicting survival in stage I melanoma based on tumor progression. *J. Natl. Cancer Inst.* 81:1893, 1989.

Creagan, E. T., et al. A prospective randomized controlled trial of megestrol acetate among high risk patients with resected malignant melanoma. *Am. J. Clin. Oncol.* 12:152, 1989.

Dutcher, J. P., et al. A phase II study of interleukin-2 and lymphokine-activated killer cells in patients with metastatic malignant melanoma. *J. Clin. Oncol.* 7:477, 1989.

Ghussen, F., et al. The role of regional hyperthermic cytostatic perfusion in the treatment of extremity melanoma. *Cancer* 61:654, 1988.

Khayat, D., et al. Fotemustine: an overview of its clinical activity in malignant melanoma. *Melanoma Res.* 2:147, 1992.

Kirkwood, J., et al. A randomized controlled trial of high-dose IFN alfa-2b for high risk melanoma. The ECOG Trial EST 1684. *Proc. Am. Soc. Clin. Oncol.* 12:390, 1993.

Legha, S. S., Buzaid, A. C. Role of recombinant IL2, in combination with interferon-alfa and chemotherapy in the treatment of advanced melanoma. *Semin. Oncol.* 20:27, 1993.

Morton, D., et al. Technical details of intraoperative lymphatic mapping of early stage melanoma. *Arch. Surg.* 127:392, 1992.

Nathanson, L. (ed.), *Current Research and Clinical Management of Melanoma.* Boston: Kluwer Academic, 1993. Pp. 1–388.

Nathanson, L., et al. Chemohormone therapy of metastatic melanoma with megestrol acetate plus dacarbazine, carmustine, and cisplatin. *Cancer* 73:98, 1994.

Safai, B. Cancers of the Skin. In V. T. Devita, S. Hellman, and S. A. Rosenberg (eds.), *Cancer: Principles and Practice of Oncology* (4th ed.). Philadelphia: Lippincott, 1993. Pp. 1567–1611.

Primary and Metastatic Brain Tumors

Jane B. Alavi

I. Occurrence and tumor characteristics

A. Primary brain tumors

1. **Incidence.** Primary tumors of the brain result in 2–3% of all deaths caused by cancer. The overall incidence in the United States is about 5/100,000, but in children under age 14 the incidence is 6.5/100,000. These tumors account for about 20% of all cancers in children.

2. **Histology.** Most intracranial neoplasms arise from meningeal or neuroectodermal tissue. Meningiomas (which arise from the meninges) are generally benign and encapsulated and can be removed surgically. They are rarely malignant (sarcomatous), and chemotherapy has no role in their treatment. Gliomas account for two-thirds of primary brain tumors. They arise from astrocytes (astrocytoma and glioblastoma), oligodendroglia (oligodendroglioma), and the ependymal cells that line the ventricles (ependymoma). Medulloblastomas and primitive neuroectodermal tumors (pineoblastoma and cerebral neuroblastoma) arise from unknown precursor cells, are highly malignant, and have a propensity to spread via the cerebrospinal fluid (CSF) to the spinal cord.

   The astrocytomas occur with a broad range of histologic differentiation. The well-differentiated tumors can often be cured by surgery. The more highly malignant types—anaplastic astrocytoma and glioblastoma—are not curable. During childhood, two-thirds of the neoplasms are found in the cerebellum or brainstem, and the common histologic types are medulloblastoma, ependymoma, and low-grade astrocytoma. Fewer than 20% are glioblastoma. In contrast, primary tumors in adults are nearly always supratentorial, more than 50% are glioblastomas, and about 18% are meningiomas.

3. **Staging.** The astrocytomas remain localized to the brain throughout the disease course. Thus, staging is not necessary. The prognosis depends on the degree of histologic malignancy. For medulloblastomas, staging should include MRI of the spine and cytology examination of CSF.

B. Metastatic (secondary) brain tumors.
The overall incidence of metastatic tumors to the brain is higher than the incidence of primary brain tumors in adults. Approximately 20% of patients with cancer are found to have brain metastases at autopsy. The most common primary sites are the lung (all cell types) and breast. Metastases from melanoma, colorectal carcinoma, unknown primaries, and renal carcinoma occur less frequently.

Some rare tumors, such as choriocarcinomas, give rise to brain metastases with unusual frequency. Most brain metastases are found in the cerebral hemispheres, few are found in the cerebellum or midbrain, and most are multiple at the time of diagnosis. Meningeal metastases are seen less frequently, and the primary tumors are usually breast or lung cancers, lymphoma, or melanoma.

II. Approach to therapy: primary and metastatic brain tumors

A. Primary tumors

1. **Surgery.** Surgical removal depends on the location of the lesion, its size, and its propensity to infiltrate surrounding areas of the brain. Because gliomas tend to infiltrate normal brain tissue surrounding the obvious tumor mass, it is unusual to cure patients with surgery alone without resultant unacceptable neurologic deficits.

2. **Radiation therapy.** This form of therapy has a major role in the treatment of gliomas. The tumor dose must exceed 5000 cGy to achieve control. Partial brain irradiation is usually adequate. In the case of medulloblastomas, radiotherapy is applied to the entire neuraxis after surgical extirpation of the primary lesion because these tumors tend to metastasize by shedding cells into the CSF.

3. **Chemotherapy.** Chemotherapy is used to treat patients with the more malignant gliomas, including the anaplastic astrocytomas, anaplastic oligodendrogliomas, and glioblastoma multiforme. Because of the highly malignant features of medulloblastoma, chemotherapy is often used to treat this tumor.

4. **Supportive care.** Because of their location in the central nervous system (CNS), intracranial tumors can cause serious neurologic symptoms, including seizures, headaches, and impairment of mental, motor, and sensory function. This dysfunction is the result of the combined effects of the tumor and a variable degree of surrounding cerebral edema. Therapy is therefore directed toward reducing the edema as well as reducing the size of the malignant tumor mass.

B. Metastatic tumors

1. **Surgery.** Because metastatic cancers often do not extensively infiltrate the surrounding normal brain parenchyma, they can sometimes be easily resected. However, this measure should be attempted only when the metastasis is solitary as revealed by computed tomography (CT) or magnetic resonance imaging (MRI) and when the patient's cancer is under good control systemically. In these circumstances, surgery followed by radiotherapy results in a longer survival period than is produced by radiotherapy alone (40 versus 15 weeks for lung cancers).

2. **Radiation therapy.** Whole-brain irradiation is employed for metastatic cancers.

3. **Chemotherapy.** Chemotherapy probably has little

role in the treatment of cerebral metastases. The exception to this is that metastases from breast cancer sometimes respond well to the usual regimens for breast tumors. On the other hand, malignant meningeal infiltrates, also called *carcinomatous meningitis,* may respond to a combination of radiation therapy and intrathecal chemotherapy.

4. **Evaluation for a primary tumor.** Occasionally, a patient will present with brain metastases as the first manifestation of cancer. In most cases there is little benefit gained by an extensive search for the primary site, if the history, physical examination, chest x-ray film, blood cell count, and chemistry profile do not give a clue, since the prognosis for patients with brain metastases is generally quite poor. An exception to this rule should be made if the patient is a younger male in whom metastatic testicular cancer (and occasionally other germ cell tumors) can be cured despite brain metastases. In the younger male, measuring alpha-fetoprotein and beta-human chorionic gonadotropin (HCG) levels is warranted. In addition, small-cell lung cancer sometimes responds well to chemotherapy and radiation therapy. Therefore, it is reasonable to perform a chest CT scan and to biopsy any lung tumor, if the patient has a good performance status.

III. Chemotherapy
A. General considerations
1. **Special characteristics of primary brain tumors.** The blood supply to brain tumors is not homogeneous owing to poorly vascularized areas of central necrosis. The tumor vessels lack the normal blood-brain barrier, but at the more rapidly growing outer edge of the tumor the blood-brain barrier is mostly intact. Therefore, it has usually been assumed that the most effective chemotherapeutic agents are those that are lipid-soluble or with a relatively low molecular weight, such that they are able to cross the normal blood-brain barrier and achieve an adequate intracerebral concentration. Another requirement for the use of brain tumor chemotherapy is that it be able to achieve cell kill in a heterogeneous population of tumor cells as is found in malignant gliomas. An additional consideration is that a large percentage of the cells in gliomas appear to be in a resting state (G_0) and thus are relatively insensitive to cell cycle–active agents.

2. The two major **aims of therapy for gliomas** are to **reduce the neurologic deficit and to prolong useful and comfortable life** by reducing the tumor mass and associated edema. Surgical decompression, when possible, and radiation therapy are standard treatments. Adjuvant chemotherapy has been shown to prolong the survival of patients with anaplastic astrocytoma. Either carmustine (BCNU) or the PCV regimen (procarbazine, lomustine [CCNU], and vin-

cristine) is commonly used, starting simultaneously with or immediately after radiation, and continued for approximately 1 year.

There is little evidence that adjuvant chemotherapy improves the survival time (median of < 1 year) for glioblastoma. Survival has been shown to depend more on certain prognostic factors such as patient age, performance status at diagnosis, and the extent of surgical resection.

3. **Quality of life.** Quality of life is a complex issue with neurologic tumors because it depends largely on the type of deficit induced by the tumor (e.g., hemiparesis, aphasia, and inability to read or write). Treatment has been shown to improve quality of life somewhat.

4. **Response evaluation.** Responses are sometimes difficult to analyze because of symptoms due to edema, seizures, steroid therapy, and a fixed neurologic deficit from surgery. Nonetheless, regular neurologic examination with a scoring of the neurologic deficit and CT or MRI scans of the brain usually enable the physician to make an objective determination of response. Scans are repeated every 2–3 months for the first year and less frequently thereafter.

B. **Specific chemotherapy agents**

1. **Nitrosoureas.** Nitrosoureas have been the most effective drugs against malignant gliomas and medulloblastomas. As first-line agents, these drugs result in responses in 30–50% of patients, with a median duration of about 6 months. When administered to patients with glioma as an adjuvant to radiation therapy, carmustine or lomustine appears to prolong survival minimally, compared with radiation therapy alone. The major benefit may be to young and middle-aged adults or to those with anaplastic astrocytoma rather than glioblastoma.

    a. **Carmustine (BCNU).** This is given usually at a dose of 80 mg/m² IV daily for 3 days every 6–8 weeks.

    b. **Lomustine (CCNU).** Lomustine may be given at 130 mg/m² PO once every 6–8 weeks.

    c. **Duration.** Two cycles are usually administered for patients with recurrent tumors. If a response is observed clinically or by CT, the drug is continued until progression is noted or a total dose of 1200 mg/m² (of either drug) has been reached.

    d. **Precautions.** These drugs may produce severe and delayed myelotoxicity. Some investigators decrease the dose by 25% in patients over the age of 60. All patients should have frequent blood cell counts during treatment, and subsequent doses should be lowered if there is a significant nadir: white blood cell (WBC) count less than 2000/μl or platelet count less than 75,000/μl. Treatment to cumulative doses in excess of 1200 mg/m² may be associated with pulmonary fibrosis that is usually irreversible and sometimes fatal. Less common toxicities are hepatotoxicity, renal toxicity, and phlebitis or pain in the arm used for treatment.

2. **Combinations.** Vincristine and procarbazine are sometimes given together with a nitrosourea. The PCV regimen is a combination of procarbazine (60 mg/m^2 orally on days 8–21), lomustine (110 mg/m^2 orally on day 1), and vincristine (2 mg IV on days 8 and 29), repeated every 6–8 weeks. Other combination schedules have been used without clear advantage. Vincristine can be used at a dose of 1–2 mg/m^2 (maximum 2 mg) IV weekly for up to 4 weeks; procarbazine can be given at a dose of 100 mg/m^2 PO daily for 2 weeks followed by a 2-week rest. Doses of the latter should be reduced if given with a nitrosourea.

C. **Medulloblastoma: special considerations.** There is some evidence that adjuvant chemotherapy benefits high-risk patients (those with incomplete tumor resection, brain stem involvement, seeding to the subarachnoid space, or positive CSF cytology). One successful regimen consists of vincristine 1.5 mg/m^2 (maximum 2 mg) weekly during radiation therapy, followed by a 6-week break. This is then followed by lomustine 75 mg/m^2 PO on day 1, cisplatin 68 mg/m^2 IV on day 1, and vincristine 1.5 mg/m^2 (maximum 2 mg) IV weekly for weeks 1–3 (days 1, 8, and 15). Cycles of the three-drug combination are repeated every 6 weeks for a total of 8 cycles. This treatment results in considerable toxicity, especially pancytopenia and peripheral neuropathy. Patients must be followed very closely.

D. **Investigational therapy**
   1. **Recurrent glioma.** In most patients with recurrent tumor after radiation therapy and primary chemotherapy with a nitrosourea, second-line chemotherapy offers little benefit. However, if the patient is young and has a good performance status, phase II trials of several available agents can be considered. Partial objective and symptomatic response rates to salvage chemotherapy are usually 15–25%, but complete responses are almost never observed. The drugs with activity include cisplatin (60–90 mg/m^2), carboplatin (350–500 mg/m^2 every 3–4 weeks), and etoposide (100–120 mg/m^2/day for 3 days).
   2. **Newer approaches.** Newer modalities for brain tumors include administration of drugs into the internal carotid artery in order to achieve higher level doses. Intracarotid carmustine has been associated with severe ophthalmic and cerebral toxicity and cannot be recommended. Cisplatin by the intraarterial route does produce a large number of responses, but there is not yet evidence that this prolongs survival. Very-high-dose systemic chemotherapy with autologous bone marrow rescue is another investi-

gational approach. Interferons do not appear to be effective. Interleukins and lymphokine-activated killer (LAK) cells are being evaluated, but thus far there is little to suggest that biologic treatments are useful. Second surgical resection or bradytherapy may be used for localized recurrences.

E. **Meningeal carcinomatosis.** This is treated with radiation therapy to the symptomatic areas of the CNS (e.g., to the brain for cranial nerve dysfunction) together with intrathecal chemotherapy.

1. The most commonly used agent is **methotrexate** 12 mg/m^2 (maximum 15 mg) per dose once or twice a week until the cytologic examination shows clearing of the CSF, then once a month as maintenance.

2. **Alternative agents.** Thiotepa 2–10 mg/m^2, and cytosine arabinoside 30 mg/m^2 are alternatives.

3. **Administration.** Each of these chemotherapy agents should be freshly prepared in preservative-free diluent. Because drugs administered into the lumbar intrathecal space do not always reach the upper region of the spinal cord, it is preferable to give the agents into an Ommaya reservoir, which may be implanted under the scalp and connected by a catheter, through a burr hole, to the frontal horn of the lateral ventricle. This method permits easy access to the CSF, and achieves good drug levels throughout the CSF pathways. If the lumbar intrathecal route is used, it is recommended that the volume injected be larger than the volume withdrawn (e.g., withdraw 5 ml for analysis and inject 10 ml).

4. **Complications.** Complications of intrathecal chemotherapy include painful arachnoiditis and leukoencephalopathy. The latter is more likely to occur if the Ommaya catheter tip becomes lodged in the brain tissue rather than the lateral ventricle. Bone marrow suppression is not usually severe unless the patient undergoes spinal irradiation or systemic chemotherapy as well. Oral leucovorin can be given after the intrathecal methotrexate (10 mg leucovorin PO q6h × 6–8 doses, starting 24 hours after the methotrexate) to prevent marrow toxicity.

IV. **Treatment of cerebral edema**

A. **Corticosteroids.** These are usually started soon after the diagnosis of a brain tumor is established. Dexamethasone 10 mg IV followed by 4–10 mg q6h PO or IV reduces or eliminates the lethargy, headaches, visual blurring, and nausea caused by cerebral edema and also often reduces some of the focal neurologic signs and symptoms such as hemiparesis or dysphagia.

The corticosteroid dose may be tapered and stopped after radiation therapy is complete—and resumed if symptoms recur. The dose should be held at a level that maximizes therapeutic benefit and minimizes unwanted side effects (e.g., gastric irritation, sleeplessness, mood swings, cushingoid body features, increased appetite, and proximal myopathy). It is also advisable to suggest that patients take an antacid with the steroid and that they watch for the occurrence of oral and vaginal thrush, which can be effectively treated with nystatin (suspension or suppositories) or clotrimazole (lozenges or suppositories).

B. **Treatment of refractory cerebral edema**
  1. **When moderate doses of dexamethasone** do not effectively control cerebral edema, the dose may be increased transiently to 40 mg IV q4–6h. This dose should usually not be maintained longer than 48–72 hours.
  2. **An osmotic diuretic** in an urgent situation acts more rapidly than a corticosteroid.
     a. **Mannitol** 75–100 gm (as a 15–25% solution) is given by rapid infusion over 20–30 minutes and repeated at 6- to 8-hour intervals as needed.
     b. **Cautions and duration.** Careful monitoring of electrolytes, fluid intake and output, and body weight is essential to avoid dehydration. The osmotic diuresis may be discontinued when there is an improvement in the signs and symptoms of the cerebral edema and when the corticosteroids or other measures to reduce cerebral edema have taken effect.

V. **Seizure control.** Because the occurrence of seizures is common in patients with cerebral neoplasms, many physicians recommend starting all such patients on anticonvulsant therapy with phenytoin 300 mg/day, regardless of whether the patient has already experienced a seizure. Other oncologists treat only if the patient has had seizures or has undergone craniotomy. Anticonvulsants are used for every patient who has had a craniotomy, regardless of the seizure history. For those on long-term anticonvulsant therapy, it is important to check drug levels at intervals, especially after dosages of other medications are changed or new medications are added, because interaction between drugs occur and the therapeutic range is narrow.

Seizures are a particular problem after cisplatin therapy. They result from falling phenytoin levels and hypomagnesemia. The blood level of phenytoin should be checked daily for several days and magnesium should be replaced. If a patient cannot tolerate phenytoin or has poor seizure control, the best alternative is carbamazepine. The usual dose is 200 mg PO qid, but higher doses may be necessary and should be adjusted according to the anticonvulsant blood level. Phenobarbital 30 mg PO qid is another alternative.

Selected Readings

Boogard, W., et al. Meningeal carcinomatosis in breast cancer. Prognostic factors and influence of treatment. *Cancer* 67:1685, 1991.

Burger, P. C., et al. Glioblastoma multiforme and anaplastic astrocytoma. Pathologic criteria and prognostic implications. *Cancer* 56:1106, 1985.

Duffner, P. K., et al. Primitive neuroectodermal tumors of childhood. *J. Neurosurg.* 55:376, 1981.

Grossman, S. A., et al. Decreased phenytoin levels in patients receiving chemotherapy. *Am. J. Med.* 87:505, 1989.

Hubbard, J. L., et al. Adult cerebellar medulloblastoma: the pathological, radiographic, and clinical disease spectrum. *J. Neurosurg.* 70:536, 1989.

Kornblith, P. L., and Walker, M. Chemotherapy for malignant gliomas. *J. Neurosurg.* 68:1, 1988.

Kovnar, E. H., et al. Preirradiation cisplatin and etoposide in the treatment of high-risk medulloblastoma and other malignant embryonal tumors of the central nervous system: a phase II study. *J. Clin. Oncol.* 8:330, 1990.

Levin, V. A., et al. Superiority of post-radiotherapy adjuvant chemotherapy CCNU, procarbazine, and vincristine (PCV) over BCNU for anaplastic astrocytomas: NCOG 6G61 final report. *Int. J. Radiat. Oncol. Biol. Phys.* 18:321, 1990.

Mellet, L. B. Physicochemical consideration and pharmacokinetic behavior in delivery of drugs to the central nervous system. *Cancer Treat. Rep.* 61:527, 1977.

Packer, R. J., et al. Improved survival with the use of adjuvant chemotherapy in the treatment of medulloblastoma. *J. Neurosurg.* 74:433, 1991.

Patchell, R. A., et al. A randomized trial of surgery in the treatment of single metastases to the brain. *N. Engl. J. Med.* 322:494, 1990.

Shapiro, W. R., et al. Randomized trial of three chemotherapy regimens and two radiotherapy regimens in postoperative treatment of malignant glioma. *J. Neurosurg.* 71:1, 1989.

Shapiro, W. R., and Shapiro, J. R. Principles of brain tumor chemotherapy. *Semin. Oncol.* 13:56, 1986.

Sposto, R., et al. The effectiveness of chemotherapy for treatment of high grade astrocytoma in children: results of a randomized trial. *J. Neurooncol.* 7:165, 1989.

Tirelli, U., et al. Etoposide (VP-16-213) in malignant brain tumors: a phase II study. *J. Clin. Oncol.* 2:432, 1984.

Trojanowski, T., et al. Quality of survival of patients with brain gliomas treated with postoperative CCNU and radiation therapy. *J. Neurosurg.* 70:18, 1989.

Walker, M. D., et al. Randomized comparison of radiotherapy and nitrosoureas for malignant glioma after surgery. *N. Engl. J. Med.* 303:1323, 1980.

Wasserstrom, W. R., Glass, J. P., and Posner, J. B. Diagnosis and treatment of leptomeningeal metastasis from solid tumors: experience with 90 patients. *Cancer* 49:759, 1982.

Weiss, R. M., Poster, D. S., and Penta, J. S. The nitrosoureas and pulmonary toxicity. *Cancer Treat. Rev.* 8:111, 1981.

Zimm, S., et al. Intracerebral metastasis in solid-tumor patients: natural history and results of treatment. *Cancer* 48:384, 1981.

Soft-Tissue Sarcomas

Robert S. Benjamin

I. Classification and approach to treatment
A. Types of soft-tissue sarcomas.
The soft-tissue sarcomas are a group of diseases characterized by neoplastic proliferation of tissue of mesenchymal origin. Thus, they differ from the more common carcinomas, which arise from epithelial tissue. Sarcomas can arise in any area of the body and from any origin; however, they most commonly arise in the soft tissue of the extremities, trunk, retroperitoneum, or head and neck area. There are at least 21 different types of sarcomas, classified according to lines of differentiation toward normal tissue. For example, rhabdomyosarcoma shows evidence of skeletal muscle fibers with cross-striations, liposarcoma shows fat production, and angiosarcoma shows vessel formation. Precise characterization of the types of sarcoma is often impossible, and these tumors are called *unclassified sarcomas*. All of the primary bone sarcomas may arise from soft tissue, leading to such diagnoses as extraskeletal osteosarcoma, extraskeletal Ewing's sarcoma, and extraskeletal chondrosarcoma. An increasingly common diagnosis at present is malignant fibrous histiocytoma. This tumor is characterized by a mixture of spindle (or fibrous) cells and round (or histiocytic) cells arranged in a storiform pattern with frequent areas of pleomorphic appearance and frequent giant cells.

B. Metastases.
Metastatic spread of all sarcomas tends to be through the blood rather than through the lymphatic system. The lungs are by far the most frequent site of metastatic disease. Local sites of metastasis by direct invasion are the second most common area of involvement, followed by bone and liver. (Liver metastases are common with leiomyosarcomas of gastrointestinal origin, however.) Central nervous system (CNS) metastases are extraordinarily rare.

C. Staging.
Staging of sarcomas is complex and demands an expert sarcoma pathologist. Tumors are staged according to two systems, the American Joint Committee for Cancer Staging (AJCC) system and the Musculoskeletal Tumor Society staging system.

1. The AJCC staging system
a. The primary determinant of stage is **tumor grade.**
(1) Grade 1 tumors are stage I,
(2) Grade 2 tumors are stage II, and
(3) Grade 3 tumors are stage III.

Any tumor with lymph node metastases is automatically stage III, and any tumor with gross invasion of bone, major vessel, or major nerve is stage IV.

b. Further division of stages I–III into A and B are based on **tumor size.**

(1) A = tumor smaller than 5 cm, and

(2) B = tumor size 5 cm or larger.

In stage III, lymph node metastases are classified as IIIC; in stage IV, local invasion is called IVA; and IVB represents distant metastases.

2. **The Musculoskeletal Tumor Society staging system**

   a. The Musculoskeletal Tumor Society stages sarcomas according to grade and compartmental localization. The Roman numeral reflects the tumor grade.

      (1) Stage I: low grade

      (2) Stage II: high grade

      (3) Stage III: any-grade tumor with distant metastases

   b. The letter reflects compartmental localization. Compartments are defined by fascial planes.

      (1) Stage A: intracompartmental (i.e., confined to the same soft-tissue compartment as the initial tumor)

      (2) Stage B: extracompartmental (i.e., extending outside of the initial soft-tissue compartment into the adjacent soft-tissue compartment or bone)

   c. A stage IA tumor is a low-grade tumor confined to its initial compartment, a stage IB tumor is a low-grade tumor extending outside the initial compartment, and so forth.

D. **Evaluation.** Patients are evaluated and followed according to the plan in Table 21-1.

E. **Primary treatment**

   1. **Surgery and radiotherapy.** Treatment of the primary tumor involves surgery with or without radiation therapy. If radiation therapy is not used, surgery must be radical. While this may often involve amputation, more and more frequently at present, complete excision of the involved muscle group from origin to insertion is performed.

   2. **Adjuvant chemotherapy.** The role of adjuvant chemotherapy is controversial, with both positive and negative results reported. A recent meta-analysis indicated a highly significant decrease in the risk of disease recurrence (either local or distant) and death for patients treated with adjuvant chemotherapy; thus, some investigators believe that adjuvant therapy is clearly indicated for patients whose histologic type, grade, or location is known to convey a poor prognosis.

F. **Prognosis.** Prognosis is related to stage with a 5-year survival rate of 75% for AJCC stage I, 55% for stage II, and 29% for stage III. The survival rate for stage IV disease is less than 10%; however, a definite fraction of patients in this category can be cured. The majority of patients with stage IV disease, if left untreated, die within 6–12 months; however, there is great variation in actual survival and patients may go on with slowly progressive disease for many years.

G. **Treatment response.** Response to treatment is measured in the standard fashion for solid tumors.

1. **Complete remission.** This implies complete disappearance of all signs and symptoms of disease.

2. **Partial remission.** There is a 50% or greater decrease in measurable disease, calculated by comparing the sum of the products of perpendicular diameters of all lesions before and after therapy. When disease is not measurable in two dimensions but can be followed objectively by magnetic resonance imaging, x-ray, ultrasound, or computed tomography (CT), a definite decrease in the amount of metastatic disease confirmed by two independent investigators is the equivalent of a partial response, as calculated by a 50% decrease in measurable tumor.

3. **Stable disease or improvement.** Lesser degrees of tumor shrinkage are categorized by some physicians as stable disease and by others as improvement or minor response. Stable disease implies a smaller than 25% increase in disease for at least 8 weeks. For all response categories, no new disease must appear during response.

4. **Progression.** New disease in any area or a 25% or more increase in measurable disease constitutes progressive disease.

5. **Survival.** All patients whose disease responds objectively to chemotherapy survive longer than do patients with progressive disease, and the degree of prolongation of survival is directly proportional to the degree of antitumor response that can be measured.

II. **Chemotherapy**

A. **General considerations and aims of therapy.** Although there are numerous types of soft-tissue sarcomas, there are few differences among them regarding responsiveness to a standard soft-tissue sarcoma regimen. Chondrosarcomas and leiomyosarcomas of gastrointestinal origin respond less frequently than do the other soft-tissue sarcomas. In contrast, in a fraction of patients, two tumors—Ewing's sarcoma and rhabdomyosarcoma—particularly in the pediatric age group, are responsive to dactinomycin, vincristine, or etoposide. The other tumors are not. The goal of therapy for patients with advanced disease is primarily palliative, although a small fraction (about 20%) of patients who achieve complete remission are, in fact, cured. The first aim, therefore, is to achieve complete remission. Several investigators, including the author, have shown that the prognosis is the same whether complete remission is obtained by chemotherapy alone or by chemotherapy with adjuvant surgery, that is, surgical removal of all residual disease. Short of complete remission, partial remission causes some palliation with relief of symptoms and pro-

Table 21-1. Soft-tissue sarcoma evaluation

Tests	Initial	During treatment	Follow-up (if no evidence of disease)
History and physical examination	X	Prior to each treatment	Yr 1: q2mo; yr 2, 3: q3mo; yr 4: q4mo; yr 5: q6mo; then yearly
CBC, differential, and platelet counts*	X	Twice weekly	Yearly
Electrolytes*	X	Prior to each treatment	—
Chemistry profile*	X	Prior to each treatment	q4mo
Urinalysis	If giving ifosfamide	Prior to each treatment	—
PT, APTT, fibrinogen	X	—	—
Chest x-ray	X	Prior to each treatment	Same as for history and physical examination
CT scan chest	If chest x-ray film appears normal	To confirm chest x-ray findings (if initially abnormal) or for surgical planning	If chest x-ray becomes equivocal

		Preoperatively	
MRI primary (if not intraabdominal)	X		—
Ultrasound primary	—		Yr 1: q4mo; yr 2, 3: q6mo
CT abdomen and pelvis	If myxoid liposarcoma or retroperitoneal or pelvic primary tumor	If baseline, every 3rd cycle	If baseline, yr 1: q4mo; yr 2, 3: q6mo
ECG	If cardiac history		—
Cardiac nuclear scan (for ejection fraction)	If cardiac history	If doxorubicin dose to exceed standard limits for schedule	Yearly for 2 yrs, then as clinically indicated
Central venous catheter	X		—
Bone marrow	If small-cell tumor		—
Bone scan	If indicated by history		—
Plain film	If indicated by history		—

CBC = complete blood cell count; PT = prothrombin time; APTT = activated partial thromboplastin time; CT = computed tomography; MRI = magnetic resonance imaging; ECG = electrocardiography.
*Required more frequently if patient is on a medical treatment program.
Note: Tests may be ordered more frequently based on clinical indications.

longation of survival by approximately 1 year. Any degree of improvement or stabilization of previously advancing disease will likewise increase survival.

B. Effective drugs. The most important chemotherapeutic agent is doxorubicin (Adriamycin), which forms the backbone of all combination chemotherapy regimens. Ifosfamide, a newly released analog of cyclophosphamide that has documented activity even in patients who are refractory to combinations containing cyclophosphamide, is usually included in front-line chemotherapy combinations. It is always given together with the uroprotective agent mesna to prevent hemorrhagic cystitis. Dacarbazine (DTIC), a marginal agent by itself, adds significantly to doxorubicin in prolonging remission duration and survival as well as increasing the response rate. Cyclophosphamide adds marginally, if at all, but is included in some effective regimens.

The key to effective sarcoma chemotherapy is the steep dose-response curve for doxorubicin. At a dose of 45 mg/m^2, the response rate is lower than 20% compared with a 37% response rate at a dose of 75 mg/m^2. A similar dose-response relationship exists for ifosfamide and for combination chemotherapy, and the regimens with the best reported results are those utilizing the highest doses.

C. Primary chemotherapy regimen. The most effective primary chemotherapy regimens include doxorubicin and dacarbazine (ADIC), with or without the addition of cyclophosphamide (CyADIC) or ifosfamide and mesna (MAID). The CyADIC regimen is a modification of the standard CyVADIC regimen, which includes vincristine. Since analysis has shown that vincristine makes no significant contribution and produces neurotoxicity, its addition at a dose of 2 mg maximum or 1.4 mg/m^2 weekly for 6 weeks and then once every 3–4 weeks is recommended only for rhabdomyosarcoma and Ewing's sarcoma.

By giving doxorubicin and dacarbazine by continuous 72- or 96-hour infusion with the two drugs mixed in the same infusion pump, nausea and vomiting are markedly reduced, and the chemotherapy can be continued until a cumulative doxorubicin dose of 800 mg/m^2 is reached, with less cardiac toxicity than with standard doxorubicin administration and a cumulative dose of 450 mg/m^2.

1. The **continuous-infusion CyADIC** regimen is as follows.

  a. Cyclophosphamide 600 mg/m^2 IV on day 1, *and*

  b. Doxorubicin by continuous 96-hour infusion, 60 mg/m^2 IV (15 mg/m^2/24 hours for 4 days), *and*

  c. Dacarbazine by continuous 96-hour infusion, 1000 mg/m^2 IV (250 mg/m^2/24 hours for 4 days) mixed in the same bag or pump as the doxorubicin. Doses should be divided into 4 consecutive 24-hour infusions.

  Repeat cycle every 3–4 weeks.

2. The **continuous-infusion ADIC** regimen is as follows.
   a. Doxorubicin by continuous 96-hour infusion, 90 mg/m^2 IV (22.5 mg/m^2/24 hours for 4 days), *and*
   b. Dacarbazine by continuous 96-hour infusion, 900 mg/m^2 IV (225 mg/m^2/24 hours for 4 days) mixed in the same bag or pump as the doxorubicin. Doses should be divided into 4 consecutive 24-hour infusions.
   Repeat cycle every 3–4 weeks.
3. The **MAID** regimen is as follows.
   a. Mesna by continuous 96-hour infusion, 10,000 mg/m IV (2500 mg/m^2/24 hours for 4 days).
   b. Doxorubicin by continuous 72-hour infusion, 60 mg/m^2 IV (20 mg/m^2/24 hours for 3 days).
   c. Ifosfamide by continuous 72-hour infusion, 6000 mg/m^2 IV (2000 mg/m^2/24 hours for 3 days). Doses should be divided into 3 consecutive 24-hour infusions. (Some investigators prefer to infuse ifosfamide over 2 hours rather than 24 hours because of higher single-agent activity with the shorter infusions.)
   d. Dacarbazine by continuous 72-hour infusion, 1000 mg/m^2 IV (333.3 mg/m^2/24 hours for 3 days) mixed in the same bag or pump as the doxorubicin. Doses should be divided into 3 consecutive 24-hour infusions.
   Repeat cycle every 3–4 weeks.
4. **Dose modification.** Doses of doxorubicin, cyclophosphamide, ifosfamide, and mesna should be increased or decreased by 25% for each course of therapy in order to achieve a lowest absolute granulocyte count of approximately 500/μl. The maximum doxorubicin dose is limited to 800 mg/m^2, at which point therapy should be discontinued unless cardiac biopsy specimens indicate that it is safe to continue. With Ewing's sarcoma and rhabdomyosarcoma, therapy may be continued and dactinomycin, 2 mg/m^2 in a single dose or 0.5 mg/m^2 daily for 5 days, may be substituted for the doxorubicin with continuation of the regimen for a total of 18 months.
5. **An alternative regimen for children with rhabdomyosarcoma** is an alternating regimen, using ifosfamide and etoposide alternating with the so-called VAdriaC regimen. Vincristine 1.5 mg/m^2 is given weekly for the first 2 cycles of VAdriaC and then on day 1 only. Doxorubicin is given at 60–75 mg/m^2 as a 48-hour continuous infusion, and cyclophosphamide 600 mg/m^2 is given daily for 2 days (with mesna). After 3 weeks, ifosfamide is given at a dose of 1800 mg/m^2 daily for 5 days (with mesna) and etoposide is given at a dose of 100 mg/m^2 daily for 5 days. Chemotherapy cycles are alternated for 39 weeks.
6. **A less intensive, older but still effective regimen for children with good-prognosis rhabdo-**

myosarcoma is the so-called pulse VAC regimen. Dactinomycin is given at a total dose of 2.0–2.5 mg/m² by divided daily injection over 5–7 days (e.g., 0.5 mg/m² daily for 5 days) repeated every 3 months for a total of 5 courses. Cyclophosphamide pulses of 275–330 mg/m² daily for 7 days are begun at the same time, but are given every 6 weeks with vincristine, 2 mg/m² on days 1 and 8 of each cyclophosphamide cycle. Cyclophosphamide cycles are terminated prematurely if the white blood cell counts fall below 1500/μl. Chemotherapy continues for 2 years. (The necessity of the 2-year duration of the chemotherapy program is not certain.)

D. Secondary chemotherapy. Secondary chemotherapy for patients with sarcoma is relatively unrewarding, with response rates lower than 10% for almost all conventional drugs or regimens tested. The best commercially available drug is ifosfamide, which if not used in primary treatment produces a response in about 20% of patients. Methotrexate, with a response rate of about 15% regardless of schedule, is the only other active agent. Patients who do not respond to primary chemotherapy and ifosfamide should be entered in a phase II study of a new agent to see if some activity can be established, since other reasonably good alternatives do not exist.

E. Complications of chemotherapy. Side effects of sarcoma chemotherapy can be classified into three categories: life-threatening, potentially dangerous, and unpleasant.

   1. Life-threatening complications of chemotherapy are infection or bleeding. Since thrombocytopenia lower than 20,000/μl rarely occurs with this type of chemotherapy, bleeding is rare. Approximately 20% of patients will have documented or suspected infection related to drug-induced neutropenia at some time during their treatment courses. These infections are rarely fatal if treated promptly with broad-spectrum, bactericidal antibiotics at the onset of the febrile neutropenia episode.

   2. Potentially dangerous side effects of chemotherapy include the following.

   a. Mucositis, which occurs in fewer than 25% of patients, may interfere with oral intake or may act as a source of infection.

   b. Granulocytopenia predisposes the patient to infection but because of its brevity, rarely causes infection.

   c. Thrombocytopenia is usually insignificant.

   d. Cardiac damage from doxorubicin rarely causes clinical problems at the doses recommended, with usually reversible congestive heart failure occurring in fewer than 5% of patients.

   e. Renal insufficiency is a rare complication of ifosfamide. Fanconi's syndrome, particularly manifested by a significant loss of bicarbonate, is a dose-related complication of ifosfamide, occurring in about 10% of patients at standard ifosfamide doses.

f. CNS toxicity of ifosfamide is rarely a serious complication. Patients frequently demonstrate minor confusion, disorientation, or difficulty with fine movements. Somnolence and coma are rarely seen in patients without hypoalbuminemia and/or acidosis.

g. Hemorrhagic cystitis, a rare complication of cyclophosphamide therapy, used to be the dose-limiting toxicity of ifosfamide. It can be prevented in most cases by administration of another agent, mesna, before and after each ifosfamide dose, allowing higher doses of ifosfamide to be used.

3. Unpleasant but rarely serious problems include nausea and vomiting (primarily from dacarbazine and ifosfamide) and alopecia (from doxorubicin, cyclophosphamide, and ifosfamide).

F. Special precautions

1. Ifosfamide. Patients must be kept well hydrated with an alkaline pH in order to prevent CNS toxicity and minimize nephrotoxicity. Sodium bicarbonate or sodium acetate should be added to IV fluids at an initial concentration of 100 mEq/liter and fluid administration should be adjusted to produce a urine output of at least 2 liters/day and to maintain the serum bicarbonate concentration at 25 mEq/liter or higher.

2. Doxorubicin. Avoid extravasation. Continuous infusions must (and short infusions should) be administered through a central venous catheter. Attention to cumulative dose administered (varying according to the schedule of administration) is critical to minimize the risk of cardiac toxicity.

Selected Readings

Antman, K. H., et al. Phase II trial of ifosfamide with mesna in previously treated metastatic sarcoma. *Cancer Treat. Rep.* 69:499, 1985.

Antman, K. H., et al. An intergroup phase III randomized study of doxorubicin and dacarbazine with or without ifosfamide and mesna in advanced soft tissue and bone sarcomas. *J. Clin. Oncol.* 11:1276, 1993.

Benjamin, R. S., et al. The Chemotherapy of Soft Tissue Sarcomas in Adults. In R. G. Martin, A. G. Ayala (eds.), *Management of Primary Bone and Soft Tissue Tumors*. Chicago: Year Book, 1977. Pp. 309–316.

Elias, A. Response to mesna, doxorubicin, ifosfamide, and dacarbazine in 108 patients with metastatic or unresectable sarcoma and no prior chemotherapy. *J. Clin. Oncol.* 7:1208, 1989.

Lindberg, R. D., et al. Conservative Surgery and Radiation

Therapy for Soft Tissue Sarcomas. In R. G. Martin, A. G. Ayala (eds.), *Management of Primary Bone and Soft Tissue Tumors*. Chicago: Year Book, 1977. Pp. 289–298.

Russell, W. O., et al. A clinical and pathological staging system for soft tissue sarcomas. *Cancer* 40:1562, 1977.

Zalupski, M. M., et al. Defining the Role of Adjuvant Chemotherapy for Patients with Soft Tissue Sarcoma of the Extremities. In S. E. Salmon (ed.), *Adjuvant Therapy of Cancer VII*. Philadelphia: Lippincott, 1993. Pp. 385–392.

Bone Sarcomas

Robert S. Benjamin

There are four major sarcomas of bone, each differing somewhat in clinical behavior, chemotherapy responsiveness, and prognosis. All present as painful bony lesions, and all metastasize preferentially to lung and then to other bones. The prognosis of untreated sarcomas of the bone is inversely proportional to their chemotherapy responsiveness. The sarcomas will be considered in order of greatest to least chemotherapeutic responsiveness: Ewing's sarcoma, osteosarcoma, malignant fibrous histiocytoma of bone, and chondrosarcoma.

Response to treatment is evaluated according to the usual criteria used for solid tumors and identical to that reported in Chapter 21 for soft-tissue sarcomas. Angiography is particularly helpful in defining the response of primary bone tumors to chemotherapy, and the angiographic response correlates well with pathologic tumor destruction. Complete resection and examination of the total specimen often are required to determine response to therapy in a primary lesion and to confirm complete remission.

I. **Staging.** Bone tumors are staged exclusively according to the criteria of the Musculoskeletal Tumor Society.
  A. The Roman numeral reflects the **tumor grade.**
    1. Stage I: Low grade
    2. Stage II: High grade
    3. Stage III: Any-grade tumor with distant metastasis
  B. The companion letter reflects **tumor compartmentalization.**
    1. Stage A: Confined to bone
    2. Stage B: Extending into adjacent soft tissue
  C. Thus, a stage IA tumor is a low-grade tumor confined to bone, and a stage IB tumor is a low-grade tumor extending into soft tissue, and so forth. Patients are evaluated and followed according to the plan in Table 22-1.

II. **Ewing's sarcoma**
  A. **General considerations and aims of therapy**
    1. **Tumor characteristics.** Ewing's sarcoma is a highly malignant, small round-cell tumor of bone. It occurs most commonly in the second decade, with 90% of patients under age 30. There is a slight predominance of males. The most common locations are the pelvis or the diaphysis of long tubular bones of the extremities. Often systemic symptoms of fever and leukocytosis suggest infection. Radiographically, the predominant feature is osteolysis, although sclerosis does occur. Frequently, the periosteal reaction has the so-called onion skin pattern with layering of subperiosteal new bone, frequently with spicules radiating out from the cortex. Prognosis, until recently, was extremely poor, with a 5-year survival rate lower than 10% and almost one-half of the patients dead within 1 year of diagnosis. Since Ewing's sar-

Table 22-1. Primary bone sarcoma evaluation

Tests	Prior to therapy	On initial treatment	Pre-operative	On subsequent treatment	Follow-up
History and physical examination	X	Prior to each treatment	X	Prior to each treatment	Yr 1: q2mo; yr 2, 3: q3–4mo; yr 4: q4mo; yr 5: q6mo; then yearly
CBC, differential, and platelet counts[a]	X	Twice weekly	X	Twice weekly	Yearly
Chemistry profile[a]	X	Prior to each treatment	X	Prior to each treatment	Yr 1–4: q4mo; yr 5: q6mo; then yearly
Creatinine clearance	X	For methotrexate	—	For methotrexate	—
Electrolytes, Mg[a]	X	Prior to each treatment	X	Prior to each treatment	—
Urinalysis	If ifosfamide	Prior to each treatment	X	Prior to each treatment	—
PT, APTT, fibrinogen	X	Prior to each intraarterial (IA) treatment and qd while on IA treatment	X	—	—

Plain films of primary tumor	X	q2 cycles	X	q3mo	X	Yr 1: q4–6mo; then yearly
CT of primary tumor	X	After 2–4 cycles	X	—	X	At end of treatment for head and neck or pelvic primaries
MRI of primary tumor	—	For surgical planning only	—	—	—	—
Bone scan	X	—	X	—	X	—
Sestamibi[b] scan	X	After 2–4 cycles	X	If needed to assess response	X	—
Chest x-ray	X	Prior to each treatment	X	Prior to each treatment	X	Yr 1: q2mo; yr 2, 3: q3–4mo; yr 4: q4mo; yr 5: q6mo; then yearly
CT of chest	If chest x-ray appears normal	If chest x-ray is equivocal or for surgical planning	—	If chest x-ray is equivocal or for surgical planning	—	If chest x-ray is equivocal or for surgical planning
Angiogram	—	Prior to each preoperative treatment	—	—	—	—

Table 22-1. (continued)

Tests	Prior to therapy	On initial treatment	Pre-operative	On subsequent treatment	Follow-up
Bone marrow	Only for small-cell tumors with metastases	—	—	—	—
ECG	If cardiac history	—	If cardiac history	—	—
Cardiac scan	If cardiac history	—	—	If doxorubicin dose exceeds standard limits for schedule	—
Central venous catheter	X	—	—	—	—
Bone tumor conference	X	—	—	—	If further multidisciplinary decisions are required

CBC = complete blood cell count; PT = prothrombin time; APTT = activated partial thromboplastin time; CT = computed tomography; MRI = magnetic resonance imaging; ECG = electrocardiogram.
[a]Required more frequently if patient is on a medical treatment program.
[b]Name of the thallium-technetium isotope used for scanning. Trade name is Cardiolyte.
Note: Tests may be ordered more frequently based on clinical indications.

coma is a high-grade tumor by definition, and since it is almost always accompanied by a soft-tissue mass, it usually is staged as IIB or IIIB depending on the demonstration of metastatic disease in lung, bone, or both.

2. **Primary treatment.** For this reason and because of the mutilative surgery involved in resection of the primary lesion, radiotherapy has been the primary modality for local tumor control. As techniques for limb salvage surgery have become more widely practiced, attempts to utilize surgery rather than radiation therapy are again increasing.

B. Chemotherapy

1. **CyVADIC regimen.** Perhaps the best chemotherapeutic regimen for Ewing's sarcoma is the continuous infusion CyVADIC regimen, which is mentioned in Chapter 21 (sec. **II.C.**).

   a. Cyclophosphamide 600 mg/m^2 IV on day 1.

   b. Vincristine 1.4 mg/m^2 (2 mg maximum) IV weekly for 6 weeks, then on day 1 of each cycle.

   c. Doxorubicin (Adriamycin) 60 mg/m^2 IV by 96-hour continuous infusion through a central venous catheter (15 mg/m^2/24 hours for 4 days).

   d. Dacarbazine (DTIC) 1000 mg/m^2 IV by 96-hour continuous infusion (250 mg/m^2/24 hours for 4 days) mixed in the same bag or pump as the doxorubicin. Doses should be divided into 4 consecutive 24-hour infusions.

   Repeat cycle every 3–4 weeks.

2. **Dose modifications.** Courses are repeated with a 25% increase or decrease in the doses of cyclophosphamide and doxorubicin depending on morbidity. Courses are repeated in 3–4 weeks as soon as recovery to 1500 granulocytes and 100,000 platelets occurs. Complications are as described in Chapter 21 (sec. **II.E.**), with the addition of peripheral neuropathy from vincristine. When the cumulative dose of doxorubicin has reached 800 mg/m^2, therapy is discontinued.

3. **Alternative regimens.** Alternative regimens omit dacarbazine; vary doses of cyclophosphamide up to 1500 mg/m^2; give dactinomycin with, or in place of, doxorubicin; and in some patients, add other drugs. A common regimen at present alternates two regimens every 3 weeks: ifosfamide plus etoposide and vincristine; doxorubicin plus cyclophosphamide, with dactinomycin substituted for doxorubicin after a cumulative (bolus) dose of 375 mg/m^2 (VAdCA). In a recent intergroup study, this regimen was superior to VAdCA alone. The schedule of drug administration is as follows.

   a. Initial combination

      (1) Ifosfamide 1800 mg/m^2 IV daily × 5 (with mesna), *and*

      (2) Etoposide 100 mg/m^2 daily IV × 5.

    b. Three weeks later, start
      (1) Vincristine 1.5 mg/m^2 IV on day 1, *and*
      (2) Doxorubicin (Adriamycin) 75 mg/m^2 IV on day 1, *and*
      (3) Cyclophosphamide 1200 mg/m^2 IV on day 1.
    c. Three weeks later, return to the first regimen, and so forth. At a cumulative doxorubicin dose of 375 mg/m^2, substitute dactinomycin 1.25 mg/m^2. Chemotherapy continues for a total of 1 year.

4. Responses. The majority of patients with metastatic disease will obtain complete remission; however, almost all patients will experience relapse and ultimately die of disease. When chemotherapy is used in the therapy of primary disease with surgery or radiation, prognosis depends on the size and location of the primary tumor. Patients with large flat-bone lesions have a lower than 30% cure rate compared with a 60–70% cure rate for those patients with long-bone lesions, which are generally smaller. An alarming complication of the chemotherapy-radiation therapy combination is a high frequency of second malignancies in cured patients, with 4 of 10 patients in one series developing secondary sarcomas within the radiated fields. This complication is another reason for considering surgical intervention rather than radiation, since chemotherapy is required for cure whether or not the primary lesion can be controlled with radiation.

5. Secondary chemotherapy. Occasional responses have been seen with etoposide (VP-16), other alkylating agents (especially ifosfamide), the nitrosoureas, and cisplatin. A combination of etoposide and ifosfamide is now frequently used in patients for whom those drugs were not used in initial therapy. High-dose ifosfamide (14 gm/m^2 divided over 3–7 days, either as a 2-hour infusion with each dose or as a continuous infusion) with mesna or high-dose doxorubicin (90 mg/m^2) plus dacarbazine (900 mg/m^2) as a 96-hour continuous infusion is occasionally effective at producing brief remissions in patients for whom these agents were not used or were used at substantially lower doses during initial therapy. Nonetheless, secondary responses are extremely poor, and the survival of a relapsed patient with Ewing's sarcoma is measured in weeks.

6. High-dose chemotherapy. The standard chemotherapy used for Ewing's sarcoma is accompanied by severe but transient myelosuppression. The availability of hematopoietic growth factors to reduce infectious complications provides an added measure of safety, but is not routinely required. Our policy has been to use growth factors only in patients who have had febrile-neutropenic episodes during a previous course of chemotherapy rather than to reduce the doses of the myelosuppressive drugs.

Bone marrow transplantation or peripheral stem cell rescue programs are being investigated in patients presenting with poor prognostic features (large pelvic primary tumors, metastatic disease) but are not yet demonstrated to improve prognosis. Such regimens have been tried with negative results in patients relapsing after standard chemotherapy and have been demonstrated to have no significant benefit. Clearly, this approach should not be used in patients with relapse.

III. Osteosarcoma

A. General considerations. Osteosarcoma is a tumor with a poor prognosis in the absence of effective chemotherapy. It is the most common primary bone sarcoma. Frequently, it affects patients 10–25 years old and tends to be located around the knee in about two-thirds of patients, with two-thirds of those tumors involving the distal aspect of the femur. As with other sarcomas of bone, pulmonary metastases are most common, followed by bone metastases. Since conventional osteosarcoma is a high-grade tumor by definition, and since it is accompanied by a soft-tissue mass in 90% or more of patients, it is usually staged as IIB or IIIB depending on the demonstration of metastatic disease in lung and/or bone.

B. Role of chemotherapy. Chemotherapy is usually employed in the adjuvant situation and its value preoperatively has been conclusively demonstrated. Patients who show a complete response to preoperative chemotherapy with tumor destruction of at least 90% have significantly improved survival. Response rates in evaluable tumors range from 30 to 80%. Cure of primary disease with adjuvant chemotherapy is 50–80%.

C. Effective agents. The four major standard single agents in the treatment of osteosarcoma are cisplatin, doxorubicin, ifosfamide, and high-dose methotrexate. In addition, the combination of bleomycin, cyclophosphamide, and dactinomycin (BCD) has been effective.

D. Recommended regimen. A variety of regimens may be recommended based on preliminary, or more extensive, evaluation.

1. Doxorubicin and cisplatin

    a. Doxorubicin 90 mg/m^2 IV by 96-hour continuous infusion through a central venous catheter, *and*

    b. Cisplatin 120 mg/m^2 intraarterially (IA) (for primary tumor) or IV on day 6.

Repeat every 4 weeks.

Three to 4 courses of therapy should be administered preoperatively. Postoperative therapy depends on the response of the primary tumor. Patients with tumor necrosis of 90% or more should continue on the same regimen for 6 postoperative courses or until a cumulative doxorubicin dose of 800 mg/m^2 is reached. If cisplatin must be discontinued earlier, substitute dacarbazine 750 mg/m^2 IV over 96 hours (ADIC).

2. Following primary chemotherapy, if there is less

than 90% tumor necrosis at surgery, switch to the **alternative regimen** as follows.

    a. High-dose methotrexate 12 gm/m^2 IV every 2 weeks for 4 weeks with leucovorin rescue (see sec. **III.E.2.**).

    b. Three weeks later, administer ifosfamide 2 gm/m^2 IV over 2 hours for 5 consecutive days with mesna 1200 mg/m^2 IV in 3 divided doses each day (i.e., 400 mg/m^2 IV q4h × 3) or by continuous infusion after a loading dose of 400 mg/m^2 mixed with the first ifosfamide dose. Three weeks later repeat the course.

    c. Three weeks later administer a 96-hour continuous infusion of doxorubicin 75 mg/m^2 plus dacarbazine 750 mg/m^2 (ADIC). Three to 4 weeks later, repeat the course.

    d. Three to 4 weeks later, repeat the entire cycle of 2 courses of methotrexate, 2 courses of ifosfamide, and 2 courses of ADIC. End with 2 more courses of high-dose methotrexate.

  3. An **alternative approach** to alternating cycle chemotherapy is as follows.

    a. High-dose methotrexate 12 gm/m^2 IV weekly for 4 weeks with leucovorin rescue (see sec. **III.E.2.**).

    b. Three weeks later, administer BCD for 2 consecutive days.

      (1) Bleomycin 12 units/m^2 IV daily on days 1 and 2, *and*

      (2) Cyclophosphamide 600 mg/m^2 IV daily on days 1 and 2, *and*

      (3) Dactinomycin 450 μg/m^2 IV daily on days 1 and 2.

    c. Three weeks later, repeat high-dose methotrexate weekly for 2 weeks.

    d. One week later, give doxorubicin 45 mg/m^2 IV daily for 2 consecutive days.

    e. Three weeks later, repeat high-dose methotrexate weekly for 2 weeks.

  Repeat the cycles using the sequence of BCD, high-dose methotrexate, doxorubicin, and high-dose methotrexate for 5 courses.

E. Special precautions in administration

  1. Cisplatin. Prehydration is necessary, with overnight infusion of IV fluids at 150 ml/hour or 1 liter of fluid over 2 hours (for adults), followed by at least 6 liters of fluid containing potassium chloride (KCl), at least 20 mEq/liter, and magnesium sulfate (MgSO$_4$), at least 4 mEq/liter, for the first day or 2 following cisplatin administration. The addition of mannitol, 50 ml of a 20% solution prior to cisplatin followed by 200 ml of a 20% solution mixed with normal saline in a total volume of 1 liter to run simultaneously with the cisplatin over 2–3 hours, is preferred by many investigators. Particular care in electrolyte balance, including frequent determinations of magnesium levels, is necessary. In the presence of severe hypomagnesemia, magnesium sulfate, up to 1–2 mEq/kg, may be infused over 4 hours.

2. **High-dose methotrexate.** Pretreatment creatinine clearance rate should be at least 70 ml/min.

a. **Methotrexate administration and alkalinization of urine.** Before administration of high-dose methotrexate, 0.5 mEq/kg of sodium bicarbonate is infused IV over 15–30 minutes in an attempt to create an alkaline urine. Allopurinol 300 mg daily for 3 days is given starting 1 day before the methotrexate infusion. Methotrexate is dissolved in no more than 1000 ml of 5% dextrose in water with a final concentration of approximately 1 gm/100 ml. The total dose ranges from 8 gm/m^2 for patients over 40 years old to 12 mg/m^2 for children and young adults. The dose should be increased on subsequent courses if an immediate postinfusion methotrexate level is less than 10^{-3} M. Sodium bicarbonate 50 mEq is added per liter of methotrexate solution, which is infused over 4 hours. Following completion of the methotrexate infusion, 10 ml/kg of an IV infusion of 5% dextrose in water with 50 mEq/liter of bicarbonate is given over 2 hours if the patient is unable to drink or if the 24-hour methotrexate levels of the previous high-dose methotrexate treatment have been higher than 1.5×10^{-5} M. The IV infusion is then discontinued and the patient is encouraged to drink sufficient fluid to produce approximately 1600 ml/m^2 of alkaline urine for the first 24 hours, and 1900 ml/m^2 daily for the next 3 days. Sodium bicarbonate 14–28 mEq every 6 hours PO is administered to ensure alkaline urine. The pH of the urine is measured, and if it is < 7, an extra dose of bicarbonate is administered.

b. **Leucovorin rescue.** Twenty-four hours after the start of the methotrexate infusion, leucovorin 15–25 mg is administered PO q6h for at least 10 doses, or IM if the oral medication is not tolerated.

c. **Serum methotrexate levels.** These levels should be followed and should fall approximately 1 log/day. When methotrexate concentration falls below 1×10^{-7} M, leucovorin may be safely discontinued. IV hydration is required whenever oral intake is inadequate to produce sufficient urine output as previously defined, for abnormal serum methotrexate concentration, for persistent vomiting, or for early toxicity.

3. **Ifosfamide.** Patients must be kept well hydrated with an alkaline pH in order to prevent central nervous system (CNS) toxicity and minimize nephrotoxicity. Sodium bicarbonate or sodium acetate should

be added to IV fluids at an initial concentration of 100 mEq/liter and fluid administration adjusted to produce a urine output of at least 2 liters/day and to maintain the serum bicarbonate concentration at 25 mEq/liter or higher.

F. **Complications.** Complications of chemotherapy depend on the drugs. For doxorubicin and cyclophosphamide, the major complication is infection owing to neutropenia. Other complications include stomatitis, nausea and vomiting, and delayed cardiac toxicity, as discussed in the management of soft-tissue sarcomas (see Chap. 21, sec. **II.E.**). Dactinomycin causes similar side effects but not cardiac toxicity. Methotrexate predominantly causes stomatitis, but it may cause myelosuppression and renal, hepatic, and CNS abnormalities. Cisplatin and dacarbazine cause severe nausea and vomiting. In addition, cisplatin nephrotoxicity is primarily a tubular defect, with hypomagnesemia as the most prominent manifestation, but hypocalcemia, hypokalemia, and hyponatremia also occur. Delayed cumulative nephrotoxicity can cause impaired glomerular function as well. Ototoxicity may occur but is less common. Delayed neurotoxicity also occurs. Both cisplatin and methotrexate can, by causing renal toxicity, exacerbate their other side effects. Ifosfamide produces myelosuppression, nausea and vomiting, and alopecia, similar to doxorubicin. Hemorrhagic cystitis, once the dose-limiting toxicity, is rarely seen since the use of mesna has become routine. The most serious toxicities of ifosfamide are nephrotoxicity and CNS toxicity. Nephrotoxicity in the form of Fanconi's syndrome is a frequent problem, the morbidity of which can be minimized by the routine use of alkaline infusions and correction of electrolyte levels with oral replacement therapy. Only rarely does the nephrotoxicity progress to renal failure. Correction of acid-base balance and hypoalbuminemia can essentially prevent the CNS toxicity.

G. **Recurrence and treatment of refractory disease.** Patients with osteosarcoma who are refractory to a combination of doxorubicin and cisplatin may respond to high-dose methotrexate, patients refractory to high-dose methotrexate may respond to doxorubicin-cisplatin, and patients refractory to both may respond to ifosfamide or, rarely, to BCD. However, treatment of refractory disease is usually disappointing, and participation in studies of new agents is indicated for patients whose disease cannot be resected. Surgical resection of pulmonary metastases remains the only viable secondary therapy for the majority of patients. For this reason, careful follow-up for detection of metastases while they are still at the stage of resectability is indicated.

H. **High-dose chemotherapy.** The standard chemotherapy used for osteosarcoma is accompanied by severe but transient myelosuppression. The availability of hematopoietic growth factors to reduce infectious complications provides an added measure of safety, but is not routinely required. Our policy has been to use growth factors only in patients who have had febrile-neutropenic episodes during a previous course of chemotherapy rather than to reduce the doses of the myelosuppressive drugs.

Bone marrow transplantation or peripheral stem cell rescue programs are being investigated in patients presenting with poor prognostic features (poor-prognosis histologic subtypes, pelvic primary tumors, metastatic disease, etc.), but are not yet demonstrated to improve prognosis.

IV. **Malignant fibrous histiocytoma of bone.** This recently reported entity, characterized by a purely lytic lesion in bone, has an exceptionally poor prognosis when treated with surgery alone, although the number of reported patients is small. It may be extremely difficult to distinguish from fibroblastic osteosarcoma, and may be best considered as a fibroblastic osteosarcoma with minimal (i.e., no detectable) osteoid production. The tumor responds well to the CyADIC regimen for soft-tissue sarcomas, with more than one-half of patients obtaining at least partial remission. In addition, cisplatin at a dose of 120 mg/m^2 every 4 weeks has caused remissions, even in patients who did not respond to primary therapy. A particularly attractive approach for patients with large, unresectable primary tumors is the use of cisplatin given by the intraarterial route. Complete tumor destruction in 1 patient and a good partial remission in a second patient are the reported results among 3 patients so treated. Systemic doxorubicin may be added as for osteosarcomas (see sec **III.D.1.**). Alternatively, responses have been seen after high-dose methotrexate–based regimens for osteosarcomas (see sec. **III.D.2.**). After local tumor destruction, surgery may be employed to remove residual disease. Because of the primary poor prognosis, adjuvant chemotherapy with the continuous-infusion CyADIC regimen is recommended until an 800 mg/m^2 cumulative doxorubicin dose has been reached.

V. **Chondrosarcoma.** The chemotherapy for chondrosarcoma is totally inadequate and no regimen can be recommended except for the rare patients with mesenchymal chondrosarcoma, a subtype that may respond to CyADIC chemotherapy or cisplatin, or with dedifferentiated chondrosarcoma, which should be treated the same way as osteosarcoma. The vast majority of patients, those with conventional chondrosarcoma, are candidates only for surgical management. Metastatic disease should be treated with phase II protocols in an attempt to determine some effective type of chemotherapy that may be recommended in the future.

Selected Readings

Benjamin, R. S., et al. Chemotherapy for metastatic osteosarcoma. Studies by the M.D. Anderson Hospital and the Southwest Oncology Group. *Cancer Treat. Rep.* 62:237, 1978.

Benjamin, R. S., et al. Preoperative Chemotherapy for Osteosarcoma: A Treatment Approach Facilitating Limb Salvage with Major Prognostic Implications. In S. E. Jones and S. E. Salmon (eds.), *Adjuvant Therapy of Cancer IV.* New York: Grune & Stratton, 1984. Pp. 601–610.

Chawla, S. P., et al. Adjuvant Chemotherapy of Primary Malignant Fibrous Histiocytoma of Bone—Prolongation of Disease-free and Overall Survival. In S. E. Jones and S. E. Salmon (eds.), *Adjuvant Therapy of Cancer IV.* New York: Grune & Stratton, 1984. Pp. 621–629.

Gehan, E. A., et al. Osteosarcoma: The M. D. Anderson Experience, 1950–1974. In W. D. Terry and D. Windhorst (eds.), *Immunotherapy of Cancer: Present Status of Trials in Man.* New York: Raven, 1978.

Grier, H. et al. Improved outcome in non-metastatic Ewing's sarcoma (EWS) and PNET of bone with the addition of ifosfamide (I) and etoposide (E) to vincristine (V), Adriamycin (Ad), cyclophosphamide (C), and actinomycin (A): a Childrens Cancer Group (CCG) and Pediatric Oncology Group (POG) report. *Proc. Am. Soc. Clin. Oncol.* 13:421, 1994.

Rosen, G., et al. The Successful Management of Metastatic Osteogenic Sarcoma: A Model for the Treatment of Primary Osteogenic Sarcoma. In A. T. van Oosterom, F. M. Muggia, and F. J. Cleton (eds.), *Therapeutic Progress in Ovarian Cancer, Testicular Cancer and the Sarcomas.* Hingham: Leiden University Press, 1980. Pp. 249–365.

Acute Leukemias

Neil A. Lachant

The acute leukemias are a heterogeneous group of disorders characterized by the abnormal proliferation and accumulation of hematopoietic progenitor cells. The appellation *acute* is now a historical anachronism, since it refers to the short natural history of the disease prior to the modern chemotherapeutic era. Great therapeutic advances have been made since the early 1960s, so that many individuals can now be cured of these otherwise fatal illnesses. Unfortunately, however, an unacceptable high proportion of affected individuals still die. Many questions remain unanswered as to the optimum way to treat these disorders. Therefore *all individuals with acute leukemia should be considered candidates for well-designed randomized, prospective studies.*

I. **Diagnosis and classification.** Acute leukemia is a clonal disorder that arises in a hematopoietic stem cell and ultimately gives rise to a state of functional bone marrow failure. The acute leukemias are arbitrarily divided into acute nonlymphocytic (ANLL) and acute lymphocytic (ALL) forms based on the stem cell of origin. Although the peripheral smear may be highly suggestive of acute leukemia, the diagnosis is made by examining the bone marrow. Classification into the ANLL and ALL categories is usually based on the morphologic, histochemical, enzymatic, and immunologic (antigenic) characteristics of the blast cells. Occasionally, electron microscopy, cytogenetics, and molecular biologic techniques aid in establishing the diagnosis. The principles used to diagnose and classify acute leukemia are briefly presented below.

A. **Acute nonlymphocytic leukemia.** The French–American–British (FAB) system is the most widely used for the diagnosis and subclassification of ANLL. Normally, myeloblasts (monoblasts cannot be distinguished morphologically from myeloblasts) and promyelocytes constitute fewer than 5% of the nucleated cells in the marrow. In general, the diagnosis of ANLL is established by demonstrating that leukemic cells (myeloblasts, promyelocytes, monoblasts, promonocytes, megakaryoblasts) constitute more than 30% of the nucleated marrow cells (or > 30% of the nonerythroid nucleated cells in the case of erythroleukemia). Classically, histochemical stains have been used to demonstrate that cells are of nonlymphoid origin. Common histochemical stains that are "positive" in nonlymphoid cells are Sudan black B and peroxidase (myeloblasts, promyelocytes), "nonspecific" esterases which are inhibited by sodium fluoride (monoblasts), and "block positive" periodic acid-Schiff (pronormoblasts in erythroleukemia). Antigens commonly demonstrated by immunologic techniques include My 7 (CD13) and My 9 (CD33) on myeloblasts and monoblasts; My 4 (CD14) on monoblasts; and von Willebrand factor, GP IIIa (CD61), and GPIIb/IIIa (CD41) on megakaryoblasts. Electron microscopy is critical for demonstrating the presence of myeloperoxidase and platelet peroxidase in the FAB M_0 and M_7 variants, respectively. A simplified version of the FAB classification system is as follows: M_0—myelocytic leukemia without maturation; M_1—myelocytic leukemia with minimal differentiation; M_2—myelocytic leukemia with maturation; M_3—promyelocytic leukemia; M_4—myelomonocytic leukemia; M_5—monocytic leukemia; M_6—erythroleukemia; and M_7—megakaryoblastic leukemia.

B. **Acute lymphocytic leukemia.** Whereas mature lymphocytes may account for up to 25% of the nucleated cells in the adult bone marrow, recognizable lymphoblasts are not a component of normal marrow. In general, the diagnosis of ALL is established by demonstrating that leukemic lymphoblasts constitute more than 25% of the nucleated marrow cells. Because of its lack of reproducibility, the morphologic subclassification of ALL by the FAB system has been abandoned. In general, ALL is subclassified according to B cell or T cell lineage based on immunophenotyping. Immunologic markers classically suggesting B cell lineage are the common ALL antigen (CALLA, CD10) ("common" or prepre-B cell ALL), intracytoplasmic mu heavy chains (pre-B cell ALL), and surface membrane immunoglobulin (B cell ALL). Ia and B4 (CD19) are common generic markers for cells of B lineage, while B1 (CD20) is seen in more mature B lineage cells. T cell ALL arises from stage I (prothymocyte) and stage II thymocytes. Immunologic markers classically suggesting T cell lineage are T11 (CD2, sheep red blood cell receptor), T10 (CD38, panthymocyte), and T9 (CD71, transferrin receptor). The enzyme terminal deoxynucleotidal transferase (TdT) can be demonstrated in cells of early B cell (prior to pre-B cell) and T cell (through thymocyte) lineage.

C. **Acute mixed-lineage (AMLL) and stem cell leukemias.** With the expansion of immunophenotyping panels and the increased use of electron microscopy and gene rearrangement studies for the characterization of acute leukemia, increasing degrees of infidelity of myeloid and lymphoid markers can be demonstrated. Minimal deviation from the expected markers is not uncommon and may produce well-defined syndromes that do not alter the basic cellular lineage (e.g., My^+ ALL, $CD7^+$ AML, TdT^+ AML). There are no consensus guidelines for the diagnosis of AMLL; rather the diagnosis rests on the vague "unequivocal demonstration" of myeloid and lymphoid characteristics (e.g., myeloperoxidase positivity plus two lymphoid markers) either on the same cells or on two different subpopulations. In stem cell leukemia, the cells express only rudimentary hematopoietic markers (e.g., Ia antigen, TdT, CD34). The identification of entities such as My^+ ALL, AMLL, and stem cell leukemia may be of prognostic importance and have therapeutic implications.

II. Initial support. Once the diagnosis of acute leukemia has been established, the next 24–48 hours are usually spent preparing the patient for the initiation of cytotoxic chemotherapy. The following issues need to be addressed in almost all individuals facing induction chemotherapy, as those individuals who are in the best overall shape are best able to tolerate the rigors of induction chemotherapy.

    A. Hydration and correction of electrolyte imbalance. Dehydration needs to be corrected and adequate urine output maintained to prevent renal failure due to the deposition of cellular breakdown products. In the absence of cardiac disease, normal saline with or without 5% dextrose is infused to maintain the urine output at more than 100 ml/hour. The concomitant use of loop diuretics may be necessary in individuals with congestive heart failure. Although a variety of electrolyte problems may occur in individuals with acute leukemia, hypokalemia is the most troublesome, particularly in individuals with ANLL. Parenteral potassium replacement should be given even in individuals with ANLL who are normokalemic, as a normal serum potassium level does not reflect the diminished potassium stores of most of these individuals.

    B. Prevention of uric acid nephropathy. Hyperuricemia is common at presentation and may also occur with the tumor lysis caused by chemotherapy. Allopurinol is the mainstay of preventing uric acid nephropathy. The usual initial adult dose is 300 mg (150 mg/m^2) bid for 2–3 days, which is then decreased to 300 mg once a day. Allopurinol is often stopped after 10–14 days to lessen the risk of rash and hepatic dysfunction. If chemotherapy needs to be initiated urgently, allopurinol at a dose of 600 mg bid is well tolerated for 1–2 days. With the advent of allopurinol, the role of urine alkalinization has become less clear. Although urine alkalinization increases uric acid solubility, it decreases the solubility of urinary phosphates and may promote phosphate deposition in individuals susceptible to the tumor lysis syndrome (e.g., B cell ALL and T cell lymphoblastic leukemia). A commonly employed method of urine alkalinization is to hydrate the patient with 0.5 N saline to which two syringes of sodium bicarbonate (44 mEq $NaHCO_3$/syringe) have been added per liter.

    C. Blood product support. Most individuals with acute leukemia present with bone marrow failure, so symptomatic anemia and thrombocytopenia must be corrected (see Chap. 32).

    D. Fever or infection. Individuals frequently have a fever or an infection at initial diagnosis. The approach to fever and infection is discussed in Chapter 31. *The cardinal rule is that all individuals with acute leukemia and fever have an infection until proved otherwise.* Given the additional myelo- and immunosuppressive effects of chemotherapy, severe infections should be treated aggressively prior to initiating chemotherapy.

E. **Vascular access.** Because of the need for several sites of venous access for at least 1 month, a multiple-lumen implantable catheter must be placed as soon as possible (see Chap. 40).

F. **Suppression of menses.** A serum human chorionic gonadotropin (β-hCG) assay (pregnancy test) should be done in all premenopausal women prior to initiating chemotherapy. Because menorrhagia may occur owing to the severe thrombocytopenia that is seen during induction chemotherapy, preventing menses becomes desirable. Medroxyprogesterone (Provera) may be used for hormonal support of the progestational endometrium. Medroxyprogesterone 10 mg bid PO should be started 5–7 days before the presumed starting time of the next menstrual period. It may be increased to 10 mg tid or higher if breakthrough bleeding occurs. Depo-Provera is contraindicated in the thrombocytopenic and neutropenic individual.

G. **Psychosocial support.** Individuals with acute leukemia are usually previously healthy individuals who have suddenly had to accept their own imminent mortality. Intensive psychologic support by the health care team, family, and religious leaders is critical for maintaining the patient's sense of well-being (see Chap. 38).

H. **Optimization of comorbid disease.** Individuals with good performance status are best able to tolerate chemotherapy. Comorbid disease (e.g., heart failure, diabetes, chronic lung disease) should be aggressively treated prior to initiating induction chemotherapy.

III. **Therapeutic principles of and approach to therapy for acute leukemia**

A. **Therapeutic aim.** The goals of chemotherapy are to eradicate the leukemic clone and reestablish normal hematopoiesis in the bone marrow. Two important principles need to be remembered: (1) Long-term survival is seen only in individuals in whom a complete response is attained; and (2) with the exception of bone marrow transplantation (BMT) as salvage therapy, the response to initial therapy predicts the fate of the individual with acute leukemia. Although leukemia therapy is toxic, and infection is the major cause of death during therapy, the median survival time of untreated (or unresponsive) acute leukemia is 2–3 months, and most untreated individuals die of bone marrow failure. The doses of chemotherapy are never reduced because of cytopenias, as lowered doses still produce the unwanted side effects (further marrow suppression) without having as great a potential for eradicating the leukemic clone and ultimately improving marrow function.

B. **Forms of chemotherapy**

1. **Induction chemotherapy** is initial intensive chemotherapy given in an attempt to eradicate the leukemic clone and to induce a remission (complete response).

2. **Postinduction (postremission) chemotherapy** is further chemotherapy given after a complete re-

sponse (CR) has been obtained in an attempt to further eradicate the residual, but nondetectable, leukemic cells. Given the generally high induction rate for acute leukemia, future advances are likely to be made through improved postinduction chemotherapy. Therefore, all individuals should be candidates for experimental protocols evaluating options for postinduction therapy.

  a. Maintenance. Low doses of drugs designed for outpatient use given for up to 3 years.

  b. Consolidation. Repeated courses of the same drugs at the same or similar doses used to induce the remission, given soon after the remission has been achieved. Consolidation requires further acute hospitalization.

  c. Intensification. Intensive courses of drugs given at increased dosages to take advantage of steep dose–response relationships (e.g., high-dose cytarabine) or of putatively non-cross-resistant drugs. Intensification is given soon after the remission has been achieved and requires further acute hospitalization.

C. Definition of response. The criteria are based on the peripheral blood counts and the status of the bone marrow at the time of marrow recovery, not at the time of marrow aplasia.

  1. Complete response (complete remission, CR) is the return of the complete blood count (CBC) to "normal"—absolute neutrophil count (ANC) of more than $1500/\mu l$, and platelet count of more than $100,000/\mu l$ in conjunction with a normal bone marrow (i.e., normal cellularity, $< 5\%$ blasts or promyelocytes/promonocytes, and an absence of obvious leukemic cells, [e.g., containing Auer rods]).

  2. Partial response is the persistence of gross residual leukemia: 5–25% leukemic cells in the bone marrow.

IV. Therapy of adult ANLL

A. General plan of therapy. The day that induction chemotherapy is started is arbitrarily called day 1. Bone marrow aspiration and biopsy are repeated on approximately days 12–14. If the bone marrow is severely hypoplastic with fewer than 5% residual blasts or if the bone marrow is aplastic, no further chemotherapy is given and the patient is supported until bone marrow recovery occurs (usually 1–3 weeks). If there is residual leukemia at day 14, a second course of chemotherapy at attenuated doses is given. A bone marrow examination is repeated 2 weeks later (approximately days 26–28). For those patients with residual disease at day 28, a third course of chemotherapy may be given and the same evaluation process repeated. Once a CR has been documented, the potential benefit of further postinduction therapy should be determined on an individual basis.

B. Induction. The same chemotherapeutic regimens are used to treat the various subtypes of ANLL (M_0–M_7).

Factors that influence the choice of the chemotherapeutic program to be employed include the individual's cardiac function, age, and performance status. The initial drug doses outlined below are based on the presence of normal hepatic function. They are not modified based on peripheral blood counts.

1. **De novo ANLL.** Individuals who develop ANLL de novo have the best response to chemotherapy. Therapeutic options vary depending on the clinical situation. Cytarabine (ara-C) is the most active agent for ANLL and is the agent around which most active regimens are built.

   a. **Normal cardiac function.** The two most commonly used programs are "7 + 3" and "DAT." Both will produce remission rates of 65–70% "across the board," and should be considered equivalent.

      (1) **"7 + 3"** is the combination of a 7-day infusion of cytarabine and 3 days of an anthracycline or anthracenedione. Although idarubicin may have a marginal advantage by inducing more remissions after a single cycle of therapy compared to daunorubicin and may have a slightly higher CR rate based on small studies, the use of idarubicin is not a substantial advance. Thus, although many investigators have strong personal biases about the choice for induction therapy, I would consider daunorubicin, idarubicin, and mitoxantrone as essentially equivalent choices based on current data. All three should be considered potentially cardiotoxic.

         (a) Cytarabine 100 mg/m²/day continuous IV infusion on days 1–7, *and*

         (b) Daunorubicin 45 mg/m² IV push on days 1–3, *or*
         Idarubicin 12 mg/m² IV push on days 1–3, *or*
         Mitoxantrone 12 mg/m² IV push on days 1–3.

      If there is residual leukemia in the bone marrow specimen obtained on day 14, but there has been good cytoreduction, the second course of chemotherapy is attenuated to a 5-day infusion of cytarabine and 2 days of the anthracycline or anthracenedione ("5 + 2"). There is no dose modification for the second course based on blood cell counts. The dose of cytarabine and daunorubicin for the second cycle may be decreased if hepatic dysfunction develops and is believed to be due to drug toxicity (see sec. **IV.B.1.a.(2)**, DAT). If there has been little cytoreduction in the day 14 bone marrow specimen, 4 doses of high-dose cytarabine (HDAC) (see sec. **IV.B.1.b.**) would be a reasonable alternative to "5 + 2."

(2) DAT is the following combination.

Cytarabine 25 mg/m^2 IV bolus, followed by 200 mg/m^2/day continuous IV infusion on days 1–5, *and*

Daunorubicin 60 mg/m^2 IV push on days 1–3, *and*

Thioguanine 100 mg/m^2 PO q12h on days 1–5.

If there is residual leukemia in the day 14 bone marrow specimen, a second course of DAT is initiated at full doses. There is no dose modification based on blood cell counts. Drug dosage for the second cycle may be modified if hepatic dysfunction has developed (regardless of cause) (50% reduction of both daunorubicin and thioguanine for bilirubin 1.5–3.0 mg/dl or transaminase 150–300 IU/ml and 75% reduction for bilirubin > 3.0 or transaminase > 300).

(3) Other agents. HDAC (see sec. **IV.B.1.b.**) with or without an anthracycline has been shown to be active for the induction of ANLL. There is no evidence to suggest that HDAC is superior to the "7 + 3" regimen. Although etoposide is active in relapsed/refractory ANLL, its addition to the "7 + 3" regimen at a dose of 75 mg/m^2/day on days 1–7 ("7 + 3 + 7") does not improve the CR rate compared to "7 + 3." In addition, the risk of secondary acute leukemia from topoisomerase inhibitors needs to be considered in individuals who are potentially long-term survivors.

b. Impaired cardiac function. The use of an anthracycline or an anthracenedione is contraindicated for induction therapy in individuals with severe underlying cardiac disease, particularly if the patient has had a recent myocardial infarction or has an ejection fraction of less than 50%. The choice of therapy in this situation is **HDAC** which consists of cytarabine 3 gm/m^2 IV infusion over 1–2 hours q12h for 12 doses. Unique complications include ulcerative keratitis and neurotoxicity. Because ara-C is secreted in tears, ulcerative keratitis can be prevented by instilling eyedrops (saline, methylcellulose, or steroid) q2h while awake and Lacri-Lube Ophthalmic Ointment (Allergan Pharmaceuticals) at bedtime starting at the time HDAC is initiated and continuing for 2–3 days after the last dose of HDAC. Neurotoxicity (e.g., cerebellar dysfunction, somnolence) occurs more frequently in older individuals and as the number of doses of HDAC increases. Renal and hepatic dysfunction contribute to the development of neurotoxicity. Neurotoxicity increases as the infusion time increases. Thus, 1–2-hour infusions are recommended compared to the original rate of 2–3 hours.

2. **ANLL in the elderly.** Given that the median age at presentation is approximately 60 years, ANLL in the "elderly" individual is a common problem. Owing to the effects of comorbid disease and "old age" on normal physiology, elderly individuals are less able to withstand the inherent toxicity of induction chemotherapy compared to "younger adults." The decision to forgo therapy in an elderly patient with ANLL should not be made a priori based solely on age; rather, the decision to treat or not to treat should be based on more substantive factors, such as the presence of comorbid disease, performance status prior to diagnosis, quality of life prior to diagnosis, and projected long-term survival. In general, 40–50% of elderly individuals can achieve a CR to chemotherapy. When a decision is made to treat the elderly patient with ANLL, many investigators would recommend that modified doses of induction chemotherapy be used. The role of growth factors (e.g., G-CSF) to stimulate earlier marrow recovery in order to allow elderly patients to better tolerate full doses of induction chemotherapy is currently under investigation; this approach should be considered experimental given the theoretical potential for selectively stimulating the growth of the leukemic clone.

a. **Modified "7 + 3"** attenuates the dose of daunorubicin. Full-dose idarubicin and mitoxantrone have not been shown to be superior to full-dose daunorubicin in the elderly, nor have they been compared to attenuated-dose daunorubicin. A modified "7 + 3" regimen is recommended.

Cytarabine 100 mg/m^2/day IV continuous infusion on days 1–7, *and*
Daunorubicin 30 mg/m^2 IV push on days 1–3.

b. **Modified DAT**

Cytarabine 100 mg/m^2/day SQ bid on days 1–5, *and*
Daunorubicin 50 mg/m^2 IV push on day 1, *and*
Thioguanine 100 mg/m^2 PO bid on days 1–5.

c. **Modified HDAC** decreases the cytarabine dose to try to diminish the dose-limiting neurotoxicity. Modified HDAC is generally believed to be more toxic than the "7 + 3" regimen. Although the optimum dose and schedule are not known, 1.5–2.0 gm/m^2 q12h for 8–12 doses is commonly used.

d. **Low-dose cytarabine.** Low-dose ara-C should not be considered as first-line therapy but should be reserved for individuals who truly are not candidates for more intensive therapy. Low-dose ara-C is 10 mg/m^2 given SQ bid for 10–21 days.

3. **Secondary ANLL.** In general, secondary ANLL (e.g., arising after prior irradiation, chemotherapy with alkylating agents or topoisomerase inhibitors, or evolving from a myelodysplastic syndrome or myeloproliferative disorder) has been thought not to respond as well to standard induction chemotherapy as does de novo ANLL. The advisability of chemotherapy needs to be assessed in each individual situation. Recent data suggest that secondary ANLL with normal cytogenetics has a response rate similar to that of de novo ANLL. Therapeutic options include supportive care, "7 + 3," and HDAC plus daunorubicin (45 mg/m^2 IV on days 1–3).

4. **ANLL during pregnancy.** The fortunes of both the mother and the fetus must be considered when discussing the therapeutic options for a pregnant woman who develops ANLL. Therapeutic abortion must be considered if ANLL develops during the first trimester. If therapeutic abortion is not an option or if ANLL develops during the second or third trimester, induction chemotherapy may be undertaken. Except for a modest increase in fetal deaths and an increased risk of premature labor, "7 + 3" and DAT appear to be well tolerated by both the patient and the fetus. However, the long-term effects of in utero exposure are not yet known, as these exposed individuals are now just reaching their third decade of life.

C. **Postinduction therapy.** The fact that most patients with ANLL relapse despite attaining a CR suggests that further postinduction therapy is indicated to eradicate the residual but undetected leukemic clone. Although the optimum form remains to be defined, almost all patients with ANLL benefit from some form of postinduction therapy. As with induction therapy, the type of postinduction therapy should be determined on an individual basis. Relative contraindications to postinduction therapy include complications during induction (e.g., posttransfusion hepatitis with persistent hepatic dysfunction, persistent systemic fungal infection), poor tolerance of induction by the elderly, and pregnancy. Individuals with ANLL in first remission should be considered candidates for experimental protocols examining postinduction therapy options.

1. **Maintenance.** Given the rigors of further intensive, cytoreductive chemotherapy, maintenance is generally the treatment of choice for elderly (> 60 years old) individuals as well as younger individuals who did not tolerate induction well. In general, remission duration is 12–15 months, and overall survival time is 18–24 months with maintenance chemotherapy. Approximately 15–20% of individuals treated with maintenance therapy remain long-term disease-free

survivors. Maintenance may be initiated when the peripheral blood counts have returned to normal, marrow cellularity is normal, infections have cleared, and mucositis has resolved. In general, maintenance is of no additional value after consolidation therapy. Maintenance may be alternating blocks of drugs or repetitive courses of the same drugs.

a. **Alternating courses.** A commonly used program of alternating blocks of drugs has been devised by Cancer and Acute Leukemia Group B (CALGB). Each of the four courses is given on a monthly basis during the cycle. Two cycles are given. If a bone marrow examination shows that the patient is still in a CR at the end of the second cycle, no further therapy is given. Minimal blood counts for initiating maintenance are an ANC of more than 2000/μl and a platelet count of more than 100,000/μl. Each cycle consists of the following four courses.

Course 1:	Cytarabine 100 mg/m^2 SQ bid on days 1–5, *and*
	Thioguanine 100 mg/m^2 PO bid on days 1–5.
Courses 2 and 4:	Cytarabine 100 mg/m^2 SQ bid on days 1–5, *and*
	Vincristine 2 mg IV on days 1 and 8, *and*
	Prednisone 40 mg/m^2 PO on days 1–5 (100 mg maximum).
Course 3:	Cytarabine 100 mg/m^2 SQ bid on days 1–5, *and*
	Daunorubicin 45 mg/m^2 IV on days 1 and 2.
	This course may require support for pancytopenia.

Once maintenance has been started, the next course may be given in 4 weeks, provided that infection and mucositis from the previous course have cleared, the ANC is more than 2000/μl, and the platelet count is more than 100,000/μl. If the ANC and platelet count are below the minimum, repeat them in 1 week and use the following criteria.

Dose (%)	ANC/μl	Platelets/μl
100	> 2000	> 100,000
50	1000–1999	50,000–99,999
0	< 1000	< 50,000

Dose adjustments for hematologic toxicity should also be based on nadir blood counts or the development of grade 4 bleeding or infection during the previous course.

Dose (%)	Nadir ANC/μl	Nadir platelets/μl
100	> 1000	> 50,000
50	< 1000	< 50,000

b. Repetitive courses. A program of repetitive courses of the same drugs may also be used. The course is repeated every week for 2 years. Minimal blood counts for initiating maintenance are an ANC of more than 1500/μl and a platelet count of more than 100,000/μl. The drugs used are

Thioguanine 40 mg/m² PO bid on days 1–4, *and* Cytarabine 60 mg/m² SQ on day 5.

Once maintenance has been started, dose adjustments for hematologic toxicity may be based on blood counts obtained at the start of the course.

Dose (%)	ANC/μl	Platelets/μl
100	> 1500	> 100,000
50	1000–1499	50,000–99,999
0	< 1000	< 50,000

c. Cytarabine and daunorubicin produce similar results according to recent data from CALGB.

Cytarabine 100 mg/m²/day continuous IV infusion on days 1–5 monthly for 4 months, *then* Cytarabine 100 mg/m² SQ bid on days 1–5, *and* Daunorubicin 45 mg/m² IV on day 1 both monthly for 4 months.

d. Birth control. Given the potential teratogenic effects of cytotoxic chemotherapy, appropriate measures for preventing conception must be addressed with women who are undergoing maintenance therapy and who may still be in their reproductive years. Although there are no clear data linking maintenance chemotherapy in the male partner to teratogenic effects in the fetus, it appears prudent to suggest that appropriate birth control measures be undertaken in this situation as well.

2. Consolidation. When taken in toto, the current published data do not suggest that consolidation offers a distinct advantage (improved survival or improved cost-benefit ratio) compared to maintenance. While consolidation with 1–3 cycles of "7 + 3" or DAT without maintenance has been empirically recommended by some investigators in the past, consolidation has fallen out of favor for individuals who are good candidates for intensification. Whether consolidation offers an advantage in elderly individuals with good performance status compared to maintenance is unproved.

3. Early intensification. Early intensification represents the best strategy devised thus far for postinduction chemotherapy. Uncontrolled series suggest that 40–50% of individuals will be in a continuous CR 5 years after intensification with HDAC with or without daunorubicin, while randomized controlled studies suggest this rate may be closer to 30–50% at 3–4 years. There is approximately 5% mortality with HDAC or HDAC plus daunorubicin. Amsacrine appears to increase the toxicity of HDAC without a significant increase in benefit. Intensification is the best postinduction chemotherapeutic option currently available for individuals under the age of 40 or 50 years. Intensification should be strongly considered in individuals between the ages of 50 and 60. Because of the significant morbidity and mortality, intensification is not recommended outside of the experimental setting for individuals older than 60 years. Intensification should be initiated when the peripheral blood counts have returned to normal (ANC > 1500/μl and platelet count > 100,000/μl), marrow cellularity is normal, infections have cleared, and mucositis has resolved. The most tolerable intensification programs are based on HDAC. The optimum regimen is not known. Options include the following.

a. HDAC

Cytarabine 3 gm/m^2 IV infusion over 3 hours q12h on days 1, 3, and 5 for 4 monthly courses, *or*
Cytarabine 3 gm/m^2 IV infusion over 2–3 hours q12h on days 1–6 (12 doses) for 1–3 courses.

b. HDAC + daunorubicin has been used in two different programs.
   (1) Cytarabine 3 gm/m^2 IV infusion over 1 hour q12h on days 1–6, *and*
      Daunorubicin 30 mg/m^2 IV on days 7–9 are given for 1–3 cycles.

   (2) Cycle 1: Cytarabine 3 gm/m^2 IV infusion over 2 hours q12h days 1–4, *and*
                Daunorubicin 45 mg/m^2 IV on days 1–3.
        Cycle 2: Cytarabine 200 mg/m^2/day continuous IV infusion on days 1–5, *and*
                Daunorubicin 45 mg/m^2 IV on days 1–3.

c. HDAC + multiple agents

Cycle 1: Cytarabine 3 gm/m^2 IV infusion over 2 hours q12h on days 1–4, *and*
         Mitoxantrone 10 mg/m^2 IV on days 1–3.
Cycle 2: Etoposide 200 mg/m^2/day on days 1–5, *and*
         Mitoxantrone 10 mg/m^2 IV on days 1–3.
Cycle 3: Cytarabine 2 gm/m^2 IV infusion over 2 hours q12h on days 1–4, *and*
         Daunorubicin 45 mg/m^2 IV on days 1–3.

D. Relapsed ANLL. Given the current state of the art, cytotoxic chemotherapy offers essentially no chance for long-term survivorship for the individual with relapsed ANLL. Given the palliative nature of further chemotherapy at this point, a realistic appraisal of the situation should be offered to the patient in order to develop a plan that can optimize both the quantity and the quality of meaningful life. A long first remission portends a better chance of attaining a substantial second remission. Unfortunately, second remissions tend to be short with median durations in the range of 4–6 months. Individuals with relapsed ANLL should be considered prime candidates for experimental protocols or BMT. Depending on prior therapy, age, and perceived ability to tolerate another induction, chemotherapeutic options using commercially available drugs would include the following.

1. **"7 + 3."** Up to 50% of individuals induced with the "7 + 3" regimen followed by maintenance will respond to a repeat course of "7 + 3."

2. **HDAC.** Fifty to 70% of individuals will respond to a form of HDAC. Although HDAC combination regimens may have a slightly higher response rate, their increased toxicity may not make them significantly better than single-agent HDAC. Options include **HDAC**, *or* **HDAC plus anthracycline**, *or* **HDAC** (3 gm/m^2 IV infusion over 2 hours q12h on days 1–4) **plus mitoxantrone** (10 mg/m^2/day IV on days 2–5 or 2–6), *or* **fludarabine** (30 mg/m^2/day IV infusion over 30 minutes on days 1–5) **plus HDAC** (2 gm/m^2/day IV infusion over 4 hours starting 3.5 hours after the fludarabine is finished on days 1–5).

3. **Etoposide** (100 mg/m^2/day IV on days 1–5) **and mitoxantrone** (10 mg/m^2/day IV on days 1–5) represent a very active and well-tolerated combination that is commonly used for relapsed/refractory leukemia.

4. **High-dose etoposide** (70 mg/m^2/hour continuous IV infusion for 60 hours) **and high-dose cyclophosphamide** (50 mg/kg (1850 mg/m^2)/day IV infusion over 2 hours on days 1–4) is a highly toxic but active regimen that does not require bone marrow support. It is active in HDAC-resistant ANLL (30% CR). (For details, see Brown's article listed in Suggested Readings.)

E. Role of BMT in ANLL. The role and timing of BMT in the management of adult ANLL have been the subjects of much speculation and controversy due to the reporting of uncontrolled results (see Chap. 2). Individuals who are potential candidates for BMT should be enrolled in prospective, randomized studies to further define its use.

1. **Allogeneic transplantation.** Although allogeneic BMT receives much fanfare in the medical literature and the lay press, it has been estimated that in reality at most 10% of individuals with ANLL are candidates for a BMT from a human leukocyte antigen (HLA)-compatible sibling. Although allogeneic BMT

has been considered an option for individuals under the age of 40–45 years, many centers will now take patients up to 55 years old. For individuals with ANLL in second remission, allogeneic BMT is the treatment of choice since it offers a 20–30% chance of long-term survivorship. Recent randomized studies suggested that the use of BMT in patients in their first remission does not improve the overall survival rate compared to individuals treated with postinduction chemotherapy followed by BMT during the second remission should they experience relapse. As the "community standard," BMT should be considered as the optimum form of salvage therapy to be used in patients in second remission or early relapse. However, eligible patients should continue to be entered into randomized prospective clinical trials that examine the use of allogeneic BMT.

2. **Autologous transplantation.** Autologous BMT is the use of the recipient's own bone marrow. The most obvious benefit of using the person's own bone marrow is the absence of the risk of graft-versus-host disease, while the obvious disadvantage is the potential to reinfuse leukemic cells. As methods of bone marrow purging improve and new technology (e.g., polymerase chain reaction) allows for the better detection of residual leukemia, autologous BMT may become the best form of early intensification.

3. **Relapse.** Relapse after BMT in patients in their first remission occurs after approximately 20% of allogeneic transplantations and 40% of autologous BMTs. Salvage of these individuals is difficult, especially if relapse occurs within 3 months after transplantation. Although 35% of individuals may achieve a remission with subsequent "7 + 3" reinduction, long-term leukemia-free survival is rare. A second allogeneic BMT can be considered in individuals who have achieved a second remission after reinduction chemotherapy and whose disease has relapsed at least 6 months after the initial BMT. For individuals who are not candidates for a second BMT, preliminary data suggest that G-CSF (5 μg/kg SQ daily) can stimulate the normal hematopoietic clone in posttransplantation chimerics.

V. **Therapy of adult ALL**
  A. **Overview.** All adults have high-risk ALL compared to children. Although 75–85% of adults with ALL can attain a CR, only 20–35% remain disease-free. The emphasis in recent years has been on the development of therapeutic regimens that contain more intensive induction and postremission therapies. These regimens have usually been developed as complete programs without testing the contributions of the individual components. With the advent of these more aggressive regimens, long-term disease-free survival has improved. Whether this is due to a true improvement in chemotherapy as opposed to

the biases of patient selection and better supportive care is not clear. Given the lessons learned from the "evolution" of therapy for diffuse large-cell lymphoma in the 1980s and 1990s, these improved regimens (and the components thereof) need to be tested in rigorous, randomized prospective trials. All patients with ALL should be considered as candidates for chemotherapy in well-designed, randomized, prospective studies.

B. **Prognostic features.** As opposed to ANLL where chemotherapy is the same regardless of FAB classification, prognostic features are now being used to determine the intensity of induction and postremission chemotherapy for adult ALL. The variables most commonly used include immunophenotype, cytogenetics, white blood cell count, and age. Since the cutoff values for prognostic features vary between studies and institutions, it is the concepts of standard risk and high risk that are most important.

C. **General plan.** The general plan of therapy for adult ALL is somewhat different from that of ANLL. Adults with ALL should be stratified according to known risk factors at the time of diagnosis and started on a regimen appropriate for the perceived risk of failure. The day that induction chemotherapy is started again is arbitrarily called day 1. As opposed to ANLL, the bone marrow in adult ALL has usually been checked for residual leukemia only at the time of marrow recovery. Newer more aggressive protocols do base therapeutic decisions on the status of day 14 bone marrow. Once a CR has been attained, the form of central nervous system (CNS) prophylaxis and postinduction therapy should be determined on an individual basis if not already done at the time of induction (e.g., assignment to a risk category based on the results of cytogenetic analysis not available at the time of initiation of induction).

D. **Standard-risk ALL.** Standard-risk ALL consists of disease that is CALLA$^+$, does not express "myeloid" antigens, does not have the Philadelphia chromosome (Ph1), and occurs in younger adults who have a white blood cell count less than 30,000–60,000/μl.

1. **Normal cardiac function**
   a. **Induction.** In the presence of normal cardiac function, adults with ALL are usually treated with an anthracycline-containing program. Regimens for the induction of adult ALL are built around vincristine, prednisone, and daunorubicin (VPD). L-Asparaginase is commonly added. The overall response rate is 75–85%. Although L-asparaginase proved to be of value in the pre-anthracycline era, its role in anthracycline-based programs is unclear. Given the significant toxicity of L-asparaginase, many investigators no longer recommend its use. There are a number of variations on the basic VPD program described here. Some options are shown in parentheses.

Vincristine 2 mg IV on days 1, 8, 15, (22), *and*

Prednisone 40 or 60 mg/m^2 PO on days 1–28 or days 1–35, followed by rapid taper, *and*

Daunorubicin 45 mg/m^2 IV on days 1–3 (and day 14 if residual leukemia is present in bone marrow),

(*and* L-asparaginase 500 IU/kg [18,500 IU/m^2] IV on days 22–32).

b. CNS prophylaxis is given as 6 doses of intrathecal (IT) methotrexate and whole-brain irradiation starting on approximately day 36 (see sec. **V.K.**).

c. Maintenance for adult ALL usually consists of methotrexate and 6-mercaptopurine. Pulses of vincristine and prednisone are often given as "reinforcement" since they have relatively little toxicity. Maintenance is usually started once the marrow suppression and the oral toxicity of the CNS prophylaxis have cleared. Maintenance may be given in a pulse or a continuous manner. Although allopurinol is usually not needed during maintenance, the dose of 6-mercaptopurine should be decreased by 75% when given concomitantly with allopurinol.

(1) Pulse maintenance is an 8-week cycle consisting of 3 courses of methotrexate and 6-mercaptopurine given every 2 weeks, followed by a 2-week pulse of vincristine and prednisone.

Methotrexate 7.5 mg/m^2 PO on days 1–5, weeks 1, 3, and 5, *and*

Mercaptopurine 200 mg/m^2 PO on days 1–5, weeks 1, 3, and 5, *and*

Vincristine 2 mg IV on day 1, weeks 7 and 8, *and*

Prednisone 40 mg/m^2 PO on days 1–7, weeks 7 and 8.

Oral methotrexate should be taken in a single daily dose, since splitting the daily dose will significantly increase the mucositis. Approximately 3 doses of IT methotrexate will need to be given once maintenance has started. The schedule should be coordinated so that the IT methotrexate is given on day 1 of the 5 scheduled days of oral methotrexate. On those day 1s when IT methotrexate is given, the oral methotrexate is not given. Pulse maintenance is given for 3 years.

Dose adjustments for hematologic toxicity from the methotrexate and 6-mercaptopurine should be made based on blood cell counts obtained prior to the start of each course.

Dose	ANC/μl	Platelets/μl
100%	≥ 2000	≥ 100,000
75%	1500–1999	75,000–99,999
50%	1000–1499	50,000–74,999
0%	< 1000	< 50,000

(2) **Continuous maintenance** consists of continuous daily 6-mercaptopurine with weekly doses of methotrexate. Two weeks of vincristine and prednisone as described already may be added every 10–12 weeks.

Mercaptopurine 50 mg/m² PO every day, *and*
Methotrexate 20 mg/m² IV or PO every week.

Dose adjustments for hematologic toxicity from the methotrexate and 6-mercaptopurine should be made based on blood cell counts obtained periodically during the course.

Dose	WBC/μl	Platelets/μl
100%	≥ 2500	≥ 100,000
66%	2000–2499	75,000–99,999
33%	1500–1999	50,000–74,999
0%	< 1500	< 50,000

    d. Intensification with cytarabine and daunorubicin given as "7 + 3" and "5 + 2" does not improve remission duration or overall survival compared to pulse maintenance in randomized prospective trials.

2. ALL in the elderly. Although elderly individuals are often considered a poor risk because of their comorbid disease and the increased incidence of the Ph1 chromosome, they cannot tolerate more intensive therapy. Thus, they are usually treated as a standard risk. In general, full doses of induction therapy are used in elderly individuals with ALL. Some investigators will decrease the dose of vincristine by 50%.

3. Impaired cardiac function

    a. Induction. The use of an anthracycline is contraindicated for induction therapy in individuals with underlying cardiac disease. Vincristine, prednisone, and asparaginase in the doses described already represent suboptimal therapy. An active program is MOAD, which is given in sequential 10-day courses (minimum 3, maximum 5) until remission is achieved. Once a CR has been attained, 2 additional courses of MOAD are given.

Methotrexate 100 mg/m² IV on day 1 (increase by 50% courses 2 and 3, and by 25% each additional course until mild toxicity is achieved), *and*
Vincristine 2 mg IV on day 2, *and*

L-Asparaginase 500 IU/kg (18,500 IU/m^2) IV infusion on day 2, *and*

Dexamethasone 6 mg/m^2/day PO on days 1–10.

b. Consolidation therapy is repeated every 10 days for 6 courses.

Methotrexate (final dose from induction) IV on day 1, *and*

L-Asparaginase 500 IU/kg (18,500 IU/m^2) IV infusion day 2.

c. Cytoreduction begins on day 30 of the last consolidation cycle of methotrexate/asparaginase. Cytoreduction is given monthly for 12 months.

Vincristine 2 mg IV on day 1, 30 minutes prior to methotrexate, *and*

Methotrexate 100 mg/kg (3.7 gm/m^2) IV infusion over 6 hours on day 1, *and*

Leucovorin 5 mg/kg (185 mg/m^2) divided into 12 doses starting 2 hours after the methotrexate infusion over days 1–3, *and*

Dexamethasone 6 mg/m^2/day PO on days 2–6.

d. Maintenance begins on day 30 of the last course of cytoreduction. It is repeated weekly until relapse.

Vincristine 2 mg IV on day 1, *and*

Dexamethasone 6 mg/m^2/day PO on days 1–5, *and*

Methotrexate 15 mg/m^2 PO weekly, *and*

Mercaptopurine 100 mg/m^2 PO daily.

E. T cell lymphoblastic leukemia. This form of leukemia comprises 20–25% of adult ALL. Although it previously had a poor prognosis with standard induction and maintenance chemotherapy, with the advent of more intensive chemotherapy regimens, T cell ALL has become a potentially curable malignancy. There was a 100% response rate, with 59% of responders projected to have long-term disease-free survival with the following regimen.

1. Induction

Daunorubicin 60 mg/m^2 IV on days 1–3, *and*

Vincristine 2 mg IV on days 1, 8, 15, and 22, *and*

Prednisone 60 mg/m^2 PO on days 1–28, *and*

L-Asparaginase 6000 IU/m^2 IM on days 17–28.

If a bone marrow examination on day 14 shows residual leukemia, a single dose of daunorubicin 50 mg/m^2 is given. If a bone marrow examination on day 28 shows residual leukemia, additional induction therapy is given:

Daunorubicin 50 mg/m^2 IV on days 29 and 30, *and*

Vincristine 2 mg IV on days 29 and 36, *and*

Prednisone 60 mg/m^2 PO on days 29–42, *and*

L-Asparaginase 6000 IU/m^2 IM on days 29–35.

2. **CNS prophylaxis** consists of cranial radiation (1800 cGy) and 6 weekly doses of IT methotrexate.
3. **Consolidation therapy** is given monthly for 9 months if the ANC is higher than 1000/μl and the platelet count is higher than 100,000/μl.

   a. **Treatment A** is given in months 1, 3, 5, and 7.

   Daunorubicin 50 mg/m^2 IV on days 1 and 2, *and*
   Vincristine 2 mg IV on days 1 and 8, *and*
   Prednisone 60 mg/m^2 PO on days 1–14, *and*
   L-Asparaginase 12,000 IU/m^2 IM on days 2, 4, 7, 9, 11, and 14.

   b. **Treatment B** is given in months 2, 4, 6, and 8.

   Teniposide 165 mg/m^2 IV on days 1, 4, 8, and 11, *and*
   Cytarabine 300 mg/m^2 IV on days 1, 4, 8, and 11.

   c. **Treatment C** is given in month 9.

   Methotrexate 690 mg/m^2 continuous IV infusion over 42 hours, *and*
   Leucovorin 15 mg/m^2 every 6 hours × 12 doses starting at 42 hours.

4. **Maintenance** is continued for 30 months.

   Methotrexate 20 mg/m^2 PO weekly, *and*
   Mercaptopurine 75 mg/m^2 PO daily.

F. **B cell ALL.** B cell ALL (FAB L$_3$, Burkitt cell) in the adult previously had a very dismal prognosis. Short-term, dose-intensive regimens with the potential to produce long-term disease-free survival have now been reported. Although the numbers of reported individuals are somewhat small, French POG LMB86 produced an 86% CR rate, with 4 long-term survivors out of 7 adults with B cell ALL. Long-term responses were seen with maintenance, as well as after autologous and allogeneic BMT.

1. **Induction**

   Vincristine 2 mg/m^2 IV on day 1, *and*
   Cyclophosphamide 600 mg/m^2 IV on day 2, *and*
   Cyclophosphamide 1200 mg/m^2 IV on days 5–7, *and*
   Daunorubicin 60 mg/m^2 IV on days 5–8, *and*
   Etoposide 150 mg/m^2 IV on days 5–8, *and*
   Prednisone 60 mg/m^2 PO on days 1–8.

2. **Intensification**

   Methotrexate 3000 mg/m^2 on day 1, *and*
   Leucovorin on day 2 (see Chap. 10 for details), *and*
   Vincristine 2 mg/m^2 IV on day 1.

3. **CNS prophylaxis** consists of 8 doses of double IT therapy (methotrexate and cytarabine), as well as cranial radiation (2400 cGy).
4. **Maintenance** is monthly reinduction for 4 months.

G. **Ph1$^+$ ALL.** Ph1$^+$ ALL accounts for 25–30% of adult ALL and as much as 50% of CALLA$^+$ ALL. Overall, Ph1$^+$-

ALL has the worst prognosis. Although Ph1$^+$ ALL has a 50–70% induction rate, long-term responses are rare even with aggressive regimens as described for T cell lymphoblastic leukemia (see sec. **V.E.**). Since cytogenetic analysis is not usually available in a timely manner and not all institutions can examine for *bcr-c-abl* rearrangement on site, individuals with Ph1$^+$ ALL are usually treated with standard induction therapy or with an appropriate experimental protocol. Those who attain a CR should be offered BMT if possible. If not, they should be viewed as candidates for aggressive or novel postinduction experimental protocols.

H. My$^+$ ALL. My$^+$ ALL generally has been shown to have a worse prognosis than My$^-$ ALL in adults. An intuitive approach to improve the outcome in face of lineage infidelity has been to combine the "7 + 3" regimen as used for ANLL with vincristine and prednisone as used for adult ALL. However, neither the combined induction approach nor the use of cytarabine/daunorubicin ("7 + 3" followed by "5 + 2") intensification after standard ALL induction have improved the outcome for My$^+$ ALL.

I. Relapsed ALL. Although a second remission can usually be achieved in adults with ALL, it tends to be short-lived. No regimen is distinctly superior to the others. Individuals with relapsed ALL should be considered prime candidates for experimental protocols or BMT. Chemotherapeutic options using commercially available agents are shown.

1. **"7 + 3"** (cytarabine and daunorubicin) as used for the induction of ANLL is active in ALL. Vincristine and prednisone may be added.

2. **HDAC** as a single agent has modest activity in ALL, with a CR rate of approximately 34% and a median remission duration of 3.6 months in data from combined studies. The addition of idarubicin or mitoxantrone increases the response rate to 60% with a median response time of 3.4 months.

3. **Cytarabine (intermediate dose) and fludarabine** comprise an active noncardiotoxic combination. The median response duration is 5.5 months. Neurotoxicity is low. A second course can be given in 3 weeks if needed.

   a. Induction

   Cytarabine 1 gm/m^2 IV over 2 hours/day on days 1–6, *and*

   Fludarabine 30 mg/m^2/day IV over 30 minutes 4 hours prior to cytarabine, on days 2–6.

   b. Consolidation is given monthly for 2 or 3 courses.

   Cytarabine 1 gm/m^2 IV over 2 hours/day on days 1–4, *and*

   Fludarabine 30 mg/m^2/day IV over 30 minutes 4 hours prior to cytarabine, on days 1–4.

c. Maintenance

Mercaptopurine 50 mg PO tid, *and*
Methotrexate 20 mg/m² PO per week.

4. **Sequential methotrexate and L-asparaginase** is another option. Stomatitis is dose-limiting. Twenty-three percent of treated patients had allergic reactions to L-asparaginase.
   a. **Induction**

   Methotrexate 50–80 mg/m² IV on day 1, *and*
   L-Asparaginase 20,000 IU/m² IV 3 hours after methotrexate on day 1, followed by
   Methotrexate 120 mg/m² IV on day 8, *and*
   L-Asparaginase 20,000 IU/m² IV on day 9.

   Repeat day 8 and 9 doses for methotrexate and asparaginase every 7–14 days until remission is attained.
   b. **Maintenance** is repeated every 2 weeks.

   Methotrexate 10–40 mg/m² IV on day 1, *and*
   L-Asparaginase 10,000 IU/m² IV on day 1.

5. **Etoposide and cytarabine** are given every 3 weeks for up to 3 courses until marrow hypoplasia and remission are achieved. They are then repeated monthly until relapse.

   Etoposide 60 mg/m² IV every 12 hours on days 1–5, *and*
   Cytarabine 100 mg/m² IV bolus every 12 hours on days 1–5.

J. **BMT.** As with adult ANLL, the role of BMT in the management of adult ALL is constantly in evolution (see Chap. 2). Eligible candidates should be entered into randomized prospective trials to further define the use of BMT in adult ALL.
   1. **Allogeneic BMT.** Allogeneic transplantation has been compared to chemotherapy in randomized prospective trials. For standard-risk patients, the outcome is similar. Thus, for standard-risk patients, BMT should be considered as salvage therapy in second remission. BMT should be considered the postremission treatment of choice in Ph1⁺ ALL, and strongly considered for other high-risk individuals.
   2. **Autologous BMT.** Autologous transplantation in patients in first remission appears to offer no advantage over chemotherapy in the prospective trials reported to date. Autologous transplantation in second remission can lead to a significant prolongation of leukemia-free survival.
   3. **Relapse after BMT.** Although up to 50% of individuals can attain another remission with reinduction chemotherapy (vincristine and prednisone plus daunorubicin and/or L-asparaginase), fewer than 10%

are leukemia-free after 3 years. If a second remission can be attained with chemotherapy, a second BMT may improve survival, especially in those who have had relapse more than 1 year after the initial transplantation.

K. CNS prophylaxis. In the era prior to prophylaxis of the CNS, more than 50% of children and adults would experience relapse solely in the CNS. Treatment of the CNS sanctuary after a CR has been attained has dramatically decreased the risk of CNS relapse. The timing of CNS prophylaxis depends on the intensity of postremission therapy and the perceived risk of developing CNS leukemia. Two equivalent options exist.

1. Cranial irradiation and intrathecal (IT) methotrexate. Cranial irradiation with IT methotrexate has been the classic method of CNS prophylaxis. It has usually been initiated within 2 weeks of attaining a CR when classic maintenance is given.

a. Cranial irradiation is usually given to the cranial vault (anteriorly to posterior pole of the eye and posteriorly to C2) in 0.2-Gy fractions for a total of 18–24 Gy. The spine is not irradiated because marrow toxicity will significantly limit the ability to give further chemotherapy. Common acute complications of radiation include stomatitis, parotitis, alopecia, marrow suppression, and headaches. Long-term complications include dental caries. Like children, young adults may develop learning disorders, impaired growth, and leukoencephalopathy.

b. IT methotrexate. Methotrexate is used instead of radiation for prophylaxis of the spinal cord. A commonly used program is 12 mg/m^2 (maximum 15 mg) of preservative-free methotrexate diluted in preservative-free saline or Elliot's B solution given IT once a week for 6 weeks. Some investigators also give 10 mg of hydrocortisone succinate IT to try to prevent lumbar arachnoiditis, since the latter may limit the ability to give all 6 of the planned courses of IT methotrexate. After cerebrospinal fluid (CSF) is obtained for appropriate studies, 5 ml of CSF is withdrawn into a syringe containing methotrexate diluted in 10 ml of vehicle. This produces a final methotrexate concentration of 1 mg/ml or less (higher concentrations increase the risk of arachnoiditis). The IT methotrexate is then given in an "in and out" manner. One to 2 ml of the methotrexate solution is injected into the spinal canal. One-half to 1 ml of spinal fluid is then withdrawn back into the syringe. This "in and out" process is repeated until all of the methotrexate has been given. It is used to ensure that the methotrexate is actually given into the subarachnoid space. Leucovorin 5 mg may be given orally every 6 hours for 4 doses to ameliorate the mucositis, although this

usually is not needed unless the patient is getting concurrent systemic methotrexate. Complications of methotrexate include chemical arachnoiditis and leukoencephalopathy.

2. **Chemoprophylaxis.** Given the toxicity of whole-
brain irradiation for individuals younger than 25
years, other strategies of CNS prophylaxis have been
developed. The combination of systemic intermedi-
ate- to high-dose methotrexate with IT methotrexate
is considered to be as effective as cranial irradiation
with IT methotrexate. HDAC used for intensification
is also an active adjunct to IT methotrexate.

VI. **Mixed lineage and stem cell acute leukemia** represent
interesting management problems. Although large series of
these patients are not usually reported, they are generally
thought to have a poor prognosis. An intuitive approach to
induction that is often used with these diseases of unclear
lineage is to combine "7 + 3" as used for ANLL with vincristine and prednisone as used for adult ALL. Given the
partial lymphoid nature of these cells, CNS prophylaxis
should be given. The best form of postremission therapy is
unclear. BMT would be an appropriate option during remission.

VII. **Management problems.** Although individuals receiving
therapy for acute leukemia often have a "predictable"
course, certain clinical manifestations require further individualization of the therapeutic approach.

A. **CNS leukemia.** Leukemic involvement of the CNS
bodes poorly for the adult with acute leukemia given the
morbidity of the associated neurologic dysfunction, the
inability to control CNS leukemia on a long-term basis,
and the common association with active marrow disease.
CNS involvement occurs most frequently with hyperleukocytosis and the monoblastic, B cell, and T cell lymphoblastic leukemias.

1. **Diagnosis.** Although the occurrence of CNS involvement in ALL at diagnosis is well recognized, there is
a 10% risk of occult CNS involvement at the time of
diagnosis in adult ANLL. Thus in all cases of acute
leukemia a lumbar puncture should be performed at
or shortly after the time of diagnosis. In individuals with high peripheral blast counts and no CNS
symptoms, it is usually prudent to perform the lumbar puncture after chemotherapy has decreased the
blast count. In this way, contamination of the CSF
specimen in the event of a traumatic lumbar puncture is prevented. Common clinical features of CNS
leukemia include headache, altered sensorium, and
cranial nerve palsy (especially cranial nerve VI).
Features suggestive of CNS involvement indicate the
need for an immediate lumbar puncture because (1)
neurologic dysfunction is most amenable to therapy
within the first 24 hours, and (2) infectious meningitis must be excluded in the immunocompromised
host. The diagnosis of CNS leukemia is made by
finding 5 or more blast cells on a cytospin prepara-

tion of 1 ml of CSF. Essentially all individuals with CNS leukemia have an elevated CSF protein level as well; however, in the absence of infection, this finding by itself is suggestive but not diagnostic of CNS leukemia.

2. **Treatment.** Although the therapy of CNS leukemia is usually only palliative, it should be initiated as soon as possible. The rapid initiation of therapy may reverse or prevent cranial nerve palsies, which are a morbid complication for both patients and caretakers. The treatment for CNS leukemia is usually concomitant cranial irradiation and IT chemotherapy. Cranial irradiation is usually given to a total of 30 Gy in 1.5–2.0 Gy fractions. IT chemotherapy is given in the manner described under CNS prophylaxis (sec. **V.K.**). IT chemotherapy is repeated every 3–4 days with appropriate laboratory studies being done with each lumbar puncture. When blast cells are no longer seen on the cytospin preparation, two more doses of IT drug are given, usually followed by a monthly "maintenance" IT injection. IT methotrexate (12 mg/m^2 IT, maximum 15 mg) with oral leucovorin (5 mg PO q6h × 4 doses starting at the time of the lumbar puncture) is most commonly used for ALL. Ara-C (50 mg IT) is most commonly used for ANLL. The addition of 10 mg of IT hydrocortisone succinate may ameliorate chemical arachnoiditis and have some antileukemic effect as well. Some investigators advocate instilling IT ara-C and methotrexate at the same time or alternating doses of ara-C and methotrexate. Some investigators advocate the routine use of an intraventricular reservoir for treating individuals with CNS leukemia.

B. **Hyperleukocytosis** (blast counts > 100,000/μl) predisposes to rheologic problems.

1. **Leukostasis** (vascular plugging) occurs almost exclusively with ANLL. Cerebral and cardiopulmonary dysfunction due to vascular obstruction, vessel wall necrosis with hemorrhage, or both are the most common clinical manifestations. Hyperleukocytosis is an oncologic emergency. Given the increased risk of early death with hyperleukocytosis, therapy should be rapidly initiated as soon as the diagnosis is made. If the patient is hemodynamically stable, leukapheresis is the most rapid way to lower the blast count. The goal of the leukapheretic session is to lower the blast count to less than 100,000/μl if possible. With very high blast counts (>200,000/μl), decreasing the blast count by 50% may have to be the initial goal, as mathematic modeling suggests that prolonged leukapheresis after a "3-liter exchange" does not significantly decrease the blast count further. Leukapheresis may be repeated daily. Systemic chemotherapy should be initiated immediately after emergent leukapheresis or if leukapheresis is contraindicated. Hydroxyurea 3–5 gm/m^2/day split into 3 doses daily

is most commonly used. Hydroxyurea is stopped at the time more specific induction chemotherapy is initiated. In patients presenting with hyperleukocytosis, an allopurinol dose of 600 mg bid is well tolerated for the first 2 days followed by 300 mg bid for 2–3 days.

2. **Hyperviscosity.** Blood viscosity increases as the blast count rises. Fortunately, concomitant anemia produces a decrease in viscosity. Aggressive red blood cell (RBC) transfusion in individuals with hyperleukocytosis may precipitate symptoms of hyperviscosity. RBC transfusions should be used judiciously with a blast count of more than 200,000/µl, especially in patients with ANLL. Unless the patient is symptomatic due to anemia, a packed cell volume (hematocrit) of 20–25% is a reasonable goal.

C. **Acute promyelocytic leukemia (APML)** is an uncommon (approximately 5%) form of ANLL that presents unique management challenges.

1. **Promyelocytic coagulopathy.** Hypergranular promyelocytic leukemia predisposes to the development of a devastating coagulopathy that is due to a combination of disseminated intravascular coagulation (DIC) and primary hyperfibrinolysis. Pooled data through the late 1980s suggest that under the best of circumstances with cytotoxic induction chemotherapy, 5% of these individuals would die of CNS hemorrhage within the first 24 hours of hospitalization and that another 20–25% would die of CNS hemorrhage during induction chemotherapy. With intensive supportive care, the most recent studies suggest that approximately 10% of individuals will die of hemorrhage during induction chemotherapy. If looked for *carefully, essentially all* individuals with APML will have clinical or laboratory features of DIC. Even with severe thrombocytopenia, bleeding stops quickly at the site of bone marrow examination in the usual patient. Prolonged oozing (1–2 hours) at the bone marrow site is a telltale sign of DIC. Subtle laboratory signs suggestive of an underlying consumptive coagulopathy in APML include a prolongation of only the prothrombin time (> 0.1 second) or a normal fibrinogen titer (fibrinogen is an acute-phase reactant that is normally elevated in acute leukemia at presentation).

2. **Therapy.** Therapy for APML has represented the most exciting recent advancement in the treatment of acute leukemia. All-*trans*-retinoic acid (ATRA) is a unique chemotherapeutic agent since it is able to induce a high rate of clinical remission by promoting cell maturation without producing marrow hypoplasia.

a. **Induction therapy.** Induction therapy consists of either anthracycline-based chemotherapy (e.g., "7 + 3") or ATRA. Although the initial results with ATRA are promising, further randomized prospective studies are needed to define the roles of ATRA and standard chemotherapy.

(1) **Anthracycline-based** chemotherapy can induce a remission in 75–80% of individuals with APML. Death during induction is usually due to bleeding or infection. Drug resistance is rare.

(2) **ATRA (Tretinoin)** (45 mg/m^2/day, divided into 2 doses with food) can induce a remission in 85–90% of individuals with APML. Since hemorrhagic death is rare in individuals treated with ATRA alone, the "retinoic acid syndrome" (RAS) and infection become the major causes of death during induction. Induction and maintenance with single-agent ATRA results in a short remission duration. Given that APML is the form of ANLL with the highest rate of long-term survivorship, the current trend has been to use ATRA induction to decrease the risk of early hemorrhagic death followed by intensification with a cytarabine/anthracycline combination to maximize leukemic cell kill once the risk of hemorrhage has returned to normal. The one randomized prospective trial published to date compared induction plus intensification with cytarabine/daunorubicin to induction by ATRA followed by the same cytarabine/daunorubicin chemotherapy. Although the median follow-up time was short, there was no difference in the remission rate or overall survival between the two treatment arms. The incidence of early death was also similar. The coagulopathy did resolve sooner after ATRA than after chemotherapy. Given the rarity of APML, it is imperative that all eligible patients be entered into the current Eastern Cooperative Oncology Group (ECOG)-coordinated Intergroup trial which is comparing induction therapy with ATRA followed by chemotherapy, to chemotherapy alone.

The RAS has been seen in 20–25% of individuals beginning 2–21 days after starting ATRA treatment. It is a "capillary leak" syndrome that is mediated in part by interleukin-2. The cardinal clinical manifestations are fever and dyspnea. Subsequent evaluation may show arterial hypoxemia, pulmonary infiltration, pleural and pericardial effusions, and renal and cardiac failure. Prevention is the best therapy for RAS. Although a rising white blood cell count is a risk factor for the RAS, it may occur with a count below 5000/μl. If the white blood cell count is greater than 5000–10,000/μl prior to initiating ATRA, hydroxyurea (see sec. **VII.B.1.**) should be used to lower the count to the target range. If the white blood cell count rises to more than 10,000/μl during ATRA therapy, hydroxyurea (see sec. **VII.B.1.**), cytarabine (100 mg/m²/day continuous IV infusion on days 1–5), or induction chemotherapy should be started. Regardless of the white blood cell count or the risk of neutropenic sepsis, at the first sign of dyspnea or fever, dexamethasone 10 mg IV bid should be initiated, as this appears to be the best treatment for established RAS.

b. **Therapy of promyelocytic coagulopathy.** The first rule of managing DIC is to treat the underlying cause. Thus, once the patient has been stabilized, the rapid initiation of induction therapy is the cornerstone of the management of APML (ideally within 24 hours of diagnosis). If induction chemotherapy is used, lysis of the leukemic promyelocytes will transiently exacerbate the clinical and laboratory manifestations of DIC. Intensive blood product support is usually necessary. Reasonable transfusion goals would be to keep the platelet counts above 50,000/μl (especially if heparin is used or there is a significant elevation of the fibrin degradation products, which may impair platelet function) and the fibrinogen concentration higher than 150 mg/dl. Platelet and cryoprecipitate transfusions may be needed as often as every 2–4 hours in order to maintain hemostasis. The most controversial aspect of the management of APML is the role of heparin in controlling the DIC. Given that APML is an uncommon form of ANLL, it is not possible to assess the efficacy of heparin in the usual randomized prospective manner. Thus, all of the available data are based on retrospective analyses.

(1) **Supportive care.** Retrospective single-institution data suggest that aggressive replacement with coagulation factors and platelets can control the coagulopathy in APML, with an acute hemorrhagic death rate of 10–15%.

(2) **Heparin.** The goal of therapy with heparin is to slow the rate of consumption of coagulation factors and platelets, and thus prevent the development of microvascular thromboses and an uncontrolled hemorrhagic state. Even if heparin does not decrease the risk of initial fatal hemorrhage, control of the consumptive coagulopathy should translate into a decreased need for replacement with co-

agulation factors and platelets, and hence a decreased risk from the morbidity and long-term mortality associated with multiple transfusions (e.g., viral infection, alloimmunization). If heparin is to be used, it should be initiated immediately if the patient has clinical or laboratory evidence of DIC. If even subtle laboratory signs of DIC are absent, then heparinization probably can be delayed until the time when chemotherapy is to be initiated. Since the goal of heparin therapy is to control the clinical manifestations of DIC, the heparin dose should be adjusted by monitoring the platelet count and the fibrinogen titer every 4–6 hours initially depending on the severity of the DIC, and not by aiming for an arbitrary partial thromboplastin time as is done with thromboembolic disease. A reasonable initial heparin dose is a 500 units/hour (7 units/kg) by constant infusion given without an initial heparin bolus. The duration of heparin therapy is empiric. The heparin can usually be tapered and stopped within 7–10 days as the manifestations of DIC subside.

(3) **Antifibrinolytic therapy.** Individuals who have uncontrolled coagulopathy despite aggressive transfusion therapy and heparin, and those with disproportionate fibrinolysis may benefit from epsilon-aminocaproic acid (EACA) given as either 1 gm PO every 2 hours or as a 3–4-gm IV bolus followed by continuous IV infusion at 1 gm/hour. Tranexamic acid 6 gm/24 hours by continuous IV infusion for up to 6 days has also been suggested. Given that an underlying consumptive coagulopathy is present, concomitant heparin may be needed to prevent life-threatening thrombosis.

3. **Residual disease.** Residual disease is not uncommonly found in the bone marrow after the second attempt at induction therapy for APML. Although residual disease in other forms of ANLL needs further vigorous treatment if long-term survivorship is to be attained, data suggest that "promyelocytic maturation" and bone marrow recovery may occur in individuals with residual APML. Thus, the benefits of further cytotoxic therapy need to be addressed in each individual.

D. **Extramedullary leukemia.** Infiltration of organs outside the marrow may occur with acute leukemia. Diffuse organ infiltration (e.g., multiple skin nodules and gum infiltration with acute monoblastic leukemia) is best treated with systemic chemotherapy. Isolated accumulations of leukemic cells may occur with ANLL (granulocyte sarcoma, chloroma) and less often with ALL (lymphoblastoma). These foci are best treated with local irradiation at curative doses (30 Gy). Although most commonly associated with active marrow disease, chloromas and lymphoblastomas may occur as a sole site of relapse or as an initial presentation in association with a normal bone marrow. In either case, they universally herald the subsequent development of leukemic infiltration of the bone marrow. An intuitive approach is to treat these individuals with "adjuvant" induction chemotherapy.

VIII. Growth factors. Growth factors (e.g., G-CSF, GM-CSF) hold the promise of an increased response to therapy in acute leukemia. Growth factors have the potential to decrease the risk of neutropenic infection, increase the dose intensity of chemotherapy (especially in the elderly), modulate the chemosensitivity of the leukemic cells, and decrease the overall cost of antileukemic therapy. Conversely, they are expensive and can also theoretically offer the leukemic clone a growth advantage. When taken in toto, the trials published to date do not conclusively support the use of growth factors as adjuncts to chemotherapy in acute leukemia. Under most circumstances, their use should be within the context of a randomized prospective trial.

Selected Readings

Ball, E. D., and Rybka, W. B. Autologous bone marrow transplantation for adult acute leukemia. *Hematol. Oncol. Clin. North Am.* 7:177, 1993.

Brown, R. A., et al. High-dose etoposide and cyclophosphamide without bone marrow transplantation for resistant hematologic malignancy. *Blood* 76:473, 1990.

Cassileth, P. A., et al. Varying intensity of postremission therapy in adult myeloid leukemia. *Blood* 79:1924, 1992.

Christiansen, N. P. Allogeneic bone marrow transplantation in the treatment of adult acute leukemias. *Hematol. Oncol. Clin. North Am.* 7:177, 1993.

Ellison, R. R., et al. The effects of postinduction intensification treatment with cytarabine and daunorubicin in adult acute lymphocytic leukemia: a prospective randomized clinical trial by Cancer and Leukemia Group B. *J. Clin. Oncol.* 9:2002, 1991.

Estey, E. H. Use of colony-stimulating factors in the treatment of acute myeloid leukemia. *Blood* 83:2015, 1994.

Fenaux, P., et al. Effect of all transretinoic acid in newly diagnosed acute promyelocytic leukemia. Results of a multicenter randomized trial. *Blood* 11:3241, 1993.

Frenkel, S. R., et al. All-*trans* retinoic acid for acute promyelocytic leukemia: results of the New York study. *Ann. Intern. Med.* 120:278, 1994.

Grignani, F., et al. Acute promyelocytic leukemia: from genetics to treatment. *Blood* 83:10, 1994.

Hirsch-Ginsberg, C., et al. Advances in the diagnosis of acute leukemia. *Hematol. Oncol. Clin. North Am.* 7:1, 1993.

Ho, A. D., et al. Combination of mitoxantrone and etoposide in refractory acute myelogenous leukemia—an active and well-tolerated regimen. *J. Clin. Oncol.* 6:213, 1988.

Holzer, D. F. Therapy of the newly diagnosed adult with acute lymphoblastic leukemia. *Hematol. Oncol. Clin. North Am.* 7:139, 1993.

Kantarjian, H. Adult acute lymphoblastic leukemia: critical review of current knowledge. *Am. J. Med.* 97:176, 1994.

Kumar, L. Leukemia: management of relapse after allogeneic bone marrow transplantation. *J. Clin. Oncol.* 12:1710, 1994.

Linker, C. A., et al. Treatment of adult acute lymphoblastic leukemia with intensive cyclical chemotherapy: a follow-up report. *Blood* 78:2814, 1991.

Mayer, R. J., et al. Intensive postremission chemotherapy in adults with acute myeloid leukemia. *N. Engl. J. Med.* 331:896, 1994.

Schwartz, B. S., et al. Epsilon-aminocaproic acid in the treatment of patients with acute promyelocytic leukemia and acquired alpha-2-plasmin inhibitor deficiency. *Ann. Intern. Med.* 105:873, 1986.

Stone, R. M., and Mayer, R. J. The approach to the elderly patient with acute myeloid leukemia. *Hematol. Oncol. Clin. North Am.* 7:65, 1993.

Stone, R. M., and Mayer, R. J. Treatment of the newly diagnosed adult with de novo acute myeloid leukemia. *Hematol. Oncol. Clin. North Am.* 7:47, 1993.

Suki, S., et al. Fludarabine and cytosine arabinoside in the treatment of refractory or relapsed acute lymphocytic leukemia. *Cancer* 72:2155, 1993.

Welborn, J. L. Impact of reinduction regimens for relapsed refractory acute lymphoblastic leukemia in adults. *Am. J. Hematol.* 45:341, 1994.

Wolff, S. N., et al. High-dose cytarabine and daunorubicin as consolidation therapy for acute myeloid leukemia in first remission: long-term follow-up and results. *J. Clin. Oncol.* 9:1260, 1989.

Chronic Leukemias

Carol S. Palackdharry

In the chronic leukemias there is excessive proliferation of functionally mature, differentiated cells. This contrasts with the acute leukemias and myelodysplastic syndromes where there is abnormal proliferation of immature cells with impaired differentiation. Thus, the chronic leukemias are postulated to be diseases caused by impaired signal transduction and regulation of cell proliferation, rather than impaired differentiation. This chapter briefly covers four chronic leukemias: chronic myelogenous leukemia (CML), chronic lymphocytic leukemia (CLL), hairy cell leukemia (HCL), and adult T cell leukemia/lymphoma (ATLL).

I. **Chronic myelogenous leukemias (CML, chronic granulocytic leukemia)**

A. **Diagnosis.** CML is a clonal myeloproliferative disorder of a hematopoietic stem cell. Its incidence peaks in the fifth and sixth decades of life and declines thereafter. The hallmark presentation is leukocytosis in which cells at all stages of myeloid differentiation are present. These myeloid cells typically have low or absent leukocyte alkaline phosphatase activity. At diagnosis, splenomegaly is common and small numbers of peripheral blasts may be present. Patients commonly have anemia, thrombocytosis, and a white blood cell (WBC) count of more than $100 \times 10^3/\mu l$. Because molecular studies on peripheral blood can be performed, the bone marrow is examined for prognosis rather than for diagnosis.

CML involves the marrow myeloid, erythroid, megakaryocytic, and rarely, lymphocytic cell lines. The disease is characterized by the presence of the Philadelphia chromosome (Ph), which is the result of a reciprocal translocation involving chromosomes 9 and 22 [t(9;22)(q34;q11)]. This translocation transposes the c-*abl* protooncogene on chromosome 9 to the breakpoint cluster region (*bcr*) on chromosome 22, creating a hybrid oncogene, *BCR-ABL*. This oncogene produces a fusion protein with tyrosine kinase activity which is thought to be responsible for the transformation of normal cells into CML cells. In approximately 90% of patients, routine cytogenetics will demonstrate this translocation. For patients with the morphologic picture of CML but negative findings on cytogenetic analysis, Southern blot analysis of *bcr* gene rearrangement can identify a subset of Ph-negative, rearrangement-positive patients (additional 5%). The natural history and treatment for the 5% of patients with myeloproliferative disorders without any evidence for a translocation are different from those with the translocation.

B. **Natural history.** CML characteristically has a biphasic or triphasic course. The median survival time after diagnosis with conventional therapy and routine supportive care is 3–4 years. During the indolent, or chronic phase, the disease is easily controllable with therapy. Even with standard treatment, it progresses to an accelerated phase which can last up to 1.5 years. The exact definition of accelerated phase remains controversial. However, standard criteria are being developed and include circulating blasts of more than 15%, circulating blasts plus promyelocytes of more than 30%, peripheral basophils of more than 20%, and cytogenetic evolution. Cytogenetic analysis during transformation may demonstrate clonal evolution with new DNA abnormalities, including more than one Philadelphia chromosome or loss of the original Philadelphia chromosome. Approximately 25% of patients will die of complications during the accelerated phase, while 25% will progress into the blastic phase (blast transformation) without going through a definable accelerated phase. Blast transformation is the final phase and in most patients represents a terminal event either from complications of therapy or from complications of marrow failure. About 67% will transform to an acute nonlymphocytic leukemia (ANLL, AML) which is usually refractory to standard antileukemic treatment. The remaining 33% will transform to an acute lymphocytic leukemia (ALL), which may have a better prognosis since some remissions are obtained with appropriate treatment.

C. **Therapy.** Transplantation of allogeneic bone marrow (AlloBMT) from a sibling or of bone marrow from a matched unrelated donor (MUD) is currently the only known potentially curative therapy for CML. Therapy with interferon alpha (IFN-α) is providing encouraging results for patients unable to undergo transplantation. Standard chemotherapy with hydroxyurea prolongs survival of patients with CML, but does not prevent disease evolution.

1. **Bone marrow transplantation.** All patients in the accelerated or blastic phases of CML who are candidates for AlloBMT (age < 55, related matched or one antigen–mismatched donor) should be offered this procedure. The overall disease-free survival rate may correlate with the patient's disease state at the time of AlloBMT, but is approximately 40% at 5 years. There continue to be late relapses, possibly due to the primitive stem cell involved. The timing of AlloBMT during the chronic phase is more controversial because of the risks of the procedure, with an average transplantation-related mortality of 30%.

MUD transplantations are yielding encouraging results, especially in young patients (< 30) with complete human leukocyte antigen (HLA) matches. The overall 2-year disease-free survival rate is approximately 30%, depending on the patient's age and degree of HLA matching. However, this procedure is associated with significant transplant mortality (50–60%) and is still considered investigational. For most patients, a trial of interferon is warranted prior to consideration of MUD transplantation unless disease progression has occurred and the patient is younger than 30 with an HLA-identical donor.

Autologous bone marrow transplantation (ABMT) remains investigational in CML. This procedure appears to prolong survival, although it does not appear curative. Follow-up of ongoing studies will help clarify the role of ABMT. This approach should be considered in the context of a clinical trial for patients who did not respond to interferon and do not have matched related donors (or unrelated donors, if young).

2. **IFN-α**
   a. **Responses.** A number of clinical trials have confirmed the high complete hematologic remission rate (55–80%), with a substantial rate of cytogenetic remissions (20–60%), with the use of high-dose IFN-α. Response rates appear to be dose-dependent, with the highest responses seen at 5×10^6 units/m^2 SQ daily. Maturing results from initial trials demonstrate a median survival time of 5–6 years, with 25% of patients maintaining durable cytogenetic remissions; with conventional hydroxyurea therapy, there are no major cytogenetic responses and the median survival time is about 4 years.
   b. **Side effects.** Most patients experience self-limited flulike symptoms (fever, chills, anorexia) during the first few weeks of therapy, which is not considered dose-limiting. This can be minimized by starting at 50% dosage (2.5×10^6 units/m^2 SQ daily) for the first week and by giving the dose at bedtime with acetaminophen. Using hydroxyurea to reduce initial WBC counts to 20,000/μl also decreases early side effects. However, there are a number of dose-limiting late side effects, including depression, fatigue, neurotoxicity, and hepatitis. Antidepressants may be required in some patients. Other dose-limiting complications include immune-mediated hemolysis or thrombocytopenia, collagen vascular syndromes, and immune-mediated nephrotic syndrome or hypothyroidism. Rare cases of cardiac toxicity are reported.
   c. **Recommendations** (taken after Kantarjian). For patients who are not marrow transplantation candidates, give an initial trial of IFN-α. If there is a cytogenetic response with some reduction in Ph-positive cells by 6 months, IFN-α is continued indefinitely until the cytogenetic response is lost. By 12 months, there should be less than 65% Ph-positive cells to qualify for a response. For those patients who have grade 3 or 4 toxicity, therapy is temporarily held and when the toxicity abates, dose reductions of 50% are given. If there is persistent grade 2 toxicity that does not improve with supportive therapy, the dose is re-

duced by 25%. Other indications for dose reduction are a WBC count less than $2.0 \times 10^3/\mu l$ or platelet count less than $60 \times 10^3/\mu l$.

Were it not for the significant side effects associated with IFN-α, this therapy would more widely be considered the treatment of choice for older patients and for younger patients who do not have a matched related donor for AlloBMT. Because of cost and the IFN-α–associated side effects, however, many clinicians (and patients) still prefer chemotherapy.

3. **Chemotherapy in the chronic phase.** Therapy should be initiated in patients at the time of diagnosis. The goal of palliative chemotherapy is to lower the WBC count into the normal range ($< 10,000/\mu l$). Two agents are currently utilized. Recently, hydroxyurea was shown to provide a survival advantage when compared to busulfan and is currently considered the treatment of choice. In addition, busulfan therapy is associated with a higher transplantation-related mortality and should not be used in patients in whom bone marrow transplantation is a consideration.

   a. **Hydroxyurea.** In patients with a WBC count higher than $100,000/\mu l$ at diagnosis, hydroxyurea 3–5 gm PO daily is required until the WBC count falls to $30,000$–$50,000/\mu l$. At this point, lower doses can be instituted. Maintenance doses of hydroxyurea range from 500 to 2000 mg/day. It is not unusual to have to routinely adjust the maintenance dose. An increase in the required dose may herald evolution of the disease.

   b. **Busulfan.** This drug inhibits stem cell proliferation. Given the therapeutic advantage of hydroxyurea, busulfan is now considered second-line chemotherapy. The time to response is long (3–4 weeks after initiation of therapy). The initial dose is usually 4 or 8 mg PO daily. The dose should be cut in half each time the WBC count decreases by 50%. Therapy should be stopped when the WBC count reaches $20,000/\mu l$ since counts will continue to fall 1–2 weeks after discontinuing therapy. Busulfan therapy is associated with a number of long-term side effects including pulmonary fibrosis, skin pigmentation, and an addisonian-like wasting syndrome.

4. **Therapy in aggressive phase.** Outside the setting of bone marrow transplantation, therapy during the aggressive phase produces few responses. Interferon therapy produces far fewer responses than when this therapy is used in the chronic phase. Eligible patients in the aggressive phase should be considered for AlloBMT or experimental therapies such as ABMT, MUD transplantation, or other interferons.

5. **Splenectomy.** Symptomatic splenomegaly usually responds to therapy. Splenectomy is reserved for pa-

tients with cytopenia due to sequestration not responsive to other therapies. Radiation therapy may also be used in this situation.

6. **Therapy in blast transformation.** In most patients, this represents a terminal event. Patients with AML transformation respond poorly to any conventional AML regimen. Even AlloBMT in this setting produces poor results, with disease in most patients relapsing. Some patients who undergo ALL transformation will obtain remissions to standard ALL therapy (see Chap. 23).

7. **Leukapheresis.** Individuals with CML may develop symptoms of leukostasis (CNS changes, hypoxia, cardiac ischemia, and renal insufficiency) when the WBC count approaches $500,000/\mu l$, even without increased numbers of blasts and promyelocytes. However, when the blast and promyelocyte counts are $50,000-100,000/\mu l$, leukostasis can develop even with lower total WBC counts. Symptoms of leukostasis are absolute indications for leukapheresis, which will alleviate symptoms until hydroxyurea takes effect.

8. **CML and pregnancy.** All therapy for CML is potentially teratogenic and represents a significant risk to the fetus. Effective contraception should be discussed and offered to sexually active patients with childbearing potential. If pregnancy occurs while a female patient is taking hydroxyurea and therapeutic abortion is not an option, busulfan should be used as it appears to be less teratogenic than hydroxyurea.

II. Chronic lymphocytic leukemia

Lymphoid ontogeny results in the production of a variety of immunologically and morphologically different lymphocytes. As a result, chronic lymphoid leukemias include many types of mature clonal proliferations, including B cell chronic lymphocytic leukemia (B-CLL), T cell chronic lymphocytic leukemia (T-CLL), HCL, prolymphocytic leukemia (PLL), small cleaved cell leukemia, Sézary syndrome, ATLL, and large granular lymphocytic leukemia (LGL). This section discusses issues attendant to B-CLL, whereas HCL and ATLL are discussed separately.

A. **Diagnosis of B-CLL.** In North America and Western Europe, B-CLL is the most common chronic lymphoid malignancy, accounting for 30% of all adult leukemias. The median age at diagnosis is 64 years, after which the incidence continues to increase. There is a 2:1 male-female ratio, with only 10% of patients being diagnosed before the age of 50. Most patients are asymptomatic at the time of diagnosis, likely due to the increased use of automated cell counters and routine complete blood cell (CBC) counts.

The demonstration of B cell monoclonality (by kappa-gamma ratio analysis) with an absolute lymphocyte count (ALC) of more than $5000/\mu l$ sustained for at least 4 weeks is sufficient for diagnosis. Flow cytometric analysis of peripheral blood demonstrates clonal B-CLL cells that differ from normal B lymphocytes in their characteristic expression of the T cell antigen CD5, the common CLL antigen (cCLLa), and mouse red blood cell (RBC) receptors. Morphologically, the cells appear as mature small lymphocytes, though varying amounts of atypical prolymphocytic-like cells may be present. Examination of the bone marrow is not necessary for diagnosis, but may aid in prognosis. If flow cytometry is not available, the presence of more than 30% lymphocytes in the marrow with an ALC higher than $10,000/\mu l$ is sufficient for diagnosis.

B. Staging. Tumor burden is linked to survival. There are many proposed staging systems for CLL, of which the modified Rai (Table 24-1) and the Binet (Table 24-2) staging systems are the most widely used. Both of these systems correlate extent of disease with median survival. It is important to remember that autoimmune cytopenias are not considered part of the staging systems. Both staging systems are comparable and provide the same general guidelines for a staging work-up, which should include a thorough physical examination, a CBC count, and peripheral blood flow cytometry usually with a bone marrow examination. Computed tomography (CT) of the chest, abdomen, and pelvis to assess adenopathy, hepatomegaly, or splenomegaly not clinically detectable may also be done.

C. Prognostic factors. The major prognostic factor in CLL is the clinical stage of disease. However, a number of laboratory parameters have prognostic significance.

Table 24-1. Modified Rai staging system

Stage	Distribution (%)	Criteria	Median survival time (yrs)
Low risk	30	Lymphocytosis only (in blood and bone marrow)	10
Intermediate risk	60	Lymphocytosis plus adenopathy or lymphocytosis plus splenomegaly or hepatomegaly	6
High risk	10	Lymphocytosis plus anemia (hemoglobin < 11 gm/dl) or thrombocytopenia (platelets < 100 $\times$ $10^3/\mu l$)	2

Table 24-2. Binet staging system

Stage	Distribution (%)	No. of lymphoid areas involved[a]	Anemia or thrombo- cytopenia[b]	Median survival time (yrs)
A	60	0–2	No	9
B	30	3–5	No	5
C	10	0–5	Yes	2

[a]5 areas = cervical, axillary, inguinal, spleen, and liver. Bilaterality does not increase number of areas designated.
[b]Anemia = hemoglobin < 10 gm/dl; thrombocytopenia = platelets $< 100 \times 10^3/\mu l$.

A diffuse pattern of lymphocyte infiltration in the bone marrow as shown by histology is associated with a poor prognosis. Patients with short lymphocyte doubling times (< 12 months) also have a poor prognosis.

Approximately 55% of patients with B-CLL will have clonal DNA changes, the most common of which is trisomy 12. The role of trisomy 12 in the pathogenesis of CLL remains unclear. Other abnormalities include structural changes of the long arms of chromosomes 13 and 14. In addition, translocations involving the regions of the *bcl-1, -2,* or *-3* protooncogenes have been identified in subsets of patients with CLL. Which chromosomal changes portend a poor prognosis remains uncertain.

D. **Therapy.** Not all patients with CLL require therapy. Since no standard therapy is curative, the goal of therapy remains palliation. Patients with early-stage stable disease require no antineoplastic therapy. Standard therapy with oral alkylating agents in early-stage, stable, asymptomatic patients does not prolong survival, and may be associated with a shorter survival time. For this reason, the standard of care for early-stage stable patients remains observation.

1. **Treatment of autoimmune hemolytic anemia (AIHA) and immune thrombocytopenia.** Approximately 20–35% of CLL patients will have immune-mediated cytopenias. These disorders are thought to be due to the production of polyclonal IgG antibodies by cells other than the malignant clone. The mainstay of therapy remains prednisone at 60–100 mg/day for 3–6 weeks or until hemolysis subsides, after which the prednisone is tapered. Unresponsive patients may benefit from splenectomy, intravenous immunoglobulin, danazol, or splenic irradiation. While chemotherapy of the leukemia may be of no direct benefit, in some patients it may decrease the risk of recurrence of the autoimmune process.

2. **Treatment of progressive or advanced-stage disease.** Indications for treatment include progressive early-stage disease, B symptoms (fever, night

sweats, weight loss), bulky nodal disease or hepato-splenomegaly, and evidence of a compromised bone marrow (early disease with extensive diffuse marrow infiltrate, developing anemia or thrombocytopenia). The optimal duration of therapy is unknown. In general, therapy is discontinued when the disease is controlled and maintenance therapy is not indicated unless necessary for disease control.

a. **Single alkylating agents with or without prednisone.** Oral chlorambucil is the best tolerated and most active alkylating agent administered alone, or in combination with prednisone. It can be administered on a daily or intermittent (pulse) schedule. Prednisone appears effective in reducing adenopathy and splenomegaly, and improving anemia and thrombocytopenia. However, whether prednisone improves response rates or survival remains unclear. Its use must be balanced against the greater risk for infection with corticosteroid therapy.

  (1) **Continuous chlorambucil.** Three to 6 mg/m^2 PO is given daily. Doses should be reduced for hematologic toxicity (ANC < 1000/μl, or platelet count < 75,000/μl); dose reductions are often required as the disease responds.

  (2) **Intermittent chlorambucil.** A single dose of chlorambucil 20–30 mg/m^2 PO can be given every 2–4 weeks. An alternative approach is to give a single dose of chlorambucil 75 mg PO plus prednisone (30 mg/day for 7 days with each course of chlorambucil). This dose may be repeated in 4 weeks when the WBC count returns to pretreatment levels. This may be associated with a higher response rate and longer survival than daily dosing, but the toxicity is greater.

  (3) **Cyclophosphamide.** Cyclophosphamide is an acceptable alternative to chlorambucil. The recommended dose is 80–120 mg/m^2/day PO. Because of the risk of hemorrhagic cystitis, it should always be taken in the morning and oral hydration with 2–3 liters of fluid daily is encouraged.

b. **Combination chemotherapy.** Combinations with a variety of regimens have been used to treat advanced-stage disease, though the advantage to this approach remains unclear and many oncologists would consider these options inferior to the newer purine nucleoside analogs. Updated data from earlier promising reports with aggressive combination chemotherapy regimens fail to clearly demonstrate a survival advantage when compared to chlorambucil and prednisone. Commonly employed regimens are as follows.

(1) CVP

Cyclophosphamide 400 mg/m² PO on days 1–5 (or 750 mg/m² IV on day 1), *and*
Vincristine 1.4 mg/m² IV on day 1 not to exceed 2.0 mg, *and*
Prednisone 100 mg/m² PO on days 1–5.

Repeat every 3–4 weeks.

(2) CHOP

Cyclophosphamide 750 mg/m² IV on day 1, *and*
Vincristine 2 mg IV on day 1, *and*
Doxorubicin 50 mg/m² IV on day 1, *and*
Prednisone 100 mg.

Repeat every 4 weeks.

(3) Modified CHOP

Cyclophosphamide 300 mg/m² PO on days 1–5, *and*
Vincristine 2 mg IV on day 1, *and*
Doxorubicin 25 mg/m² on day 1, *and*
Prednisone 40 mg/m² PO on days 1–5.

Repeat every 4 weeks.

c. **Purine nucleoside analogs.** Three nucleoside analogs, fludarabine, cladribine (2-chlorodeoxyadenosine, 2-CdA), and pentostatin (2-deoxycoformycin), have demonstrated potent antitumor activity in CLL and related disorders and are currently considered either first- or second-line therapy of CLL. Of the three drugs, current studies indicate fludarabine is the most effective against CLL, with 2-CdA and pentostatin being less effective at the currently recommended doses.

(1) **Fludarabine.** The estimated overall response rate in previously untreated patients is 80%, with a 70% complete response (CR) rate. In previously treated patients, the overall response rate is 57%, with a 29% CR rate. Prednisone does not improve response rates and may increase mortality due to infection and is not recommended.

(a) **Recommended dose.** The recommended dose is 25 mg/m²/day IV on days 1–5, every 4 weeks for 4–6 months. The combination of fludarabine with other agents such as chlorambucil and low-dose cytarabine (ara-C) is currently being investigated and is not considered standard practice.

(b) **Toxicities.** Fludarabine is usually well tolerated, with its major side effects being myelosuppression, reversible neurologic dysfunction (peripheral neuropathy), muscle weakness, and hearing loss. Severe and prolonged CD4 lymphopenia is a long-term side effect and these patients must be monitored closely for associated infections. Allergic pneumonitis may masquerade as a pulmonary infection in these immunocompromised hosts. Occasional severe and nonreversible central and peripheral neurologic toxicity is seen.

- (c) **Cross-resistance.** Fludarabine and 2-CdA have similar structures. Recently, cross-resistance was confirmed with only 20% of fludarabine-refractory patients achieving a response to 2-CdA.

(2) **Cladribine (2-CdA) and pentostatin.** These appear to have less activity in CLL than fludarabine. Dosing information for these drugs can be found in sec. **III.D.**

3. **Alternative therapies.** Virtually all CLL patients will become resistant to the above-described therapies. Experimental approaches include AlloBMT, biologic response modifiers (BRMs), and monoclonal antibody (MoAB) therapy.

a. **AlloBMT.** AlloBMT is considered investigational for the treatment of CLL. Current reports on limited numbers of patients suggest a 53% disease-free survival rate with a median follow-up of 26 months. Early studies reported a high transplantation-related mortality (50%) and late relapses. More recent studies with different preoperative regimens showed a reduced early mortality to 10% and clearly prolonged survival. Though still investigational, this therapy should be considered for young patients with poor-risk disease who are refractory to fludarabine.

b. **BRMs.** Very few of the many BRM agents have reached clinical trials in CLL. Interleukin-2 appears ineffective in CLL and the response to IFN-α remains disappointing.

c. **MoABs.** There are a number of MoABs directed against CLL-associated antigens, including CD5, cCLLa, CD19, CD20, lym-1, lym-2, and CAMPATH binding protein. Encouraging results are being seen, especially with the CAMPATH binding protein MoAB. Additional data and results from the conjugated MoAB trials are needed before the usefulness of these antibodies in the treatment of CLL can be determined. These should be considered within the framework of a clinical trial for refractory patients who are not eligible for an AlloBMT trial.

E. **Complications**

1. **Infections.** Infections, particularly bacterial infections, account for up to 60% of deaths in CLL. Hypogammaglobulinemia is the factor most responsible for the susceptibility to bacterial infections. Special

attention to unusual upper respiratory tract pathogens such as *Listeria* or *Pneumocystis carinii* should be given to patients with CD4 lymphopenia. Immunizations are ineffective in CLL patients. Antibiotic or immunoglobulin prophylaxis should be considered in patients with repeated severe infections. Immunoglobulin prophylaxis is expensive. If it is done, doses of 400 mg/kg every 3 weeks significantly reduce infections and increase infection-free intervals, but a survival advantage over routine antibiotics has not been demonstrated.

2. **Richter's transformation.** This is transformation to an aggressive large-cell non-Hodgkin's lymphoma (NHL) in patients with previously existing or coexisting CLL or other indolent lymphoproliferative disorders. The exact incidence is difficult to determine but is estimated at 3–15%. Fever, marked progression of adenopathy, and an elevated lactate dehydrogenase level herald transformation, with most patients dying within 6–8 months, despite treatment.

3. **PLL transformation.** The diagnosis is heralded by the sudden appearance of prolymphocytes (>55% of the ALC) in the peripheral blood. It is usually refractory to therapy.

4. **Second malignancies.** New reports confirm a higher incidence of second malignancies in patients with CLL which does not appear to be influenced by stage of disease or treatment modality. There appears to be a combined 28% increased risk of the following malignancies: NHL, intraocular melanomas, malignant melanoma, brain tumors, and lung cancers. The explanation for this increased risk is unclear at present.

III. **Hairy cell leukemia**

A. **Diagnosis.** HCL was first identified in 1958, but because of the recent development of purine nucleoside analogs, which are very active in producing durable complete remissions, there has been a substantial body of new literature on this disease. This is now the most treatable type of chronic lymphoid malignancy.

HCL is an uncommon disorder that characteristically presents with infection due to pancytopenia, splenomegaly, and a bone marrow that is difficult or impossible to aspirate. HCL is most commonly seen in elderly men, with a male-female ratio of 5:1. Diagnosis can be made by morphologic, biochemical, and flow cytometric examination of peripheral blood cells or bone marrow elements (if obtainable).

In the majority of patients with typical HCL, the malignant cells are monoclonal B cells that are tartrate-resistant acid phosphatase (TRAP)–positive. These cells have hairlike projections, best seen on wet mounts with phase-contrast light microscopy. There is a small subset of patients with "atypical HCL," some with atypical B cell phenotypes (TRAP-negative), and isolated patients who may represent T cell variants. Variant HCL is less responsive to therapy and is not discussed. The following sections apply to typical B cell HCL.

Flow cytometric analysis has become the mainstay in differentiating HCL from other chronic lymphoid malignancies. The most specific findings are coexpression of B-ly7 with CD19, coexpression of CD11c with CD19, and moderate staining for CD25 (interleukin-2 receptor) and CD19. Most HCL cells do not express CD5. The most specific marker appears to be B-ly7, which is positive in all patients with HCL and negative in all patients with CLL.

B. Natural history. Before the advent of the purine nucleoside analogs, the prognosis for patients with HCL was poor since there was no known curative therapy. The median survival time was only 53 months. Some patients had palliation of cytopenias with splenectomy and most of them still required systemic therapy within the first year after splenectomy. Exciting new developments have made this a highly treatable and possibly curable disease.

C. Staging. There is no formal staging system for HCL, since staging does not alter therapy or outcome.

D. Treatment. Approximately 10–20% of patients with HCL will never require therapy and have stable disease without complications. These individuals are best managed by observation and are offered therapy if there is disease progression. Indications for treatment include significant cytopenias, repeated infections, massive splenomegaly, painful adenopathy, and vasculitis.

   1. Purine nucleoside analogs. These are now considered first-line therapies in the treatment of HCL. They all produce high CR rates, which appear to be durable for years. Longer follow-up will be needed to determine whether these therapies are curative. Responses appear independent of previous splenectomy or interferon therapy. The three drugs differ in their response rates, duration of remission, side effects, degree of immunosuppression, and cost of therapy.

      a. Definition of response. Because of the impressive activity seen with these drugs, a more rigorous definition of CR has been devised (Table 24-3). Documentation of response requires examination of both the bone marrow and peripheral blood.

      b. Cladribine (2-CdA). A single 7-day continuous infusion of 2-CdA consistently produced CR rates above 80% in multiple studies. The additional 20% of patients are partial responders. At this point, remissions appear durable with a median follow-up time of 16 months. The recommended dose is 4 mg/m^2 daily as a continuous IV infusion for 7 days. Recent reports suggest that SQ dosing may also be equally effective, but this is not yet the recommended route.

Table 24-3. Definition of response in hairy cell leukemia (HCL)

	Physical examination	Bone marrow	Peripheral blood
Complete remission (CR)	Absence of all signs and symptoms of HCL	Absence of hairy cells	Hemoglobin > 12 gm/dl ANC > 1500/μl Platelets > 100 × 10³/μl
Partial remission (PR)	50% reduction of all findings of HCL	1–5% hairy cells	Hemoglobin > 12 gm/dl ANC > 1500/μl Platelets > 100 × 10³/μl

ANC = absolute neutrophil count.

The major side effects are myelosuppression and associated fever. However, with longer follow-up of patients treated with 2-CdA, a lengthy period of profound CD4 and CD8 lymphopenia has been seen and can last years after treatment, rendering patients susceptible to a variety of opportunistic infections. CD4 counts should be monitored regularly. Rare side effects include late bone marrow failure, peripheral neuropathy, and disturbing isolated incidences of severe proximal myopathy.

c. **Pentostatin (2-deoxycoformycin).** Pentostatin is an inhibitor of adenosine deaminase. The overall response rate is approximately 80%, with a CR rate of more than 50%. As with 2-CdA, many remissions have been durable to date, with approximately a 15% relapse rate. The recommended dose is 4 mg/m^2 IV every 2 weeks for 6 months, or 2 cycles beyond CR. In many cases, this is given with IV hydration (1 liter) because of reports of a high frequency of renal toxicity in the higher-dose phase I studies.

As with all of the purine nucleoside analogs, pentostatin is a potent depressor of CD4 and CD8 cells, which may last for many months after discontinuation of therapy. The incidence of neurologic, renal, hepatic, and bone marrow toxicities has decreased with the above-recommended dose. Patients must be monitored closely for opportunistic infections for at least a year after therapy and should have CD4 counts monitored.

d. **Fludarabine.** Current clinical trials indicate fludarabine may have activity in HCL similar to that of 2-CdA. Results of ongoing studies will help determine the exact response and remission rates of this drug, as well as the extent and duration of long-term immunosuppression. Current data suggest fludarabine is not as active in HCL as 2-CdA or pentostatin.

2. **Splenectomy.** This is no longer considered the treatment of choice for patients with HCL since most patients will still require systemic treatment. It is reserved for patients with life-threatening thrombocytopenia due to splenic sequestration.

3. **Interferon.** Splenectomy followed by interferon therapy produces very low remission rates (< 10%) that are not usually durable. Like splenectomy, this is also no longer considered first-line therapy.

4. **Treatment failures.** There are few data on salvage therapy after treatment failure with one of the above-mentioned purine analogs. A few patients may benefit from cross-over to another purine analog, but there is expected to be a relatively high degree of cross-resistance. As a palliative measure, therapy with granulocyte colony-stimulating factor (G-CSF) may increase

the ANC into an acceptable range, thus decreasing infection complications. Sparse data suggest that HCL cells are not stimulated by G-CSF.

IV. Adult T-cell leukemia/lymphoma

A. Diagnosis. ATLL is characterized by hypercalcemia and the presence of malignant helper T cells in the skin and blood. There can be involvement of the lungs, liver, and spleen; lymphadenopathy (sparing the mediastinum); and lytic bone lesions. The initial clinical course may be chronic, but is usually followed by a rapidly progressive phase that is terminal. The disease is caused by human T cell lymphotropic virus type I (HTLV-I). HTLV-I is endemic in southwest Japan, the Caribbean, and the southeastern United States. There appears to be a lengthy latency phase necessary before the development of ATLL, with infected individuals having lifetime risk of developing ATLL of 5%. Those with the highest risk of developing ATLL were likely infected perinatally.

Diagnosis is made by the classic appearance of the T cells, which have indented or lobulated nuclei, flow cytometric studies demonstrating the CD4 phenotype, hypercalcemia, and the clinical presentation.

B. Natural history. In the early or pre-ATLL phase, the patient is usually asymptomatic. Leukemic cells can usually be identified in the peripheral blood. Studies of HTLV-I integration demonstrated these cells to be polyclonal. In 50% of patients, these cells disappear spontaneously. In others, smoldering ATLL occurs and is manifested by circulating leukemia cells (normal total WBC count) and skin involvement, without visceral involvement. In this phase, the malignant cells demonstrate clonality. This can progress to a chronic or acute phase.

In the chronic phase, an elevated WBC count reflects an increase in circulating ATLL cells. There is visceral involvement with hepatosplenomegaly and adenopathy. There is no hypercalcemia, though the serum lactate dehydrogenase level may be elevated.

The acute phase is the most common form of presentation. Up to 25% will present as lymphoma (skin lesions, adenopathy, and hepatosplenomegaly) without circulating ATLL cells. Hypercalcemia is seen in 50% of patients, with or without bone lesions, and is thought to be a paraneoplastic syndrome with elaboration of parathyroid hormone–related protein.

C. Treatment. Acute ATLL is usually resistant to standard leukemia therapy and most patients die within weeks to months. These patients should be treated with experimental protocols. Currently, there are some responders to 2-CdA infusions. Larger studies and longer follow-up will be needed to determine the extent of activity of 2-CdA. There are scattered case reports in the Japanese literature suggesting some patients respond to topical tretinoin (all-*trans*-retinoic acid, TRA), including some CRs in patients with visceral disease. Studies to confirm this using oral and topical TRA are just beginning in the United States. It is too early to confirm these findings.

Selected Readings

Cheson, B. D., et al. Neurotoxicity of purine analogs: a review. *J. Clin. Oncol.* 12:2216, 1994.

Doane, L. L., Ratain, M. J., and Golumb, H. M. Hairy cell leukemia: current management. *Hematol. Oncol. Clin. North Am.* 4:489, 1990.

Faguet, G. B. Chronic lymphocytic leukemia: an updated review. *J. Clin. Oncol.* 12:1974, 1994.

Hollsberg, P., and Hafler, D. A. Pathogenesis of diseases induced by HTLV-1. *N. Engl. J. Med.* 328:1173, 1993.

Kantarjian, H. M., et al. Chronic myelogenous leukemia: a concise update. *Blood* 82:691, 1993.

Kyle, R. A., and Tefferi, A. Multiple myeloma, chronic lymphocytic leukemia, and hairy cell leukemia. *Curr. Opin. Hematol.* 4:195, 1994.

Neely, S. M. Adult T-cell leukemia-lymphoma. *West. J. Med.* 150:557, 1989.

Palackdharry, C. S. Non-Hodgkins lymphoma: why the increasing incidence? *Oncology* 8:67, 1994.

Piro, L. D., et al. Lasting remissions in hairy-cell leukemia induced by a single infusion of 2-chlorodeoxyadenosine. *N. Engl. J. Med.* 322:1117, 1990.

Robbins, B. A., et al. Diagnostic application of two color flow cytometry in 161 cases of hairy cell leukemia. *Blood* 82:1277, 1993.

Saven, A., and Piro, L. D. Treatment of hairy cell leukemia. *Blood* 79:1111, 1992.

Myeloproliferative and Myelodysplastic Syndromes

Peter White and Carol S. Palackdharry

I. Myeloproliferative syndromes. The myeloproliferative syndromes are clonal disorders of the hematopoietic stem cell characterized by autonomous and sustained overproduction of morphologically and functionally mature granulocytes, erythrocytes, or platelets. The diagnostic label of the individual syndrome indicates the cellular element most strikingly increased, but it is not uncommon to have modest or even major elevations in other lineages (e.g., thrombocytosis and leukocytosis in polycythemia vera (P. vera)). Studies such as marrow karyotypes and isoenzyme patterns have verified the concept that the common trilineage marrow stem cell is the neoplastic cell of origin for these disorders. Bone marrow aspirates and biopsy specimens show hyperplasia of megakaryocytes and of granulocytic and erythroid precursors, but maturation is normal, without a shift toward immaturity. Also, the progeny of the neoplastic stem cells display essentially normal physiologic function in most respects, though it is not unusual to have platelet dysfunction (prolonged bleeding time, abnormal aggregation studies), which may contribute to bleeding. Chronic granulocytic leukemia is discussed in Chapter 24. The other myeloproliferative disorders are discussed here.

A. Polycythemia vera

1. Diagnosis. P. vera must be distinguished from relative or spurious polycythemia (normal red blood cell [RBC] mass, decreased plasma volume) and from secondary erythrocytosis (increased RBC mass due to hypoxia, carboxyhemoglobinemia, inappropriate erythropoietin syndromes with tumors or renal disease, etc.). The following diagnostic criteria adopted by the P. vera Study Group have proved useful.

Category A

A1 Increased RBC mass (measured with ^{51}Cr-labeled RBCs); males $\geq$ 36 ml/kg; females $\geq$ 32 ml/kg

A2 Normal arterial oxygen saturation: $\geq$ 92%

A3 Splenomegaly

Category B

B1 Thrombocytosis: platelets $\geq$ 400,000/μl

B2 Leukocytosis: white blood cell (WBC) count $\geq$ 12,000/μl (in absence of fever or infection)

B3 Elevated leukocyte alkaline phosphatase score: > 100 in absence of fever or infection

B4 Elevated serum vitamin B_{12} or unbound B_{12} binding capacity: B_{12} > 900 pg/ml; unbound B_{12} > 2200 pg/ml

P. vera is considered established if parameters A1, A2, and A3 are all present, or if A1 and A2 are present plus any two category B parameters. RBC mass and arterial oxygen saturation should routinely be determined. It is also usually advisable to perform bone marrow aspiration and biopsy, including karyotype studies (the results of which are abnormal in 10–15% of patients at diagnosis), to confirm the presence of panmyelosis (hyperplasia of all nonlymphoid elements), and to assess iron stores and fibrosis. Measurements of serum B_{12} and unsaturated B_{12} binding capacity levels and imaging studies to evaluate for splenomegaly (detectable by physical examination alone in 70% of P. vera patients) are helpful in questionable cases, but are not needed routinely. Serum erythropoietin levels should be measured when the diagnosis is not straightforward: Patients with P. vera should have a subnormal level; elevated values should prompt a search for occult tumor, renal disease, and other causes of secondary erythrocytosis.

2. **Aims of therapy.** Thrombosis is a major cause of morbidity in P. vera, due primarily to increased blood viscosity and stasis, and leading to stroke, myocardial infarct, and venous thromboembolism. Lowering the hematocrit to 40–45% markedly reduces the risk of thrombosis. High platelet counts may also pose a risk for thrombosis, and spontaneous platelet activation occasionally causes erythromelalgia (hot, red, painful digits). It is particularly important to maintain good control of hematocrit and platelets in the elderly, and in others at increased risk for thrombosis.

3. **Treatment regimens**
   a. **Phlebotomy.** Removal of 350–500 ml of blood every other day (once or twice weekly in the elderly or in patients with cardiac disease) is the standard initial approach, to lower the hematocrit to 40–45%. The blood cell count is then checked monthly, and phlebotomy is repeated as needed to maintain the hematocrit under 45%.

   Elective surgery should be deferred until the hematocrit has been stabilized at 45% or less for 2–4 months. Rapid lowering of the hematocrit may also be achieved in surgical or thrombotic emergencies by erythroapheresis. Evaluation of platelet function (bleeding time, aggregation studies, or both) should also be carried out before major surgery or invasive diagnostic procedures are undertaken.

   b. **Myelosuppressive agents.** Persistent thrombocytosis, recurrent thrombosis, enlarging spleen, or similar problems despite adequate phlebotomy indicate the need for myelosuppressive therapy. Alkylating agents such as chlorambucil carry a high risk of producing leukemia and are no longer recommended. Currently recommended choices are as follows.

(1) **Hydroxyurea** 600–800 mg/m^2 PO daily. This drug requires weekly blood cell counts initially and dosage adjustments to maintain the hematocrit at 40–45%, the platelet count at 100,000–500,000/μl, and the WBC count at more than 3000/μl. Side effects are usually minimal.

For patients difficult to control with hydroxyurea, acceptable alternatives include the following.

(2) **Interferon alpha.** This drug appears promising, on the basis of limited short-term experience. Starting dose is 3 million units/m^2 3 times weekly but with subsequent readjustment, depending on platelet count and hematocrit. Side effects include myalgias, fever, and asthenia, usually controlled with acetaminophen. Leukemogenic effects are presumably absent, but expense is a deterrent to long-term use.

(3) **Radioactive phosphorus** (^{32}P) 2.3 mCi/m^2 IV (5 mCi maximum single dose). Repeat in 12 weeks if the response is inadequate (25% dose escalation optional). Lack of response after a third dose mandates a switch to other forms of therapy. Use of ^{32}P entails an approximately 10% risk of leukemia, and it is best reserved for use in the elderly and in patients refractory to other modalities. Supplemental phlebotomies may be required for patients with satisfactory platelet and WBC counts but a rising hematocrit.

(4) **Busulfan.** This drug appears to have less leukemogenic potential than other alkylating agents, and may occasionally be appropriate in patients not controlled by other treatments, or in the elderly. It is best given in short courses over several weeks (to avoid prolonged marrow suppression). Starting dose is 4–6 mg daily.

(5) **Anagrelide.** This is an experimental drug available on protocol only, and used specifically to control thrombocytosis. This drug also inhibits platelet function and produces mild anemia, but has no effect on the WBC count. Response is reported in 80% of patients given 4 mg daily in divided doses. Side effects include fluid retention, heart failure, tachycardia, headaches, and nausea. Its effectiveness in preventing thromboses is uncertain. Platelet counts rebound rapidly after discontinuation of the drug.

c. **Ancillary treatments.** Allopurinol 300 mg daily is commonly needed to control hyperuricemia. Pruritus is a frequent problem but usually abates with myelosuppressive therapy. Cyproheptadine

(5–20 mg daily) and cimetidine (900 mg daily) may help. Aspirin and similar antiplatelet agents are often helpful for erythromelalgia but do not protect against most thrombotic complications; they may cause bleeding.

4. **Evolution and outcome.** The median survival time for patients with P. vera is approximately 10 years. One-third of deaths are caused by thrombosis. The risk of leukemia is small in patients treated by phlebotomy alone. Approximately 10% of patients develop myelofibrosis with myeloid metaplasia (see sec. **I.C.**). Many patients progress to the "spent phase," with increasing splenomegaly and stable or falling hematocrit. Splenectomy or splenic irradiation may be indicated for massive splenomegaly in such patients.

B. Essential thrombocythemia

1. **Diagnosis.** This requires (1) a persistent elevation of the platelet count above 600,000/μl, plus (2) the absence of other known causes for reactive or secondary thrombocytosis (e.g., due to iron deficiency, malignancy, or chronic inflammatory disease). Differentiation from other myeloproliferative syndromes may be difficult. Marrow aspiration and biopsy should be performed, to demonstrate hyperplasia of megakaryocytes and granulocytes, to evaluate iron stores, and to exclude myelofibrosis. Marrow chromosome studies are desirable to show that the Philadelphia chromosome is not present, but abnormal karyotypes are found in less than 10% of patients at diagnosis. Palpable splenomegaly is present in less than 50% of patients at diagnosis. Platelet function studies may show either spontaneous aggregation or impaired response to agonists such as epinephrine. Pseudohyperkalemia is common and should be detected by comparing plasma to serum potassium levels. Microvascular occlusion may cause digital gangrene, transient ischemic attacks, visual complaints, and paresthesias. Large-vessel occlusion (myocardial infarct, cerebrovascular accident) and hemorrhagic manifestations due to platelet dysfunction are also seen.

2. **Treatment regimens.** Observation alone is considered the best course in younger asymptomatic patients with fewer than 1×10^6 platelets/μl. Therapy to lower platelet count should be undertaken in patients with a history of hemorrhagic or thrombotic complications, and in the elderly and other patients at increased risk for vascular problems. Options include the following.

   a. **Hydroxyurea** 600–800 mg/m^2 PO daily, with dosage adjustments on the basis of the weekly complete blood cell count, should achieve satisfactory response in 2–6 weeks.

   b. **^{32}P and alkylating agents** are effective but carry increased risk of secondary leukemia. Ni-

trogen mustard (mechlorethamine, 0.15–0.3 mg/
kg [6–12 mg/m²] IV) can be helpful when rapid
reduction in platelet count is needed. Busulfan
(4–6 mg daily initial dose) is appropriate in selected patients resistant to other agents, particularly the elderly.

c. **Plateletapheresis** may be indicated in emergent situations (e.g., cerebral ischemia), but the
effect is usually short-lived. On occasion, platelet
transfusion may be indicated to control hemorrhage regardless of platelet count.

d. **Anagrelide** is available only with experimental
protocols. Comments in sec. **I.A.3.b.(5).** regarding dosage, efficacy, and side effects pertain.

e. **Interferon alpha.** The majority of thrombocythemic patients will respond to this agent, at initial doses of 3–6 million units SQ daily. As noted
in sec. **I.A.3.b.(2),** side effects and expense are
potential problems and its effectiveness in reducing thrombotic and hemorrhagic complications
remains uncertain.

f. **Aspirin** 300 mg daily may control erythromelalgia and similar vasoocclusive problems but is contraindicated in patients with a history of hemorrhagic symptoms or platelet dysfunction (e.g.,
prolonged bleeding time). Aspirin may be useful
in the management of the pregnant patient,
where the preceding agents are contraindicated.

3. **Evolution and outcome.** The course is often indolent, particularly in young patients. The median survival time probably exceeds 10 years, and some patients appear to have normal life expectancy. In a
few patients the disease transforms to other myeloproliferative disorders or to acute leukemia.

C. **Agnogenic myeloid metaplasia (AMM)**
1. **Diagnosis.** This disorder of the stem cell, also
called *idiopathic myelofibrosis,* is marked by (1) an
intense reactive fibrosis of the marrow; (2) splenomegaly (frequently massive), reflecting ectopic hematopoiesis in the spleen, portal hypertension, or
both; and (3) the presence of immature granulocytes,
nucleated RBCs, and teardrop RBCs in the peripheral blood (leukoerythroblastic blood picture). Studies of marrow hematopoietic cells and circulating
blood cells have confirmed that AMM is a clonal
disorder; abnormal karyotype is demonstrable in
50–60% of patients at diagnosis. Other causes of
secondary marrow fibrosis such as metastatic carcinoma, hairy cell leukemia, and granulomatous infections must be ruled out. Postpolycythemic myelofibrosis is clinically indistinguishable, but carries a
poor prognosis, evolving to acute leukemia in 25–
50% of patients (versus 5–20% for de novo AMM).
Acute myelofibrosis is also distinct from AMM and
may be identical or closely related to acute megakaryoblastic leukemia (see Chap. 23).

2. **Treatment regimens.** The median survival time is approximately 5 years, but asymptomatic patients may do well without treatment for a number of years. Intervention is indicated for the following problems.

   a. **Anemia.** Androgens (e.g., testosterone enanthate 600 mg IM weekly or oxymetholone 50 mg qid PO for men; danazol 600 mg PO daily for women) are recommended and frequently reduce transfusion requirements. Corticosteroids (prednisone 1 mg/kg [40 mg/m^2] PO daily) should be tried if overt hemolysis is present.

   b. **Splenomegaly.** Massive splenomegaly may lead to cytopenias, portal hypertension, variceal bleeding, abdominal pain, or compression of adjacent organs. In some patients, mild splenomegaly may be accompanied by excess fatigue, sweats, and systemic complaints that merit treatment. Options for control include myelosuppressive therapy with hydroxyurea as for P. vera (see sec. **I.A.3.b.**) or busulfan 2 mg daily in older patients, splenic irradiation (e.g., 25–50 cGy daily for 3–5 days), or splenectomy (careful preoperative evaluation of hemostasis is mandatory; there is a high risk of perioperative bleeding, postoperative thrombocytosis, or sepsis). Responses to interferon alpha have been reported for AMM, but its role in management is uncertain.

   c. **Marrow failure.** Erythropoietin is helpful in improving anemia in a small percentage of patients (dose, 4000–10,000 units 3 times weekly SQ) but cannot be recommended for routine use. Allogeneic marrow transplantation (for patients < 50 years old) may prove useful.

II. **Myelodysplastic syndromes (MDSs).** These disorders, also referred to as *preleukemia* or *oligoblastic leukemia,* represent clonal abnormalities of hematopoietic stem cells. In contrast to myeloproliferative syndromes, dysplastic morphologic features are prominent, reflecting impaired maturation and functional abnormalities. Even without transformation to acute leukemia, there are fatal disorders, with death resulting from the complications of bone marrow failure (infection, bleeding, or both).

A. **Diagnosis.** The bone marrow is usually hypercellular, but hematopoiesis is ineffective, and anemia with or without other cytopenias is the rule. Occasionally, the bone marrow will be hypocellular or normocellular. Reticulocyte counts are normal or low, despite erythroid hyperplasia. Diagnostic features include dysplasia, megaloblastoid changes, or both in RBC precursors; ring sideroblasts; bilobed neutrophils (i.e., pseudo-Pelger-Huët anomaly); hypogranulation of neutrophils; monolobular or hypolobular megakaryocytes; and agranular platelets. Small numbers of blast cells may be found in the peripheral blood, as well as up to 30% in the marrow.

Transformation to acute leukemia can be diagnosed when the bone marrow blast count is greater than 30%.

The French-American-British (FAB) classification divides MDS into five categories.

1. **Refractory anemia (RA)** ($<$ 5% blasts in marrow)
2. **Refractory anemia with ring sideroblasts (RARS)** ($<$ 5% blasts, $>$ 15% ringed sideroblasts)
3. **Refractory anemia with excess blasts (RAEB)** (5–20% blasts in marrow)
4. **Refractory anemia with excess blasts "in transformation" (RAEB-T)** (20–30% blasts in marrow)
5. **Chronic myelomonocytic leukemia (CMML)** (5–20% blasts in marrow, $>$ 1000 monocytes/μl)

B. **Cytogenetics and prognostic variables**

1. **Karyotypic abnormalities.** A number of chromosomal abnormalities have been associated with MDSs, especially on chromosomes 5 and 7. Patients with 5q $-$ syndrome (female predominance, anemia with a normal or high platelet count, and monolobulated or bilobulated megakaryocytes) have a longer survival and less frequent transformation to acute nonlymphocytic leukemia (ANNL) than do patients with other DNA abnormalities. Recent studies demonstrated the translocation of chromosome 11q21 in MDSs secondary to epipodophyllotoxins and chromosome 21q22 in MDSs secondary to anthracyclines.

2. **Prognostic factors.** Several prognostic factors have been postulated. The most consistent predictors of a poor prognosis include advanced age, very low peripheral blood counts, increased blasts in the bone marrow, increased cytogenetic abnormalities, and a high ALIP (abnormal localization of immature precursors) score in the bone marrow.

C. **Clinical course.** These are fatal disorders, even without transformation to acute leukemia. Patients die from complications of bone marrow failure or acute leukemia. The median survival time for patients without transformation is only 2–4 years for RA and RARS, and less than 1 year for RAEB and RAEBT. The frequency of transformation to acute leukemia prior to death correlates with the FAB classification.

RA, RARS	10–20%
CMML	20–30%
RAEB	40–50%
RAEB-T	60–75%

Transformation into a secondary acute leukemia is usually fatal. Durable remissions are rare and in most studies involving induction chemotherapy the toxic death rate equals or exceeds the response rate.

D. **Treatment regimens**

1. **Allogeneic bone marrow transplantation (BMT).** This is the only known curative therapy for MDSs. It should be considered the treatment of choice in

young patients for whom a matched related donor is available. Improvements in supportive care have allowed some centers to perform allogeneic BMT safely in healthy patients up to age 70. Studies indicate that 30–50% of eligible patients may be cured.

2. **Supportive care.** The majority of patients diagnosed with MDS will not qualify for allogeneic BMT because of advanced age, poor health, or lack of a human leukocyte antigen (HLA)–identical sibling donor. For these patients, supportive care with antibiotics and transfusions when they are symptomatic should be considered the standard of care.

3. **Growth factors**
   a. **Erythropoietin.** Only about 20% of patients with MDS will have a meaningful increase in hemoglobin with high-dose erythropoietin. Response does not correlate well with baseline endogenous erythropoietin levels.
   b. **GM-CSF and G-CSF.** Although these factors can transiently increase the number of functioning neutrophils, studies have not demonstrated an improved survival with these therapies. A recent large randomized trial demonstrated a decreased survival rate after G-CSF treatment compared to supportive care. Given these data and the concern regarding the possible stimulation of progression to ANNL, these factors remain experimental.
   c. **Other hematopoietic growth factors.** Other factors currently being investigated include interleukin (IL)-3, IL-6, IL-11, Pixy 321, and stem cell factor. Sufficient data regarding response rates are not yet available.

4. **Hormonal therapies.** Several studies utilizing steroids have been performed. There are essentially no durable responses and an increase in infectious complications. For this reason, steroids are relatively contraindicated in MDS. Neither androgens nor danazol have been shown to prolong survival or produce meaningful responses.

5. **Cytotoxic chemotherapy.** Trials utilizing acute leukemia induction regimens to treat MDS (without transformation to ANNL) have produced response rates of 15–50%; however, the toxic death rates have equaled or exceeded response rates in the majority of trials. Similar results are seen when transformation to a secondary ANNL occurs, with a 20–40% complete response (CR) rate but 20–60% mortality with induction chemotherapy. This approach could be considered for young patients without a match for allogeneic BMT, but in the elderly patient, may result in early death.

6. **Differentiating agents**
   a. **Retinoids.** Initial promising data reporting a 20% CR with the use of isotretinoin (*cis*-retinoid acid) have not been confirmed by additional stud-

ies. Currently, neither isotretinoin nor tretinoin (all-*trans*-retinoic acid) has demonstrated a survival advantage.

    b. Low-dose cytarabine (ara-C). Studies demonstrate only a 16% CR rate in MDS; however, patients with MDS appear ultrasensitive to ara-C and toxicities are significant. Despite an increase in disease-free survival, overall survival has not been prolonged by this therapy.

    c. Vitamin D analogs. Thus far, early trials have failed to demonstrate a significant effect.

    d. 5-Azacitadine. Limited experience has not demonstrated a superior response rate compared to cytarabine.

E. Summary. For the majority of patients in whom allogeneic BMT is not feasible, MDSs represent fatal disorders. Even without transformation to ANNL, most patients die from complications of bone marrow failure. Allogeneic BMT is the only known curative modality. Supportive care is considered standard therapy outside the setting of a clinical trial for the majority of patients.

Selected Readings

Anagrelide Study Group. Anagrelide, a therapy for thrombocythemic states: experience in 577 patients. *Am. J. Med.* 92:69, 1992.

Appelbaum, F. R., et al. Bone marrow transplantation for patients with myelodysplasia: pretreatment variables and outcome. *Ann. Intern. Med.* 112:590, 1990.

Bennett, J. M., et al. Proposals for the classification of the myelodysplastic syndromes. *Br. J. Haematol.* 51:189, 1982.

Brenner, B., et al. Splenectomy in agnogenic myeloid metaplasia and postpolycythemic myeloid metaplasia: a study of 34 cases. *Arch. Intern. Med.* 148:2501, 1988.

Cheson, B. D. The myelodysplastic syndromes: current approaches to therapy. *Ann. Intern. Med.* 112:932, 1990.

Cimino, R., et al. Recombinant interferon a-2b in the treatment of polycythemia vera. *Am. J. Hematol.* 44:155, 1993.

Frenkel, E. The clinical spectrum of thrombocytosis and thrombocythemia. *Am. J. Med. Sci.* 301:69, 1991.

Murphy, S. Polycythemia vera. In W. J. Williams et al. (eds.), *Hematology* (4th ed.). New York: McGraw-Hill, 1990. Pp. 193.

Schafer, A. I. Bleeding and thrombosis in the myeloproliferative disorders. *Blood* 64:1, 1984.

Zuckerman, K. S. Myelodysplasia. *Curr. Opin. Hematol.* 4:183, 1993.

Hodgkin's Disease and Malignant Lymphomas

Richard S. Stein

Hodgkin's disease and the non-Hodgkin's lymphomas (NHLs) constitute a diverse spectrum of lymphoproliferative malignancies that share a number of important clinical features. They commonly present as solitary or generalized adenopathy, and for both diseases accurate clinical staging is the basis for rational therapeutic planning. Nevertheless, important clinical differences exist. With Hodgkin's disease contiguous spread of tumor from node to node is the rule, and most patients present with disease limited to the lymph nodes (or to the lymph nodes and spleen). Many of these patients are candidates for curative radiation therapy. In contrast, most patients with NHLs present with advanced disease. Furthermore, whereas Hodgkin's disease is curable regardless of stage (advanced Hodgkin's disease is curable by chemotherapy), only certain histologic types of NHL are curable when disseminated. Radiation therapy plays a very limited role in NHL. For these reasons, Hodgkin's disease and the major histologic types of NHL must be considered separately.

I. Hodgkin's disease

A. Incidence and histologic types.
Hodgkin's disease accounts for approximately 1% of newly diagnosed malignancies in the United States. The average age of new patients is 32 years, and the incidence curve is bimodal: One peak occurs near age 25 and another at age 55. Four major histologic types of Hodgkin's disease exist: lymphocyte predominance (10% of cases), nodular sclerosis (60% of cases), mixed cellularity (20% of cases), and lymphocyte depletion (10% of cases). Nodular sclerosis Hodgkin's disease is commonly seen in young adults and is frequently associated with a large mediastinal mass. Lymphocyte-depleted Hodgkin's disease is usually associated with symptomatic disease (see sec. **I.B.**) and frequent involvement of the bone marrow. Nevertheless, the critical variable with respect to the therapy of Hodgkin's disease is not the histologic type but the stage of disease.

B. Staging

1. **Modified Ann Arbor staging system.** The modified Ann Arbor staging system is used for patients with Hodgkin's disease. Clinically, patients are placed in one of four stages and are further classified as to the presence or absence of symptoms: A denotes that no symptoms are present; B denotes that any or all of the following are present: fever, night sweats, and unexplained weight loss of 10% or more of body weight. In addition, the subscript E (e.g., II_E) may be used to denote involvement of an extralymphatic site primarily or by direct extension,

rather than by hematogenous spread, e.g., mediastinal mass extending to involve the lung. Stage III
Hodgkin's disease is subdivided into stages III$_1$ and
III$_2$ based on evidence that the clinical approaches to
these two substages should be different. The modified Ann Arbor staging system is as follows.

Stage I—involvement of a single lymph node region.

Stage II—involvement of two or more lymph node
regions on the same side of the diaphragm.

Stage III$_1$—involvement of lymph node regions on
both sides of the diaphragm. Abdominal disease is
limited to the upper abdomen: spleen, splenic hilar, celiac, or porta hepatis nodes.

Stage III$_2$—involvement of lymph node regions on
both sides of the diaphragm. Abdominal disease
includes paraaortic, mesenteric, iliac, or inguinal
nodes, with or without disease in the upper abdomen.

Stage IV—diffuse or disseminated involvement of
one or more extralymphatic tissues or organs, with
or without associated lymph node involvement.

2. **Staging tests.** Staging must be performed with consideration of therapeutic options and not just to complete a "checklist." When performing staging tests,
one should remember that Hodgkin's disease tends
to spread in a contiguous manner. Considering that
the thoracic duct makes the left supraclavicular area
and the abdomen contiguous sites, it is not surprising that abdominal disease is found in 40% of patients with left supraclavicular presentations and in
only 8% of patients with presentations in the right
supraclavicular nodes. Additionally, one should consider that staging tests are designed to establish a
baseline extent of disease so that completeness of remission can be evaluated following completion of
therapy. Procedures used for the staging of Hodgkin's disease are as follows.

   a. **History taking.** Symptoms to watch for are fever, night sweats, and weight loss.

   b. **Complete physical examination.** Attention
   must be paid to lymph nodes and spleen.

   c. **Laboratory tests.** Complete blood count (CBC)
   (including a platelet count), erythrocyte sedimentation rate, serum alkaline phosphatase, and
   tests of liver and kidney function must be performed.

   d. **Chest x-ray film.** Computed tomography (CT) of
   the chest is useful in establishing the baseline dimensions of a mass when the chest x-ray film
   demonstrates abnormalities. Although the chest
   CT is often obtained as a routine staging test, the
   clinical value of detecting minimal chest disease
   that might be missed by routine chest x-ray films
   alone is not established.

   e. **Lymphangiogram.** The lymphangiogram is useful in that it can detect normal-size nodes in which the internal architecture has been disrupted by Hodgkin's disease. These nodes may not be identified by CT of the abdomen. However, performance of lymphangiography may be limited by the fact that many institutions lack radiologists to perform or interpret the test results. In patients in whom a lymphangiogram cannot be obtained, and in whom a CT scan of the abdomen appears normal, staging laparotomy (see sec. **I.B.2.h.**) should be considered to rule out retroperitoneal disease, if radiation therapy is planned as the only therapy. Since lymphangiography can be associated with embolization of lipid dye to the lungs, the procedure should not be performed in patients with pulmonary Hodgkin's disease or a large mediastinal mass. Omission of the lymphangiogram is of little clinical consequence since these patients are candidates for chemotherapy anyway.

f. **CT of the abdomen.** This test is routinely performed as part of staging and is very helpful when the results are positive. It has eliminated the need for performing isotope scans of the liver and spleen.

g. **Bone marrow biopsy** may be omitted in patients who are in clinical stages IA or IIA after the above-mentioned staging procedures have been performed.

h. **Staging laparotomy.** Staging laparotomy may be of value when clinical staging is equivocal, especially when the therapeutic plan is to give radiation therapy alone. However, one can often compensate for uncertain staging by omitting laparotomy and proceeding with chemotherapy in the absence of a laparotomy. Relative indications for staging laparotomy in patients who are candidates for radiation therapy include mixed cellularity Hodgkin's disease, Hodgkin's disease involving the left supraclavicular or left cervical nodes, and inability to perform a lymphangiogram. Staging laparotomy should include inspection, liver biopsies (wedge biopsy of left lobe plus needle biopsy of both lobes), and biopsies of the splenic, hilar, celiac, porta hepatis, mesenteric, paraaortic, and iliac lymph nodes. Ovariopexy is often performed as part of laparotomy to move the ovaries out of the radiation port. This is of value *only* if pelvic radiation is given and *only* if the radiation therapists are willing to shield the ovaries. (Some radiotherapists are concerned about damage caused by radiation scatter and are unwilling to shield the ovaries after ovariopexy.) At institutions where therapeutic plans rarely include total nodal radiation therapy, because chemotherapy is given to patients requiring more than mantle and upper abdominal radiation therapy, ovariopexy is not routinely performed as part of laparotomy.

C. Therapy of Hodgkin's disease

1. General considerations.

Therapy of Hodgkin's disease must be considered on a stage-by-stage basis. The incidence of the various stages of Hodgkin's disease is presented in Table 26-1 with an estimated cure rate for each stage. In general, limited stages of Hodgkin's disease are treated with radiation therapy (stages IA and IIA), and advanced stages (IVA and IVB) are treated with combination chemotherapy. The optimal therapy for the intermediate stages of Hodgkin's disease remains somewhat controversial. There is a trend at many institutions to treat patients with stage III disease with combination chemotherapy.

While it would be nice to state that therapy has become a less complex problem over the last few years, in truth, decisions regarding the choice of optimal therapy have become more complex. Although effective therapies for all stages of Hodgkin's disease exist, new data indicate that late complications of radiation therapy for Hodgkin's disease include breast cancer, lung cancer, hypothyroidism, thyroid cancer, coronary artery disease, and valvular heart disease. While the incidence of each of these complications is fairly low, the cumulative risk of all these complications makes it legitimate to consider either chemotherapy or chemotherapy plus limited-dose radiation therapy as an approach to limited-stage Hodgkin's disease. Unfortunately, there are no data showing that long-term overall survival of patients with limited-stage Hodgkin's disease can be improved by this alteration of therapy, leaving the clinician faced with uncertainty over the optimal therapeutic approach to limited-stage disease after decades of "knowing" that radiation therapy was the optimal approach.

While chemotherapy has clearly been established as optimal treatment for advanced-stage disease,

Table 26-1. Hodgkin's disease: incidence of stages and results of therapy

Stage	Incidence (%)	Potential cure rate (%)
IA	10	95
IIA	30	85
IB, IIB	10	70
III$_1$A	15	85
III$_2$A	10	65
III	15	60
IVA, IVB	10	60

clinical trials have not resolved the question of which chemotherapy regimen represents optimal therapy.

Prior to initiating chemotherapy, patients should be placed on allopurinol 300 mg/day to avert the hyperuricemia that may follow tumor lysis. It may be discontinued after the first cycle of chemotherapy or after the first 2 weeks of radiotherapy.

2. **Radiotherapy.** With respect to radiation therapy, studies have shown that the optimal dose for local control is 36–40 Gy given over 3.5–4.0 weeks. With modern equipment, adequate radiation can be administered to involved areas while shielding adjacent tissues. Nevertheless, radiation injury such as radiation pneumonitis or pericarditis occurs infrequently. Similarly, inappropriate overlapping of radiation ports can result in damage to the overtreated area. If this damage involves radiation myelitis, the results can be disastrous owing to resultant paraplegia. Because of the common occurrence of hypothyroidism, and the less common occurrence of thyroid cancer in patients who receive radiation to the thyroid gland, we monitor thyroid-stimulating hormone (TSH) levels yearly in these patients. Patients with elevated levels of TSH, even if euthyroid, are placed on thyroid replacement therapy to limit stimulation of the radiated thyroid gland by elevated levels of TSH. See Figure 26-1 for standard radiation therapy ports.

3. **Stages IA and IIA.** Patients with stage IA disease are most commonly treated with mantle irradiation when the disease occurs above the diaphragm (as it does in 90% of patients) or with pelvic radiotherapy when the disease presents in an inguinal node. Patients with stage IIA disease above the diaphragm are most commonly treated with mantle plus para-aortic-splenic radiotherapy. There is no firm evidence that adding chemotherapy or modifying the ports leads to either improved results or significantly decreased toxicity in these patients.

4. **Stage II$_E$ disease with bulky mediastinal mass.** Patients with bulky mediastinal masses (disease diameter 9 cm or more than one-third of the chest diameter) present a special problem. When treated with radiotherapy alone, these patients have a risk of relapse approaching 50%. Since combined-modality therapy creates a risk of inducing acute nonlymphocytic leukemia, our approach is to treat these patients with combination chemotherapy, and then to give low-dose radiation therapy (20 Gy) only to patients with residual disease, and only to the area of residual disease. Unfortunately, there are no data showing that overall survival using this approach is superior to that with other approaches, such as the initial use of radiation therapy with chemotherapy given only to the patients who relapse following radiotherapy alone.

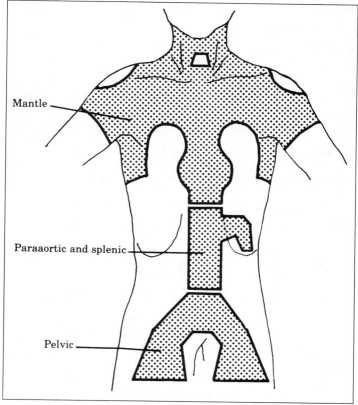

Fig. 26-1. Standard radiation therapy ports used for the treatment of Hodgkin's disease. For disease presenting above the diaphragm, the mantle plus paraaortic and splenic ports would be regarded as extended field therapy. The use of all three ports would be considered total nodal irradiation. (Reprinted by permission from J. R. Salzman and H. S. Kaplan. Effect of prior splenectomy on hematologic tolerance during total lymphoid radiotherapy of patients with Hodgkin's disease. *Cancer* **27:472, 1972.)**

5. **Stages IB and IIB.** In view of the limited number of patients with these stages of disease, available data do not allow firm treatment recommendations to be made. These patients are most commonly treated with extended field radiotherapy or combined-modality therapy, i.e., radiation therapy plus 3–6 cycles of a combination regimen such as MOPP or ABVD (Table 26-2), or MOPP/ABV (Table 26-3). Dose adjustments for MOPP appear in Table 26-4. A discussion of the relative merits of the chemotherapy options for advanced-stage Hodgkin's disease is

Table 26-2. MOPP and alternatives to MOPP chemotherapy

Regimen	Dosage
MOPP	Mechlorethamine 6 mg/m² IV on days 1 and 8
	Vincristine (Oncovin) 1.4 mg/m² (not to exceed 2.5 mg) IV on days 1 and 8
	Procarbazine 100 mg/m² PO on days 1–14
	Prednisone 40 mg/m² PO on days 1–14, cycles 1 and 4 only
	Repeat cycle every 28 days for 6 cycles minimum. Complete remission should be documented prior to discontinuing therapy.
BVCPP	Carmustine 100 mg/m² IV on day 1
	Vinblastine 5 mg/m² IV on day 1
	Cyclophosphamide 600 mg/m² PO on day 1
	Procarbazine 100 mg/m² PO on days 1–10
	Prednisone 60 mg/m² PO on days 1–10
	Repeat every 28 days.
ABVD	Doxorubicin (Adriamycin) 25 mg/m² IV on days 1 and 15
	Bleomycin 10 units/m² IV on days 1 and 15
	Vinblastine 6 mg/m² IV on days 1 and 15
	Dacarbazine 150 mg/m² on days 1–5
	Repeat every 28 days.
BCAVe	Bleomycin 2.5 units/m² IV or IM on days 1, 28, and 35
	Lomustine (CCNU) 100 mg/m² PO on day 1
	Doxorubicin (Adriamycin) 60 mg/m² IV on day 1
	Vinblastine 5 mg/m² IV on day 1
	Repeat every 42 days.
ABDIC	Doxorubicin (Adriamycin) 45 mg/m² IV on day 1
	Bleomycin 5 units/m² IV or IM on days 1 and 5
	Dacarbazine 200 mg/m² IV on days 1–5
	Lomustine (CCNU) 50 mg/m² PO on day 1
	Prednisone 40 mg/m² PO on days 1–5
	Repeat every 28 days.

Table 26-3. MOPP/ABV for Hodgkin's disease

Drug	Dose
Mechlorethamine	6 mg/m² IV on day 1
Vincristine (Oncovin)	1.4 mg/m² IV on day 1 (not to exceed 2 mg)
Procarbazine	100 mg/m² PO on days 1–7
Prednisone	40 mg/m² PO on days 1–14
Doxorubicin	35 mg/m² IV on day 8
Bleomycin	10 units/m² IV on day 8
Vinblastine	6 mg/m² IV on day 8
	Repeat every 28 days.

Table 26-4. Sliding scale of MOPP dose adjustment for myelotoxicity

Blood counts on day of treatment			Dose (%)			
WBC count/μl		Platelet count/μl	M	O	P	P
>4000	*and*	>100,000	100	100	100	100
3000–4000	*and*	>100,000	50	100	50	100
2000–3000	*or*	50,000–100,000	25	100	25	100
1000–2000	*and/or*	<50,000	25	50	25	100
<1000	*and*	<50,000	0	0	0	0

found in the discussions on stages IIIA, IVA, and IVB disease.

6. **Stage IIIA.** Therapy for stage IIIA disease has become less controversial in the past decade, although total consensus regarding the optimal treatment for these patients has not been obtained. Therapeutic options include total nodal radiotherapy alone, combination chemotherapy alone, or combined-modality therapy, i.e., radiotherapy plus chemotherapy.

With the demonstration that combined-modality therapy is associated with a 4–7% risk of acute non-lymphocytic leukemia, the use of total nodal radiotherapy in conjunction with combination chemotherapy fell from favor. Additionally, studies in the early 1980s established that total nodal radiotherapy was adequate therapy only for patients with limited, i.e., stage III_1, disease. For patients with stage III_2 disease, the use of radiotherapy alone was associated with a significant increase in mortality due to unacceptably high relapse rates, and the inability of these patients to tolerate salvage chemotherapy. Since demonstration that stage III_2 disease is present often requires a staging laparotomy, the simplest approach to stage III disease is to treat all stage III patients with combination chemotherapy, and this has become the most frequent approach to patients with stage IIIA disease.

7. **Stage IIIB, IVA, and IVB.** Combination chemotherapy is the standard therapy for these stages of Hodgkin's disease although the optimal chemotherapy regimen for advanced Hodgkin's disease remains a subject of controversy.

In 1970, the demonstration that MOPP chemotherapy could cure advanced Hodgkin's disease was one of the major events of the modern chemotherapy era, as it was the first demonstration that a previously incurable advanced disease could be cured by use of combination chemotherapy. This has provided the rationale for the use of combination chemotherapy in medical oncology.

a. Dose and duration of the therapy. The optimal chemotherapy regimen for use in Hodgkin's disease has not been established, and concerns about choosing the "best" regimen should not obscure the following principles. Drugs should be administered in accordance with prescribed doses and schedules and not modified for toxicities such as nausea and vomiting (which should be controlled symptomatically with antiemetics). Full doses should be given despite bone marrow involvement with Hodgkin's disease. Vincristine should be decreased only in the presence of ileus, motor weakness, or numbness involving the entire fingers, not just the fingertips. Six cycles of chemotherapy represent the standard duration of therapy, but it is not an absolute, and the policy is to treat until a complete remission is documented (usually after four cycles), and then for two additional cycles. If tests are equivocal, it is better to treat with additional cycles and reevaluate than to prematurely discontinue therapy.

b. Response to MOPP chemotherapy. When MOPP was administered in optimal fashion in one study, 81% of patients achieved a complete remission. Of these patients, 66% (representing 53% of the total series) remained in complete remission for 5 years, and an identical percentage remained in complete remission for 10 years. Thus 5-year disease-free survival is probably equivalent to cure. It should also be noted that the figure 53% is a minimal estimate for the cure of advanced Hodgkin's disease, as many patients who experience a complete remission and then relapse may still be cured with later salvage therapy.

c. Alternatives to MOPP induction therapy. Many efforts have been made to develop combination regimens that are more effective and less toxic than the standard MOPP regimen. Some of these regimens represent minor variations of the MOPP regimen, and others are combinations of non-cross-resistant drugs (see Table 26-2). The latter regimens may be used for MOPP failures but may also be considered as initial therapy.

Another approach to advanced disease is to use a hybrid regimen that integrates both the MOPP and ABV regimens (ABVD without dacarbazine) into the chemotherapy cycle. Based on the Goldie-Coldman model of development of tumor resistance, initial studies alternated 1 month of MOPP with 1 month of ABVD. More recent approaches involve giving the drugs included in MOPP on day 1 and giving ABV on day 8 (Table 26-3). Using supplemental radiotherapy to single areas of residual adenopathy, this regimen has been associated with complete remission rates of 97.5% and a 3-year relapse-free survival rate of 90.5% in uncontrolled trials.

Several large controlled trials investigated whether or not alternating or hybrid regimens are superior to the "standard" MOPP regimen. The results of worldwide trials are still equivocal. In a cooperative group trial, MOPP–ABVD (alternating monthly cycles of each regimen) was found to be significantly superior to MOPP with respect to complete remission rate and failure-free survival; survival was improved, but not significantly in the MOPP–ABVD group. One limitation of this study was that MOPP, as given in this study, was somewhat attenuated as compared to standard MOPP. Additionally, the ABVD arm of the study was not significantly different from MOPP–ABV.

Thus, standard MOPP, ABVD, MOPP–ABVD (alternating months), as well as the hybrid MOPP–ABV appear to be reasonable choices for initial combination chemotherapy in patients with advanced Hodgkin's disease. In patients who are most concerned about fertility, ABVD is the treatment of choice.

Although some investigators proposed combining chemotherapy with radiotherapy for advanced disease, there is no evidence that the standard use of this approach can improve survival enough to justify the potential leukemogenic risk of this practice. In selected patients with bulky disease, however, it is reasonable to consider supplementing combination chemotherapy with local radiation therapy to sites of bulky disease.

8. **Salvage therapy** for treatment failures. Relapse of Hodgkin's disease does not mean death, as salvage therapy is capable of producing cures. However, the chance of curing a patient with Hodgkin's disease who has relapsed is greater if the recurrence is nodal than if it is visceral. Also, the chance of salvaging a patient with Hodgkin's disease is greater when the initial stage of disease was limited than when it was relatively advanced.

For patients with limited nodal relapses following radiation therapy, additional irradiation may be considered. Alternatively, chemotherapy may be used in these patients and in those who relapse following chemotherapy. It has been appreciated that patients who relapse following initial radiotherapy may achieve a complete remission and may be potentially cured with combination chemotherapy. It has also been shown that patients who achieve a complete remission with MOPP therapy and who remain in remission for more than 1 year may have remis-

sion reinduced with MOPP therapy at the time of relapse and may be cured by this salvage therapy. In
past years, many of these patients, who were not
truly MOPP-resistant, were treated with one of the
regimens listed in Table 26-2 as salvage therapy. Inclusion of these relatively favorable patients in studies of such newer regimens as salvage therapy has
led to overestimating the value of these regimens as
salvage therapy in the patient who is truly MOPP-
resistant.

Because of the heterogeneity of patient groups
studied in reports of salvage therapy, it has not
been established that any one salvage regimen is optimal. However, in patients truly resistant to primary treatment, the possibility of cure with salvage
regimens such as ABVD or BCAVe is probably 15%
or less. Furthermore, the use of regimens such as
MOPP–ABV as primary therapy, by exposing patients to multiple agents, clearly decreases the possibility that they will respond to salvage therapy.

For this reason, high-dose chemotherapy in conjunction with reinfusion of autologous bone marrow
has been widely studied as primary or secondary salvage treatment in patients with Hodgkin's disease.
CBV (cyclophosphamide, carmustine [BCNU], etoposide) and BEAM (BCNU, etoposide, cytosine arabinoside, and melphalan) have been the most widely
studied regimens.

Controlled trials comparing preparative regimens
for autologous transplantation have not been conducted, and in view of the heterogeneity of treated
patients with respect to variables such as prior
therapy, sensitivity to therapy, site of relapse, and
disease-free interval, it is impossible to compare the
various studies meaningfully. Nevertheless, it appears that long-term disease-free survival may be
achieved in 30–50% of patients undergoing salvage
high-dose therapy in conjunction with autologous
bone marrow reinfusion. Patients who achieved long
disease-free intervals with standard therapy, especially if they have good performance status and remain sensitive to standard chemotherapy, have an
even better prospect of long-term disease-free survival.

While high-dose therapy with autologous bone
marrow reinfusion has become a standard approach
to salvage therapy, the optimal timing of such treatment, i.e., at the time of first relapse versus after a
trial of salvage chemotherapy, has not yet been resolved. Additionally, the role of peripheral blood
stem cells or growth factors as an alternative to autologous bone marrow transplantation has not been
completely evaluated.

While the use of granulocyte and granulocyte-
macrophage colony-stimulating factors (G-CSF and

GM-CSF, respectively) is expected to reduce the morbidity of these high-dose approaches to relapsed Hodgkin's disease, they are unlikely to impact significantly on mortality. At the present time, the mortality associated with high-dose therapy in conjunction with autologous bone marrow reinfusion is only 5–10%, and the major cause of death is relapse of disease, not therapy-related mortality.

9. **Treatment of symptoms.** Fever, and occasionally pruritus, may be disabling for some patients with Hodgkin's disease. The basic approach to these problems is to treat the disease. However, in patients with resistant disease, that approach may not be successful. Indomethacin 25–50 mg tid may be helpful in these patients. Anecdotal experience also supports the use of other nonsteroidal and anti-inflammatory agents in these patients.

10. **Follow-up.** Hodgkin's disease patients who achieve a complete remission and who show relapse usually do so at previous sites of disease. Our policy for follow-up is to see the patient every 2 months for the first year, every 3 months for the next year, every 4 months for the third year, every 6 months for the fourth year, and yearly thereafter. Follow-up evaluation for possible relapse is limited to physical examination and chest x-ray films (for patients with mediastinal involvement at presentation). If a patient who presented with B symptoms (see sec. **I.B.1.**) develops recurrent symptoms, we would add an abdominal CT to the evaluation, recognizing that the ability of CT to detect retroperitoneal disease is limited. Areas suspicious for clinical relapse should be confirmed by biopsy before proceeding with treatment.

Because of the risk of acute leukemia, we obtain complete blood cell counts at the time of each visit in patients who received combination chemotherapy. Monitoring for hypothyroidism was discussed in the section on radiation therapy. While elevated sedimentation rates or lactate dehydrogenase (LDH) levels may provide hints of relapse, we have not used these tests for follow-up monitoring in our practice.

II. Non-Hodgkin's lymphoma

A. **Introduction.** The NHLs are a group of malignancies that involve lymphocytes. The disorders included in NHLs differ in many basic characteristics. At the time of presentation some types of lymphoma, e.g., small cleaved cell lymphoma (poorly differentiated lymphocytic lymphoma), are almost always disseminated and have a high incidence of bone marrow and hepatic involvement. Other lymphomas, e.g., diffuse large noncleaved cell lymphoma (diffuse "histiocytic" lymphoma), may be limited to one or two lymph node areas in 30% of patients and involve the bone marrow at presentation in fewer than 20% of patients. In most adult lymphomas the malignant cell is a B lymphocyte. In a few cases the malignant cell is a T lymphocyte. Some types of lymphoma (primarily nodular lymphomas) have a slow, indolent course that initially responds to therapy but eventually progresses to a fatal outcome. Other types of lymphoma (mostly diffuse large cell lymphomas) have a rapidly fatal course in the absence of therapy but may be cured by combination chemotherapy.

In these circumstances, accurate classification of lymphomas is essential for scientific and clinical purposes. Ideally, one would want a classification system to divide lymphomas into entities that were both scientifically and clinically meaningful, i.e., a classification system that would define entities that were relatively homogeneous from a morphologic, immunologic, and clinical point of view. One would also want a classification system that could be widely used by pathologists so results could be compared from one institution to another, enabling clinicians to apply the results of studies to individual patients secure in the knowledge that the term used in the study meant the same thing to the academic pathologist writing the paper as to the local pathologist reviewing a particular case. Unfortunately, such an ideal classification system does not exist, and what is commonly used, the "New Working Formulation," is an attempt to use pathologic and immunologic principles to classify lymphomas into broad prognostic categories. The good news for clinicians is that this approach may facilitate treatment decisions. The bad news is that classification of lymphomas remains a suboptimal situation in which diverse disorders may be "lumped" together in the interests of simplifying care. Because the confusion over classification systems often prevents understanding the clinical state of the art with respect to lymphoma, a brief consideration of the classification of lymphomas is relevant prior to a discussion of therapy.

1. Classification—historical perspective. During the 1960s Rappaport divided lymphomas on the basis of whether the predominant cell was small (poorly differentiated lymphocytic lymphoma), large ("histiocytic" lymphoma), or a mixture of the two (mixed cell lymphoma). Lymphomas were also categorized as nodular or diffuse, although in many cases it was a continuum and not an absolute distinction. Entities such as diffuse "histiocytic" lymphoma were defined.

This system predated the understanding that there were B cells and T cells, and that most adult lymphomas involved the cells usually found in normal follicular centers. The Lukes-Collins classification system attempted to classify lymphomas on the basis of cell of origin and, by definition, define immunologically homogeneous entities. Several problems limited the adoption of this system. First, several systems considering immunologic features were simultaneously advocated by various hematopathologists, creating an atmosphere of confusion. Second, while attempting to define lymphomas by immune origin, as many as 25% of cases were "unclassified" in the "newer" Lukes-Collins system unless fresh tissue was available for the study of surface markers or until techniques to detect gene rearrangements were developed. Third, although the Rappaport system clearly had limitations, because of its widespread use by the mid-1970s there was concordance among pathologists regarding the classification of cases with respect to the Rappaport classification. Lacking a history of practical experience, none of the newer systems, including that of the Lukes-Collins system, had this level of agreement among pathologists with respect to cases. Fourth, although the Lukes-Collins system emphasized that a disorder such as "histiocytic" lymphoma was actually many disorders (i.e., large noncleaved cell lymphoma, large cleaved cell lymphoma, immunoblastic sarcoma of B cells, peripheral T cell lymphoma), there was no evidence that any or all of these hematopathologic distinctions were of clinical significance. Thus although the Lukes-Collins system appeared to be a scientific step forward, concerns over its practical application led to confusion.

2. **Classification—New Working Formulation.** In this context the National Cancer Institute created a working panel of hematopathologists who created the New Working Formulation. This classification system put the ideas of the Lukes-Collins system (and other immunologically oriented systems) into the mainstream; but instead of emphasizing the creation of many entities based on "cell of origin," the New Working Formulation defined broad categories of lymphoma based on general clinical prognosis, specifically low grade, intermediate grade, and high grade. The following is only a slight oversimplification.

Low-grade lymphomas are indolent lymphomas, e.g., chronic lymphocytic lymphoma and follicular (nodular) small cleaved cell lymphoma. In asymptomatic patients, even with widespread disease, they may require no initial treatment. These disorders are associated with a high response rate, but after a prolonged clinical course (often 5 to 10 + years) they are invariably fatal. *Intermediate-grade lymphomas* are more aggressive lymphomas that are associated with a fatal course within months (or occasionally a few years) in the absence of therapy but that have a high response rate and probably a cure rate approaching 50% with combination chemotherapy. This category includes diffuse small cleaved cell lymphoma and diffuse large noncleaved cell lymphoma, the most frequently seen subset of "histiocytic" lymphoma. *High-grade lymphomas* are those lymphomas associated with a high growth fraction, rapidly progressive clinical course in the absence of effective therapy, and a response rate to most chemotherapy regimens generally lower than that seen with intermediate grade lymphomas. The New Working Formulation is presented in Table 26-5 and represents more of a framework for clinical trials and therapeutic decisions than a pathologic classification system.

B. Staging

1. **Limited versus advanced disease.** The Ann Arbor staging system for Hodgkin's disease (see **I.B.**) is also used for NHLs. However, in contrast to Hodgkin's disease, which arises at an extranodal site in fewer than 1% of patients, approximately 10–20% of NHL cases arise at extranodal sites. Furthermore, the clinical applicability of the four stages of Hodgkin's disease to NHL is limited. For practical purposes there may be only two stages: limited disease (stage I) and advanced disease (stages II, III, and IV). With the exception of low-grade lymphomas, it is established that radiotherapy has no role in the curative therapy of stage II NHL and that chemotherapy is required in these patients. (As will be noted, even for stage I intermediate-grade lymphoma, the role of radiotherapy has generally been supplanted by chemotherapy.)

2. **Special considerations** apply to the staging of patients with NHL.

    a. **When performing a physical examination** special care must be given to sites such as Waldeyer's ring, epitrochlear nodes, femoral nodes, and popliteal nodes, which are rarely involved by Hodgkin's disease.

    b. **Bone marrow biopsy** is a key diagnostic procedure in NHLs owing to the high incidence of involvement, especially in small cleaved cell lymphoma.

    c. **Abdominal CT** is of greater value in NHLs than in Hodgkin's disease. In Hodgkin's disease involved abdominal nodes are small and may be missed by CT, whereas lymphangiography can detect small nodes in which the internal architecture is disrupted. With NHLs, retroperitoneal masses are often large and easily detected by CT. In addition, whereas mesenteric nodes are rarely involved in Hodgkin's disease, they are involved in approximately 70% of patients with nodular NHLs and may be detected by CT but are not opacified by lymphangiography. As for Hodgkin's disease, tests that are performed for purposes of staging establish a baseline so patients can be evaluated for a complete remission when therapy has been given with curative intent.

    d. **Gallium scan** may be helpful in identifying loci

Table 26-5. New Working Formulation for non-Hodgkin's lymphoma

Low grade
　Small lymphocytic consistent with CLL or plasmacytoid cell
　Follicular, predominantly small cleaved cell
　　Diffuse areas
　　Sclerosis
　Follicular, mixed, small cleaved cell and large cell
　　Diffuse areas
　　Sclerosis

Intermediate grade
　Follicular, predominantly large cell
　　Diffuse areas
　　Sclerosis
　Diffuse small cleaved cell
　Diffuse mixed, small cleaved cell and large cell
　　Sclerosis
　　Epithelioid cell component
　Diffuse large cell
　　Cleaved cell
　　Noncleaved cell
　　Sclerosis

High grade
　Large cell, immunoblastic
　　Plasmacytoid
　　Clear cell
　　Polymorphous
　　Epithelioid cell component
　Lymphoblastic
　　Convoluted cell
　　Nonconvoluted cell
　Small noncleaved cell
　　Burkitt's
　　Follicular areas

Miscellaneous
　Composite
　Mycosis fungoides
　Histiocytic
　Extramedullary plasmacytoma
　Unclassifiable
　Other

Source: Modified from the Non-Hodgkin's Lymphoma Pathologic Classification Project. National Cancer Institute-sponsored study of classification of non-Hogdkin's lymphomas: summary and description of a working formulation for clinical usage. *Cancer* 49:2112, 1982.

of disease, and if the results are positive can be a sensitive marker for residual disease.

e. **Peripheral blood cell counts** are generally an insensitive way to determine marrow involvement, but if abnormal strongly point to marrow infiltration with lymphoma.

f. **Prognostic indicators.** The serum LDH is an important prognostic indicator in patients with aggressive histologies. It is used together with stage, performance status, number of extranodal disease sites, and age in the international prognostic index. Newer molecular biomarkers such as *bcl-2* and P-53, and multidrug resistance (MDR) expression are under active investigation as prognostic indicators and may soon complement clinical indicators.

C. **Radiation therapy of non-Hodgkin's lymphomas: general considerations.** Because most patients with NHLs have disseminated disease, radiotherapy plays a more limited role in NHLs than in Hodgkin's disease. However, the value of radiotherapy should not be overlooked. With most histologic types of nodular lymphoma, doses of 44 Gy can achieve control of local disease. Because disease occurs outside of treatment fields, e.g., bone marrow disease, irradiation is rarely curative. However, when patients with nodular lymphoma have large masses, local radiotherapy may be the most effective means of palliation. A dose-response curve for large cell lymphoma is less well established, although radiotherapy may play a role in palliating patients with large cell lymphoma who have become refractory to chemotherapy. Although 30% of patients with large cell lymphoma have stage I or II disease, the role of radiotherapy in these patients is not firmly established.

Radiotherapy has been associated with cure rates exceeding 80% in stage I large cell lymphomas *only* when patients have been staged by laparotomy. Rather than subject these patients to a laparotomy, the usual approach is to treat clinical stage I patients with six cycles of a chemotherapy regimen such as CHOP (Table 26-6) or three cycles of CHOP with involved field radiotherapy. These approaches are associated with cure rates exceeding 90%. Stage II patients with large cell lymphoma are considered as having advanced disease and are treated the same as patients with stage III or IV disease.

D. **Therapy of non-Hodgkin's lymphoma: Low, intermediate, and high grade**

1. **Low-grade lymphoma** predominantly small cleaved cell lymphoma—nodular* (SCC-N), also called poorly differentiated lymphocytic lymphoma—nodular. Patients with this type of lymphoma generally have widespread disease at presentation. Nevertheless, the median survival time of patients with SCC-N has

---

*"Nodular" in these sections (**D.1–3.**) is equivalent to "follicular" in the New Working Formulation (see Table 26-5).

Table 26-6. Combination chemotherapy for the clinically indolent lymphomas

Regimen*	Dosage
CVP	Cyclophosphamide 400 mg/m² PO on days 1–5 Vincristine (Oncovin) 1.4 mg/m² IV on day 1 (not to exceed 2.0 mg) Prednisone 100 mg/m² PO on days 1–5 Repeat every 21 days.
COPP	Cyclophosphamide 600 mg/m² IV on days 1 and 8 Vincristine (Oncovin) 1.4 mg/m² IV on days 1 and 8 (not to exceed 2.5 mg) Procarbazine 100 mg/m² PO on days 1–10 Prednisone 40 mg/m² on days 1–14 Repeat every 28 days.
CHOP	Cyclophosphamide 750 mg/m² IV on day 1 Doxorubicin (Adriamycin) 50 mg/m² IV on day 1 Vincristine (Oncovin) 1.4 mg/m² IV on day 1 (not to exceed 2.0 mg) Prednisone 100 mg PO on days 1–5 Repeat every 21 days.
CNOP	Cyclophosphamide 750 mg/m² IV on day 1 Mitoxantrone (Novantrone) 10 mg/m² IV on day 1 Vincristine (Oncovin) 1.4 mg/m² IV on day 1 (not to exceed 2.0 mg) Prednisone 100 mg PO on days 1–5 Repeat every 21 days.

*These regimens employ a sliding scale for myelotoxicity similar to that used for the MOPP regimen (see Table 26-2). The alphabetic abbreviations used for these regimens consider doxorubicin (Adriamycin) as hydroxyldaunomycin.

ranged from 4 to 8 years in most series. Combination regimens such as those in Table 26-6 have produced complete remissions in up to 80% of patients. However, such remissions are not durable, and these regimens are associated with considerable toxicity (myelotoxicity, nausea, vomiting, alopecia, and neurotoxicity). Because therapy is palliative and there is no proof that survival is improved by the early use of combination chemotherapy, many clinicians use a policy of "watchful waiting," as might be employed for chronic lymphocytic leukemia. Nevertheless, it should be noted that some clinicians still advocate the early use of combination chemotherapy for these patients in the hope of having a favorable impact on individual patients.

Patients with minimal symptoms or moderate lymphadenopathy may be treated with chlorambucil, either 2–4 mg/m² PO daily or 30 mg/m² PO every 2 weeks, with or without prednisone. In patients with enlarging nodes or spleen, cytopenias, fever, sweats, weight loss, or visceral involvement other than bone marrow or microscopic liver involvement, one would generally initiate therapy with one of the simple chemotherapy regimens shown in Table 26–6. In many patients years elapse before such treatment is required.

For patients who relapse following initial therapy, several options are available. If initial therapy has been low-dose chlorambucil, for example, a regimen such as CHOP or CNOP would be reasonable. If a regimen such as CHOP or CNOP has been used, one can consider fludarabine 25 mg/m^2 IV as a 15–30-minute infusion daily for 5 days. This drug, which has recently been approved for chronic lymphocytic leukemia, is also effective in low-grade lymphoma. Additionally, interferon alpha 2–10 × 10^6 units/m^2 IM 3 times a week has been shown to be effective in patients with low-grade lymphoma. While its inclusion in primary therapeutic regimens has not been consistently associated with improved survival, it is a reasonable option for salvage therapy. The combination chemotherapy regimen DHAP (Table 26-7), generally used in refractory intermediate-grade lymphomas, is also a therapeutic option for relapsed low-

Table 26-7. Salvage chemotherapy regimens for non-Hodgkin's lymphoma

Regimen	Drugs and dosage
DHAP	Dexamethasone 40 mg PO or IV push on days 1–4
	Cytarabine 2 gm/m^2 over 3 hours q12h for 2 doses on day 2 starting after cisplatin infusion ended. If age < 70, reduce cytarabine dose to 1 gm/m^2 per dose.
	Cisplatin 100 mg/m^2 CIV over 24 hours on day 1
	Repeat every 3–4 weeks (depending on marrow recovery) for 4 cycles beyond maximum response (total = 6–10 cycles).
DICE	Dexamethasone 10 mg IV bolus q6h on days 1–4
	Ifosfamide 1 gm/m^2 (maximum 1.75 gm) IV in 100 ml of saline over 15–20 minutes on days 1–4
	Cisplatin 25 mg/m^2 IV in 250 ml of saline over 60 minutes on days 1–4
	Etoposide 100 mg/m^2 IV over 1 hour on days 1–4
	Mesna 200 mg/m^2 in 50 ml of saline IV over 5–10 minutes 1 hour prior to each ifosfamide infusion on days 1–4. Starting immediately after first ifosfamide infusion, give a continuous infusion of mesna 900 mg/m^2/24 hours, given as 300 mg/m^2 in 1 liter of saline over each 8 hours. Continue mesna infusion for 12 hours after last dose of ifosfamide.
	Repeat every 3–4 weeks for 2 cycles beyond maximum response (6 maximum).

Table 26-7. (continued)

Regimen	Drugs and dosage
EPOCH	Etoposide 50 mg/m^2/24 hours CIV on days 1–4
	Vincristine 0.4 mg/m^2/24 hours CIV on days 1–4
	Doxorubicin 10 mg/m^2/24 hours CIV on days 1–4
	Cyclophosphamide 750 mg/m^2 IV on day 6
	Prednisone 60 mg/m^2 PO on days 1–6
	Trimethoprim-sulfamethoxazole 1 double-strength tablet PO bid on days 1–3 each week
	Repeat cycle on day 21 if ANC > 1000/μl. Reduce cyclophosphamide dose by 25% on day 1 if ANC 1000–1500/μl or ANC nadir < 500 μl; reduce by 50% if both pertain. If subsequent ANC nadir > 500 μl returns, reescalate dose as dictated by day 1 counts.
	If ANC < 1000 μl, hold therapy and repeat count in 1 week.
	Repeat for 2 cycles beyond maximum response (6 minimum).
ESHAP	Etoposide 60 mg/m^2 IV on days 1–4
	Methylprednisolone 500 mg IV on days 1–4
	Cytarabine 2 gm/m^2 IV over 2 hours on day 5 after cisplatin infusion ends
	Cisplatin 25 mg/m^2/24 hours CIV on days 1–4
	Repeat every 3–4 weeks until maximum response (minimum 6 cycles).
MINE	Mesna 1.33 gm/m^2 mixed with ifosfamide over 1 hour on days 1–3, followed by 500 mg PO 4 hours after the ifosfamide
	Ifosfamide 1.33 gm/m^2 IV over 1 hour on days 1–3
	Mitoxantrone 8 mg/m^2 IV over 15 minutes on day 1
	Etoposide 65 mg/m^2 over 1 hour on days 1–3
	Repeat every 21 days for 6 cycles if complete response attained; for partial response, change to ESHAP when maximum response attained.

CIV = continuous venous infusion over 24 hours; ANC = absolute neutrophil count.

Note: Dose modifications vary among regimens, but usually include delay of a new cycle if the ANC is < 1000/μl, reduction of the more myelosuppressive agents by 25% for an ANC of 1000–1500/μl, and full doses if the ANC is > 1500/μl. Reduction may also be indicated if the ANC nadir is < 500/μl, particularly if the patient had a febrile episode. These guidelines should be modified as indicated by the clinical situation.

grade lymphoma when patients are refractory to standard regimens.

For disease associated with long-term survival despite recurrent disease there is no one best clinical algorithm for all patients, and palliative treatments should be individualized based on extent of disease, clinical pace of disease, and age of the patient.

An alternative approach to low-grade lymphomas involves the use of very-high-dose chemotherapy and total body radiation in conjunction with autologous bone marrow transplantation. This approach is limited by the fact that bone marrow involvement is common in low-grade lymphomas. Even when genetic markers such as *bcl-2* are used to confirm complete purging of tumor cells, lymphoma may not be completely eliminated from the bone marrow. Use of this approach as salvage therapy has provided long-term disease-free survival in some patients with low-grade lymphoma who remain sensitive to standard chemotherapy.

Clinical studies also have shown long-term disease-free survival in many patients when high-dose therapy and autologous bone marrow reinfusion are used to consolidate first remissions in patients with low-grade lymphoma. However, the ultimate value of this approach to low-grade lymphoma is unknown. Long-term survival is the rule in patients with low-grade lymphoma even without this aggressive approach. Therefore, the long-term survival rates seen following high-dose therapy and autologous marrow reinfusion may represent long-term palliation rather than cure. Further follow-up of patients will be necessary to learn the value of this approach in low-grade lymphoma (i.e., curative or palliative) as well as to determine the role of purging, and the optimal timing of this approach (i.e., as salvage or as consolidation of remission).

2. **Intermediate-grade lymphomas**
    a. **Small cleaved cell—diffuse.** The disease initially described by Rappaport as "poorly differentiated lymphocytic lymphoma diffuse" (PDL-D) has been shown to be composed of two disorders. One group of patients have a disease similar to small cleaved cell nodular lymphoma, which is indeed composed of small cleaved lymphocytes. This disease is similar to SCC-N but tends to be associated with a shorter survival. Although it is not known whether initial chemotherapy produces results superior to "watchful waiting" in this group of patients, the general tendency is to treat at the time of diagnosis with either CHOP or a more aggressive regimen (Table 26-8). The other group of patients included in the Rappaport category PDL-D have a T cell lymphoma generally equivalent to T cell acute lymphocytic leukemia that is often associated with a large me-

Table 26-8. Chemotherapy regimens for diffuse histiocytic lymphoma

Regimen	Dosage
BACOP	Bleomycin 5 units/m^2 IV on days 15 and 22 Doxorubicin (Adriamycin) 25 mg/m^2 IV on days 1 and 8 Cyclophosphamide 650 mg/m^2 IV on days 1 and 8 Vincristine (Oncovin) 1.4 mg/m^2 IV on days 1 and 8 (not to exceed 2.0 mg) Prednisone 60 mg/m^2 PO on days 15–28 Repeat every 28 days.
COMLA	Cyclophosphamide 1500 mg/m^2 IV on day 1 Vincristine (Oncovin) 1.4 mg/m^2 IV on days 1, 8, and 15 (not to exceed 2.5 mg) Methotrexate 120 mg/m^2 IV on days 22, 29, 36, 43, 50, 57, 64, and 71 Leucovorin 25 mg/m^2 PO q6h for 4 doses starting 24 hours after each methotrexate dose Cytarabine 300 mg/m^2 IV on days 22, 29, 36, 43, 50, 57, 64, and 71 Repeat every 91 days.
m-BACOD	Methotrexate 200 mg/m^2 IV on days 8 and 15 Leucovorin 10 mg/m^2 PO q6h for 8 doses starting 24 hours after methotrexate Bleomycin 4 units/m^2 IV on day 1 Doxorubicin (Adriamycin) 45 mg/m^2 IV on day 1 Cyclophosphamide 600 mg/m^2 IV on day 1 Vincristine (Oncovin) 1 mg/m^2 IV on day 1 Dexamethasone 6 mg/m^2 PO on days 1–5 Repeat every 21 days.
ProMACE/MOPP	Prednisone 60 mg/m^2 PO on days 1–14 Methotrexate 1.5 gm/m^2 IV on day 14 Leucovorin 50 mg/m^2 IV q6h for 5 doses starting 24 hours after methotrexate Doxorubicin (Adriamycin) 25 mg/m^2 IV on days 1 and 8 Cyclophosphamide 650 mg/m^2 IV on days 1 and 8 Etoposide 120 mg/m^2 IV on days 1 and 8 Cycles are given every 28 days. ProMACE is given for a variable number of cycles based on tumor response; then MOPP therapy is given for approximately the same number of cycles.

Table 26-8. (continued)

Regimen	Dosage
MACOP-B	Methotrexate 400 mg/m² IV weeks 2, 6, and 10; one-fourth of dose as IV bolus, then three-fourths over 4 hours
	Leucovorin 15 mg PO q6h for 6 doses, starting 24 hours after each methotrexate dose
	Doxorubicin (Adriamycin) 50 mg/m² IV weeks 1, 3, 5, 7, 9, and 11
	Cyclophosphamide 350 mg/m² IV weeks 1, 3, 5, 7, 9, and 11
	Vincristine (Oncovin) 1.4 mg/m² IV weeks 2, 4, 6, 8, 10, and 12
	Bleomycin 10 units/m² IV weeks 4, 8, and 12
	Prednisone 75 mg/day PO for 12 weeks; taper to 0 during weeks 10–12
	Trimethoprim-sulfa 1 double-strength tablet PO bid × 12 weeks

diastinal mass. These patients clearly have a high-grade lymphoma and are discussed in that section.

b. **Large cleaved cell lymphoma (LCCL) or "mixed cell" lymphoma.** These lymphomas, in which large cleaved cells are often the predominant cell, are generally mixtures of large cleaved cells and small cleaved cells. Large noncleaved cells are often present. Classification of these lymphomas is also complicated by the fact that most of them have both a nodular and a diffuse pattern.

When watchful waiting is employed in this group of patients, therapy is generally initiated within less than a year, so most clinicians treat these patients at the time of diagnosis. Nevertheless, there has not been a consistent demonstration that the patients have a curable disease when aggressive chemotherapy is employed. Optimal therapy for this group of patients is clearly undefined. Some clinicians prefer minimal therapy on the grounds that treatment is palliative, as in SCC-N. Other clinicians believe that these patients should receive CHOP or one of the other regimens (see Table 26-8) used for large noncleaved (transformed) cell lymphoma, as some of these lymphomas behave in an aggressive fashion and prospective identification of these cases is not possible.

There is less concordance among pathologists regarding classification of mixed cell lymphomas or large cleaved cell lymphomas than for any other NHL. Because these lymphomas are mixtures of cell types and are generally both nodular and diffuse, what is one pathologist's "large cleaved cell—nodular" or "mixed cell—nodular" lymphoma may be interpreted as "large noncleaved cell—diffuse" by another. Fortunately, this confusing disorder represents only 5–10% of adult NHLs.

c. **Large noncleaved (transformed) cell lymphoma, immunoblastic sarcoma of B cells, and peripheral T cell lymphoma**

(1) **Immunologic and pathologic subtypes.** These disorders represent most of the cases previously considered "diffuse histiocytic" lymphoma and now entered into studies of "diffuse large cell lymphoma," or "intermediate-grade lymphoma." Exact percentage breakdowns are not known, but T cell lymphomas comprise only 5–10% of "large cell lymphomas," and approximately 10% are immunoblastic sarcoma of B cells. Controversy still exists as to whether the immunologic subtype of "large cell" lymphoma is clinically important. Some studies found immunologic subclassification to be clinically insignificant, whereas others found that such subclassification is a major prognostic variable in this group of patients. These differences may reflect differences in the use of the pathologic classification systems, or an interaction between prognosis and therapy. Another methodologic issue relates to the recent identification of T cell–rich B cell lymphomas. In the past, lymphomas composed primarily of T cells have been presumed to be T cell lymphomas. The ability to identify cells in tissue sections has enabled hematopathologists to determine that some lymphomas in which the predominant cell is a T cell are composed of malignant B cells and reactive T cells. As a result, the entire literature on whether T cell lymphoma has a worse prognosis than B cell lymphoma must be reassessed. In our experience, T cell–rich B cell lymphomas have a prognosis similar to that for other intermediate-grade B cell lymphomas, while T cell lymphomas have a worse prognosis and appear to require a more aggressive therapeutic approach.

(2) **Combination chemotherapy: historical perspective.** In the era of single-agent chemotherapy, the lymphomas classified as "diffuse histiocytic" were associated with a median survival time of 6 months, with approximately 5–10% of patients surviving for

2 years. The demonstration that COPP chemotherapy (see Table 26-6) could produce complete remissions in approximately 40% of patients, with 35% of patients continuing as long-term relapse-free survivors, was a major clinical advance. Numerous regimens have replaced COPP since the early 1970s, but all of these regimens (see CHOP, Tables 26-6 and 26-8) can be interpreted relative to the COPP study.

(a) COPP showed that "histiocytic" lymphoma was curable. As noted above, there is suggestive evidence that certain subsets, e.g., LCCL and possibly peripheral T cell lymphoma (PTCL), are less curable than other subsets.

(b) The COPP study showed that approximately 80% of complete remissions are associated with cure. Patients with LCCL and PTCL also appear to have higher rates of relapse after achieving a complete remission.

(c) The COPP study showed that the 2-year relapse-free survival rate is a good estimate of cure. Late relapses occur but are rare. Because patients with large masses may have some residual mass (either fibrosis or residual disease) on completion of therapy, the complete remission rate may be an overestimate of the cure rate based on "wishful thinking." The 2-year relapse-free survival rate is more meaningful because if the residual mass represents persistent disease, it will be clinically evident within 2 years.

(d) The complete remission rate reported for newer regimens (see Table 26-8) increased from the 40% observed with COPP to 80+% with regimens such as MACOP-B. However, in a large-scale randomized trial comparing the apparently obsolete regimen, CHOP, to newer regimens such as m-BACOD, or MACOP-B, complete remission and long-term survival rates were not significantly different between regimens. While this result was surprising to many investigators, there are several reasons why apparent improvement with newer regimens might prove to be more artifactual than real.

These lymphomas are a heterogeneous group clinically and immunologically, and the patients in different studies may not be comparable. First, as therapies have become more aggressive, the median age of the patients in the studies has decreased because older patients are excluded (reasonably so) as being too old to tolerate toxic therapies. Second, whereas chemotherapy studies initially included only patients with stage III and IV disease, patients with stage II disease are now routinely treated with chemotherapy. Because a lower tumor burden appears to be a favorable prognostic feature, these patients favorably bias results of clinical trials. Third, as noted above, the natural history of LCCL (mixed cell lymphoma) is not firmly established. These lymphomas tend to be both nodular and diffuse and may behave somewhat like indolent lymphomas. Inclusion of these patients in studies of large cell diffuse lymphoma may create a favorable bias, as these patients may have a high response rate and may relapse beyond the point at which one is looking for relapses in large cell diffuse lymphoma.

(3) **Combination chemotherapy: current recommendations.** In view of the recently completed randomized trial, CHOP has re-emerged as standard therapy for intermediate-grade lymphoma. Nevertheless, one should recognize that with further follow-up and further data analysis, one of the regimens listed in Table 26-8 may yet prove to have value in certain subsets of intermediate-grade lymphomas. Additionally, further studies of dose intense regimens are ongoing, and it is conceivable that regimens even more dose-intensive than those compared to CHOP in the aforementioned randomized trial will prove to be clinically superior to CHOP.

(4) **Salvage therapy.** As primary therapies have become more aggressive and more effective, patients who fail such therapy represent a less and less favorable group of patients. As a result, it is not surprising that salvage chemotherapy of these lymphomas has not produced outstanding results. Some investigators have claimed response rates above 50% with salvage therapy, but complete response rates are generally in the 20–30% range, and long-term relapse-free survival has been observed in fewer than 5% of patients treated in most salvage studies. Salvage regimens generally include drugs such as cisplatin, high-dose cytosine arabi-

noside, etoposide, or ifosfamide. Individual investigators often prefer a particular salvage regimen based on personal experience (i.e., perceived toxicity, response of previous patients) (see Table 26-7). However, there is no evidence to suggest that any salvage regimen is truly superior to the other regimens.

Additionally, very-high-dose chemotherapy in conjunction with total body radiotherapy and reinfusion of autologous bone marrow has been extensively studied as salvage therapy in patients with intermediate-grade lymphoma. Response rates to this approach have generally depended on responses to prior therapy. In patients who respond to primary therapy, and who remain sensitive to standard salvage regimens, response rates near 60% may be seen, with 3-year disease-free survival observed in approximately 30% of patients. The 3-year disease-free survival rate is approximately 15% in patients who initially respond to treatment, but who are resistant to conventional salvage therapy. In patients who are refractory to primary therapy and salvage therapy, long-term disease-free survival is rare. With a mortality of 5–10% associated with this approach, many clinicians justifiably exclude these latter patients with resistant disease from trials involving autologous transplantation.

Recent studies suggested that adequate stem cells can be collected from peripheral blood, allowing this technique to substitute for collection of bone marrow stem cells. Some controversy exists as to whether the cells collected from peripheral blood represent true "stem cells" or "committed progenitor cells." This issue is likely to be resolved within the next few years. However, while peripheral blood stem cells might seem to be an optimal source of cells for patients with bone marrow involvement, sophisticated techniques of measuring minimal residual tumor have suggested that when the bone marrow is involved, so is the peripheral blood, and further studies in this area are needed.

(5) **Lymphoma in the elderly.** The incidence of lymphoma increases with age. Thus, the clinician is often faced with the elderly patient with an aggressive lymphoma. Although there are no strict guidelines, elderly individuals are often defined as those 70 years or older or between 60 and 70 years old with significant comorbid disease. As with

acute leukemia, elderly individuals should not empirically be denied potentially curative therapy due to age bias. Elderly individuals with good performance status and well-controlled comorbid disease make excellent candidates for potentially curative chemotherapy. Unfortunately, the optimum regimen or intensity of therapy has not been defined since these "non-Cadillac" patients have often been excluded from the practice-defining studies for the treatment of lymphoma or the reported response data have not been stratified according to patient age in the studies that included elderly participants. Recent reports have started to address the issue of aggressive lymphoma in the elderly. Based on long-term experience, CHOP or CNOP should be the standard to which new regimens should be compared. Some investigators recommend giving these regimens on an every-4-week schedule to lessen the risk of severe neutropenia and thrombocytopenia, while others may empirically add G-CSF. Intensive therapy of short duration (DOCE, P-VABEC) appears to produce similar results with acceptable toxicity. More recent regimens are built around daily oral VP-16 (Vanderbilt VP-16, PEN). These regimens contain fewer intravenous medications and are less myelosuppressive, which results in fewer costly and time-consuming trips to the chemotherapy center (Table 26-9). The curative potential of these VP-16-based regimens is not known. Ultimately, they may prove to be good palliation for the "poor-risk" patient. The final choice of regimens is usually based on the personal experience of the clinician (i.e., previous toxicity, response of previous patients), as well as the clinician's estimate of how much toxicity is appropriate for each individual patient.

3. **High-grade lymphomas**
   a. **Peripheral T cell lymphoma.** Although there is not unanimity on this point, there is considerable evidence that when patients with peripheral T cell lymphoma are correctly identified, their chance of being cured with "standard" regimens such as CHOP is significantly less than that for patients with intermediate-grade lymphomas. No standard therapy for these patients exists, but we recommend "high-intensity/brief-duration" therapy in these patients (see Table 26-10). Fortunately, when separated from patients with T cell–rich B cell lymphomas, these patients probably represent only 5% of adult NHLs.

Table 26-9. Regimens for treatment of aggressive lymphoma in the elderly

Regimen	Drugs and dosage
DOCE	Doxorubicin 40 mg/m^2 IV weeks 1, 2, 7, and 8
	Vincristine 1.2 mg/m^2 IV weeks, 1, 4, and 7
	Cyclophosphamide 300 mg/m^2 IV weeks 1, 4, and 7
	Etoposide 50 mg/m^2 IV on day 1 of week 4, then 100 mg/m^2 PO on days 2, 3, 4, and 5 (of week 4)
	Trimethoprim-sulfamethoxazole 1 double-strength tablet bid continuously weeks 1–8
	Prednisone 50 mg PO for 10 days beginning weeks 1, 4, and 7
	Ketoconazole 200 mg PO for 10 days beginning weeks 1, 4, and 7
	Cimetidine 600 mg PO bid for 10 days beginning weeks 1, 4, and 7
	This regimen is given for 8 weeks only.
	Delay treatment 1 week if ANC is < 500/µl.
	Reduce dose of doxorubicin, cyclophosphamide, and etoposide by 50% if ANC is 500–999/µl; give full dose if ANC is ≥ 1000/µl.
	Reduce vincristine by 33% for abnormal buttoning or writing, by 50% for moderate motor neuropathy, omit for severe motor neuropathy.
P-VABEC	Doxorubicin 30 mg/m^2 IV weeks 1, 3, 5, 7, and 11
	Etoposide 100 mg/m^2 IV weeks 1, 3, 5, 7, 9, and 11
	Cyclophosphamide 350 mg/m^2 IV weeks 1, 3, 5, 7, 9, and 11
	Vincristine 1.2 mg/m^2 IV weeks 2, 4, 6, 8, 10, and 12
	Bleomycin 5 mg/m^2 IV weeks 2, 4, 6, 8, 10, and 12
	Prednisone 50 mg PO for 12 weeks
	Delay first three drugs by 1 week if ANC is < 1000/µl or platelet count is < 80,000/µl; delay latter three if ANC is < 500/µl or platelet count is < 50,000/µl.
	Regimen may be discontinued after 8 weeks, depending on tolerance.
Vanderbilt Prolonged VP-16	Etoposide 50 mg/m^2 PO for 21 days
	Methotrexate 40 mg/m^2 IV weeks 1 and 3, followed 24 hours later by leucovorin 15 mg PO q6h for 4 doses
	Prednisone 60 mg PO for 7 days starting weeks 1 and 6
	Cyclophosphamide 500 mg/m^2 IV bolus week 6
	Mitoxantrone 12 mg/m^2 IV bolus week 6
	Vincristine 1 mg/m^2 IV week 6
	A second cycle of the 8-week regimen is repeated weeks 9–15.
PEN	Prednisone 50 mg PO on days 1–14
	Etoposide 50 mg PO on days 1–14
	Mitoxantrone (Novantrone) 8 mg/m^2 IV on day 1
	Repeat every 4 weeks.

b. **Small noncleaved (transformed) cell lymphoma.** This category of lymphoma includes both Burkitt's and non-Burkitt's lymphoma. In the United States, the Burkitt's type tends to occur in younger patients, and to be associated with more gastrointestinal disease and a lower incidence of bone marrow involvement. Both are high-grade lymphomas. They are relatively resistant to standard chemotherapy, with median survival times of 6–10 months being reported. Our preliminary results suggest that high-intensity/brief-duration therapy (Table 26-10) can improve the long-term disease-free survival rate to 50%, although these results are closely tied to stage. Patients with central nervous system (CNS) disease, bone marrow involvement, or markedly elevated serum LDH levels have an especially poor prognosis. Due to the aggressiveness of this disease, it is reasonable to consider other therapeutic alternatives such as the use of very-high-dose chemotherapy along with total body radiation therapy, and autologous bone marrow transplantation as consolidation therapy.

c. **Lymphoblastic lymphoma.** This entity has been frequently observed in children and may be regarded as a variant of T cell acute lymphoblastic leukemia. Mediastinal masses are common, and CNS disease and marrow involvement are frequently observed. Patients may be treated with any of the protocols in use for acute lymphoblastic leukemia. In 1986, Coleman reviewed the Stanford experience with a complex regimen including a CHOP-like induction, CNS prophylaxis, consolidation with methotrexate and L-asparaginase, and consolidation with methotrexate and 6-mercaptopurine. The 5-year survival rate was 19% in high-risk patients (marrow involvement,

Table 26-10. High-intensity/brief-duration therapy for non-Hodgkin's lymphoma

Cyclophosphamide 1500 mg/m^2 IV on days 1, 2, and 29

Etoposide 400 mg/m^2 IV on days 1, 2, and 3

Etoposide 100 mg/m^2 on days 29, 30, and 31

Doxorubicin (Adriamycin) 45 mg/m^2 IV on days 29 and 30

Vincristine 1.4 mg/m^2 IV on days 8, 22, 36, and 50

Bleomycin 10 units/m^2 IV on days 8, 22, 36, and 50

Methotrexate 200 mg/m^2 IV on days 15 and 43

Leucovorin 15 mg/m^2 PO q6h × 6 doses, starting 24 hours after each methotrexate dose

Prednisone 60 mg/m^2 PO on days 1–7 and 29–35

CNS involvement, LDH > 300 IU/liter), and 94% in patients without these features. As with small transformed cell lymphoma, we have employed high-intensity/brief-duration therapy in these patients, but the number of patients so treated is inadequate to draw firm conclusions. The role of high-dose therapy in conjunction with autologous bone marrow transplantation as consolidation or as salvage also requires further investigation.

E. **Special considerations in therapy**

1. **CNS prophylaxis.** Involvement of the CNS by NHL has been associated with bone marrow involvement. However, in the majority of patients, small transformed cell lymphoma and lymphoblastic lymphoma are the histologic types of lymphoma involved. In patients with these high-grade lymphomas and bone marrow involvement, we recommend cranial irradiation and intrathecal methotrexate as would be used in acute lymphoblastic leukemia. In patients with intermediate-grade lymphoma and bone marrow involvement, consideration of CNS prophylaxis is reasonable. However, there has never been a prospective trial showing that approach to decrease the incidence of CNS complications or to improve survival.

2. **Extranodal lymphomas.** NHLs arise at extranodal sites in 10–20% of patients. In the past, these patients were most often treated with radiation therapy. However, with the demonstration that chemotherapy was a rational approach to *nodal* stage I NHL, many of these patients have been treated with chemotherapy. The optimal approach to extranodal NHL is unknown. However, NHL occurs frequently enough at some extranodal sites to raise specific considerations with respect to treatment.

a. **Lymphomas of the CNS.** In patients who do not have acquired immunodeficiency syndrome (AIDS), these lymphomas are most often large transformed cell lymphoma or immunoblastic lymphoma. Radiation therapy alone has generally been associated with a median survival time of less than a year in these patients, even when high doses of radiation are employed. Recent trials employing chemotherapy, i.e., high-dose methotrexate, prior to radiation therapy have produced better results. However, randomized trials to compare chemotherapy plus radiation therapy to radiation therapy alone have not yet been performed.

In patients who are positive for human immunodeficiency virus (HIV), large noncleaved cell lymphoma, immunoblastic lymphoma, and small noncleaved cell lymphoma are all common. Because of the limited prognosis of these patients

due to HIV infection, they generally have been
treated with radiation therapy alone. The role of
chemotherapy in patients whose lymphomas develop early in the course of HIV infection is yet to
be established.

b. **Gastric lymphomas.** These lymphomas are
most commonly large noncleaved cell lymphoma.
Because of the risk of perforation during therapy, it is often recommended that these patients
undergo resection prior to definitive treatment.
However, that recommendation dates to a period
when bulky tumors were discovered at surgery
and when radiotherapy was the most commonly
used modality. The relevance of that recommendation in an age where the diagnosis is often
made at endoscopy and when minimal tumor can
be detected by CT is not known. We do not believe
that gastrectomy should be employed routinely
prior to chemotherapy of gastric lymphomas.

3. **Unique hematopathologic issues in lymphoma.**
Since treatment of NHL is based on histologic classification, the routine treatment of NHL depends on
accurate hematopathologic diagnosis. Some complex
issues in hematopathologic diagnosis require consideration in this review.

a. **Anaplastic large cell lymphoma, Ki-1 lymphoma.** These lymphomas primarily involve
lymph nodes, but can also be associated with dermal lesions. The majority of these lymphomas are
T cell lymphomas, but some have been identified
as B cell lymphomas. The importance of this entity is that anaplastic large cell lymphoma and
Ki-1 lymphoma may be mistaken for Hodgkin's
disease, malignant histiocytosis, metastatic carcinoma, or malignant melanoma. With respect to
responsiveness to therapy, there is no evidence
that these lymphomas behave differently than
other intermediate-grade lymphomas.

b. **Angioimmunoblastic lymphadenopathy.** This
lymphoproliferative disorder is characterized by
lymphadenopathy, hepatosplenomegaly, and nonspecific hyperglobulinemia. In many patients,
this disorder evolves to an aggressive form of T
cell lymphoma. Criteria have not been established that would allow clinicians or pathologists
to distinguish patients who will have a benign
clinical course from those in whom lymphoma
will develop. Our approach is to treat benign
forms of the disease with corticosteroids. In the
face of clinical change, i.e., progressive adenopathy, organomegaly, or weight loss, we recommend
repeat biopsy to assess for evolution to lymphoma. We recommend high-dose therapy (as
used in other high-grade lymphomas) for these
patients once malignant disease is documented.

However, since the median age for this condition is 60 years, patients may be unable to tolerate regimens more aggressive than CHOP.

   c. T cell–rich B cell lymphomas. The importance of identifying these large cell diffuse lymphomas in which the malignant cell is a B cell, while the predominant cell is a T cell has already been noted (see sec. **D.2.c.(1).**).

Selected Readings

Armitage, J. O. Bone marrow transplantation in the treatment of patients with lymphoma. *Blood* 73:1749, 1989.

Canellos, G. P., et al. Chemotherapy of advanced Hodgkin's disease with MOPP, ABVD, or MOPP alternating with ABVD. *N. Engl. J. Med.* 327:1478, 1992.

Coleman, C. N., et al. Treatment of lymphoblastic lymphoma in adults. *J. Clin. Oncol.* 4:1628, 1986.

Connors, J. M., and Klimo, P. MACOP-B chemotherapy for malignant lymphomas and related conditions: 1987 update and additional observations. *Semin Hematol.* 25(suppl. 2):41, 1988.

Fisher, R. I., et al. Comparison of a standard regimen (CHOP) with three intensive chemotherapy regimens for advanced non-Hodgkin's lymphoma. *N. Engl. J. Med.* 328:1002, 1993.

Greer, J. P., et al. Peripheral T-cell lymphoma: a clinicopathologic study of 42 cases. *J. Clin. Oncol.* 2:788, 1984.

Klimo, P., and Connors, J. M. An update on the Vancouver experience in the management of advanced Hodgkin's disease treated with the MOPP/ABV hybrid program. *Semin. Hematol.* 25(suppl. 2):34, 1988.

Lister, T. A., and Crowther, D. Staging for Hodgkin's disease. *Semin. Oncol.* 17:696, 1990.

Longo, D. L. The use of chemotherapy in the treatment of Hodgkin's disease. *Semin. Oncol.* 17:716, 1990.

Martelli, M., et al. P-VABEC: a prospective study of a new weekly chemotherapy regimen for elderly aggressive non-Hodgkin's lymphoma. *J. Clin. Oncol.* 11:2362, 1993.

Mauch, P., et al. Influence of mediastinal adenopathy on site and frequency of relapse in patients with Hodgkin's disease. *Cancer Treat. Rep.* 66:809, 1982.

McMaster, M. L., et al. Effective treatment of small non-cleaved cell lymphoma with high-intensity, brief-duration chemotherapy. *J. Clin. Oncol.* 9:941, 1991.

Non-Hodgkin's Lymphoma Pathologic Classification Project. National Cancer Institute sponsored study of classification of non-Hodgkin's lymphomas: summary and description of a working formulation for clinical usage. *Cancer* 49:2112, 1982.

O'Reilly, S. E., et al. In search of an optimal regimen for elderly patients with advanced-stage diffuse large-cell lymphoma: results of a phase II study of P/DOCE chemotherapy. *J. Clin. Oncol.* 11:2250, 1993.

Philip, T., et al. High-dose therapy and autologous bone marrow transplantation after failure of conventional therapy in adults with intermediate grade or high grade non-Hodgkin's lymphoma. *N. Engl. J. Med.* 316:1493, 1987.

Portlock, C. S., et al. "Good risk" non-Hodgkin's lymphomas: approaches to management. *Semin. Hematol.* 20:25, 1983.

Stein, R. S., et al. Anatomic substages of stage III-A Hodgkin's disease: followup of a collaborative study. *Cancer Treat. Rep.* 66:733, 1982.

The International Non-Hodgkin's Lymphoma Prognostic Factors Project: a predictive model for aggressive non-Hodgkin's lymphoma. *N. Engl. J. Med.* 329:987, 1993.

Multiple Myeloma and Other Plasma Cell Dyscrasias

Martin M. Oken

I. Introduction

A. Types of plasma cell dyscrasias. Plasma cell dyscrasias or plasma cell neoplasms are a group of conditions characterized by unbalanced proliferation of cells that normally synthesize and secrete immunoglobulins. They range from malignant neoplasms such as multiple myeloma to monoclonal gammopathy of undetermined significance, a usually benign condition that is sometimes termed *benign monoclonal gammopathy*. Associated with the abnormal cellular proliferation in nearly all instances is the production of homogeneous monoclonal immunoglobulin, referred to either as myeloma protein or M protein, or of excessive quantities of homogeneous polypeptide subunits of a monoclonal protein. The latter usually appear as monoclonal free light chains excreted into the urine. Frequently both whole immunoglobulin M protein and free light chains are produced. The plasma cell dyscrasias discussed in this chapter are multiple myeloma, macroglobulinemia (Waldenström's macroglobulinemia), heavy-chain diseases, amyloidosis, and monoclonal gammopathy of undetermined significance.

B. M protein. Unlike most neoplastic diseases, which are followed objectively by serial evaluation of palpable or radiographically measurable tumor masses, most plasma cell dyscrasias are best followed by serial measurements of the monoclonal protein (M protein) elaborated by the tumor. Effective use of this tumor marker is important for the proper evaluation of the disease course of most plasma cell dyscrasias and is usually essential to the determination of response to treatment. The basic immunoglobulin unit comprises two identical heavy chains with a molecular mass of 55,000 daltons linked to two identical light chains with molecular masses of 22,500 daltons. The heavy chains are either γ, α, μ, δ, or ε corresponding to IgG, IgA, IgM, IgD, and IgE, respectively. The light chains exist as either κ or λ subtypes. Serum M protein is a monoclonal whole immunoglobulin and therefore possesses only one heavy-chain type and one light-chain type. Urine M protein consists of free light chains or, in the case of some heavy-chain diseases, free heavy-chain fragments of single specificity. Serum M protein may be quantitatively evaluated by either serum protein electrophoresis or determining the concentration of the individual immunoglobulins (particularly IgG, IgA, and IgM) by radial immunodiffusion or nephelometry. Urinary M protein, usually in the form of free light chain, should be characterized by immunoelectrophoresis as monoclonal κ or λ light chain and then followed sequentially, expressed as urinary light-chain excretion in grams per 24 hours. This characterization requires determination of 24-hour urine protein excretion and scanning the urine protein electrophoresis to determine the percentage of urine protein present as free monoclonal immunoglobulin light chain.

II. Multiple myeloma

A. General considerations and aims of therapy

1. **Diagnosis.** Multiple myeloma is a neoplasm of malignant plasma cells invading bone and bone marrow, causing widespread skeletal destruction, bone marrow failure, and problems related to quantitatively abnormal serum or urinary M proteins. The diagnosis of multiple myeloma requires histologic documentation by the demonstration of increased numbers (usually > 10%) or abnormal, atypical, or immature plasma cells in the bone marrow in addition to finding serum or urinary M protein or characteristic osteolytic bone lesions. Some patients have multiple plasmacytomas of bone with intervening normal areas of bone marrow. In these patients a random bone marrow aspirate and biopsy may fail to reveal the tumor, and biopsy of specific bone lesions may be necessary to establish the diagnosis. A recently described variant is polyneuropathy, organomegaly, endocrinopathy, monoclonal gammopathy (POEMS) syndrome. Patients with POEMS have a better survival than do those with multiple myeloma.

2. **Incidence.** The annual incidence of multiple myeloma is 4/100,000 population with a peak occurrence between ages 60 and 70. Although as many as 4% of patients with myeloma have indolent or smoldering disease at diagnosis, and an additional 5% have an isolated plasmacytoma of bone, most patients with multiple myeloma require chemotherapy of their disease soon after diagnosis.

3. **Effect of treatment.** The goal of therapy is to improve the duration of survival and to diminish or prevent the serious manifestations of this disease, such as bone pain, pathologic fractures, severe anemia, renal failure, or hypercalcemia. Treatment produces an objective response in at least 50% of patients as determined by a sustained 50% decline in the levels of serum or urine M protein. Temporary, sometimes long-lasting, alleviation of symptoms occurs in nearly all patients exhibiting an objective response to treatment and in some additional patients with lesser degrees of objective improvement. Median survival times usually reported for treated patients range from 2 to 3 years and are strongly influenced by response to treatment and by the initial tumor load.

4. **Prognostic factors.** Table 27-1 presents a clinical staging system developed to estimate myeloma tu-

Table 27-1. Myeloma clinical staging system

Stage	Criteria	Myeloma cell mass (cells/m²)

I	All of the following
	1. Hemoglobin >10 gm/dl
	2. Serum calcium value normal (≤12 mg/dl)
	3. On x-ray film, normal bone structure or solitary bone plasmacytoma only
	4. Low M component production rates
	  a. IgG value <5 gm/dl
	  b. IgA value <3 gm/dl
	  c. Urine light-chain M component on electrophoresis <4 gm/24 hours
		$<0.6 \times 10^{12}$ (low)

II	Fitting neither stage I nor III	0.6×10^{12} to 1.2×10^{12} (intermediate)

III	One or more of the following
	1. Hemoglobin <8.5 gm/dl
	2. Serum calcium value > 12 mg/dl
	3. Advanced lytic bone lesions
	4. High M-component production rates
	  a. IgG value >7 gm/dl
	  b. IgA value >5 gm/dl
	  c. Urine light-chain M component on electrophoresis >12 gm/24 hours
		$>1.2 \times 10^{12}$ (high)

	Subclass of any stage	
A	Serum creatinine <2 mg/dl	
B	Serum creatinine ≥2 mg/dl	

Source: Modified from B. G. M. Durie and S. E. Salmon. A clinical staging system for multiple myeloma: correlation of measured myeloma cell mass with presenting clinical features, response to treatment and survival. *Cancer* 36:842, 1975.

mor cell mass utilizing readily obtained clinical findings. Severe anemia, hypercalcemia, advanced osteolytic lesions, and extremely high M protein production rates are all associated with a high tumor burden and a poor survival prognosis. Renal failure, although not well correlated with tumor burden, is associated with poor prognosis. Advanced age, poor performance status, high serum lactate dehydrogenase (LDH), and plasmablastic subtype have also been established as adverse prognostic signs.

The serum level of β_2-microglobulin correlates with the myeloma tumor burden but is of little value for serially monitoring patients with myeloma. Serum β_2-microglobulin usually falls during response to therapy and may increase during relapse, but it has been inconsistent in detecting fulminant progression in which the serum or urinary M proteins may fail to reflect the increasing tumor mass. The plasma cell labeling index is a reflection of the proportion of myeloma cells that are synthesizing DNA. Patients with a labeling index higher than 3% who have a high cell mass have a particularly poor survival prognosis. A low labeling index has been associated with more indolent disease and particularly with a stable plateau phase during an objective response to therapy.

When pretreatment plasma cell labeling index is combined with serum B_2-microglobulin, one can assign half the patients either to a very favorable prognostic group in which both values are low and the prognosis approaches 6 years, or to a very poor prognostic group in which both values are high and the survival prognosis is under 2 years. The remaining patients have an intermediate and less well-defined prognosis. Others have used serum levels of C-reactive protein (CRP) as a reflection of interleukin (IL)-6 activity and have combined this with β_2-microglobulin level to produce an index that divides myeloma patients into low-, intermediate-, and high-risk groups with observed median survival times of 54, 27, and 6 months, respectively.

B. Initial treatment

1. **General measures.** Complications of myeloma, e.g., hypercalcemia and renal failure, may be present at the time of diagnosis (see **II.C.**). These complications should be promptly identified and treated before the start of chemotherapy. Patients who present with smoldering or indolent, asymptomatic stage IA disease may be followed with observation alone until evidence of progression appears. Most patients have more advanced or progressive disease at diagnosis and require chemotherapy. Patients should be maintained on allopurinol 300 mg/day PO through the first 2 months of chemotherapy to prevent urate nephropathy. A general supportive care regimen

emphasizing ambulation and hydration should be maintained throughout the initial treatment.

2. **Standard induction chemotherapy** recommendations are based on an Eastern Cooperative Oncology Group (ECOG) prospective, randomized clinical trial comparing moderate (MP) therapy (see **b.,** below) to a more intensive regimen (VBMCP) (see **a.,** below). In that study VBMCP yielded an objective response rate of 72%, in contrast to 51% objective responses with MP. Median survival time was similar for the two treatments at 28–30 months, but 26% of VBMCP patients survived 5 years compared with a 19% five-year survival rate with MP.

   a. **Most patients** should receive VBMCP. With this regimen the prednisone schedule is frequently individualized so that slowly responding patients with persistent generalized bone pain or severe anemia may receive low-dose prednisone each day of the first two or three cycles in addition to the higher scheduled prednisone dose on days 1–14.

      The **VBMCP regimen** consists of the following.

      Vincristine 1.2 mg/m^2 IV on day 1 (up to 2.0 mg) *and*
      Carmustine (BCNU) 20 mg/m^2 IV on day 1 *and*
      Melphalan 8 mg/m^2 PO on days 1–4 *and*
      Cyclophosphamide 400 mg/m^2 IV on day 1 *and*
      Prednisone 40 mg/m^2 PO on days 1–7 (all cycles), 20 mg/m^2 PO on days 8–14 (cycles 1–3 only)
      Repeat cycle of VBMCP every 35 days for at least 1 year.

   b. **Patients over 70 years old who have poor performance status,** defined as partially or completely bedridden (ECOG grades 2–4), do not tolerate VBMCP. These high-risk patients, who comprise 10–15% of myeloma patients, should instead be treated with MP according to the following schedule.

      Melphalan 8 mg/m^2 PO on days 1–4 *and*
      Prednisone 60 mg/m^2 PO on days 1–4
      Repeat cycle every 28 days for at least 1 year.

      Because of the similarity in median survival data between VBMCP and MP, the later regimen can also be considered an alternative to VBMCP even for some patients not in the above high-risk group if a less aggressive approach is required. Because of erratic absorption of melphalan in most patients, some investigators recommend cautiously escalating the dose of melphalan on subsequent cycles of chemotherapy until a dose is reached that produces moderate nadir leukocyte counts of 2000–3000 cells/μl. For reliable absorption, melphalan should be taken on an empty stomach.

3. **Alternative induction chemotherapy.** VBMCP + interferon (IFN) alpha (rIFN-α2) represents a promising alternative approach to induction therapy. With this regimen, two initial cycles of VBMCP are given followed by alternating 3-week cycles of rIFN-α2 with 3-week cycles of VBMCP. The rIFN-α is administered at 5×10^6 units/m^2 SQ 3 times a week × 10 doses each IFN cycle, for a total treatment duration of 2 years. A complete remission rate of 30% has been observed with this regimen, leading to the controlled comparison of VBMCP + rIFNα2 to VBMCP alone now being conducted by the ECOG.

   Another induction regimen giving comparable results to VBMCP is comprised of alternating cycles of vincristine, melphalan, cyclophosphamide, and prednisone with vincristine, BCNU, doxorubicin (Adriamycin), and prednisone (VMCP/VBAP). This and a similar regimen lacking VP are described more fully in two selected readings (Durie, 1986; Mac-Lennan, 1992). A third regimen, VAD, is described later as a salvage treatment option. It may be used as an induction regimen when autologous transplantation is contemplated since it lacks alkylating agents and is therefore less damaging to marrow stem cells.

4. **Bone marrow and peripheral blood stem cell transplantation.** Allogeneic bone marrow transplantation following high-dose therapy can cure myeloma in approximately 30% of suitable candidates. At present, these represent only a small portion of patients with myeloma. Nevertheless, marrow transplantation should be discussed with every patient under age 55 who has a matched donor. In patients with poor prognostic factors it is reasonable to consider it during first remission.

   High-dose therapy followed by autologous transplantation with bone marrow or peripheral blood stem cells as rescue is less likely to be curative, but with growth factor support can be carried out with relative safety and merits consideration as consolidation therapy during first remission or after relapse in patients with responsive disease. Its precise role is yet to be determined and is the subject of ongoing clinical trials. The most commonly used preparative regimens are high-dose melphalan with or without total body radiation. A role for purging the graft of potentially malignant cells seems intuitively likely but proof of its efficacy in preventing recurrence remains an unmet challenge.

5. **Duration of therapy and the role of maintenance therapy.** Although no study has conclusively demonstrated benefit by continuing chemotherapy beyond 1 year in responding patients, several investigators have noted earlier reemergence of active myeloma after early cessation of therapy. Therefore one acceptable approach is to continue the induction

regimen for a total duration of 2 years or to maximal response but to decrease its frequency to one cycle every 6–8 weeks during the second year while continuing to follow M protein production carefully. It is probably safe to stop treatment at 1 year in patients who started therapy with stage I disease and whose disease has remained stable, in plateau phase, for at least 6 months. These patients should be observed carefully, with reevaluation of serum and urine M protein once every 3 months.

Six randomized studies evaluated maintenance therapy with IFN after at least 1 year of induction chemotherapy. Of these, four showed significant improvement in response duration but only one showed significant improvement in survival. The regimens used were rIFN-α2 2–3 $\times$ 10^6 units/m^2 SQ 3 times a week. Based on these recent findings, IFN maintenance deserves consideration as an acceptable maintenance approach in patients with initial disease control by standard induction therapy. Preliminary results suggest that IFN maintenance might also have a role in maintaining remissions consolidated by intensification therapy with autologous stem cell rescue.

6. **Role of radiotherapy.** Solitary plasmacytoma of bone is best treated by local radiation therapy and may not require chemotherapy for months to years. Radiotherapy is also useful as palliative therapy for patients with extraskeletal plasmacytomas, large lytic lesions threatening fracture of long bones, spinal cord or root compression by plasma cell tumor, and certain pathologic fractures. Repeated local irradiation should be avoided where possible in patients with disseminated myeloma, as chemotherapy is the only treatment demonstrated to improve survival while controlling systemic manifestations of the disease. Excessive use of radiation therapy can impair marrow reserves and render the patient less able to tolerate subsequent chemotherapy.

C. **Complications of disease or therapy.** Chemotherapy for multiple myeloma typically causes myelosuppression, and packed red blood cell transfusions are often required during the early weeks of treatment and the late refractory period. Toxicity of each chemotherapeutic agent is described in Chapter 10. In addition to these problems, several complications characteristic of multiple myeloma may occur.

1. **Hypercalcemia.** This common complication of multiple myeloma is believed to result from the liberation of bone calcium stimulated by osteoclast-activating factor released by the tumor cells. Presenting symptoms may include anorexia, nausea, vomiting, constipation, and polyuria progressing to lethargy, confusion, coma, and death. Dehydration and potentially reversible renal failure frequently occur during

hypercalcemic crises. Control of hypercalcemic crises of multiple myeloma is usually accomplished with saline hydration (initially 200–300 ml/hour IV), furosemide (20–40 mg q4–6h) once the hypovolemia has been corrected, and prednisone (40–80 mg PO daily for 3–7 days). When hypercalcemia occurs in previously untreated patients, prompt initiation of chemotherapy of the myeloma, in addition to these measures, usually produces effective, durable control. In some patients oral inorganic phosphates, calcitonin, pamidronate, or, more exceptionally, plicamycin may be needed and can be used on the following schedules.

   a. **Inorganic phosphate,** e.g., Neutra-Phos or Fleet Phospho-Soda, at a dose equivalent to 0.5 gm of phosphorus PO qid (diluted in water to reduce diarrhea). This may be useful for chronic control of hypercalcemia in some patients.

   b. **Pamidronate** 60–90 mg is given as a 24-hour IV infusion that can be repeated at 7–30-day intervals if needed.

   c. **Calcitonin** 100–300 units SQ q8–12h for up to 2–3 days. Calcitonin is usually given with prednisone 10–20 mg PO 2–3 times daily to prolong its effectiveness.

   d. **Plicamycin (mithramycin)** 1.0 mg/m^2 IV every 3–7 days. This agent is myelosuppressive and can cause hemostatic disorders and nausea. Its long-term or repeated use in myeloma patients should be avoided except refractory instances of hypercalcemia.

   e. **Hemodialysis** is effective but seldom needed for hypercalcemia.

2. **Infection.** Myeloma patients are highly susceptible to respiratory and urinary tract infections with common gram-positive and gram-negative bacterial pathogens. Deficiency of normal immunoglobulins, diminished bone marrow reserves, and immobilization due to skeletal disease are important predisposing factors. The weeks immediately following initiation of chemotherapy are a particularly high-risk period for infection. Prompt evaluation of fever or other manifestations of infection is essential. Antibiotic coverage for gram-positive and gram-negative organisms should be instituted while awaiting culture results from patients whose clinical pictures suggest infection. Infection prophylaxis with antibiotics during the first 2 months of chemotherapy may be of help. Use of trimethoprim-sulfamethoxazole (1 double-strength tablet bid) or ciprofloxacin (500 mg bid) is under study in this setting. Granulocyte colony-stimulating factor (G-CSF) 5 μg/kg/day SQ will hasten neutrophil recovery by 1–3 days in neutropenic febrile patients. More dramatic reduction in the duration of neutropenia may be seen

when this agent is used from 24 hours after cytotoxic therapy until full recovery from nadir neutropenia has occurred. Such prophylactic use of G-CSF is justified in patients with prior prolonged neutropenia or infection or who pose exceptionally high risk for infection due to age, intercurrent illness, chemotherapy regimen, or prior history of infection during chemotherapy.

3. **Hyperviscosity** may present as central nervous system (CNS) impairment, congestive heart failure, ischemia, or bleeding tendency. It is more characteristic of Waldenström's macroglobulinemia than of multiple myeloma, but it may be seen in patients with extremely high IgG or IgA concentrations or in patients whose M protein tends to form aggregates. The treatment for symptomatic hyperviscosity is plasmapheresis.

4. **Renal dysfunction** may be caused by myeloma kidney, amyloidosis, pyelonephritis, hypercalcemia, hyperuricemia with urate nephropathy, hyperviscosity syndrome, plasma cell infiltration of both kidneys (rare), and renal tubular acidosis. Most of these problems are at least partially reversible if recognized and treated promptly. Renal failure may also result from radiographic contrast material, particularly in a patient whose renal function is already compromised or who is dehydrated. Hypercalcemia and hyperuricemia are especially common potential causes of reversible renal failure and should be ruled out at the onset of the evaluation of a patient with myeloma. In patients with severe renal failure, hemodialysis should be considered as long as chemotherapy offers the potential for a prolonged remission.

5. **Skeletal destruction** is a major cause of disability and immobilization in multiple myeloma. Radiation therapy or surgery, or both, may be needed to treat fractures or to prevent impending fractures of weight-bearing bones. The role of fluoride, calcium, and vitamin D in promoting skeletal repair during remission is under study.

6. **Anemia.** For patients with refractory disease and chronic symptomatic anemia, treatment with recombinant human erythropoietin (r-HuEPO) will frequently diminish or eliminate the transfusion requirement and return the hemoglobin to asymptomatic levels. A schedule of 150–250 units/kg SQ 2 times a week may be used.

7. **Leukemia.** Acute nonlymphocytic leukemia (ANLL) develops in about 4% of myeloma patients who receive chemotherapy. The incidence of ANLL is appreciably greater in patients surviving 4 years or more after the start of chemotherapy. Leukemia in this setting appears to be caused by the interaction of a carcinogenic drug with a predisposed host. ANLL

complicating multiple myeloma is usually preceded by sideroblastic anemia as part of a myelodysplastic syndrome.

D. Recurrence and treatment of refractory disease. Objective responses to chemotherapy have a median duration of about 2 years. Response duration is influenced by the degree of reduction of tumor burden as reflected by the degree of reduction of myeloma proteins in the serum and urine. Eventually, virtually all patients develop recurrent or refractory disease. These patients pose a difficult clinical problem because of the small number of chemotherapeutic agents with proved activity in myeloma. Patients relapsing months or years after last receiving chemotherapy can frequently be reinduced with the original regimen.

1. **Treatment of patients refractory to melphalan.** Patients refractory to melphalan or melphalan + prednisone regimens may still respond to other alkylating agents. Two regimens that may be considered are as follows.
   a. **VBMCP** (see sec. **II.B.2.a.**)
   b. **BCP** may be effective in patients who absorbed oral melphalan poorly.

   Carmustine (BCNU) 75 mg/m^2 IV on day 1 *and*
   Cyclophosphamide 400 mg/m^2 IV on day 1 *and*
   Prednisone 75 mg PO on days 1–7
   Repeat every 4 weeks.

   Treatment with these alkylating agent-based regimens can be expected to yield objective responses in about 20% of patients refractory to prior MP therapy. These regimens remain useful as conservative treatment choices for patients in their first relapse or for some patients who have failed initial MP therapy.

2. **Alternative regimens** not based on standard dose alkylating agents include the following.
   a. **VAD**

   Vincristine 0.4 mg/day as a continuous IV infusion on days 1–4 *and*
   Doxorubicin (Adriamycin) 9.0 mg/m^2/day as a continuous IV infusion on days 1–4 *and*
   Dexamethasone 40 mg PO on days 1–4, 9–12, 17–20

   Repeat cycle every 28–35 days until four cycles beyond occurrence of maximum reduction in myeloma protein. Maximum cumulative doxorubicin dose is 540 mg/m^2. To avoid problems related to adrenal steroid excess, the frequency of dexamethasone courses should be decreased once clinical response is reached.
   b. **High-dose cyclophosphamide.** Cyclophosphamide 600 mg/m^2 IV is given on days 1–4, with this dosage repeated in 1–2 months. This aggressive regimen effectively produces pain relief of more

than 1 month's duration and yields short-term objective responses in more than 30% of patients refractory to prior treatments. Because the regimen is highly myelotoxic (it is employed without dose modification), its use should generally be limited to patients with active, markedly symptomatic refractory disease in institutions equipped to render intensive support, including platelet transfusion and infectious disease consultation. The prophylactic use of G-CSF is reasonable with this regimen. A recommended schedule is filgrastrim 5 μg/kg SQ daily starting 24 hours after chemotherapy and continuing through the nadir until the granulocyte count exceeds 8–10,000/μl. Simultaneous use of plicamycin with high-dose cyclophosphamide should be avoided.

    c. Interferon alpha-2 (rIFNα2) 5 $\times$ 10^6 units/m^2 SQ 3 times a week. This regimen produces clinical benefit in 35% of patients by objective and symptomatic standards but full objective responses (50% decrease in serum myeloma protein) in only 10%.

    d. Autologous bone marrow transplantation has been employed after preparative regimens such as high-dose melphalan plus total body irradiation to induce good-quality responses in some patients with relapsed myeloma. There are issues related to marrow purge, the intensity of antitumor therapy, age range, expense, and the presence or absence of cure potential for this approach in myeloma.

III. Waldenström's macroglobulinemia

A. General considerations and aims of therapy.
This neoplasm is characterized by the proliferation of plasmacytoid lymphocytes that elaborate a monoclonal IgM. In contrast to multiple myeloma, skeletal destruction does not occur, but hepatosplenomegaly and lymphadenopathy are common. The major problems are hyperviscosity syndrome, severe anemia, and occasionally pancytopenia. The median survival time is only about 5 years from diagnosis partly owing to the advanced age of most affected patients (60–75 years old), as well as to the common association with second neoplasms (20% of patients) and chronic or recurrent infections (25% of patients). The primary aims of therapy are to control complications and to decrease their incidence. Although response to chemotherapy has, not surprisingly, been associated with a more favorable median survival, the actual role of chemotherapy in prolonging survival in this disease has not been fully defined.

B. Treatment

    1. Anemia. Most patients with macroglobulinemia are anemic; however, erythropoietin or transfusions should generally be reserved for those with symptomatic anemia. Overtransfusion is dangerous because of the important contribution of red blood cells to whole blood viscosity.

2. **Hyperviscosity.** Hyperviscosity syndrome requires plasmapheresis for acute management and chemotherapy with alkylating agents for long-term control.

3. **Chemotherapy.** In general, chemotherapy is withheld until symptomatic disease or progressive cytopenias occur.

   a. Standard chemotherapy

     Chlorambucil 2–6 mg PO daily *or*
     Cyclophosphamide 50–100 mg PO daily
     (Prednisone 40–60 mg PO on days 1–4 every 4 weeks may be added.)

   b. Alternatively, a high-dose intermittent chlorambucil-prednisone regimen may be used every 2–3 weeks.

     Chlorambucil 30 mg/m^2 PO on day 1 *and*
     Prednisone 40 mg/m^2 PO on days 1–4

   c. VBMCP is described in sec. **II.B.2.a.**

4. **Disease variants.** Some patients with IgM monoclonal proteins have clinical chronic lymphocytic leukemia (CLL) or lymphoma and should have their treatment directed at that disease. Rare patients with macroglobulinemia have prominent skeletal disease, and their disease should be approached as IgM myeloma and treated similarly to other multiple myelomas.

IV. Heavy-chain diseases comprise a group of rare plasma cell dyscrasias in which the abnormal clone of plasma cells or B lymphocytes elaborates an abnormal polypeptide consisting of anomalous γ, α, or μ heavy chains with deleted segments.

  A. Gamma heavy-chain disease presents as a lymphoma usually with lymphadenopathy, hepatosplenomegaly, and involvement of Waldeyer's ring. The latter may lead to characteristic palatal edema. Bone marrow involvement is the rule. Treatment by local radiotherapy or lymphoma-directed chemotherapy regimens is sometimes effective.

  B. Alpha heavy-chain disease appears to be the most common of the heavy-chain diseases and occurs mainly in people under the age of 50. Its most common clinical presentation is in the enteric form with chronic diarrhea, malabsorption syndrome, and marked lymphoplasmacytic infiltration of the small bowel mucosa. Remissions have been reported using lymphoma chemotherapy regimens and occasionally antibiotics alone.

  C. Mu heavy-chain disease is rare, usually presenting as CLL, and it should be managed as such.

V. Amyloidosis. Only primary amyloidosis with or without associated plasma cell or lymphoid neoplasms is considered in this section. With these disorders the amyloid substance consists of fragments of immunoglobulin light chains and is therefore termed an *amyloid L chain protein* (AL-protein). This type of amyloid characteristically infiltrates the tongue, heart, skin, ligaments, and muscle and occasionally the kidney, liver, and spleen. In patients with documented lymphomas or plasma cell neoplasms, treatment is for the underlying neoplasm, but the decline in the amount of amyloid is often minimal. With primary amyloidosis without a demonstrable underlying neoplasm, treatment with MP has been shown to be of moderate benefit when tested in a randomized double-blind study, although the exact role of chemotherapy for this disease is not yet clear.

VI. **Monoclonal gammopathy of undetermined significance** has been found in up to 3% of persons over 70 years of age. It has been termed *benign monoclonal gammopathy*; however, because approximately 20% of patients with this finding progress to more severe plasma cell dyscrasias, the term *monoclonal gammopathy of undetermined significance* has been introduced as more appropriate. With this condition, patients usually have an M spike of less than 2.0 gm/dl, no bone lesions, no conclusive evidence of myeloma on bone marrow aspirate or biopsy, no anemia or bone marrow failure, and stability of the clinical picture and M protein studies over a period of follow-up. The serum β_2-microglobulin and the plasma cell labeling index are both low. Once initial stability has been demonstrated, these patients should be followed at yearly intervals with evaluation of hemoglobin levels and M protein status. No treatment is indicated unless progression to myeloma or symptomatic macroglobulinemia occurs.

Selected Readings

Barlogie, B., Smith, L., and Alexanian, R. Effective treatment of advanced multiple myeloma refractory to alkylating agents. *N. Engl. J. Med.* 310:1353, 1984.

Bataille, R., et al. C-reactive protein and beta 2-microglobulin produce a simple and powerful myeloma staging system. *Blood* 80:733, 1992.

Case, D. C., Lee, B. J., and Clarkson, B. D. Improved survival times in multiple myeloma treated with melphalan, prednisone, cyclophosphamide, vincristine and BCNU: M-2 protocol. *Am. J. Med.* 68:897, 1977.

Durie, B. G., et al. Improved survival duration with combination chemotherapy induction for multiple myeloma: a Southwest Oncology Group Study. *J. Clin. Oncol.* 4:1227, 1986.

Durie, B. G. M., and Salmon, S. E. A clinical staging system for multiple myeloma: correlation of measured myeloma cell mass with presenting clinical features, response to treatment and survival. *Cancer* 36:842, 1975.

Durie, B. G. M., Salmon, S. E., and Moon, T. E. Pretreatment tumor mass, cell kinetics and prognosis in multiple myeloma. *Blood* 55:364, 1980.

Fernand, J. P., et al. The role of autologous blood stem cells in support of high-dose therapy for multiple myeloma. *Hematol. Oncol. Clin. North Am.* 6:451, 1992.

Gahrton, G., et al. Allogeneic bone marrow transplantation in multiple myeloma. *N. Engl. J. Med.* 325:1267, 1991.

Greipp, P. R., et al. Value of beta-2 microglobulin level and plasma cell labeling indices as prognostic factors in patients with newly diagnosed myeloma. *Blood* 72:219, 1988.

Greipp, P. R., et al. Plasma cell labeling index and beta 2-microglobulin predict survival independent of thymidine kinase and C-reactive protein in multiple myeloma. *Blood* 81:3382, 1993.

Kyle, R. A., and Lust, J. A. Monoclonal gammopathies of undetermined significance. *Semin. Hematol.* 26:176, 1989.

Lenhard, R. E., et al. High-dose cyclophosphamide: an effective treatment for advanced refractory multiple myeloma. *Cancer* 53:1456, 1984.

MacLennan, I. C., et al. Combined chemotherapy with ABCM versus melphalan for treatment of myelomatosis. The Medical Research Council Working Party for Leukemia in Adults. *Lancet* 339:200, 1992.

Mandelli, F., et al. Maintenance treatment with recombinant interferon alfa-2b in patients with multiple myeloma responding to conventional induction chemotherapy. *N. Engl. J. Med.* 322:1430, 1990.

Mirallis, G. D., Fallon, J. R., and Talley, N. J. Plasma-cell dyscrasia with polyneuropathy. *N. Engl. J. Med.* 327:1919, 1992.

Oken, M. M. Standard treatment of multiple myeloma. *Mayo Clin. Proc.* 69:781, 1994.

Oken, M. M. Multiple myeloma. *Med. Clin. North Am.* 68:757, 1984.

Metastatic Cancer of Unknown Origin

Martin M. Oken

In approximately 5 percent of patients with newly diagnosed cancer (excluding nonmelanoma skin cancer), the primary site remains unknown despite a detailed history and physical examination, routine blood chemistries, complete blood cell count, urinalysis, chest x-ray film, and histologic evaluation of biopsy specimens. The problem of metastatic cancer of unknown origin raises difficult questions for both diagnosis and treatment. While the median survival time of patients with cancer of unknown origin is less than 6 months, subgroups of patients who have a far better outlook with proper management have been defined. A major responsibility of the clinician is to identify those patients who might benefit from active intervention while not consuming the remaining days of the other patients' lives with futile or unnecessary diagnostic procedures.

I. General considerations and aims of therapy

A. Histology and presenting clinical manifestations.

Adenocarcinoma and undifferentiated carcinoma each comprise up to 40% of all cancers of unknown origin. Fewer than 15% of cancers of unknown origin are squamous cell carcinomas, and only 2–5% are malignant melanoma. Other histologies that may present as cancer of unknown origin include lymphomas, germ cell tumors, and neuroendocrine carcinomas. These histologies are particularly important to identify because they represent tumors that might be effectively managed with systemic chemotherapy. Nearly 50% of all patients with unknown primary tumors and well over 50% of those with adenocarcinoma present with hepatomegaly, abdominal mass, or other abdominal symptoms. Lymphadenopathy is the presenting clinical manifestation in 15–25% of patients. Lower cervical or supraclavicular lymph nodes usually contain adenocarcinoma or undifferentiated carcinoma, and middle to high cervical adenopathy generally represents squamous cell carcinoma (SCC). Between 10 and 20% of patients present with manifestations of bone, lung, or pleural involvement, whereas fewer than 10% present with evidence of central nervous system (CNS) disease. Most of the latter group are eventually found to have either lung or gastrointestinal tract primary carcinomas. Two presentations of advanced carcinoma of unknown primary site have been recognized as more treatable than others: (1) poorly differentiated carcinoma or adenocarcinoma, especially with predominant sites of involvement in the mediastinum, retroperitoneum, lymph nodes, or lungs; and (2) adenocarcinoma in women predominantly involving the peritoneal surfaces. In these instances, platinum-based chemotherapy regimens designed specifically for germ cell or ovarian cancers have produced many useful objective responses and occasional long-term disease-free survival.

B. **Sites of origin.** It is sometimes possible to predict the most likely primary sites from the histology and location of the metastatic lesion of unknown origin. The pancreas and the lung are the most common ultimately determined sites of origin. Together they represent over 40% of the adenocarcinomas of unknown origin. Colorectal, gastric, and hepatobiliary carcinomas each represent about 10% of the cancers of unknown origin.

In general, adenocarcinomas or undifferentiated carcinomas presenting with hepatic metastases or left supraclavicular adenopathy are eventually demonstrated to be of gastrointestinal origin. SCCs that present in the supraclavicular or low cervical lymph nodes are usually from lung primary carcinomas, whereas similar lesions of higher cervical nodes are more likely to have originated from occult primary lesions in the head and neck region.

The pattern of metastatic involvement associated with occult primary tumors differs from that associated with overt primary tumors. For example, occult lung cancer rarely involves bone, a common site of metastasis from overt lung cancer; however, bone metastases appear to be more common in patients with gastrointestinal cancer who have occult primary tumors than in those who have overt primary tumors.

C. **Aims of diagnostic evaluation.** The first objective in the management of a patient newly diagnosed with cancer of unknown origin is to plan the appropriate diagnostic evaluation. There are three chief aims of this evaluation.

1. Identify a tumor in which cure or effective disease control is possible.
2. Determine if the tumor is regionally confined or widely metastatic.
3. Identify any complication for which immediate local therapy is indicated.

D. **Goal of treatment.** In patients with tumors for which effective systemic therapy is available and in patients with disease regionally confined to peripheral lymph nodes alone, active management with the goal of prolongation of life through extended-disease control or cure should be considered. These patients represent about 25% of patients with occult primary tumors. For the remaining patients, the chance of prolonging life is less likely, and treatment should be directed toward palliation of symptoms and preservation of the best possible quality of life. Whether to employ systemic therapy depends largely on the patient's general condition and desire for active therapy.

II. **Diagnostic evaluation**

A. **Analysis of the biopsy specimen.** If possible, the pathologist should receive fresh, unfixed material to allow electron microscopy, histochemistry, immunohistology, and hormone receptor studies to be done, if needed, after routine examination. Careful review of the biopsy material should be undertaken to classify the tumor conclusively as SCC, adenocarcinoma, or other identifiable histology. Up to 40% of cancers of unknown origin are undifferentiated or poorly differentiated tumors based on evaluation of hematoxylin and eosin–stained material. Electron microscopy may be useful for the further classification of these tumors through the identification of desmosomes and intercellular bridges (SCC); tight junctions, microvilli, and acinar spaces (adenocarcinoma); premelanosomes (amelanotic melanoma); neurosecretory granules (small-cell or neuroendocrine carcinoma); and absence of junctions (lymphoma). Immunohistochemical studies on the tumor may be used to demonstrate the presence of prostatic acid phosphatase or prostate-specific antigen (prostate carcinoma), the beta subunit of human chorionic gonadotropin (β-hCG) (germ cell tumors), alpha-fetoprotein (germ cell tumors or hepatocellular carcinoma), or monoclonal immunoglobulin (lymphoma, plasmacytoma). Immunoglobulin or T cell receptor gene rearrangements may be helpful for identifying tumors of lymphoid origin. Undifferentiated carcinomas or adenocarcinomas in women should be evaluated for estrogen and progesterone receptors. Mucin positivity is helpful for eliminating the possibility of renal cell carcinoma.

Clearly the use of many of these specialized studies must be balanced against their expense. If judiciously applied, they can aid in the identification of some of the undifferentiated or poorly differentiated tumors of unknown origin and help to focus their subsequent diagnostic evaluation and management.

One exception to the policy of seeking a definitive histologic diagnosis as the first step in evaluating a tumor of unknown origin occurs when the patient presents with a potentially resectable neck mass (other than supraclavicular adenopathy) and no other apparent lesion. In these patients, a head and neck primary tumor should be sought by detailed head and neck examination, x-ray films of the sinuses, and if necessary, panendoscopy under general anesthesia to include laryngoscopy, bronchoscopy, esophagoscopy, and nasopharyngoscopy with blind biopsy of the base of the tongue, piriform sinuses, nasopharynx, and tonsillar fossae if no gross primary tumor is found. A computed tomography (CT) scan of the head and neck may also be of value. If this work-up reveals nothing abnormal, biopsy of the neck mass is undertaken. This order of evaluation is chosen so that if a resectable squamous cell cancer of the head and neck is found, the neck mass can be removed as part of the curative procedure.

B. Squamous cell carcinoma. For SCCs with apparent involvement of only one lymph node group, the possibility of long-term survival exists if proper treatment is carried out. The diagnostic evaluation depends on the lymph node region involved. The most common lymph node presentation for SCCs of unknown origin is in the cervical or supraclavicular region. Cervical lymph node metastases above the supraclavicular region usually originate from head and neck primary lesions. The diagnostic approach to these lesions is discussed in sec. **II.A.** Because surgery, irradiation, or both are employed with curative intent if disease is localized to this region, distant metastases should be ruled out with a bone scan, a chest x-ray film, and in some instances a chest CT scan. SCC of supraclavicular lymph nodes is usually of lung or esophageal origin and seldom represents regionally confined disease. Evaluation is the same as that discussed in the last paragraph in sec. **II.B.** for disease that extends beyond regional lymph nodes.

SCC in axillary or inguinal lymph nodes is rarely associated with an occult primary lesion. Regional skin and the lungs should be examined as possible primary sites with axillary disease, whereas the skin, anus, and genitalia should be carefully examined when the presentation is SCC in inguinal nodes.

SCC with generalized lymphadenopathy or more commonly, with disease that extends beyond lymph nodes represents disease that cannot be satisfactorily controlled by present-day techniques. The search for the primary lesions should consist mainly of a chest x-ray film and careful physical examination of the appropriate organs. Serum chemistry values including the calcium level should be determined. Further diagnostic studies are needed only if indicated by signs, symptoms, or abnormalities on the initial studies.

C. **Adenocarcinoma and poorly differentiated carcinoma.** Women with adenocarcinoma or poorly differentiated carcinoma of unknown origin should undergo mammography, careful pelvic examination, and hormone receptor evaluation of the tumor. In men, serum acid phosphatase, prostate-specific antigen, β-hCG, and alpha-fetoprotein should be determined to help rule out prostate and germ cell tumors, respectively. All patients should have stools and urine examined for occult blood, and the serum should be tested for abnormalities in the liver chemistry, creatinine, and electrolytes. With disease apparently confined to axillary lymph nodes, mammography is particularly important in women and should be considered in some men as well. Undifferentiated carcinoma found only in mid to high cervical lymph nodes should be evaluated in the same manner as described in sec. **II.B.** for cervical SCC.

Traditional contrast studies, such as intravenous pyelogram, barium enema, and upper gastrointestinal series, are not indicated unless specifically suggested by signs or symptoms (e.g., occult blood in the stool). Abdominal CT scan with intravenous contrast material is a reasonable option in view of the frequency with which it detects carcinoma of the pancreas or hepatobiliary cancer in this setting.

D. Malignant melanoma. The finding of malignant melanoma confined to a single lymph node group and without a detectable primary lesion represents stage II disease and is associated with a 30% five-year survival rate following lymphadenectomy. Evaluation to exclude more extensive disease should include a history, physical examination (emphasizing skin and ophthalmoscopic examination), chest x-ray film, liver chemistry analysis, liver scan, and brain CT scan.

III. Treatment

A. General strategy. The importance of identifying tumors that may be treated effectively, such as lymphomas, germ cell tumors, trophoblastic tumors, and breast, prostate, ovarian, and neuroendocrine carcinomas, is readily apparent. Once identified, these lesions should be treated as described in their respective chapters. In patients whose primary lesion remains obscure, a therapeutic distinction must be made between those with disease confined to one lymph node region and those with more widespread disease or involvement of visceral organs. In the former, some may be treated with curative intent, whereas in the latter the aims of treatment are palliative.

B. Squamous cell carcinoma. Patients with SCC confined to cervical lymph nodes above the supraclavicular region should receive full-course radiotherapy to a field extending from the base of the skull to the clavicles. Alternatively, they may be treated with radical lymph node dissection followed by radiation therapy. In either case, the irradiation is designed to include any possible head and neck primary carcinoma. Survival of patients so treated is at least as good as that for patients with known head and neck primary lesions. More limited lymph node dissection or regional irradiation may also be indicated for SCC confined to axillary or inguinal nodes.

More widespread SCCs of unknown origin are treated with a palliative intent. No treatment except for local radiotherapy to symptomatic lesions is the standard approach. In patients who are symptomatic or who have progressive disease and desire chemotherapy, regimens designed mainly for head and neck cancer should be considered.

1. MBP

Methotrexate 40 mg/m^2 IM on days 1 and 15 *and*
Bleomycin 10 units IM on days 1, 8, and 15 *and*
Cisplatin 50 mg/m^2 IV on day 4

Repeat every 3 weeks.

2. DF

Cisplatin 100 mg/m^2 IV on day 1 *and*
Fluorouracil 1000 mg/m^2 as a continuous 24-hour IV infusion for 4 days (days 1–4)

Repeat every 3 weeks.

Do not use these regimens if the serum creatinine level is more than 1.5 mg/dl. Bleomycin cumulative dose should not exceed 300 units. Use proper hydration with cisplatin as described in Chapter 10.

C. **Adenocarcinoma and poorly differentiated carcinoma.** In women, if these carcinomas are confined to unilateral axillary lymph nodes, they should be considered possible breast cancer and treated accordingly as stage II disease (see Chap. 15 on breast cancer). A woman with adenocarcinoma or poorly differentiated carcinoma predominantly confined to the peritoneal surface should be considered for a cisplatin-based ovarian cancer regimen. Undifferentiated carcinoma confined to middle or high cervical lymph nodes should be treated actively as SCC (see sec. **III.B.**).

Patients with more advanced adenocarcinoma or poorly differentiated carcinoma in whom the evaluation previously described in sec. **II.C.** does not suggest breast, prostate, or other highly treatable primary lesions should be managed according to the histology. Cisplatin-based combination chemotherapy is valuable in the treatment of poorly differentiated carcinoma and poorly differentiated adenocarcinoma. In these patients, the combination of bleomycin, cisplatin, and etoposide may produce a more than 60% objective response rate and more than 20% complete response rate, with up to a 13% long-term survival rate. This regimen is fully described in Chapter 17 on germ cell neoplasms.

Patients with widespread adenocarcinoma that is well differentiated should generally be treated palliatively with local radiotherapy given as needed for symptomatic lesions. For patients in whom symptomatic or progressive disease suggests the need for systemic chemotherapy, the DM regimen may produce partial responses in about one-third of patients.

Doxorubicin (Adriamycin) 50 mg/m^2 IV on days 1 and 22
   and
Mitomycin 20 mg/m^2 IV on day 1

Repeat every 42 days.

This regimen is worthy of consideration in patients with good performance status, as occasional durable responses have occurred. Responding patients show improvement within two cycles, and chemotherapy should be stopped after two cycles if no improvement is seen. Do not exceed a cumulative doxorubicin dosage of 550 mg/m^2.

D. **Malignant melanoma.** For disease confined to a single lymph node group, radical lymph node dissection yields long-term survival in 30% of treated patients. Treatment of disseminated melanoma is discussed in Chapter 19.

E. **Neuroendocrine carcinoma.** Poorly differentiated neuroendocrine carcinoma represents 13% of poorly differentiated carcinomas or adenocarcinomas. The diagnosis is secured by recognition of neurosecretory granules on electron microscopy. Localized lesions are uncommon and should be treated with surgery or radiation therapy. Metastatic disease frequently responds to platinum-based chemotherapy, e.g., etoposide plus cisplatin, such as used for carcinoma of the lung.

Selected Readings

Altman, E., and Cadman, E. An analysis of 1539 patients with cancer of unknown primary site. *Cancer* 57:120, 1986.

Greco, F. A., Vaughn, W. K., and Hainsworth, J. D. Advanced poorly differentiated carcinoma of unknown primary site: recognition of a treatable syndrome. *Ann. Intern. Med.* 104:547, 1986.

Hainsworth, J. D., Dial, T. W., and Greco, F. A. Curative combination chemotherapy for patients with advanced poorly differentiated carcinoma of unknown primary site. *Am. J. Clin. Oncol.* 11:138, 1988.

Hainsworth, J. D., Johnson, D. H., and Greco, F. A. Poorly differentiated neuroendocrine carcinoma of unknown primary site: a newly recognized clinicopathologic entity. *Ann. Intern. Med.* 109:364, 1988.

Hainsworth, J. D., Johnson, D. H., and Greco, F. A. Cisplatin-based combination chemotherapy in the treatment of poorly differentiated carcinoma and poorly differentiated adenocarcinoma of unknown primary site: results of a 12-year experience. *J. Clin. Oncol.* 10:912, 1992.

Levine, M. N., Drummond, M. F., and Labelle, R. J. Cost effectiveness in the diagnosis and treatment of carcinoma of unknown primary origin. *Can. Med. Assoc. J.* 133:977, 1985.

McMillan, J. H., Levine, E., and Stephens, R. H. Computer tomography in the evaluation of metastatic adenocarcinoma from an unknown primary site. *Radiology* 143:143, 1983.

Moertel, C. G. Adenocarcinoma of unknown origin. *Ann. Intern. Med.* 91:646, 1979.

Neumann, K. H., and Nystrom, J. S. Metastatic cancer of unknown origin: nonsquamous cell type. *Semin. Oncol.* 9:427, 1982.

Silverman, C., and Marks, J. E. Metastatic cancer of unknown origin: epidermoid and undifferentiated carcinomas. *Semin. Oncol.* 9:435, 1982.

Strand, C. M., et al. Peritoneal carcinomatosis of unknown primary site in women: a distinctive subset of adenocarcinoma. *Ann. Intern. Med.* 11:213, 1989.

Woods, R. L., et al. Metastatic adenocarcinomas of unknown primary site: a randomized study of two combination chemotherapy regimens. *N. Engl. J. Med.* 303:87, 1980.

HIV-Associated Malignancies

Lynne Jahnke and Jamie H. Von Roenn

I. **Introduction.** Human immunodeficiency virus (HIV)–related malignancies are increasing in incidence as patients are living longer with HIV infection. Multiple antiretroviral agents that can delay the destruction of the immune system are now available. Effective prophylaxis has been developed to prevent the opportunistic infections that were once commonplace and uniformly fatal. Approximately 40% of HIV-infected individuals develop malignancy at some time during the course of their illness. Since these malignancies are often very treatable, a patient's overall prognosis is usually as much dependent on the degree of immune impairment as it is on the stage or type of malignancy.

Currently, four malignancies are considered acquired immunodeficiency syndrome *(AIDS)–defining illnesses.* These include *Kaposi's sarcoma* (KS), *primary central nervous system lymphoma* (PCNSL), *non-Hodgkin's lymphoma* (NHL), and *cervical cancer.* Although other malignancies appear to have an increased incidence in HIV-infected individuals (e.g., squamous cell anal cancer and Hodgkin's disease), their precise relationship to the HIV infection has not yet been established. The management of any cancer in an HIV-infected patient requires an integrated team approach. In addition to the therapy for the malignancy, attention must be paid to the prophylaxis and treatment of infection, maintenance of general health and nutrition, and psychosocial support.

II. **Kaposi's sarcoma**

A. **Background.** KS is the most common HIV-associated malignancy. It is 300 times more common in HIV-infected individuals than in other immunocompromised patients. The fact that more than 95% of HIV-related KS occurs in bisexual or homosexual men and the recent observation of KS in a handful of well-studied homosexual men without HIV infection has led many investigators to suspect that a sexually transmitted cofactor contributes to the development of KS. While the prevalence of KS in HIV-infected individuals has remained stable at 25–35%, the incidence of KS as the AIDS-defining illness has decreased from about 33% of patients in the early 1980s to only 14% in 1992. This is because KS is now more often seen as a late, non-AIDS-defining manifestation of HIV infection.

B. **Presentation and detection.** The natural history of KS is extremely variable. KS most often presents as a brownish-purple macule or plaque on the skin or mucous membranes. Lesions are frequently symmetric and follow Langer's lines. KS can present anywhere, but it has a predilection for the retroauricular area, soles of the feet, nose, genitalia, and periorbital areas. In addition to their cosmetic unacceptability and their associated social stigma, the lesions of KS can cause significant morbidity and organ dysfunction. Dermal lymphatic involvement can cause painful and disfiguring lymphedema. Oral lesions can interfere with speech and eating, and can occasionally cause respiratory compromise. Gastrointestinal involvement, present in up to 50% of patients, is often asymptomatic, but can cause pain, diarrhea, and bleeding. Pulmonary involvement is the most common life-threatening manifestation of KS. It may be difficult to differentiate from opportunistic infection, since the chest x-ray (CXR) film may show a reticulonodular or nodular infiltrate, with or without pleural effusions. Bronchoscopy is useful to visualize the characteristic lesions of KS. However, biopsy is rarely done because there is a significant risk of bleeding in these highly vascular tumors. Gallium scan is a useful tool in differentiating KS from an opportunistic pulmonary infection.

   C. Staging. Since KS is a multicentric tumor, it does not fit easily into the usual TNM categorization. Because the overall prognosis is more closely related to the degree of underlying immune dysfunction than to site(s) of disease involvement, the AIDS Clinical Trials Group (ACTG) developed a staging system that reflects various prognostic factors (Table 29-1). Patients are defined as a "good" or "poor" risk on the basis of tumor burden, sites of involvement, CD4 lymphocyte count, history of opportunistic infections, systemic symptoms, and performance status.

   The initial evaluation of a patient with KS should include a careful physical examination, including a rectal examination with testing for the presence of blood. The history should focus on the rate of progression of new KS

Table 29-1. AIDS Clinical Trials Group (ACTG) staging for epidemic Kaposi's sarcoma

	Good risk (0)—all of the following:	Poor risk (1)—any of the following:
Tumor (T)	Confined to skin, minimal oral disease, or both	Edema/ulcers Extensive oral, visceral/gastrointestinal disease
Immune status (I)	CD4 count $\geq$ 200/μl	CD4 count < 200/μl
Systemic illness (S)	No prior OI or thrush No "B" symptoms	Prior OI or thrush "B" symptoms Performance status < 70% Other HIV-related illnesses

OI = opportunistic infection.

lesions, lesion-associated symptoms (pain, edema, disfigurement), as well as a history of HIV-related opportunistic infections, "B" symptoms (see Chap. 26, sec. **I.B.1**), and the rate of decline in CD4 lymphocyte counts. Even though the lesions are characteristic, a biopsy should be done to exclude other cutaneous processes. A baseline CXR study is important to look for asymptomatic visceral disease. Computed tomographic (CT) scans are not indicated unless the patient's symptoms suggest abdominal disease. Upper endoscopy and colonoscopy are not indicated in the absence of clinical gastrointestinal bleeding. Medications should be reviewed to ensure that patients are receiving appropriate prophylaxis, as well as to identify potentially myelosuppressive drugs that may complicate the use of chemotherapeutic agents (e.g., trimethoprim-sulfamethoxazole, sulfadiazine, zidovudine).

D. **Treatment.** Effective treatment of KS is dependent on clear communication between the physician and patient in regard to the risks and benefits of the proposed therapy as well as their own overall expectations. KS is not a curable tumor, and treatment has not clearly been shown to prolong survival. The first decision to be made is whether or not to initiate therapy. There are three generally accepted indications to initiate treatment for KS: cosmesis, palliation of symptoms, and visceral disease. In general, local therapies are used for minimal or slowly progressive disease, while systemic therapy is indicated for bulky, rapidly progressing or life-threatening disease (Table 29-2). The determination of appropriate therapy is based on an evaluation of both tumor and immune status.

1. **Local therapy.** Limited numbers of small lesions can be treated by excision, radiotherapy, cryotherapy, or intralesional injection. Surgery is occasionally useful for an isolated pedunculated lesion. Cryotherapy with liquid nitrogen can lead to hypopigmentation, which may be cosmetically unacceptable to dark-skinned individuals. Intralesional therapy with vinblastine or interferon can be effective, but is limited by the need for multiple injections (Table 29-3). After injection into oral lesions, patients typically slough the oral mucosa in 24–48 hours, for which narcotic analgesics should be empirically provided. Intralesional interferon alpha is occasionally effective, even in patients for whom systemic interferon failed.

2. **Systemic therapy**
   a. **Biologic response modifiers.** Interferon alpha is the best studied biologic response modifier. A clear-cut dose-response relationship has not been established. Responses have been reported with doses ranging from 1 million units per day to 36 million units 3 times per week (see Table 29-4 for recommended dosing). Immune function, as measured by CD4 lymphocyte counts, is the best pre-

Table 29-2. Treatment guidelines for Kaposi's sarcoma (KS)

Status of KS	Status of HIV disease	KS treatment options
Minimal cutaneous disease	CD4 count < 200/µl, prior OI, or "B" symptoms	Observation or local therapy
	CD4 count ≥ 200/µl, no prior OI, and no "B" symptoms	Observation, interferon, or local therapy
Cosmetically disturbing disease	Any	Local therapy
Extensive cutaneous disease	CD4 count < 200/µl, prior OI, or "B" symptoms	Chemotherapy
	CD4 count ≥ 200/µl, no prior OI, and no "B" symptoms	Interferon or chemotherapy
Localized bulky or painful disease	Any	Radiation therapy
Tumor-associated edema	Any	Radiation therapy or chemotherapy
Symptomatic visceral disease	Any	Chemotherapy

OI = opportunistic infection.
Source: Adapted from S. E. Krown, P. L. Myskowski, J. Paredes. Medical management of AIDS patients. Kaposi's sarcoma. *Med. Clin. North Am.* 76:235, 1992.

Table 29-3. Intralesional therapy for Kaposi's sarcoma

Vinblastine (0.2 mg/ml)	0.1 ml/0.5 cm of surface area of lesion (maximum 4 ml)
Interferon alpha	3–5 × 10⁶ units 3 times per week for 4 weeks

Note: Appropriate local anesthesia should be given prior to injection.

dictor of response to interferon. Patients with CD4 lymphocyte counts higher than 400 cells/µl have an overall response rate of 45% while patients with CD4 lymphocyte counts lower than 100 cells/µl respond less than 10% of the time. Although it may take up to 8 weeks to respond, the responses are often durable, with a median response duration of 1–2 years. Interferon in combination with zidovudine shows a modest improvement in response rate but at the expense of increased toxicity. Ongoing trials are evaluating interferon in combination with other less myelosuppressive antiretroviral agents.

Table 29-4. Selected systemic treatment regimens for Kaposi's sarcoma

Biologic response modifiers
1. Interferon alpha 10 × 10^6 units SQ per day, *or*

Single-agent chemotherapy
1. Doxorubicin 20 mg/m^2 IV q2wk
2. Etoposide 150 mg/m^2 PO on days 1–3, repeat q28d
3. Vincristine 2 mg/m^2 IV q2wk (maximum 2.0 mg)

Combination chemotherapy
1. **ABV**
   Doxorubicin 10–20 mg/m^2 IV on day 1 *and*
   Bleomycin 10 mg/m^2 IV on day 1 *and*
   Vincristine 1–2 mg (total) IV on day 1
   Repeat every 2 weeks.
2. **BV**
   Bleomycin 10 mg/m^2 IV on day 1 *and*
   Vincristine 2 mg (total) IV on day 1
   Repeat every 2 weeks.

     b. Chemotherapy. Single-agent chemotherapy with etoposide, vincristine, vinblastine, bleomycin, cyclophosphamide, or doxorubicin has shown a range of response rates from 26 to 84% (see Table 29-4 for doses). Combination chemotherapy is more effective than a single agent for treating tumors that are rapidly progressive, have associated edema, or involve the viscera. The best-studied regimen is doxorubicin (Adriamycin), bleomycin, and vincristine (ABV). Commonly seen toxicities include neutropenia, peripheral neuropathy, and mucositis. Bleomycin and vincristine without doxorubicin are perhaps less effective but may be a suitable alternative for patients for whom hair loss is unacceptable, and cosmesis of visible skin lesions is the primary end point of treatment. Liposomal anthracyclines (e.g., DaunoXome [liposomal daunorubicin] and DOX-SL [Stealth liposomal doxorubicin hydrochloride]) are currently being studied and may cause less toxicity than doxorubicin. Also under investigation are antiangiogenesis compounds, all-*trans*-retinoic acid, and interleukin (IL)-4.

     Patients often require growth factor support between cycles. Granulocyte colony-stimulating factor (G-CSF) 5 μg/kg SQ given on days 7–12 of a 14-day treatment cycle is often sufficient to preserve adequate neutrophil counts in order to prevent infection and allow timely administration of sequential therapy. An absolute neutrophil count of 750/μl is adequate to deliver standard ABV therapy.

     The duration of treatment is variable. Treatment should be continued until the maximal response is obtained; however, intercurrent illness often interrupts therapy. Although lesions will typically progress after therapy is discontinued, an effective maintenance therapy has not yet been defined.

III. Non-Hodgkin's lymphoma

A. Background. HIV-seropositive individuals have a 5–10% lifetime risk of developing NHL. For a small proportion of patients (2–3%), NHL is the AIDS-defining event. But for most, NHL is a late manifestation of HIV infection, arising in the milieu of prolonged immunosuppression, HIV-associated NHLs (HIV-NHL) are aggressive B cell lymphomas similar to those seen in other immunocompromised individuals. Among the high-grade histologic subtypes, 60% are small noncleaved and 40% are large cell immunoblastic.

B. Presentation and detection. The most common presentations for HIV-NHL are constitutional symptoms (fevers, night sweats, and weight loss), or a rapidly enlarging mass. Extranodal presentations are common and occur in 75–95% of patients. The most common extranodal sites of involvement are the gastrointestinal tract, bone marrow, central nervous system (CNS), and liver. Very unusual sites have been seen as well, including the ear lobe, heart, and bile ducts. Seventy-five percent of patients present with advanced disease (stage III or IV).

C. Staging. The Ann Arbor staging classification is commonly used to stage HIV-related NHL (see Chap. 26). However, no direct correlation between stage and prognosis exists. The recently described "International Index" by Shipp and colleagues for defining prognosis in aggressive NHL has not yet been applied to HIV-NHL. Histologic subtype also is not clearly correlated with prognosis. Prognosis is more closely related to immune function and prior AIDS-defining illness. In one study, patients with CD4 lymphocyte counts below 100 cells/μl had a median survival time of 4.1 months, while patients with CD4 lymphocyte counts above 100 cells/μl had a median survival time of 24 months. Similarly, in a retrospective review of 60 patients, two prognostic subgroups were identified based on immune function, performance status, and bone marrow involvement (Table 29-5).

Complete staging evaluation should include CT scans of the head, chest, abdomen, and pelvis; bilateral bone marrow biopsies; and lumbar puncture (LP) with cerebrospinal fluid (CSF) sent for protein and cytologic evaluation. Even in the absence of bone marrow involvement, 40% of patients will have CNS involvement; therefore, all patients should undergo CSF evaluation regardless of clinical stage.

D. Treatment

  1. General approach. The best therapy for HIV-NHL remains to be defined. Fortunately, many clinical trials are ongoing to improve our understanding and

Table 29-5. Prognostic stratification for HIV non-Hodgkin's lymphoma

Good prognosis: median survival time = 11.3 months
   No prior AIDS diagnosis
   Karnofsky performance status > 70%, *and*
   No bone marrow involvement
Poor prognosis: median survival time = 4.0 months
   Prior AIDS diagnosis, *or*
   Karnofsky performance status < 70%, *or*
   Bone marrow involvement

Source: From A. M. Levine, et al. Human immunodeficiency virus-related lymphoma, prognostic factors predictive of survival. *Cancer* 68:2466, 1992.

treatment of this disease. Therapy must be tailored to the overall condition of each individual patient. In contrast to non-HIV-related lymphoma where dose intensity is important, increased dose intensity is associated with decreased survival in HIV-NHL. Patients treated with dose-intensive therapy have an increased incidence of opportunistic infections and an increased rate of CNS relapse. Using a variety of "standard" lymphoma regimens, complete responses are seen in approximately 50% of patients, of whom 25–50% experience relapse within 6 months after completing therapy. Overall, the median survival time is 5–6 months. Half of the deaths are due to intercurrent opportunistic infections and half are due to progressive lymphoma.

Despite these grim statistics, we believe that most patients with HIV-NHL should be given a trial of chemotherapy. While not curative of the lymphoma in most individuals, chemotherapy may temporarily palliate symptoms and improve the overall quality of life. The relatively low-dose regimens described here are well tolerated with appropriate supportive care and follow-up. If there is no response after two cycles of chemotherapy or the performance status declines, discontinuation of chemotherapy is an appropriate consideration.

   2. **Systemic therapy.** In patients who are not eligible for a randomized clinical trial, standard-dose CHOP and low-dose m-BACOD are reasonable therapeutic options (Table 29-6). Growth factor support is usually needed as this patient population often has decreased bone marrow reserve secondary to the HIV infection itself, bone marrow infiltration by lymphoma, or concurrent drug therapies. Dideoxyinosine (DDI) or dideoxycytidine (DDC) may be substituted for zidovudine, which should be stopped during therapy to prevent additive bone marrow suppression. Aggressive prophylaxis against opportunistic infections is important. Regardless of CD4 lymphocyte count, all patients should receive pro-

Table 29-6. Selected chemotherapy regimens for HIV non-Hodgkin's lymphoma

Low-dose m-BACOD
Bleomycin 4 mg/m² IV on day 1, *and*
Doxorubicin 25 mg/m² IV on day 1, *and*
Cyclophosphamide 300 mg/m² IV on day 1, *and*
Vincristine 1.4 mg/m² IV on day 1 (maximum 2 mg), *and*
Dexamethasone 3 mg/m² PO on days 1–5, *and*
Methotrexate 500 mg/m² IV on day 15, *and*
Leucovorin 25 mg PO q6h × 4 doses, on day 16 beginning exactly 24 hours after methotrexate

CHOP
Cyclophosphamide 750 mg/m² IV on day 1, *and*
Doxorubicin 50 mg/m² IV on day 1, *and*
Vincristine 1.4 mg/m² IV on day 1 (maximum 2 mg), *and*
Prednisone 100 mg PO on days 1–5

Salvage chemotherapy
Cyclophosphamide 200 mg/m²/24 hours CIV on days 1–4, *and*
Doxorubicin 12.5 mg/m²/24 hours CIV on days 1–4, *and*
Etoposide 60 mg/m²/24 hours CIV on days 1–4

CIV = continuous IV infusion.

Table 29-7. Prophylaxis regimens for *Pneumocystis carinii* pneumonia

Trimethoprim-sulfamethoxazole (Bactrim DS) 1 tablet PO on Monday, Wednesday, and Friday, *or*
Pentamidine 300 mg in 6 ml of sterile water by aerosol, q4wk, *or*
Dapsone 100 mg PO twice per week*

*Exclude glucose-6-phosphate dehydrogenase deficiency by quantitative spectrophotometry in high-risk individuals prior to initiating therapy.

phylaxis for *Pneumocystis carinii* pneumonia during treatment of a high-grade lymphoma (Table 29-7).

3. **CNS prophylaxis.** Even in the absence of bone marrow involvement, the incidence of CNS relapse is so high that CNS prophylaxis is standard. The first dose of intrathecal therapy should be administered at the initial staging LP. CNS prophylaxis should include four weekly treatments of either preservative-free methotrexate (12 mg) or cytosine arabinoside (50 mg). In patients with documented meningeal disease, intrathecal therapy should be given 3 times per week until the CSF clears, then weekly for 8 weeks and monthly for 10 months. An Ommaya reservoir should be placed to facilitate therapy.

4. **Follow-up.** In this era of cost containment, repeat staging studies are often controversial. Despite this zeal to minimize testing, documentation of a complete response as early as clinically warranted is important in order to minimize the duration of therapy

in this already immunocompromised group of patients. Treatment should be continued for a minimum of four cycles, or for two cycles after attainment of a complete response.

5. **Salvage therapy.** For patients who relapse after initial treatment, we have recently been successful using infusional therapy with etoposide, cyclophosphamide, and doxorubicin (see Table 29-6). The primary toxicities associated with this regimen are neutropenia, thrombocytopenia, and alopecia. There is little gastrointestinal toxicity. In selected patients this regimen can be given in the outpatient setting. Other "salvage" lymphoma regimens could be tried if the patient's performance status suggests he or she might tolerate additional therapies.

IV. Primary CNS lymphoma

A. **Background.** PCNSL represents 10–20% of all HIV-NHLs. Unlike systemic HIV-NHL, which can occur at earlier stages of HIV infection, PCNSL typically occurs in profoundly immunocompromised patients with CD4 lymphocyte counts lower than 50 cells/µl. The Epstein-Barr virus (EBV) genome is identified in virtually all investigated patients with HIV-PCNSL. This supports the belief that EBV may have a direct etiologic role in the development of this disease.

B. **Presentation and detection.** The diagnosis of CNS lymphoma is often difficult to make. Most patients present with a focal neurologic defect. CT scan or magnetic resonance imaging of the head typically shows single or multiple contrast-enhancing masses with surrounding edema. These lesions are often in a periventricular location and may be difficult to distinguish from those of toxoplasmosis. Because CSF cytology is rarely diagnostic, stereotactic biopsy, which is invasive and expensive, becomes necessary to do if one wishes to establish a tissue diagnosis. Since 95% of HIV-positive patients with toxoplasmosis have serologic evidence for infection with *Toxoplasma,* the *Toxoplasma* titer can be used to help determine the course of action.

1. If the *Toxoplasma* titer is negative, stereotactic biopsy should be undertaken.

2. If the *Toxoplasma* titer is positive and the patient is clinically unstable or the clinician feels uncomfortable without a tissue diagnosis based on the clinical scenario, stereotactic biopsy should be undertaken.

3. If, however, the *Toxoplasma* titer is positive and the patient is clinically stable, a 2–3-week trial of empiric therapy for the presumptive diagnosis of toxoplasmosis may be appropriate. If there is no evidence of clinical or radiologic improvement in 2–4 weeks or if there is evidence for clinical decompensation, then stereotactic biopsy should be undertaken.

This approach requires close and frequent monitoring for signs of neurologic deterioration or progression.

C. **Treatment.** Whole brain radiation therapy is the standard therapy. Temporary control and improvement of neurologic deficits occur in 70% of patients. A range of radiation doses (2000–6000 cGy) has been used. In one retrospective review, survival was found to be a function of performance status, not the total radiation dose administered. The median survival time is only 2–5 months. In responding patients, the usual cause of death is opportunistic infection, not progressive lymphoma. Therefore, patients need prophylaxis for multiple infectious pathogens. Consideration has been given to using combined-modality therapy (chemotherapy + radiotherapy), based on the experience in non-HIV-related CNS lymphomas.

V. **Cervical cancer**

  A. **Background.** It was not until 1993 that cervical cancer became an AIDS-defining illness. As in non-HIV-infected women, the development of cervical squamous carcinoma has been directly linked to prior infection with human papilloma virus (HPV). While both HIV and HPV are sexually transmitted, other immunosuppressed populations also have an increased incidence of HPV infection, suggesting that immune competence is a deterrent to the development of HPV coinfection. The presence of HPV, especially types 16, 18, and 31, is correlated with a higher incidence of cervical intraepithelial neoplasia (CIN).

  B. **Presentation and detection.** The presentation is similar to non-HIV-related cervical cancer, except the disease is often more aggressive and advanced disease is more common. Routine Papanicolaou (Pap) smears may not be sensitive enough to detect this aggressive neoplasm. It has been recommended that colposcopy, not Pap smears, be the standard for following HIV-infected women at high risk for CIN. Since CIN may progress at a faster rate in HIV-infected women, annual screening may not detect "curable" disease. Women with very rapidly progressing CIN should probably be tested for HIV.

  C. **Staging.** The FIGO staging system, used for non-HIV-infected patients, is used (see Chap. 16). However, stage for stage, the prognosis appears worse in HIV-infected women who have compromised immune function.

  D. **Treatment.** In a small study, women with CD4 lymphocyte counts less than 500 cells/μl did significantly worse than women with intact immune function. Until these results are confirmed in larger trials, HIV-positive women with invasive cervical cancer should be treated in the same manner as women without HIV infection.

VI. **Other malignancies.** Hodgkin's lymphoma, testicular carcinoma, and anal cancers also are seen frequently in HIV-infected individuals. Anecdotally, these malignancies appear more aggressive than their usual counterpart in immunocompetent individuals, but no large trial has yet confirmed either increased virulence or incidence. It is interesting to speculate that EBV may play a role in the development of Hodgkin's disease. The role of HPV in the development of anal cancers has been well described. We recommend treatment of these malignancies with standard therapy. However, close attention should be paid to the prophylaxis and treatment of opportunistic pathogens, as well as the appropriate use of antiretroviral agents.

Selected Readings

Kaposi's Sarcoma

Epstein, J. B. Treatment of oral Kaposi sarcoma with intralesional vinblastine. *Cancer* 71:1722, 1993.

Epstein, J. B., et al. Oral Kaposi's sarcoma in acquired immunodeficiency syndrome. *Cancer* 64:2424, 1989.

Gill, P. S., et al. Advanced acquired immune deficiency syndrome-related Kaposi's sarcoma: results of pilot studies using combination chemotherapy. *Cancer* 65:1074, 1989.

Krown, S. E., Myskowski, P. L., and Paredes, J. Medical management of AIDS patients. Kaposi's sarcoma. *Med. Clin. North Am.* 76:235, 1992.

Krown, S. E., et al. Interferon alpha with zidovudine: safety, tolerance, and clinical and virologic effects in patients with Kaposi sarcoma associated with the acquired immunodeficiency syndrome (AIDS). *Ann. Intern. Med.* 112:812, 1990.

Lassoued, K., et al. Treatment of the acquired immune deficiency syndrome-related Kaposi's sarcoma with bleomycin as a single agent. *Cancer* 66:1869, 1990.

Laubenstein, L. J., et al. Treatment of epidemic Kaposi's sarcoma with etoposide or a combination doxorubicin, bleomycin, and vinblastine. *J. Clin. Oncol.* 2:1115, 1984.

Mitsuyasu, R. T. Interferon alpha in the treatment of AIDS-related Kaposi's sarcoma. *Br. J. Haematol.* 79(suppl. 1):69, 1991.

Non-Hodgkin's Lymphoma

A predictive model for aggressive non-Hodgkin's lymphoma. The International Non-Hodgkin's Lymphoma Prognostic Factors Project. *N. Engl. J. Med.* 329:987, 1993.

Gill, P. S., et al. AIDS-related malignant lymphoma: results of prospective treatment trials. *J. Clin. Oncol.* 5:1322, 1987.

Levine, A. M. Acquired immunodeficiency syndrome-related lymphoma. *Blood* 80:8, 1992.

Levine, A. M., et al. Human immunodeficiency virus-related lymphoma, prognostic factors predictive of survival. *Cancer* 68:2466, 1992.

Levine, A. M., et al. Low-dose chemotherapy with central nervous system prophylaxis and zidovudine maintenance in AIDS-related lymphoma. *J.A.M.A.* 266:84, 1991.

Sporano, J. A., et al. Infusional cyclophosphamide, doxorubicin, and etoposide in human immunodeficiency virus- and human T-cell leukemia virus type I-related non-Hodgkin's lymphoma: a highly active regimen. *Blood* 81:2810, 1993.

Primary CNS Lymphoma

Formentio, S. C., et al. Primary central nervous system lymphoma in AIDS: results of radiation therapy. *Cancer* 63:1101, 1989.

Goldstein, J. D., et al. Primary central nervous system lymphoma in acquired immune deficiency syndrome: a clinical and pathologic study with results of treatment with radiation. *Cancer* 67:2756, 1991.

Cervical Cancer

Maiman, M., et al. Human immunodeficiency virus infection and invasive cervical carcinoma. *Cancer* 71:402, 1993.

Maiman, M., et al. Colposcopic evaluation of human immunodeficiency virus-seropositive women. *Obstet. Gynecol.* 78:84, 1991.

Schafer, A., et al. The increased frequency of cervical dysplasia-neoplasia in women infected with the human immunodeficiency virus is related to the degree of immunosuppression. *Am. J. Obstet. Gynecol.* 164:593, 1991.

Selected Aspects of
Supportive Care of
Patients with Cancer

Critical Care Issues in Oncology and Bone Metastasis

Walter D. Y. Quan, Jr., and Roland T. Skeel

Spinal cord compression, cerebral edema, superior vena cava syndrome (SVCS), anaphylaxis, respiratory failure, tumor lysis syndrome, and bone metastasis can be major causes of morbidity and, in some cases, potential mortality in patients with cancer. Because of the critical nature of these complications of cancer and its treatment, oncologists, oncology nurses, and other oncology health professionals must be prepared to recognize the signs and symptoms of these disorders promptly, so that appropriate therapy can be instituted without delay.

I. **Spinal cord compression**

   A. **Tumors.** The most common tumors resulting in spinal cord compression are breast cancer, lung cancer, prostate cancer, and renal cancer, although it may also occur with sarcoma, multiple myeloma, and lymphoma. Purely intradural or epidural lesions are infrequent, as more than three-fourths of cases arise from either a metastasis to a vertebral body, other bony parts of the vertebra, or less commonly, direct extension from a paravertebral soft-tissue mass. Seventy percent of the bone lesions are osteolytic, 10% osteoblastic, and 20% are mixed. More than 85% of patients with bony metastases to the vertebra have lesions that involve more than one vertebral body.

   B. **Symptoms and signs.** The most frequent early symptoms seen in patients with spinal cord compression are localized vertebral or radicular pain. These are not from the cord compression per se, but from involvement of the vertebral structures and nerve roots at the level of the compression. Localized tenderness to pressure or percussion over the involved vertebrae is often seen on physical examination. Since pain is seen initially in up to 90% of patients, localized back pain, radicular pain, or spinal tenderness in a patient with cancer should evoke the clinical suspicion of the physician and prompt further evaluation to determine whether the patient has potential or early cord compression. Muscle weakness, evidenced by subjective symptoms or objective physical findings, is present in 75% of patients by the time of diagnosis. The clinician must be aware that progression of this symptom can vary from a gradual increase in weakness over several days to a precipitous loss of function over several hours that may worsen rapidly to the point of paraplegia. If muscle weakness is present, it is incumbent on the physician to act urgently to obtain consultation with the neurosurgeon and the radiotherapist. It is not appropriate to wait until the next morning! By the time there is muscle weakness, most patients also will have sensory deficits below the level of the compression and changes in bladder and bowel sphincter function. If compression is diagnosed late or if treatment is not started emergently, only 25% of patients who are unable to walk when treatment is started will regain full ambulation.

C. **Diagnosis.** Magnetic resonance imaging (MRI) is now considered the diagnostic modality of choice although high-resolution computed tomography (CT) with myelography is an alternative. Plain x-ray films and bone scans will give evidence of metastases to vertebrae, but in and of themselves are not diagnostic for spinal cord involvement.

When there is evidence of bony involvement of the spine on a plain x-ray film or a bone scan, our approach is to obtain an MRI for those patients who have subjective or objective evidence of weakness, radicular pain, paresthesia, or sphincter dysfunction, as these patients are at highest risk for spinal cord compression. Routine MRIs in patients who have completely asymptomatic bony spine metastases (without pain, tenderness, or neurologic findings on a comprehensive clinical examination) are not cost-effective. In the patients with only localized pain or tenderness to correspond with the bone scan or x-ray findings, the yield of additional tests is much lower. Thus, the clinical determination of whether or not to obtain additional invasive or costly diagnostic tests is more difficult and requires a careful assessment of all clinical features of the patient before the most appropriate decision can be made. All patients with spinal metastasis require close follow-up and they and their families must be urged to report relevant symptoms immediately.

D. **Treatment**
1. **Corticosteroids.** When a radiologic study identifies the level of cord compression or if a neurologic deficit is detected on physical examination, dexamethasone may be started to reduce spinal cord edema. A recommended dose is 10 mg IV as a loading dose, and then 4–6 mg PO or IV every 6 hours to be continued through the initial weeks of radiation therapy. Thereafter the dexamethasone therapy may be tapered.
2. **Radiotherapy**
   a. While the preferences of individual centers vary, we generally recommend the **immediate initiation of radiotherapy** once cord compression is diagnosed. This is based on both randomized and nonrandomized studies showing no significant improvement in outcome for patients treated with surgery plus radiation versus those treated with radiation alone. In addition, metastatic disease to the spine often is not totally resectable so that follow-up radiation therapy is frequently required. Third, since patients with evidence of spinal metastases frequently have either overt

or microscopic evidence of metastases elsewhere that would likely grow during the postoperative recuperation period following surgery, the use of radiotherapy instead allows the initiation of some form of systemic therapy concurrently.

b. **Radiation therapy** is most frequently given to a total dose of 40–45 Gy with daily dose fractions of 200–250 cGy. Alternatively, 400 cGy may be given initially for the first 3 days of therapy, and then subsequently decreased to standard-dose levels for the completion of the radiation course.

c. **The clinical response** to radiation is dependent not only on the degree of cord involvement and the duration of symptoms but also on the underlying cell type. In general, patients with severe deficits such as complete paraplegia or a long duration of neurologic deficit are unlikely to have return to normal function. This underscores the need to diagnose and treat these patients rapidly. Lymphoma, myeloma, and other hematologic malignancies along with breast and small-cell lung carcinoma tend to be more responsive than adenocarcinomas of the gastrointestinal tract, renal cancer, and others.

3. **Surgery.** Surgery (whether decompressive laminectomy for posterior lesions or newer anterior approaches for other lesions) still plays a crucial role in selected patients. Indications for surgery include worsening of neurologic signs or symptoms or the appearance of new neurologic findings during the course of radiation; vertebral collapse at presentation; a question of spinal stability; and disease recurrence within a prior radiation port. In selected patients, the use of surgery to remove disease in the vertebral bodies followed by stabilization can result in dramatic improvement in pain and patient function.

II. Cerebral edema

A. Clinical evaluation

1. **Neurologic signs and symptoms.** Intracranial metastases are commonly manifested by a variety of neurologic symptoms and signs including headache, change in mentation, visual disturbances, cranial nerve deficits, focal motor or sensory abnormalities, difficulty with coordination, and seizures. In the more critical condition of brain stem herniation, there may be gradual to rapid loss of consciousness, neck stiffness, unilateral or bilateral pupillary abnormalities, ipsilateral hemiparesis, or respiratory dysfunction; the specific findings will depend on whether there is uncal, central, or tonsillar herniation. Any neurologic complaint from a patient with cancer should be viewed with a high index of suspicion by members of the oncology team, especially if metastasis to the brain is commonly associated with the patient's tumor type.

The history and physical examination provide the first clue to the presence of a metastatic lesion or associated cerebral edema. In general, a history of gradual progression of neurologic symptoms prior to the development of a significant deficit is more consistent with a metastatic lesion whereas the absence of symptoms followed by the abrupt onset of a severe deficit is suggestive of a cerebrovascular event.

2. **Radiologic studies.** MRI is the imaging modality of choice, as it has greater sensitivity for detecting the presence of metastatic lesions and for determining the extent of cerebral edema compared to CT. CT is substituted for MRI in many institutions because of availability, ease of administration with shorter test time, and less cost. However, while CT is sufficient to detect the presence of cerebral edema in most patients, it is necessary to realize that CT does fail to diagnose some lesions and may underestimate cerebral edema. If CT of the brain reveals no definite abnormality in the presence of persistent neurologic findings, MRI is the recommended next step. In general, we do not believe that delaying appropriate imaging studies (either CT or MRI) to examine plain skull x-ray films or to obtain radionuclide studies in patients experiencing neurologic difficulties is warranted.

Warning: In a patient with cancer who has focal neurologic signs or symptoms, headache, or alteration in consciousness, a lumbar puncture to evaluate for possible neoplastic meningeal spread should not be done until a CT scan or MRI shows no evidence of mass, midline shift, or increased intracranial pressure. To do the lumbar puncture without this assurance could precipitate brain stem herniation, which is often rapidly fatal.

B. **Treatment**

1. **Symptomatic therapy.** Once the presence of cerebral edema is established, dexamethasone 10–20 mg IV to load followed by 6 mg IV or PO 4 times daily should be started. The rationale for the use of steroids centers around the etiology of cerebral edema. It appears that the invasion of malignant cells releases leukotrienes and other soluble mediators responsible for vasodilation, increased capillary permeability, and subsequent edema. Dexamethasone inhibits the conversion of arachidonic acid to leukotrienes, thereby decreasing vascular permeability. Additionally, steroids appear to have a direct stabilizing effect on brain capillaries. There is some evidence to suggest that patients who do not have lessening of cerebral edema with the dexamethasone dose just described may respond to higher doses (50–100 mg/day). Because of the risk of gastrointestinal bleeding and other side effects of doses higher than 32 mg daily, higher doses are usually not given for more than 48–72 hours.

Patients with severe cerebral edema leading to a life-threatening rise in intracranial pressure or brain stem herniation should also receive mannitol 50–100 gm (in a 20–25% solution) infused intravenously over approximately 30 minutes. This may be repeated every 6 hours if needed, although serum electrolytes and urine output must be monitored closely. Patients with severe cerebral edema should be intubated to allow for mechanical hyperventilation to reduce the carbon dioxide pressure to 25–30 mm Hg to decrease intracranial pressure.

2. **Therapy of the intracerebral tumor.** Once the patient has been stabilized, appropriate therapy for the cause underlying the cerebral edema should be implemented. Radiation is the usual modality for most metastases, but surgery may be considered for suitable candidates with easily accessible lesions.

3. **Nonmalignant causes** of cerebral edema such as subdural hematoma in thrombocytopenic patients and brain abscess in immunocompromised patients must always be considered.

III. **Superior vena cava syndrome.** The superior vena cava is a thin-walled vessel located to the right of the midline just anterior to the right mainstem bronchus. It is ultimately responsible for the venous drainage of the head, neck, and arms. Its location places it near lymph nodes that are commonly involved by malignant cells from lung primary tumors and lymphomas. Lymph node distension or the presence of a mass may compress the adjacent superior vena cava leading to the SVCS. Similarly, the presence of a thrombus due to a hypercoagulable state secondary to underlying malignancy or a thrombus developing around an indwelling central venous catheter may also lead to the development of this syndrome.

A. **Symptoms and signs.** Patients who develop SVCS commonly complain of dyspnea, orthopnea, paroxysmal nocturnal dyspnea, and facial, neck, and upper extremity swelling. Associated symptoms may include cough, hoarseness, and chest and neck pain. Headache and mental status changes also may be seen. A patient's symptoms may be gradual and progressive, with only mild facial swelling being present early in the course of this disorder. These early changes may be so subtle that the patient is unaware of them. Physical examination may reveal a spectrum of findings from facial edema to marked respiratory distress. Neck vein distension, facial edema or cyanosis, and tachypnea are commonly seen. Other potential physical findings include the presence of collateral vessels on the thorax, upper extremity edema, paralysis of the vocal cords, and mental status changes.

B. **Radiologic evaluation.** Patients may often be diagnosed by physical findings plus the presence of a mediastinal mass on chest x-ray films. While previously it was thought that the superior venocavogram was required to firmly establish the diagnosis and delineate the extent of obstruction, current opinion now appears to favor the use of CT instead. CT will allow for a more detailed examination of surrounding anatomy including adjacent lymphadenopathy, may differentiate between extrinsic compression and an intrinsic lesion (primary thrombus), poses less risk to the patient, aids in treatment planning for radiation therapy, and allows for possible percutaneous biopsy of a compressing mass.

SVCS may occur in patients with subclavian catheters. The injection of contrast material into these catheters is useful to determine the presence of a thrombus. It is important to remember, however, that a thrombus forms in the venous vasculature distal to the caval obstruction in most patients with SVCS secondary to external compression. Thus a clot may be primary or secondary; determination of the cause and the appropriate treatment will depend on both the clinical situation and the radiologic findings.

C. **Tissue diagnosis.** While some patients present with such severe respiratory compromise as to require emergent treatment, the majority of patients are clinically stable and may undergo biopsy for a tissue diagnosis. Tissue may be acquired through multiple methods including bronchoscopy, CT-guided biopsy, mediastinoscopy, or mediastinotomy. Thoracotomy is the most invasive option and is rarely needed. Because of increased venous pressure and dilated veins distal to the obstruction, extreme care must be taken to ensure adequate hemostasis following any biopsy procedure.

D. **Treatment.** Initially, patients with SVCS may be treated with oxygen for dyspnea, furosemide 20–40 mg IV to reduce edema, and dexamethasone 16 mg IV or PO daily in divided doses. The benefit of dexamethasone is not clear. In patients with lymphoma there is probably a lympholytic effect with resultant decrease in tumor mass; in patients with most other tumors, the effect is probably limited to decreasing any local inflammatory reaction from the tumor and from subsequent initial radiotherapy.

1. **Neoplasms.** The therapy for SVCS ultimately involves radiation therapy for most tumors but possibly chemotherapy as a single modality for particularly sensitive tumor types such as small-cell lung cancer, lymphomas, and germ cell cancers. Radiation therapy may be given in relatively high-dose fractions (e.g., 4 Gy) for several days followed by a reversion to "standard doses" thereafter. We usually continue dexamethasone for approximately 1 week after the start of radiation.

2. **Thrombi.** SVCS secondary to vascular thrombi may require the use of thrombolytic therapy. Both streptokinase (250,000 units by IV bolus over 30 minutes) and urokinase (4400 units/kg by IV bolus over 10 minutes) have been utilized. While 50–75% of patients will have resolution of clots with thrombolytic

therapy when treated within 7 days of occurrence, thrombi that have been present for longer than 7 days are unlikely to be treated successfully. Avoid thrombolytic therapy in patients with a tumor that might bleed. Anticoagulation with heparin after thrombolytic therapy is recommended; patients whose catheters become patent and functional should receive low-dose warfarin (1 mg PO daily) thereafter.

For patients with thrombi secondary to external superior vena cava pressure, thrombolytics are not usually used, but patients are commonly anticoagulated with heparin and then warfarin to prevent propagation of the clot. (See Chap. 32.)

IV. Anaphylaxis

   A. Causes. Anaphylaxis is a hyperimmune reaction mediated by the release of IgE. This emergency situation may arise in oncology patients who are exposed to serum products, bacterial products such as L-asparaginase, certain cytotoxic agents (such as paclitaxel [Taxol] or the Cremophor component of paclitaxel), antibiotics such as penicillin, iodine-based contrast material, and monoclonal antibodies (which have murine components). However, virtually any drug can lead to a hyperimmune response resulting in anaphylaxis.

   B. Clinical manifestations. Patients may display anxiety, dyspnea, and presyncopal symptoms. Urticaria, generalized itching, and evidence of bronchospasm and laryngeal edema may occur. Peripheral vasodilatation may result in significant hypotension and may lead to syncope.

   C. Management. Patients must be assessed rapidly to ensure that an open airway is present and maintained. Supplemental oxygen should be given for respiratory symptoms. Endotracheal intubation may be necessary. If severe laryngeal edema rather than bronchospasm is the cause of respiratory distress, tracheostomy or cricothyrotomy is necessary.

      1. Epinephrine 0.3–0.5 mg (0.3–0.5 ml of 1:1000 epinephrine or 3–5 ml of a 1:10,000 solution) IV is given every 10 minutes for severe reactions with laryngeal stridor, major bronchospasm, or hypotension for a maximum of 3 doses (1 mg) or until the episode resolves, whichever occurs first. For milder reactions, a dose of 0.2–0.3 ml of 1:1000 epinephrine may be given subcutaneously and repeated every 15 minutes × 2. In the event of life-threatening anaphylaxis, 0.5 mg (5 ml of a 1:10,000 solution) should be given intravenously; this dose may be repeated once in 10 minutes if needed. Because of the cardiovascular stress associated with epinephrine, its use in relatively minor allergic reactions such as pruritus alone should be avoided. Alternatively, epinephrine may be administered through the endotracheal tube if intravenous access is unavailable.

      2. Intravenous fluids (either normal saline or lactated Ringer's solution) may be given for hypotension. Hypotension unresponsive to these measures will require the use of vasopressors such as dopamine.

3. **Albuterol** or **metaproterenol aerosol treatments** can be used to treat bronchospasm.

4. **Diphenhydramine** 25 mg IV may be followed by a second dose if necessary. Blood pressure must be monitored as hypotension could result.

5. **Corticosteroids** have a slow onset of action measured in hours. While their administration may be reasonable for their later effects, they do not have a primary role in the acute management of this emergent condition. Hydrocortisone 100–500 mg IV or methylprednisolone 125 mg IV may be given for their later effects.

6. **Cimetidine** 300 mg IV may be given for urticaria; it has no significant role in acute, severe episodes, though it has a preventive role in averting reactions from paclitaxel.

V. Respiratory failure

A. Causes. The development of respiratory failure in patients with cancer may occur secondary to many potential causes.

1. Bacterial pneumonia especially in patients neutropenic due to therapy

2. Sepsis (and other causes of the systemic inflammatory response syndrome [SIRS])

3. Interstitial pulmonary spread of cancer

4. Overwhelming parenchymal pulmonary metastases

5. Radiation injury

6. Lung damage secondary to chemotherapy agents (such as bleomycin, high-dose cyclophosphamide, or methotrexate)

7. Pulmonary edema secondary to cardiac damage from cytotoxic agents (like doxorubicin) or biologic agents ("capillary leak syndrome" with interleukin [IL]-2)

8. Retinoic acid syndrome from tretinoin (all-*trans*-retinoic acid) therapy of acute promyelocytic leukemia

9. Pulmonary embolus developing from deep venous thrombosis in a debilitated patient

B. Management. The management of severe respiratory failure requires intubation and mechanical ventilation, which is usually managed by pulmonologists or critical care specialists. However, because the prognosis of most patients with advanced solid tumors who develop respiratory failure is poor, careful consideration of a patient's entire medical situation must be made. Relevant factors include the patient's underlying medical illnesses, such as concurrent cardiopulmonary disease, and their particular tumor type and potential for response to antineoplastic therapy. It is prudent—some would say imperative—to ascertain well in advance of the emergency the wishes of patients and their families regarding whether they wish intensive care unit support and full resuscitative measures.

C. Prevention. If possible, progressive steps to prevent or lessen the possibility of the development of respiratory failure should be undertaken. These include the following.

1. Careful monitoring of granulocyte counts to be aware of patients at risk for bacterial infection.
2. Routine lung auscultation of patients receiving agents with potential pulmonary toxicity followed by appropriate action in the event of pulmonary findings. This may include giving furosemide for patients who exhibit rales while receiving IL-2 and discontinuing offending agents (like bleomycin) prior to the development of serious symptoms.
3. Ensuring that patients are ambulatory or that antithrombotic precautions are taken for hospitalized patients who are bedridden.
4. Consideration of underlying cardiopulmonary disease before patients are considered to be candidates for systemic therapy is most important. Such concurrent illnesses may proscribe the selection of or modify the dosing of cytotoxic agents (such as cisplatin which requires substantial intravenous hydration) and biologic agents (like IL-2 prior to which patients' pulmonary function should be tested).

VI. Tumor lysis syndrome. This syndrome may potentially be seen with any tumor that is undergoing rapid cell turnover as a result of high growth fraction or because of high cell death due to therapy. In general, acute leukemia, high-grade lymphoma, and less commonly solid tumors such as small-cell lung cancer and germ cell cancers undergoing therapy are the most commonly associated tumor types. Tumor lysis syndrome is characterized by the metabolic abnormalities of hyperuricemia, hyperkalemia, and hyperphosphatemia leading to hypocalcemia. Severe clinical situations including acute renal failure and serious cardiac dysrhythmia including ventricular tachycardia and ventricular fibrillation may potentially develop. It is therefore important for physicians to be aware of which patients might be at risk for this syndrome, attempt to prevent its onset, monitor patient's blood chemistry values carefully, and initiate treatment promptly.

A. Prevention. It is useful to start all patients who have tumor types that predispose to this complication on allopurinol 600 mg PO daily for 1 or 2 days at least 24 hours prior to initiating chemotherapy. Thereafter, patients may receive allopurinol 300 mg PO daily.

For patients who must be treated immediately, allopurinol is started at the same dose just described, urine should be alkalinized (pH $\geq$ 7), and a "brisk diuresis" of approximately 100–150 ml of urine/hour should be maintained. This can be achieved through the use of intravenous crystalloid with 1 ampule (44.6 mEq) of sodium bicarbonate in each liter of intravenous solution. If the desired urine output is not reached, furosemide 20 mg IV may be given to facilitate diuresis. If routine monitoring of urine shows pH < 7.0, an additional ampule of sodium bicarbonate may be added to each liter of infused fluid. Acetazolamide 250 mg PO qid may also be added to keep urine alkaline.

B. **Monitoring.** During the course of chemotherapy for patients at risk of tumor lysis syndrome, serum electrolytes, phosphate, calcium, uric acid, and creatinine levels should be checked prior to therapy and at least daily thereafter. Patients at very high risk (e.g., high-grade lymphoma with large bulk) should have these parameters checked every 6 hours for the first 24–48 hours. In addition, patients who show any initial or subsequent abnormality in any of these parameters should have appropriate therapy initiated and have measurements of abnormal parameters repeated every 6–12 hours until completion of chemotherapy and normalization of laboratory values.

C. **Treatment.** Patients who have evidence of tumor lysis syndrome must have adequate hydration with half-normal saline solution. Aluminum hydroxide 30 ml orally every 4 hours is used to treat hyperphosphatemia.

Hyperkalemia may be treated in multiple ways. However, the clinician must differentiate between methods that reduce serum potassium by driving this ion intracellularly (as done with dextrose and insulin or sodium bicarbonate) versus those that lead to actual potassium loss out of the body (as with furosemide through the urine and with sodium polystyrene sulfonate resin [Kayexalate] through the gut). In addition, because of the potential cardiac arrhythmias secondary to hyperkalemia, cardioprotection should be achieved through the use of intravenous calcium.

We recommend the following.

1. For patients with mild elevation of potassium (serum K^+ no higher than 5.5 mEq/liter), increasing intravenous hydration using normal saline solution with a single dose (20 mg) of intravenous furosemide is often sufficient. An alternative to normal saline is the use of 2 ampules of sodium bicarbonate (89 mEq) in a liter of 5% dextrose/water.

2. For patients with serum potassium levels between 5.5 and 6.0 mEq/liter, increased intravenous fluids, furosemide, and oral sodium polystyrene sulfonate resin (Kayexalate) 30 gm with sorbitol may be utilized.

3. For serum K^+ levels over 6.0 mEq/liter or evidence of cardiac arrhythmia, several options may be combined. Intravenous calcium gluconate 10 ml of a 10% solution or 1 ampule is given first, followed by increased intravenous fluids, furosemide, plus 1 ampule of 50% dextrose and 10 units of regular insulin intravenously. Oral sodium polystyrene sulfonate resin (Kayexalate) with sorbitol also may be used except in patients with a history of congestive heart failure or reduced left ventricular function. Dialysis may be used for refractory hyperkalemia.

VII. **Bone metastasis.** Metastases to bone occur frequently from many types of tumors and have great potential for morbidity. Bone involvement can be a source of constant pain, limiting a patient's activity and quality of life. The consequences of spinal involvement have been discussed already. The occurrence of a pathologic fracture in a weight-bearing bone has catastrophic implications: Patients who are consequently immobilized or bedridden are predisposed to a variety of complications including deep venous thrombi, pulmonary emboli, aspiration pneumonia, and decubitus ulcers, as well as psychosocial consequences including depression.

A. **Clinical findings.** Bone involvement with metastatic disease can be manifested by a spectrum of clinical presentations. This can vary from constant aching pain through nocturnal exacerbations of pain to sharp pains brought on by pressure, weight bearing, other use, or range of motion of the affected site. Tenderness of an affected bone area may or may not be present. Tenderness or sharp pain with weight bearing often implies a greater degree of disruption of the bony architecture and thus a greater potential for fracture, particularly in a weight-bearing area.

B. **Radiologic findings.** These often depend on the tumor type involved as well as the extent of the metastases. Multiple myeloma is a prime example of a malignancy that leads to pure osteolytic lesions. Consequently, radionuclide bone scans are rarely useful in the evaluation of patients with this disease. Rather, a metastatic skeletal survey (plain x-ray films) is preferable. In contrast, prostate cancer most commonly has purely osteoblastic lesions. Therefore, a radionuclide bone scan would be the diagnostic test of choice. In general, most tumor types have the potential to yield either type of bone lesion or both. A radionuclide bone scan may be done to permit a "global view" in these patients.

The presence of "hot spots" in the spine, in weight-bearing bones such as the femur, or in other major long bones such as the humerus should lead the clinician to assess the patient further with plain x-ray films of these bones. Patients who display significant cortical thinning of long bones are at high risk for the development of pathologic fractures with great morbidity. These patients should be evaluated both by orthopedic surgery for consideration of prophylactic surgery to stabilize the affected bone and by radiation oncology for treatment of the tumor in order to allow regeneration of normal bone.

C. **Treatment**

1. **Surgery.** Because rapid return of the patient to as normal a life as possible is an overriding concern when treating patients with metastatic disease, surgical stabilization is most often the initial step in treating pathologic fractures of long bones. If the fracture is the initial manifestation of tumor relapse, biopsy confirmation can also be obtained. Whereas

fractures at sites of significant residual bony architecture can be satisfactorily stabilized with an intramedullary rod or pin, marked lytic destruction may necessitate additional structural support such as methylmethacrylate cement to fill the intramedullary canal and cortical defects. Pathologic fractures of non-weight-bearing bones can be managed by splinting (ribs) or sling immobilization (humerus or clavicle) while delivering radiotherapy to promote healing. Fixation may also be used in the upper extremities to speed recovery of function, particularly of the humerus. Surgical stabilization of the spine may also be used in selected circumstances (providing the patient has an anticipated survival time of >3 months) and can result in significant pain relief and reduction in risk for cord and nerve root compression.

2. **External beam therapy.** Radiation doses of 15–20 Gy in 3–5 fractions leads to complete relief of pain in approximately 50% of patients, with an additional 30% of patients having some decrease in pain, while 80–90% will show significant improvement with 30–40 Gy. The alleviation of symptoms can be expected within 2–3 weeks. For patients who may be expected to have more prolonged survival, higher doses over a larger number of fractions may be used. Most patients receive optimal results from courses of 30 Gy in 10 fractions (2 weeks) or 40 Gy in 15 fractions (3 weeks).

   Radiotherapy fields should include the area of evident bone involvement, as shown on x-ray film and bone scan, with a sufficient extension to prevent relapse at the portal margin. It is seldom necessary to treat the entire bone unless the entire bone is involved, as encroachment on marrow reserve may compromise any systemic chemotherapy that might also be indicated.

3. **Strontium-89 therapy.** A new approach to the therapy of bone metastases is through the use of the radioisotope strontium 89, which is given by intravenous injection (4 mCi or 40–60 μCi/kg). This isotope is highly selective for bone, is an emitter of beta radiation, and has low penetration into surrounding tissue. Strontium's affinity to metastatic bone disease is reported to be 2–25 times greater than its affinity for normal bone. This therapy is especially useful in patients with breast or prostate cancer who have many metastatic bone sites or who have received maximal external beam radiation to a specific site. Palliative effects may be seen in other types of tumors as well. Pain relief may occur as early as 1–2 weeks after the first injection. Multiple studies indicate that 10–20% of patients will experience complete pain relief while another 50–60% will have at least a moderate reduction in symptoms. Responses last 3–6 months. Patients who experience

some relief of symptoms may receive multiple doses at 3-month intervals if there has been adequate hematologic recovery (platelet count $> 60,000/\mu l$ and white blood cell count $> 2400/\mu l$).

The toxicity of strontium 89 is primarily hematologic involving both leukocytes and platelets. Approximately 10% of patients may experience a transient "flare" of their bone pain similar to what is seen with tamoxifen therapy in breast cancer. This flare reaction often foreshadows a response to treatment.

Selected Readings

Allen, K. L., Johnson, T. W., and Hibbs, G. G. Effective bone radiation as related to various treatment regimens. *Cancer* 37:984, 1976.

Bern, M. M., et al. Very low dose of warfarin can prevent thrombosis in central venous catheters. *Ann. Intern. Med.* 112:423, 1990.

Cooper, P. R., et al. A systematic approach to spinal reconstruction after anterior decompression for neoplastic disease of the thoracic and lumbar spine. *Neurosurgery* 32:1, 1993.

Escalante, C. P. Causes and management of superior vena cava syndrome. *Oncology* 7(6):61, 1993. (In this same issue are three reviews of this article which lend further perspective to this disorder.)

Garmatis, C. J., and Chu, F. C. The effectiveness of radiation therapy in the treatment of bone metastases from breast cancer. *Radiology* 126:235, 1978.

Gray, B. H., et al. Safety and efficacy of thrombolytic therapy for superior vena cava syndrome. *Chest* 99:54, 1991.

Hauser, M. J., Tabak, J., and Baier, H. Survival of patients with cancer in a medical critical care unit. *Arch. Intern. Med.* 142:527, 1982.

Johnston, F. G., Uttley, D., and Marsh, H. T. Synchronous vertebral decompression and posterior stabilization in the treatment of spinal malignancy. *Neurosurgery* 25:872, 1989.

Katin, M. J., et al. Hematologic effects of 89-strontium treatment for metastases to bone. *Proc. Am. Soc. Clin. Oncol.* 3:12, 1993.

Lippman, M., and Rumley, W. Medical Emergencies. In W. C. Dunagan and M. L. Ridner (eds.), *Manual of Medical Therapeutics.* Boston: Little, Brown, 1989. Pp. 484–485.

McAfee, P. C., and Bohlman, H. H. One-stage anterior cervical decompression and posterior stabilization with circumferential arthrodesis. *Am. J. Bone Joint Surg.* 71:78, 1989.

Porter, A. T., and Davis, L. P. Systemic radionuclide therapy of bone metastases with strontium-89. *Oncology* 8(2): 93, 1994.

Robinson, R. G. Radionuclides for the alleviation of bone pain in advanced malignancy. *Clin. Oncol.* 5:39, 1986.

Seifert, V., et al. Spondylectomy, microsurgical decompression and osteosynthesis in the treatment of complex disorders of the cervical spine. *Acta Neurochir. (Wien)* 124:104, 1993.

Weissman, D. E. Steroid treatment of CNS metastases. *J. Clin. Oncol.* 6:543, 1988.

Infections: Etiology, Treatment, and Prevention

Rodger D. MacArthur

I. **Overview.** Infection is a major source of morbidity and mortality among patients with cancer, despite recent advances in prevention and treatment. In many series, infection is the most frequent cause of death, exceeding all other causes combined. Granulocytopenia, cellular immune dysfunction, humoral immune dysfunction, and splenectomy each can predispose patients to certain types of infections. In addition, mucosal or integumentary damage, prolonged hospitalization, lack of ambulation, malnutrition, neurologic dysfunction, indwelling devices (e.g., central venous catheters and reservoirs), and local tumor effect all contribute to the risk of infection.

The majority of bacterial and fungal infections in patients with cancer arise from the patients' own flora. Environmental reservoirs also may contribute to infection in certain circumstances. Prolonged hospitalization and antibiotic use tend to favor the acquisition of resistant strains of organisms. Careful handwashing by health care workers is the most important means of reducing the occurrence of infection. Reverse isolation of patients can be justified only rarely. The prompt initiation of therapy with broad-spectrum antibiotics for documented and suspected bacterial infections is essential. The addition of antifungal therapy should be considered for patients who do not respond within a reasonable period of time to antibiotics. Daily reevaluation of all patients is critical.

II. **Reasons for infection**
   A. **Granulocytopenia**
      1. **General comments.** Acute leukemias or lymphomas after chemotherapy are prototypical malignancies in which infection resulting from granulocytopenia is seen. An increase in the incidence of infection can be expected when the granulocyte count is less than 500/μl. A substantial increase in both the incidence and the severity of infection occurs when there are fewer than 100 granulocytes/μl. Infection early in the course of granulocytopenia typically is caused by relatively nonresistant endogenous bacteria. Fungal infections and infection with resistant bacteria most often occur during prolonged periods of granulocytopenia.
      2. **Sites of infection.** Damage to skin and mucous membranes (e.g., from venipuncture, indwelling vascular devices, or chemotherapy) greatly increases the risk of infection in granulocytopenic patients. Thus, the integument, periodontium, oropharynx, sinuses, bladder, colon, and perianal area are common foci for infection. Organisms from these sites often seed the bloodstream and disseminate. Pneumonia

typically is caused by bacteria that have colonized the oropharynx.

3. **Microbiology**

   a. **Gram-negative bacteria.** *Escherichia coli, Klebsiella pneumoniae,* and *Pseudomonas aeruginosa* have predominated in the past. For unknown reasons, the incidence of infections caused by *P. aeruginosa* has decreased in recent years. Conversely, *Enterobacter* species, *Acinetobacter anitratus, Serratia marcescens, Pseudomonas cepacia,* and *Xanthomonas maltophilia* have become more common pathogens.

   b. **Gram-positive bacteria.** Infection with either *Staphylococcus epidermidis* or *Staphylococcus aureus* is now almost as common as infection with gram-negative bacteria. The increase in gram-positive infections probably is due to the increase in the use of central venous catheters. *Corynebacterium jeikeium* (formerly *C.* group JK) occasionally is found in association with catheter infections.

   c. **Fungi.** *Candida* and *Aspergillus* species and the agents of mucormycosis are the important pathogens. *Pseudallescheria boydii* is seen less frequently.

B. **Cellular immune dysfunction**

1. **General comments.** Cellular immune dysfunction and its associated infections can result either from the underlying disease or from antineoplastic agents and corticosteroids. Hodgkin's disease and acute lymphocytic leukemia (ALL) are characteristic malignancies in which cellular immune dysfunction–related infection is encountered.

2. **Microbiology**

   a. **Bacteria.** *Legionella pneumophila* is of special concern, as are the *Nocardia* species. Nocardiosis typically presents with one or more lesions in the lung, skin, and brain. Infections caused by *Salmonella* species and *Listeria monocytogenes* are considerably less frequent.

   b. **Mycobacteria.** *Mycobacterium avium* complex (MAC) is being seen with increasing frequency in patients with non-Hodgkin's lymphomas receiving intensive cytotoxic therapy. The incidence of infection with *Mycobacterium kansasii* is increased in patients with hairy cell leukemia. *Mycobacterium tuberculosis* is surprisingly uncommon in patients with cancer having altered cell-mediated immunity.

   c. **Fungi.** *Cryptococcus neoformans* is seen frequently. Meningitis is the most common presentation, but pulmonary and cutaneous infections also occur.

   d. **Viruses.** Herpes zoster virus, causing either varicella or zoster, is particularly common in this group of patients. Varicella can be life-threatening in children with ALL, causing pneumonitis, purpura fulminans, and encephalitis. Oropharyngeal or esophageal lesions due to herpes simplex virus (HSV) can predispose to infection with bacterial or fungal pathogens. Cytomegalovirus (CMV) is seen most often in patients undergoing bone marrow transplantation.

  e. **Protozoa and parasites.** *Pneumocystis carinii* is a frequent cause of pneumonia, especially in children with ALL. Infection with *Toxoplasma gondii* presents as either chorioretinitis or cerebral abscesses. *Strongyloides stercoralis* can cause diarrhea or life-threatening disseminated infections. Diffuse pulmonary infiltrates, shock, and sepsis from enteric gram-negative bacilli are the typical features of disseminated strongyloidiasis.

C. Humoral immune dysfunction

  1. **General comments.** Patients with agammaglobulinemia or hypogammaglobulinemia are susceptible to infections because they often lack opsonizing antibodies to the common encapsulated pyogenic bacteria. Many of these patients also are deficient in functional complement activity. Multiple myeloma and chronic lymphocytic leukemia are prototypical neoplasms with humoral immune dysfunction.

  2. **Microbiology.** *Streptococcus pneumoniae* predominates. In addition, decreased complement activity increases the risk of infection by *Haemophilus influenzae, Neisseria meningitidis,* and *E. coli.*

D. Splenectomy

  1. **General comments.** The spleen is the organ most efficient at removing nonopsonized bacteria. Specific opsonizing antibodies are required for effective killing of the encapsulated bacteria. Thus, splenectomized patients are at risk of overwhelming sepsis when infected with a strain of encapsulated bacteria against which they have never had an opportunity to make antibodies.

  2. **Microbiology.** Infections are usually caused by *S. pneumoniae,* and, to a lesser extent, *H. influenzae* and *N. meningitidis.*

E. Other factors

  1. **Indwelling vascular catheters.** These increase the risk of bacterial and fungal infections. The risk increases with the length of time they have been in place. Concurrent granulocytopenia magnifies the infection risk.

  2. **Nonambulation and length of stay.** These two factors have been identified as independent risk factors for infection in most studies. Other factors, such as previous antibiotic use and the presence of a Foley catheter, are correlated with nonambulation and length of stay, but are not themselves independent risk factors for infection.

3. **Malnutrition and neurologic dysfunction.** It is controversial whether malnutrition is an independent risk factor for immunosuppression. On the other hand, malnourished patients who require enteral feedings are certainly at increased risk for aspiration. Loss of the gag reflex also increases the risk of aspiration. Loss of sensation facilitates the development of cutaneous ulcers while neurogenic bladder predisposes to urinary tract infections.

4. **Local tumor effect.** Complete or partial obstruction by tumor may lead to infection behind the obstruction. Postobstructive pneumonia in a patient with bronchogenic cancer, and ascending cholangitis in a patient with an intraabdominal lymphoma, are two examples of this phenomenon.

III. Treatment of infection

A. **Clinical findings that suggest the diagnosis of infection**

1. **Symptoms**

   a. **General.** Malaise, fatigue, confusion, or other nonspecific or subtle symptoms may be the first indication of infection. Any unexplained change in the patient's condition should be evaluated clinically and microbiologically.

   b. **Localizing.** Symptoms referable to a particular organ system are particularly worrisome and demand an immediate and thorough evaluation.

2. **Signs**

   a. **Fever** is the single most important indicator of infection in patients with cancer. Often it is the only abnormal finding. *Never assume that an unexplained fever is due to the underlying malignancy.* Similarly, never rely exclusively on fever to diagnose infection: Debilitated or elderly patients occasionally are afebrile in the presence of infection.

   b. **Hypotension and shock** occur with a variety of infections; they are not specific for infections caused by gram-negative bacteria.

   c. **Tachycardia,** especially if new or unexplained, also can suggest infection.

   d. **Inflammation,** if present, suggests underlying infection. Note, however, that granulocytopenic patients often fail to show a normal inflammatory response to infection. Consequently, bacterial pneumonia can present without an identifiable infiltrate on chest x-ray film, or even without significant sputum production. Similarly, abscess formation is often minimal or absent, despite significant local or systemic infection.

3. **Leukocytosis,** especially when accompanied by an increase in neutrophils or band-form neutrophils, suggests infection. Of course, patients who are neutropenic from chemotherapy will not show this re-

sponse. Toxic granulation and Döhle's bodies in neutrophils also suggest infection.

B. Evaluation of patients with suspected infection

1. **General.** A thorough, daily evaluation of all hospitalized patients with cancer who are neutropenic is necessary to diagnose and treat infections properly. Areas that should not be overlooked include the retinae, ears and sinuses, mouth (including tapping the teeth with a tongue blade), skin, catheter sites, axillae, perineum, perianal region, and extremities. Routine rectal examinations should not be performed; however, the perirectal area should be gently palpated for areas of pain or induration.

2. **Cultures**

   a. **General approach.** Culture material from multiple sites needs to be obtained whenever infection is suspected. All culture material should be delivered promptly to the microbiology laboratory.

   b. **Blood**

      (1) **Technique.** At least two sets (one set = one aerobic and one anaerobic bottle) should be drawn. Each set should be from a different site. At least 5 ml of blood should be injected into each culture bottle.

      (2) **Central venous catheters.** If these indwelling devices are present, it is important to obtain additional culture material through each port of the device, as well as to obtain peripheral specimens in the usual manner.

      (3) **Resin bottles.** Culture bottles containing an antibiotic-binding resin or other antibiotic-binding substance should be included with each culture set for patients who are receiving antibiotics at the time of evaluation. This may increase the culture yield by approximately 10%.

   c. **Urine.** Clean-catch or straight-catheterization specimens are preferred. Urine that has been present in a closed collection system for more than an hour should not be sent for culture. If necessary, urine can be obtained from the catheter tubing using a syringe and a small-gauge needle.

   d. **Sputum**

      (1) **Spontaneously expectorated.** A good specimen should have fewer than 10 squamous epithelial cells per low-power (100×) field.

      (2) **Induced.** The yield on culture can be increased by using 3% saline solution delivered through an ultrasonic nebulizer. Three percent saline solution can cause significant bronchospasm, and should be administered cautiously only by trained personnel.

> (3) **Transtracheal aspiration.** This procedure is used rarely. More commonly, patients undergo bronchoscopy or open lung biopsy if pulmonary pathology is suspected and the first two techniques fail to provide an answer.

e. Cerebrospinal fluid (CSF)

> (1) **Criteria.** A lumbar puncture should be performed on any patient who has an abnormal or a changed finding on neurologic examination. It should be considered seriously in any patient in whom no other source can be found to explain the suspected infection.

> (2) **Studies.** CSF always should be sent for Gram's stain, bacterial and fungal cultures, bacterial antigen panel, cell count with differential, glucose (including simultaneous serum glucose) and protein measurements, and cytology. A cryptococcal antigen titer with or without an India ink preparation should be performed if the patient has reasons for cellular immune dysfunction. Acid-fast bacillus (AFB) stains and cultures are not indicated routinely, and require at least 10 ml of fluid for optimal yield.

f. Stool

> (1) *Clostridium difficile.* This toxin-producing anaerobic bacterium is a common cause of diarrhea in patients who have been on antibiotics. A mild to moderate leukocytosis, as well as a fever to 38.5°C, typically is part of the syndrome. All patients with diarrhea should have stool sent for a cytotoxic assay for *C. difficile* toxin. Rapid antigen detection tests are unreliable.

> (2) **Bacterial cultures.** A stool culture should be sent to the microbiology laboratory in patients in whom the diagnosis of infectious diarrhea is suspected. Occasionally, *Salmonella* species and *Listeria monocytogenes* are causes of nosocomial diarrhea and sepsis.

> (3) **Fecal leukocytes.** The presence of white blood cells (WBCs) in the stool suggests an invasive inflammatory process of the colon. Fecal leukocytes are seen with *Shigella* species, *Campylobacter* species, invasive *E. coli,* and, variably, *Salmonella* species and *C. difficile.* A methylene blue stain of the stool should be ordered routinely along with the culture.

> (4) **Ova and parasites.** Patients in whom diarrhea develops more than 3 days after hospitalization almost never have a parasitic cause for the diarrhea. The routine ordering of this test should be discouraged. The im-

portant exception is in regions in which *Strongyloides stercoralis* is endemic (e.g., southeastern United States).

g. Viral cultures

(1) HSV and varicella zoster virus (VZV). Suspicious vesicular lesions need to be cultured for HSV or VZV. Fluid-filled lesions should be carefully unroofed. A swab should be rubbed on the base of the lesion and sent in viral transport media to the laboratory within ½ hour. These specimens need to be inoculated promptly into tissue culture or stored at 4–9°C for no more than 18 hours. While it is reasonably easy to isolate HSV using these techniques, VZV is much harder to isolate. It may be prudent to call the hospital virology laboratory for assistance.

(2) CMV. Bone marrow transplant patients who are suspected of being infected with CMV should have blood (in an appropriately designated sodium heparin tube) and urine sent to the virology laboratory. When appropriate, induced sputum or bronchoalveolar lavage fluid also should be sent. No special transport media is required for any of these specimens, but they should be handled as described earlier.

h. Other. Biopsy or aspirate cultures from any accessible suspected site of infection should be obtained as soon as possible. The risk of complications from such procedures (e.g., infection, bleeding) must be weighed against the possible gains.

3. Imaging studies

a. Radiographs. A chest x-ray film should be obtained routinely for any patient suspected of having an infection. Sinus films may also be quite helpful. Panorex films of the teeth to look for periapical abscesses should be taken in the febrile neutropenic patient in whom a source of infection cannot be identified.

b. Computed tomography (CT). CT scans of the chest, abdomen, brain, sinuses, head and neck, spine, and other areas can add considerable information to the diagnostic work-up. The specific scan(s) ordered should be individualized to the clinical situation.

c. Ultrasonography. An echocardiogram should be obtained when endocarditis is suspected. A transesophageal echocardiogram is more sensitive, but also more invasive, than the standard transthoracic approach. Ultrasonography is very good at detecting ascites and biliary, hepatic, and pancreatic pathology. A portable (bedside) ultrasound unit can be useful in critically ill patients who are too sick to be transported to the radiology department.

  d. Nuclear medicine. Unfortunately, radionuclide scanning using indium-labeled granulocytes or gallium is often nondiagnostic. False-positive and false-negative results occur too frequently to recommend these tests on a routine basis. However, they can be useful, on occasion, to diagnose an unsuspected occult abscess.

4. Invasive studies

  a. Bronchoscopy. Bronchoalveolar lavage for fungi, CMV, and *P. carinii* should be considered for patients at risk for one of these organisms. The adequacy of the specimen can be ascertained by noting the presence of alveolar macrophages on subsequent stains. Specimens also should be sent for Gram's stain, AFB stain and culture, bacterial culture, and direct fluorescent antibody (DFA) testing for *Legionella* species. Note that many centers prefer to perform DFA testing on urine specimens because, on occasion, nonspecific debris from respiratory secretions will fluoresce and result in a false-positive interpretation.

  b. Skin biopsy. Biopsy of suspicious dermatologic lesions should be done and specimens sent for culture and silver (fungal) staining.

  c. Open lung biopsy. A persistent unexplained infiltrate on chest x-ray films often is evaluated best with this approach. Morbidity is low in patients with adequate platelet counts and normal coagulation.

  d. Bone marrow biopsy. Specimens should be sent for AFB stain and culture, and fungal stain and culture.

  e. Percutaneous liver biopsy. Occasionally this procedure is helpful if abnormalities referable to the liver are suspected based on imaging studies or serum chemistry values. It may be the only way to diagnose hepatic candidiasis with certainty. Hepatic candidiasis should be considered in the patient who has a persistent fever despite the recovery of neutrophils.

  f. Exploratory laparotomy. Even multiple imaging studies sometimes fail to reveal intraabdominal abscesses. A positive blood culture and abdominal tenderness should be a clue to this diagnosis. An exploratory laparotomy might be required if symptoms persist. Alternatively, surgery may need to be considered if intraabdominal abnormalities detected by other studies fail to resolve with therapy.

5. Miscellaneous studies

  a. A **complete blood cell count** with differential should be performed on every patient suspected of having an infection.

> **b. Liver function test results** are often abnormal in generalized sepsis or during infections involving the organ itself.
>
> **c.** A **urinalysis** can help differentiate infection from contamination: The absence of WBCs suggests the latter diagnosis. Note, however, that WBCs may be absent in neutropenic patients. Conversely, even 1 WBC in the urine of a neutropenic patient should be considered significant.
>
> **d. Sedimentation rate** is nonspecific, rarely useful, and seldom indicated in the evaluation for suspected infection.

C. Therapy

  1. Antibiotic resistance

  a. General trends. Resistance to multiple antibiotics among gram-negative and gram-positive bacteria is increasingly common. Even community-acquired organisms may show resistance to some previously dependable antibiotics. The length of time that an antibiotic has been available does not correlate reliably with resistance rates. For instance, many bacteria now are resistant to the third-generation cephalosporins, but remain sensitive to the aminoglycosides that have been available for decades. Expect resistance rates to continue to increase for the foreseeable future.

  b. Specific problem organisms

   (1) *Escherichia coli* **and** *Klebsiella pneumoniae.* Many strains of these bacteria now carry plasmids that code for resistance to all penicillins, including the extended-spectrum penicillins such as piperacillin. This resistance typically does not result from increased production of beta-lactamase, but rather occurs due to decreased outer membrane permeability. Consequently, beta-lactam/beta-lactamase inhibitor combination drugs such as ticarcillin-clavulanate are not likely to be effective alternatives.

   (2) *Enterobacter cloacae* **and** *Enterobacter aerogenes.* These bacteria become resistant to the third-generation cephalosporin antibiotics very quickly after exposure, due to greatly increased bacterial production of cephalosporinases. Therefore, it probably is prudent to avoid the cephalosporins when *Enterobacter* species are isolated or suspected.

   (3) *Staphylococcus aureus.* Methicillin resistance, which signifies resistance to all beta-lactam antibiotics, is now endemic among the staphylococci at most hospitals. Many tertiary-referral centers report resistance rates exceeding 30%. Vancomycin remains the drug of choice for covering all known or suspected infections involving gram-positive organisms, at least until the sensitivities of the infecting pathogens are known.

2. **Empiric therapy**

   a. **Timing.** Two or three oral temperature elevations above 38°C in a 24-hour period, or one elevation above 38.3°C, suggests infection. Patients with fewer than 500 neutrophils/μl should be started on antibiotics at this time. Nonneutropenic patients also may require antibiotics, but that decision should be individualized based on other findings.

   b. **Neutropenic coverage.** Prompt initiation of empiric antibiotic therapy has been shown to reduce mortality. Despite the success of monotherapy with ceftazidime or imipenem in some studies, the use of combination therapy is preferred by most infectious disease specialists for neutropenic patients. The main advantage of combination therapy is to increase the chance of empirically covering all infecting pathogens in an era of increasing bacterial resistance to antibiotics. However, combination therapy is unlikely to reduce resistance rates, and may increase the risk of side effects.

      (1) **Recommended regimens.** See Table 31-1. Two antipseudomonal antibiotics usually are included, despite the decreasing incidence of infections caused by *P. aeruginosa*. Current

Table 31-1. Recommended initial antibiotic regimens for neutropenic patients with normal renal function

Combination therapy
1. Piperacillin 3 gm q6h + tobramycin 2 mg/kg q8h, *or*
2. Ticarcillin-clavulanate 3.1 gm q6h + tobramycin as above, *or*
3. Ceftazidime 2 gm q8h + tobramycin as above

Monotherapy
1. Ceftazidime 2 gm q8h, *or*
2. Imipenem 750 mg q6h

Note: 1. Vancomycin 1 gm q12h can be *added* to any of the above regimens for better gram-positive coverage.
2. Amikacin at 8–10 mg/kg q12h can be *substituted* for tobramycin at institutions with significant bacterial resistance rates to tobramycin.
3. Tobramycin can be dosed at 5 mg/kg q24h and amikacin dosed at 15–20 mg/kg q24h, without apparent increased toxicity in recent studies.

Antifungal therapy with amphotericin
1. For candidiasis and initial empiric therapy: 0.5–0.6 mg/kg/day
2. For cryptococcosis or histoplasmosis: 0.6–0.8 mg/kg/day
3. For resistant candidiasis or persistent fever: 0.8–1.2 mg/kg/day
4. For aspergillosis: 1.0–1.5 mg/kg/day

popular combinations include a beta-lactam such as piperacillin or ceftazidime, combined with an aminoglycoside such as tobramycin or amikacin. Other regimens are possible; the one that is chosen should reflect local sensitivity patterns. Gentamicin typically is not used because of its poorer activity against *P. aeruginosa* compared to tobramycin or amikacin.

For patients who have had life-threatening allergic reactions to penicillins or cephalosporins, imipenem with or without tobramycin is recommended.

(2) **Double beta-lactam combinations.** These regimens have the potential advantage of avoiding aminoglycoside nephrotoxicity and ototoxicity. Unfortunately, cross-resistance to all beta-lactams occurs commonly with many gram-negative organisms. As noted previously, resistance to the aminoglycosides, especially tobramycin and amikacin, has been much slower to develop. Therefore, double beta-lactam combinations typically will not cover as many gram-negative organisms as will the combination of a beta-lactam and an aminoglycoside.

(3) **Duration.** Antibiotics generally should be continued for a full 14-day course in patients who remain neutropenic, even if they become afebrile during therapy. Fourteen days is a reasonable clinical compromise between stopping antibiotics as soon as neutropenic patients become afebrile versus continuing antibiotics for the entire duration of neutropenia. Patients who show recovery of their granulocyte counts to more than $500/\mu l$ can have their antibiotics discontinued after they have been afebrile for at least 72 hours.

(4) **Antifungal therapy.** Amphotericin B 0.5–0.6 mg/kg/day should be started if neutropenic patients remain febrile despite broad-spectrum antibiotic coverage for longer than 3–5 days. Patients should routinely be pretreated with 25–50 mg of meperidine IV and 650 mg of acetaminophen PO ½ hour prior to starting the amphotericin infusion to minimize febrile reactions and rigors that commonly accompany this drug. These doses may be repeated once in 2 hours if necessary. The amphotericin B infusion should be given over 2 hours; longer infusions do not minimize reactions in most patients. Liposome-encapsulated preparations, or an intravenous fat emulsion product (e.g., Intralipid) added to amphotericin B infusions, may decrease the number and severity of

side effects, but these approaches have not been compared to standard amphotericin B infusions in large clinical trials.

For patients with an initially normal creatinine clearance (or a serum creatinine < 2 mg/dl), a rise in serum creatinine concentration of up to 3 times the baseline value can be tolerated before the therapy must be held or the dose reduced. For patients who have an initial creatinine of 2–4 mg/dl, a rise of 1.5–2.0 times the baseline value is all that should be allowed prior to dose reduction or discontinuation.

Although the optimal duration of therapy is unknown, it is prudent to continue antifungal therapy at least as long as neutropenia exists, or to a minimum total dose of 500 mg. The imidazole derivatives ketoconazole, fluconazole, and itraconazole show promise, but cannot be recommended in place of amphotericin B at this time.

c. **Aminoglycoside dosing.** A loading dose of 2–3 mg/kg of tobramycin, or 8–10 mg/kg of amikacin, should be given initially. High peak serum levels (e.g., 7–8 μg/ml of tobramycin) have been shown to be beneficial in treating infections in neutropenic patients. To avoid unacceptably high trough levels, it often is necessary to decrease the dosing frequency and increase the amount given with each dose. A reasonable approach is to give slightly less than a loading dose (e.g., 1.7–2.0 mg/kg of tobramycin) with each dose, and adjust only the dosing interval by monitoring peak and trough levels. Recently, a regimen utilizing oncedaily dosing of amikacin (20 mg/kg q24h) was found to be as effective and no more toxic than a regimen utilizing thrice-daily dosing of amikacin (6.5 mg/kg q8h) in a large, multicenter trial involving febrile neutropenic patients with cancer and normal renal function.

d. **Gram-positive coverage.** The addition of an antistaphylococcal antibiotic to the initial empiric regimen should be considered in patients with indwelling vascular catheters, with integumentary damage from any cause, and at centers with high rates of gram-positive infections. Vancomycin is preferred because of its efficacy against methicillin-resistant *S. aureus, S. epidermidis,* and *C. jeikeium.*

e. **Additional coverage.** Patients at risk for pneumonia caused by *P. carinii* or the *Legionella* species should have trimethoprim-sulfamethoxazole or erythromycin, respectively, included in their antibiotic regimens, if evidence for pulmonary infection exists. Anaerobic coverage (e.g., metronidazole or clindamycin) should be considered for patients with necrotizing gingivitis or perianal tenderness.

   f. Therapeutic algorithm. The therapeutic approach to the febrile neutropenic patient is summarized in Figure 31-1.

3. Definitive therapy

   a. Antibiotics

   (1) General. Reevaluation of the empiric antibiotic regimen is mandatory when the identity and sensitivity pattern of an isolated pathogen become available.

   (2) Gram-negative infections. Although monotherapy with ceftazidime or imipenem is an option, neutropenic patients usually are treated with two antibiotics, each effective against the isolated organism.

   (3) Gram-positive infections. One antibiotic is sufficient, but coverage against gram-negative organisms should be continued in neutropenic patients, as discussed previously.

   b. Specific infections

   (1) Catheter-related sepsis. Staphylococcal infections predominate. Removal of infected indwelling intravascular devices is optimal, but not always possible. Eradication of infection often can be accomplished with long-term antibiotics alone. There is approximately a 70–80% chance of curing a gram-positive infection (e.g., *S. epidermidis*) with antibiotics administered for 3–4 weeks. The antibiotic administration should be rotated through each port of the device. The chance of success drops to 30–50% for gram-negative infections. Fungal infection or infection with *C. jeikeium* requires immediate removal of the catheter. Tunnel infections generally also require catheter removal.

   (2) *Candida* infections

   (a) Significance. Isolation of *Candida* species from sputum, urine, stool, or drainage fluid is not necessarily synonymous with infection. On the other hand, isolation of *Candida* species from three or more nonblood sites has been shown to correlate with disseminated candidiasis in neutropenic patients. Isolation of this organism from the blood is always significant and requires immediate therapy. Isolation of *Candida* species from catheter tips usually warrants at least a short course of therapy, even though the catheter has been removed. The presence of macronodular skin lesions shown on biopsy to be consistent with candidal infection is synonymous with dissemination.

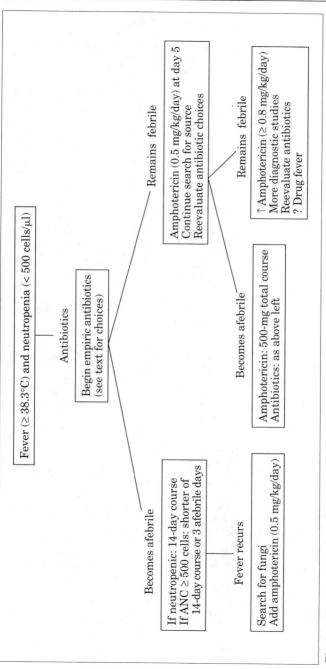

Fig. 31-1. Therapeutic approach to the febrile neutropenic patient. ANC = absolute neutrophil count.

(b) **Therapy.** Amphotericin B remains the treatment of choice. The optimum dose and duration are unknown, especially in patients who remain neutropenic. A total dose of at least 500 mg is recommended for candidemia or disseminated candidiasis. A total dose of 150 mg may be sufficient for treatment of catheter-related infections with *Candida* species in patients in whom the catheter has been removed. The addition of 5-fluoro-cytosine (flucytosine) is often synergistic, and may increase response rates. This latter agent is potentially bone marrow suppressive; serum levels should be monitored.

(c) **Dissemination.** Candidemia or other evidence of dissemination should prompt a search for deep organ involvement. Weekly funduscopic examinations are essential in such circumstances. Surgery, when feasible, may improve survival in selected patients with deep organ involvement. Patients with documented deep organ involvement are likely to require 1 gm or more of amphotericin therapy.

(3) *Aspergillus* **infections.** Even a single positive culture for one of the *Aspergillus* species warrants the initiation of therapy. Pulmonary involvement is the most common disease manifestation, but thrombosis of major blood vessels and widespread dissemination occur in neutropenic patients. Aggressive therapy is necessary to reduce mortality: Early initiation of amphotericin B at doses of 1.0–1.5 mg/kg/day is recommended. A total course of 2 gm is typical.

(4) **HSV and VZV infections.** Early initiation of therapy helps to prevent dissemination. The dose of acyclovir for herpes simplex infections in immunocompromised patients with normal renal function is 6.25 mg/kg every 8 hours, administered intravenously. Varicella zoster infections require 12.5 mg/kg of acyclovir every 8 hours. Serum levels following an oral dose average about 25% of levels obtained after an intravenous dose; for this reason, oral acyclovir typically is not used for acute HSV or VZV infections in patients with cancer. High-dose oral regimens (800 mg 5 times daily) have been tried with some success, but gastrointestinal distress is a common side effect. Foscarnet, a new intravenous antiviral agent with activity against all herpes-group viruses and human

immunodeficiency virus type 1 (HIV-1), can be used to treat resistant HSV and VZV infections (40 mg/kg every 8 hours).

(5) *Nocardia* infections. Altered cell-mediated immunity, whether intrinsic or corticosteroid-induced, is the main risk factor for infection with these organisms. The treatment of choice remains oral sulfadiazine, 6–8 gm/day. Therapy should be continued for at least 3 months, and regimens of 6–12 months are not uncommon. Trimethoprim-sulfamethoxazole (intravenous or oral), sulfisoxazole, and triple-sulfonamide combinations are likely to be as efficacious as sulfadiazine. Minocycline is an alternative for patients with sulfa allergies, and imipenem has shown impressive in vitro activity.

c. Biologic response modifiers

(1) Granulocyte transfusions have not consistently demonstrated beneficial results in controlled trials. Transfusion reactions, allosensitization to human leukocyte antigens (HLA), and transfusion-associated CMV infection occur frequently, and further limit the usefulness of this approach. An increased incidence of severe pulmonary reactions, especially when transfusions are given to patients receiving amphotericin B, has also been noted. Granulocyte transfusions are rarely recommended.

(2) Granulocyte colony-stimulating factor (G-CSF) and granulocyte-macrophage colony-stimulating factor (GM-CSF) in controlled trials have shown efficacy in reducing the depth and duration of chemotherapy-induced neutropenia in certain cancers. In addition, at least one trial showed that the use of G-CSF resulted in a 50% reduction in the number of febrile episodes and a concomitant reduction in the duration of antibiotic therapy. No survival benefit has been shown in any trial. Economic impact studies have not been completed at this time, although some modeling studies suggest that at standard doses of chemotherapy for nonhematologic malignancies, hospitalization for febrile neutropenia followed by dose reduction on subsequent cycles is equally efficacious and much less expensive than preemptive use of G-CSF.

(3) Passive immunization

(a) Monoclonal antibodies. Despite initial enthusiasm, no benefit has been demonstrated for monoclonal antibodies directed against lipid A (endotoxin), the *Enterobacteriaceae* common antigen

(ECA), or tumor necrosis factor. A large clinical trial of the interleukin (IL)-1 receptor antagonist also failed to demonstrate efficacy. Additional clinical trials of other anticytokine preparations are ongoing. However, many of these proinflammatory cytokines actually may have some beneficial effect on host defenses. Immunization with a "cocktail" of antibodies directed against different antigenic determinates ultimately may show benefit, but this approach is an elusive dream at present.

(b) Pooled immunoglobulin preparations. These preparations contain antibodies to many potential pathogens. Results of early controlled trials have been disappointing.

(4) Interleukins and interferon. Activation of monocytes and neutrophils by these substances might be expected to reduce mortality from certain kinds of infections. Unfortunately, systemic side effects might limit the usefulness of this approach.

IV. Prevention of infection

A. Environmental manipulations

1. **Handwashing and mask.** Numerous studies have confirmed that scrupulous adherence to good handwashing technique reduces infections. Handwashing is the single most important way to reduce the risk of infection. Patients should be told to remind their physicians to wash their hands before allowing them to proceed with the examination. In addition, handwashing signs should be placed outside of neutropenic patients' rooms as a reminder to all personnel.

   Masks probably do little to filter microbes, but having them outside the door for personnel or visitors who have respiratory infections serves as a reminder that they should limit their visits and the exposure of the patient to additional infectious sources.

2. **Protective isolation**

   a. **Definition.** The concept of a "total protected environment" includes the use of laminar air flow rooms; sterilization of all objects placed in those rooms; gowning, masking, and gloving of personnel before entering the rooms; decontamination of the skin and gut with antimicrobial agents; and special food preparation to reduce the number of microorganisms present on the food.

   b. **Disadvantages.** This approach is expensive and cumbersome for patients, their families, and hospital personnel, and decreases perceived quality of life. It also is difficult to justify: Recent studies did not show a significant advantage of protective isolation when compared with other preventive techniques.

3. Reservoir recognition and removal

a. **Foods.** Fresh fruits and vegetables and nonprocessed dairy products are frequently contaminated with gram-negative bacteria, especially *P. aeruginosa, E. coli,* and *K. pneumoniae.* Adherence to a cooked diet during periods of neutropenia helps to reduce the risk of infection with these organisms.

b. **Objects.** Faucet aerators, sinks, shower heads, and flowers are known to harbor bacteria. However, most epidemiologic studies did not find these objects to be significant causes of infection. No special precautions, except for good hand-washing technique, are necessary.

c. **Construction.** The incidence of infections caused by *Aspergillus* species is increased in areas of construction. Patients at risk should be moved to other areas of the hospital during periods of renovation.

B. Surveillance cultures.
Routine bacterial surveillance cultures are rarely of benefit. In centers where *Aspergillus* is a significant problem, periodic fungal cultures of the nares for this fungus might be useful for early detection.

C. Prophylaxis

1. Antibiotics

a. **Nonabsorbable agents**

(1) **Rationale.** Oral vancomycin, gentamicin, and nystatin have been used in attempts to suppress gut flora and lessen the importance of this reservoir of infection.

(2) **Disadvantages.** The combination of antibiotics is poorly tolerated by patients; increased bacterial resistance develops, especially to gentamicin; the regimens do not provide protection against bacteria originating from other body sites; and some controlled studies failed to demonstrate decreased infection rates.

(3) **Recommendations.** These oral nonabsorbable antibiotics should not be utilized.

b. **Quinolones**

(1) **Efficacy.** Both norfloxacin and ciprofloxacin have been shown to reduce the incidence of infection (but not mortality) in neutropenic patients with cancer.

(2) **Mechanism of action.** The quinolones suppress gram-negative and gram-positive aerobic gut flora, and also achieve therapeutic serum and tissue levels against many bacteria.

(3) **Recommendations.** Side effects have been minimal, and resistance has been slow to develop. Some cancer centers now routinely place patients on a regimen of 400 mg of norfloxacin twice daily prior to beginning che-

motherapy. The quinolones are not approved for use in children.

   c. **Trimethoprim-sulfamethoxazole.** The use of this agent has fallen out of favor for bacterial prophylaxis because of its potential for bone marrow suppression and other side effects. Increased bacterial resistance and breakthrough infections also have been observed.

   d. **Third-generation cephalosporins.** Several clinical studies have shown a reduction in infections by using these drugs prophylactically to "selectively decontaminate" the gut. However, the potential for increased bacterial resistance has limited the usefulness of this approach.

2. **Antifungal agents.** Prophylaxis, usually against *Candida* species, has been attempted with a number of antifungal agents. The incidence of superficial and systemic fungal infections was reduced by using fluconazole (450 mg/day) in one recent placebo-controlled study. Disadvantages include the potential for emergence of resistant strains and the lack of coverage by fluconazole against fungi such as *Aspergillus* species and the agents of mucormycosis. The routine use of antifungal prophylaxis with fluconazole is controversial at this time.

3. **Antiviral agents.** Both intravenous (6.25 mg/kg twice daily) and oral acyclovir (200–400 mg 3–5 times daily) can prevent recurrences of herpes simplex infections. Acyclovir is ineffective for treatment of CMV infections; high-dose intravenous acyclovir therapy (12.5 mg/kg 3 times daily) for 1 month following bone marrow transplantation may reduce the incidence of subsequent CMV infections. Ganciclovir, an intravenous antiviral agent with activity against all herpes-group viruses, shows promise in reducing the incidence of CMV infections in patients undergoing bone marrow transplantation.

4. **Antiparasitic agents**
   a. *Pneumocystis carinii.* Trimethoprim-sulfamethoxazole (1 double-strength tablet given twice daily on 2 or 3 consecutive days weekly) is effective prophylaxis against this organism. Monthly aerosolized pentamidine may also be of value.
   b. *Strongyloides stercoralis.* Patients living in endemic areas should have stool cultures evaluated and treatment initiated (if necessary) before immunosuppressive therapy is started.

D. Immunization
   1. **Vaccines.** Live attenuated viral vaccines should not be used in immunocompromised patients. The efficacy of vaccines against *S. pneumoniae* and *H. influenzae* in immunocompromised patients is suspect. Nevertheless, many authorities recommend their use prior to immunosuppressive therapy.

2. Biologic response modifiers

a. Pooled immunoglobulin. These preparations, given intravenously at doses of 0.1–0.2 gm/kg of body weight at monthly intervals, have been used in patients with chronic lymphocytic leukemia, multiple myeloma, and other malignancies. Controlled trials seem to indicate some reduction in bacterial infections, but the preparations are expensive, and lifelong therapy is required. Their routine use is not recommended.

b. Monoclonal antibodies. Prophylactic administration of antibodies directed against virulence determinates of gram-negative bacteria ultimately may be of value in reducing the incidence of infection. However, no benefit has been demonstrated in clinical trials to date.

3. Varicella zoster immune globulin (1 vial/10 kg of body weight, to a maximum of 5 vials) is effective in reducing morbidity and mortality in seronegative immunocompromised patients exposed to varicella. The product should be given intramuscularly within 96 hours of exposure.

E. Miscellaneous. Intravenous catheters (nonsurgically placed) should be changed at least every 72 hours. Rectal temperatures, rectal suppositories, and unnecessary rectal examinations should be avoided in neutropenic patients. Patients should be encouraged to be out of bed as much as possible.

Selected Readings

Berkman, S. A., Lee, M. L., and Gale, R. P. Clinical uses of intravenous immuno-globulins. *Ann. Intern. Med.* 112:278, 1990.

Crawford, J., et al. Reduction by granulocyte colony-stimulating factor of fever and neutropenia in patients with small-cell lung cancer. *N. Engl. J. Med.* 325:164, 1991.

Hughes, W. T., et al. From the Infectious Diseases Society of America: guidelines for the use of antimicrobial agents in neutropenic patients with unexplained fever. *J. Infect. Dis.* 161:381, 1990.

International Antimicrobial Therapy Cooperative Group of the European Organization for Research and Treatment of Cancer. Efficacy and toxicity of single daily doses of amikacin and ceftriaxone versus multiple daily doses of amikacin and ceftazidime for infection in patients with cancer and granulocytopenia. *Ann. Intern. Med.* 119:584, 1993.

Karp, J. E., Merz, W. G., and Hendricksen, C. Oral norfloxacin for prevention of gram-negative bacterial infections in patients with acute leukemia and granulocytopenia. *Ann. Intern. Med.* 106:1, 1987.

Klastersky, J., et al. Empiric antimicrobial therapy for febrile granulocytopenic cancer patients: lessons from four EORTC trials. *Eur. J. Cancer Clin. Oncol.* 24(suppl. 1):S35, 1988.

Natanson, C., et al. Selected treatment strategies for septic shock based on proposed mechanisms of pathogenesis. *Ann. Intern. Med.* 120:771, 1994.

Newman, K. A., et al. Venous access devices utilized in association with intensive cancer chemotherapy. *Eur. J. Cancer Clin. Oncol.* 25:1375, 1989.

Nichols, C. R., et al. Incidence of neutropenic fever in patients treated with standard-dose combination chemotherapy for small-cell lung cancer and the cost impact of treatment with granulocyte colony-stimulating factor. *J. Clin. Oncol.* 12:1245, 1994.

Pizzo, P. Management of fever in patients with cancer and treatment-induced neutropenia. *N. Engl. J. Med.* 328:1323, 1993.

Schmidt, G. M., et al. A randomized, controlled trial of prophylactic ganciclovir for cytomegalovirus pulmonary infection in recipients of allogeneic bone marrow transplants. *N. Engl. J. Med.* 324:1005, 1991.

Steward, W. P. Granulocyte and granulocyte-macrophage colony-stimulating factors. *Lancet* 342:153, 1993.

Disorders of Hemostasis and Transfusion Therapy

Mary R. Smith

Disorders of the hemostatic mechanisms are common in patients with malignancy. Abnormalities associated with thromboembolic events cause significantly more morbidity and mortality than disorders leading to hemorrhage.

I. **Thromboembolism in cancer**

   A. **Pathophysiology.** The thromboembolic risk associated with neoplasia reflects an imbalance between platelet number, platelet function, levels of coagulation factors, and generation of thromboplastins, compared to the levels of inhibitors of hemostasis, and fibrinolytic activity. Thrombosis may be minor and localized, or widespread and associated with multiple-organ damage. There may also be hemorrhage of varying degrees of severity in association with the thromboembolic events.

   1. **Factors that may affect the risk of thromboembolism** vary widely from patient to patient. They include the following.

      a. Specific type of tumor

      b. Nutritional status of the patient

      c. Type of chemotherapy

      d. Response of chemotherapy, e.g., tumor lysis syndrome

      e. Liver and renal function

      f. Patient immobility and venous stasis

   2. **Factors that can initiate thrombus formation** are common to many cancers.

      a. Circulating tumor cells adhere to the vascular endothelium and form a nidus for clot formation.

      b. Tumors may penetrate the vessel, destroying the endothelium and promoting clot formation.

      c. Neovascularization associated with many tumors may stimulate clotting.

      d. Arterial thrombosis associated with tumors may result from vasospasm.

      e. A systemic hypercoagulable state develops (e.g., decreased protein C).

      f. External compression of vessels by tumor masses impedes blood flow and leads to stasis and clot development.

   3. **Platelet abnormalities** associated with an increased risk of thromboembolism include thrombocytosis and increased platelet adhesion and aggregation. Tumors may produce substances that cause increased platelet aggregation with subsequent release of platelet factor 3 and ensuing acceleration of coagulation.

   B. **Clinical syndromes.** A variety of noteworthy clinical syndromes are associated with the "hypercoagulable state" of malignancy and of its treatment.

1. **Disseminated intravascular coagulation (DIC).**
   DIC is a syndrome with many signs, symptoms, and laboratory abnormalities (Table 32-1). As many as 90% of patients with metastatic neoplasms have some laboratory manifestation of DIC, but only a small fraction of these patients suffer morbidity from the coagulation process or subsequent depletion of coagulation factors and consequent bleeding due to DIC. The initiating factor for DIC is apparent in some situations, but unknown in others. Among the common initiators of DIC are the following.
   a. Thromboplastic substances in granules from promyelocytes of acute promyelocytic leukemia (DIC may worsen with therapy). There is a significant concomitant fibrinolysis in many patients.
   b. Sialic acid from mucin produced by adenocarcinomas of the lung or gastrointestinal tract.
   c. Trypsin released from pancreatic cancer.
   d. Impaired fibrinolysis associated with hepatocellular carcinoma.
   e. DIC in any patient may be fostered by sepsis or other causes of the systemic inflammatory response syndrome (SIRS).
2. **Lupus anticoagulant** in neoplastic disease. The lupus anticoagulant is an antiphospholipid antibody (IgG or IgM). Antiphospholipid antibodies are reported to be associated with a number of malignant disorders including hairy cell leukemia, lymphoma,

Table 32-1. Laboratory diagnosis of disseminated intravascular coagulation (DIC)

Laboratory tests	Acute DIC	Chronic DIC
Screening		
PT, APTT	Usually prolonged	Normal
Platelets	Usually decreased	Normal or slightly decreased
Fibrinogen	Usually decreased but may be normal[a]	Usually normal[a]
Confirmatory[b]		
Fibrin monomer	Positive	Positive
FDP	Strongly positive	Positive
D-Dimer	Positive	Positive
Thrombin time	Normal or abnormal	Usually normal
Factor assays	Decreased factors V and VIII	Normal factors V and VIII
Antithrombin III	May be reduced	Usually normal

PT = prothrombin time; APTT = activated partial thromboplastin time; FDP = fibrinogen degradation products.
[a]Fibrinogen is usually elevated in advanced malignancy or acute leukemia that is not complicated by DIC. Thus a normal fibrinogen level may actually be decreased for the physiologic state of the patient.
[b]Changes indicated are confirmatory if present; the absence of the indicated findings in some of the confirmatory tests does not exclude the diagnosis.

Waldenström's macroglobulinemia, and epithelial neoplasms. The lupus anticoagulant leads to a prolonged activated partial thromboplastin time (APTT) but is paradoxically associated with an increased risk of thrombosis.

3. **Trousseau's syndrome** (tumor-associated thrombophlebitis). Suspect the possibility of neoplasia when

   a. An unexplained thromboembolic event occurs after the age of 40.

   b. Thromboses occur in unusual sites.

   c. The thromboses affect superficial as well as deep veins.

   d. The thromboses are migratory.

   e. The thromboses tend not to respond to the "usual" anticoagulant therapies.

   f. An unexplained thrombosis occurs more than once.

4. **Thrombotic events that occur after surgery** for tumors of the lung, ovary, pancreas, or stomach.

5. **Nonbacterial thrombotic endocarditis** may be found in association with carcinoma of the lung. These thrombi are formed from accumulations of platelets and fibrin. The mitral valve is the most frequent site of origin of these thrombi, which frequently embolize.

6. **Thrombotic thrombocytopenic purpura (TTP).** TTP is a poorly understood syndrome characterized by thrombocytopenia, acute hemolysis, fever, fluctuating neurologic signs and symptoms, and acute renal failure. TTP and the hemolytic-uremic syndrome (HUS) (thrombocytopenia, hemolysis, and acute renal failure) have been associated with untreated malignancies as well as with a number of drugs used for treating malignant disease. The agent most often reported is mitomycin, but other drugs including bleomycin, cisplatin, cyclophosphamide, and vinca alkaloids may also be associated with these syndromes. TTP may be difficult to diagnose in this setting since the chemotherapy will suppress platelet production, some agents may impair renal function, and many of the features of DIC are similar to those of TTP. Careful review of the peripheral blood smear is required to identify the changes in red blood cells that one sees associated with a microangiopathic hemolytic process. The prognosis for TTP is poor, and its therapy has been varied. Plasmapheresis and transfusion with fresh-frozen plasma appear to be the best modalities of therapy.

7. **Thromboembolism associated with chemotherapy**

   a. The use of **central arterial or venous catheters** has markedly facilitated the delivery of chemotherapy, but all such catheters are associated with a significant risk of vascular thrombosis. The empiric use of low doses of warfarin (1 mg daily) decreases the risk of thrombosis without inducing a hemorrhagic state. It is not necessary to follow the prothrombin time (PT) with low-dose warfarin.

b. **Many chemotherapy agents cause significant chemical phlebitis.** The most common offending agents are mechlorethamine (nitrogen mustard), anthracyclines, nitrosoureas, mitomycin, fluorouracil, dacarbazine, and epipodophyllotoxins.

c. **L-asparaginase** inhibits the synthesis of proteins including coagulation factors. This inhibition may cause either hemorrhage or thrombosis. Patients with preexisting hemostatic disorders are at particular risk for complications when using L-asparaginase. L-asparaginase also decreases antithrombin III (AT-III) activity.

d. **Tamoxifen** has been associated with thromboembolic events. This effect may be magnified when tamoxifen is combined with chemotherapeutic agents.

e. **Estrogens** may increase the risk of thromboembolism. This is likely due, at least in part, to a decrease in protein S and an increase in coagulation factors.

f. **Superior vena cava syndrome (SVCS)** is nearly always associated with thrombosis in the thoracic venous system cephalad to the site of obstruction. SVCS may lead to upper extremity thrombosis.

C. **Principles of therapy for thrombosis associated with neoplasia**
1. **Discrete vascular thrombosis**
   a. **General guidelines.** Therapy should be directed at controlling the neoplasm. As an anticoagulant, heparin is superior to warfarin in these patients. Warfarin and antiplatelet drugs have been used with varying degrees of success in some patients with thromboembolism associated with tumors. The use of heparin, warfarin, and antiplatelet agents alone or in combination may be associated with normalization of hemostatic parameters. Despite this, patients with malignant disease are often resistant to anticoagulant therapy and may continue to have thrombotic events even while receiving what appears to be adequate anticoagulant therapy. Great care must be exercised in the use of both heparin and warfarin in patients with malignant disease since hemorrhage into areas of necrotic tumor can be hazardous. The use of anticoagulant therapy is generally contraindicated in patients with central nervous system metastases. Bulky disease is a relative contraindication, especially if central necrosis of the tumor is suspected, and particularly if the lesion is in the mediastinum or pleural spaces.

The decision to treat thromboembolism occurring in a patient with malignancy may be difficult. One must carefully weigh the risks of therapy against expected benefits. The decision will also be influenced by the patient's life expectancy, concurrent therapy, and the type of malignancy.

b. Heparin. Low doses of heparin (5000 units given subcutaneously every 12 hours) can be used to protect patients with malignant disease from thromboembolism during perioperative periods. Heparin may be used as the initial or long-term therapy for thromboembolic events in patients with malignant disease. Heparin may be administered either intravenously or by the subcutaneous route. Generally the intravenous route is preferred for initial therapy so that the anticoagulant effect begins at once and adjustment of doses can be easily achieved. An initial dose of 5000 units (70 units/kg) of heparin is given as an intravenous bolus followed by 1000–1200 units (15 units/kg)/hour as a continuous infusion. One should check the APTT 1 hour after the heparin bolus to ensure that the patient is heparinizable (i.e., not AT-III–deficient), 6 hours after beginning therapy, and 6 hours after any change in the dose of heparin. Some patients with malignant disease may appear to be "refractory to heparin"; in all likelihood this reflects low levels of AT-III due to poor production or increased consumption, both of which may occur in patients with malignant disease. (Note: Infusion therapy with L-asparaginase has been associated with reduced levels of AT-III.) As long as the AT-III activity is above 50% of normal, it is usually possible to achieve the desired anticoagulant effect if adequate doses of heparin are given. If AT-III activity is less than 50% of normal, AT-III may be replaced using AT-III concentrates or fresh-frozen plasma.

Heparin may be administered by the subcutaneous route for both the acute and the chronic management of thromboembolism associated with malignancy. Using the subcutaneous route may be less desirable when treating acute events as the onset of anticoagulant effect is somewhat slower (2–3 hours) and adjusting the therapeutic effect may be more difficult. Subcutaneous heparin can be considered for chronic therapy provided that the patient can manage the twice-daily injection and weekly monitoring of the APTT. In a patient who has been receiving intravenous heparin, one-half of the total dose of intravenous heparin received in the previous 24 hours should be given subcutaneously twice a day (e.g., 1000 units heparin/hour by intravenous infusion equals 12,000 units SQ bid). For the patient being started on subcutaneous heparin, the initial dose is 7500–10,000 units SQ bid. The partial thromboplastin time (PTT) should be checked 6 hours after the third dose of heparin. Otherwise the APTT should be checked 6 hours after a subcutaneous dose of heparin. The goal for the APTT should be similar to that of intravenous heparin, namely, 1.5–2.0 times the patient's baseline APTT.

c. **Warfarin** is often selected as the therapy of choice for chronic management of thromboembolic events associated with malignant disease. The use of warfarin in this setting is of concern, since patients with malignant disease are frequently taking multiple medications that can and often do alter the patient's response to warfarin. An additional concern about the use of warfarin in patients with malignancy is the development of purpura fulminans. This complication may be due to lower than normal protein C levels in those patients with DIC prior to initiation of warfarin therapy. Warfarin should not be used if there is laboratory evidence of DIC.

Despite these caveats, warfarin often is used for the prevention and treatment of clotting problems in patients with cancer. For most patients an international normalized ratio (INR) of 2.0–3.0 is required; for patients with mechanical prosthetic valves, recurrent systemic embolism, or lupus anticoagulant with thrombosis, an INR of 2.5–3.5 is necessary (Table 32-2). Table 32-2 also gives the recommended vitamin K_1 dose to reduce the INR to therapeutic levels in patients on warfarin with INR values higher than 4.5. Care must be taken to balance the risks of bleeding in patients with elevated INRs—with or without thrombocytopenia—against the risks of clotting and thrombosis if the reversal of the anticoagulation is too vigorous.

d. The use of **platelet-inhibiting drugs** such as aspirin, other nonsteroidal anti-inflammatory agents, or dipyridamole have met with varying degrees of success in the prevention of repeated thromboembolic events in patients with malignant disease. Care must be taken with the use of such drugs, especially in thrombocytopenic patients since the risk of bleeding associated with thrombocytopenia will be increased.

e. **Fibrinolytic therapy.** Systemic malignancy is a relative contraindication to fibrinolytic therapy.

f. **Vascular interruption** devices such as Greenfield filters may be used in patients who cannot tolerate anticoagulant therapy or who develop emboli while on adequate anticoagulant therapy.

2. **DIC.** Therapy for DIC includes the following.

a. Urgently correct shock (if present).

   b. Treat the underlying disease process.
   c. Replace depleted blood components (e.g., platelets, cryoprecipitate for fibrinogen and factor VIII, fresh-frozen plasma for other factors) if clinically significant bleeding is present.
   d. Consider the use of heparin only in the following situations.
   > **(1)** In patients with acute promyelocytic leukemia (see Chap. 23).
   > **(2)** When there is evidence of ongoing end-organ damage due to microvascular thrombosis
   > **(3)** If venous thrombosis occurs
   > These latter two complications of DIC are most likely to occur as a component of the SIRS, and the treatment of the underlying cause of the SIRS is necessary in addition to treatment with heparin. There is no evidence that chronic warfarin therapy is of value for treating the chronic DIC seen in some patients with neoplasia if thromboses are absent. Warfarin may predispose to the development of purpura fulminans in the presence of chronic DIC.

II. Bleeding in patients with cancer
   A. Tumor invasion. It is well recognized that bleeding may be a warning sign of cancer: Bloody sputum may indicate carcinoma of the lung, blood in the urine may be a sign of carcinoma of the bladder or kidney, blood in the stool may be due to carcinoma of the alimentary tract, and postmenopausal vaginal bleeding may be caused by endometrial carcinoma. In each of these instances, bleeding can be directly related to the invasive properties of cancer and disruption of normal tissue integrity.
   B. Hemostatic abnormalities. Often bleeding in patients with cancer is not due to the direct effects of the neoplasm, but to indirect effects of the cancer or its therapy on one of the components of the hemostatic system. Because of the frequency and the special management problems caused by abnormalities in the hemostatic system in patients with cancer and the frequency with which these problems occur, it is important to consider the possible causes and corrective measures in detail.
   > **1. Increased vascular fragility** may be due to chronic corticosteroid therapy, chronic malnutrition, or "senile purpura." Bleeding is usually not severe, but bruising, particularly around intravenous sites, is common. Hemostatic therapy is not necessary.
   > **2. Thrombocytopenia** may occur for a variety of reasons. Some of the more common causes are as follows.
   > > **a. Chemotherapy and radiotherapy** regularly cause depression of platelet production. Serial blood cell counts must be monitored while patients are being treated.
   > > **b. Bone marrow invasion or replacement** causing thrombocytopenia is commonly seen only

Table 32-2. Clinical indications, international normalized ratio (INR) goals, and vitamin K₁ administration for patients on warfarin

Using the INR for anticoagulation monitoring	Doses of vitamin K₁ to reduce INR in patients on warfarin		
	INR	Vitamin K₁ dosage (slow IVP)*	Time expected for response to vitamin K or to repeat INR
A. Clinical indications requiring an INR of 2.0–3.0 *Prophylaxis* Postoperative deep vein thrombosis (general surgery) Postoperative deep vein thrombosis during hip surgical procedures and fractures Myocardial infarction to prevent venous thromboembolism Transient ischemic attacks Tissue heart valves	> 4.5 but < 6	None, hold warfarin	24 hours
	> 6 but < 10	0.5–1.0 mg; may repeat dosage if INR still high at 24 hours	Reduction of INR expected at 8 hours; therapeutic INR expected at 24–48 hours

INR	Dosage	Result
> 10 but < 20	3–5 mg; may repeat dosage if INR is still high at 6–12 hours	Reductions of INR expected at 6 hours; repeat INR every 6–12 hours
> 20	10 mg; may repeat dosage if INR is still high at 6–12 hours; (consider fresh-frozen plasma)	Reduction of INR expected at 6 hours; repeat INR every 6–12 hours

Atrial fibrillation
Valvular heart disease
Recurrent deep vein thrombosis and pulmonary embolism
Arterial disease including myocardial infarction

Treatment
Venous thrombosis
Pulmonary embolism

B. Clinical indications requiring an INR of 2.5–3.5

Prophylaxis
Mechanical prosthetic valves
Recurrent systemic embolism
Lupus anticoagulant with thrombosis

*If patient is bleeding, a procedure is planned, or has just had a procedure, consider the use of fresh-frozen plasma.
Source: Modified from J. Hirsh et al. Oral anticoagulants. Mechanism of action, clinical effectiveness, and optimal therapeutic range. *Chest* 102 (suppl.):312, 1992.

with leukemias or lymphomas but may occur in other cancers that invade the bone marrow.

c. **Splenomegaly with splenic sequestration** is most common with leukemia or lymphoma.

d. **Folate deficiency with decreased platelet production** is common in patients with cancer because of poor nutrition. Dietary history should provide the clues to the diagnosis.

e. **Immune thrombocytopenic purpura (ITP).** Patients with lymphoproliferative malignancies (e.g., chronic lymphocytic leukemia (CLL), Hodgkin's disease) often develop ITP. ITP may also be the presenting symptom of a nonhematologic malignancy. Usually the ITP will improve with prednisone (1 mg/kg/day) followed by treatment of the malignancy.

f. **Drug-induced immune thrombocytopenia.** Many nonchemotherapy medications used to treat individuals with malignancy may cause immune thrombocytopenia. Offending agents to consider are heparin, vancomycin, histamine H_2-receptor antagonists, penicillins, cephalosporins, interferon, and sulfa-containing antibiotics, diuretics, or hypoglycemic agents.

g. **Graft-versus-host disease** seen after bone marrow transplantation may produce a chronic (often isolated) immune-mediated thrombocytopenia. The platelet count may respond to increased immunosuppression.

3. **Abnormalities of platelet function** must be suspected in the patient found to have a normal or near-normal platelet count but signs or symptoms of bleeding and a documented prolonged bleeding time. Most cases are secondary to drug effects, including aspirin and other nonsteroidal anti-inflammatory agents, antibiotics (e.g., ticarcillin), antidepressants (e.g., tricyclic drugs), tranquilizers, and alcohol. Consider any drug that the patient is taking as a possible offender until proved otherwise. The presence of fibrin degradation products (FDPs) is a common cause of platelet dysfunction in patients with malignancy who also have DIC. Platelet dysfunction may occur in patients with malignant paraproteinemias due to the coating of the platelet surfaces by the immunoglobulin. If renal failure develops or is present in such patients, the platelet dysfunction will be magnified.

4. **Coagulation factor deficiencies** may develop in patients with malignancy for several reasons.

a. **Acute (decompensated) DIC** depletes most clotting factors but to variable degrees.

b. **Liver failure** causes deficiency of all clotting factors except factor VIII.

c. **Malnutrition** leads to deficiency of factors II, VII, IX, and X (the vitamin K–dependent factors).

d. **Fibrinolysis** may be due to the release of urokinase in prostate cancer or secondary to DIC. This may produce hypofibrinogenemia, as well as fibrin split products which act as circulating anticoagulants.

    e. Functionally abnormal clotting factors are occasionally seen. The most commonly diagnosed abnormality is dysfibrinogenemia.

5. Acquired circulating anticoagulants may develop in patients with a number of different tumors. Many of these anticoagulants are heparinoid in nature. The most common associations are with carcinoma of the lung and myeloma. Other anticoagulants act as antithrombins; in this case the most common association is with carcinoma of the breast.

6. Chemotherapy-induced bleeding

    a. Mithramycin may lead to platelet dysfunction and a reduction in multiple coagulation factors. Hemorrhage due to these effects may occur in up to half of the patients treated with mithramycin.

    b. Anthracyclines may be associated with primary fibrinolysis or fibrinogenolysis and hemorrhage.

    c. Dactinomycin is a powerful vitamin K antagonist that causes defective synthesis of all vitamin K–dependent proteins (factors II, VII, IX, and X, protein C, and protein S).

    d. Melphalan, cytarabine, doxorubicin, vincristine, and vinblastine are all associated with platelet dysfunction.

III. Laboratory evaluation of hemostasis in patients with malignancy. About half of all patients with cancer and around 90% of those with metastases will manifest abnormalities of one or more routine coagulation parameters. These abnormalities may be minor early in the patient's disease, but as the disease progresses the hemostatic abnormalities become more pronounced. Serial coagulation tests may offer the clinician a clue to response to therapy or recurrence of malignant disease. Serial evaluations of coagulation tests are of more value in patients with no symptoms of hemostatic disruption than is a single determination.

A. Screening tests for bleeding. The following tests provide an adequate screening battery.

    1. Platelet count

    2. Bleeding time

    3. PT

    4. APTT

    5. Thrombin time

    6. Fibrinogen level

B. Interpretation of screening laboratory studies. Abnormal results of the screening tests reflect hematologic problems caused by blood vessels, platelets, or coagulation factors. The following list provides clues to the interpretation of the screening test results that help determine the most likely cause or causes of the patient's bleeding.

    1. Platelet count

        a. Normal is 150,000–450,000/μl.

      b. If thrombocytopenia is less than 100,000/μl, consider the following.

        (1) Bone marrow failure

        (2) Increased consumption of platelets

        (3) Splenic pooling of platelets

      c. Thrombocytosis with a platelet count of more than 500,000/μl.

        (1) Common in patients with neoplasms

        (2) May be seen in association with iron deficiency (e.g., secondary to gut neoplasm)

        (3) Usually poses no risk for arterial thrombosis unless the patient has a myeloproliferative disorder

2. Bleeding time. This is a useful screening test if the platelet count is normal and platelet dysfunction is suspected.

      a. A normal bleeding time requires normal platelet number, normal platelet function, and normal function of the blood vessels and connective tissues.

      b. A prolonged bleeding time may be due to thrombocytopenia, abnormal platelet function, and rarely, inadequate vessel function. The bleeding time may be spuriously prolonged in elderly individuals with "tissue paper" skin. The following formula is a rough rule of thumb to be used to estimate what the bleeding time should be in individuals who have platelet counts between 10,000 and 100,000/μl. Although it was derived using the Mielke template, the principle should still hold for contemporary bleeding time devices.

Bleeding time = 30 − (platelet count/μl ÷ 4000)

3. Prolonged PT. This is seen in the presence of the following.

      a. Deficiency of one or more of the following clotting factors: VII, X, V, II (prothrombin), or I (fibrinogen) (oral anticoagulant therapy leads to a deficiency of factors II, VII, IX, and X)

      b. Circulating anticoagulant(s) against factor VII, X, V, or II

      c. Dysfibrinogenemia

4. Prolonged APTT

      a. Deficiency of any of the following clotting factors: XII, XI, IX, VIII, X, V, II, or I. Factor XII deficiency is not associated with bleeding. Fletcher and Fitzgerald factor deficiencies (both rare) may also prolong the APTT.

      b. Circulating anticoagulants directed against the above-mentioned factors or the lupus inhibitor.

      c. Anticoagulant therapy with the following.

        (1) Heparin

        (2) Oral anticoagulants

5. Prolonged thrombin time. Prolongation of the thrombin time may be due to the following.

      a. Hypofibrinogenemia (fibrinogen < 100 mg/dl)

   b. Some forms of dysfibrinogenemia
   c. Fibrin-fibrinogen split products
   d. Heparin therapy
   e. Paraproteins
      If the thrombin time is prolonged, further studies
      to clarify the cause may be required.
   6. Low fibrinogen level. When evaluating the results
      of a fibrinogen assay, one must be familiar with the
      assay method used. Many laboratories use immuno-
      logic assays, which measure both functionally nor-
      mal and abnormal fibrinogens. If such an assay is in
      use, the thrombin time can be used to evaluate the
      functional integrity of the fibrinogen. A low func-
      tional fibrinogen level means that production is de-
      creased, consumption is increased, or a dysfibrino-
      gen is present. Fibrinogen is an acute-phase reactant
      and is often elevated with advanced malignancy. A
      fibrinogen level in the normal range may actually be
      relatively low for the patient's physiologic state, and
      thus may be a sign of DIC (see Table 32-1).
C. Laboratory findings in patients with DIC. Acute
   DIC is often associated with significant hemorrhage,
   whereas chronic DIC may be asymptomatic or associated
   with thromboses. Screening and confirmatory laboratory tests are shown in Table 32-1.
D. Additional laboratory studies. The tests listed in Table 32-3 show abnormalities that may occur in patients

**Table 32-3. Coagulation tests that may show an abnormality
in patients with cancer without clinical bleeding or thrombosis**

Test	Common result in patients with malignancy
Antithrombin III	Decreased
Beta-thromboglobulin	Increased
Cryofibrinogen	Present
D-Dimer	Increased
Factor VIII	Increased
Fibronectin	Decreased
Fibrin monomer (soluble)	Present
Fibrinogen	Increased
Fibrin(ogen) degradation products	Present
Fibrinopeptide A	Increased
Fibrinopeptide B	Increased
Plasmin	Increased
Plasminogen	Decreased
Platelet count	Increased or decreased
Platelet factor 4	Increased
Protein C	Decreased

with cancer who lack clinical signs of hemostatic derangements.

IV. Treatment of hemorrhagic syndromes in patients with malignant disease

A. Transfusion therapy

1. **General guidelines**
   a. The use of blood products must not be undertaken casually. Consider carefully the factors that will influence the use of blood products, including the following.
      (1) Alternative forms of therapy that could control bleeding, e.g., topical measures or desmopressin (DDAVP).
      (2) How symptomatic is the patient? One must take care not to "treat" an abnormal laboratory test in an asymptomatic patient. Patients with chronic DIC may demonstrate prolongation of both the PT and APTT and mild to moderate thrombocytopenia. If there is no demonstrable bleeding, there is no need to consider transfusion therapy.
   b. Use the specific blood component needed by the patient.
   c. Minimize complications of transfusion by using the following.
      (1) Only the amount and type of blood product indicated for the patient in the specific clinical setting.
      (2) Special filters, irradiated blood, or both when indicated.

2. **Blood component therapy**
   a. **Platelet transfusions**
      (1) **Available forms of platelets for transfusion.** Platelets may be ordered and transfused in various ways. Since most individuals with an underlying malignancy have the potential for needing long-term platelet support, platelet products should be leukocyte-depleted from the initiation of transfusion (see sec. **IV.A.3.**). In general, individuals needing platelet support can be started with random donor platelets. Given the added expense and the limited pools of platelet pheresis donors in many centers, single-donor and human leukocyte antigen (HLA)–matched platelets should be reserved for individuals who have become refractory to random-donor platelets (see sec. **IV.A.2.a.(4)**). There are no solid data to suggest that starting with platelet pheresis products decreases the incidence of alloimmunization. Conversely, individuals who are candidates for bone marrow transplantation should receive single-donor platelets (if available) from the initiation of platelet therapy. Individuals who are candidates for transplan-

tation with bone marrow from an HLA-matched sibling should not receive apheresis products from the potential donor prior to the transplantation.

(a) **Random-donor platelets.** Six units (usually pooled in one bag) are given each day as needed.

(b) **Single-donor platelets and HLA-matched platelets.** These come as a single pack, but represent the apheresed platelets from 3–4 liters of blood from a single donor.

(2) **Check platelet count** 1 and 24 hours after platelet transfusion to estimate survival of platelets in the patient. The expected 1-hour posttransfusion rise in platelets is 15,000 platelets/μl divided by the patient's body surface area in square meters for each unit of random-donor platelets. (Thus, for a person of 2 m^2, 6 units should produce a rise of 45,000/μl (6 × 15,000/2).)

(3) **Criteria for transfusing platelets**

(a) For patients with **reduced platelet production,** criteria for transfusion are shown in Table 32-4.

(b) **Increased platelet destruction.** Platelet transfusions are of limited benefit in patients with thrombocytopenia due to increased destruction due to either antibodies or consumption. If potentially life-threatening bleeding complicates thrombocytopenia due to increased destruction, platelet transfusions may be given; however, small increments in the platelet count usually occur. Intravenous gamma globulin (1 gm/kg IV daily × 2 days) given prior to the platelet transfusion may improve the response.

(c) **Dysfunctional platelets.** One must stop any drugs known to cause platelet dysfunction. Although the use of platelet transfusions should be considered, pharmacologic methods of enhancing platelet function such as desmopressin should be utilized if possible. (See sec. **IV.B.1.**)

(4) **Refractoriness to platelet transfusions** (platelet rise < 5000/μl after 6 units of random-donor platelets) is a common problem in multiply transfused individuals. Alloimmunization is the most difficult form to treat and therefore is best prevented (see sec. **IV.A.3.**). Apparent refractoriness to platelet transfusions may be due to shortened platelet life span from fever, septicemia, DIC, splenomegaly, drugs, or bleeding.

Table 32-4. Guidelines for platelet transfusion in patients with reduced platelet production

Platelet count	Recommendation
0–5000/μl	Transfuse with platelets even if there is no evidence of bleeding.
6000–10,000/μl	Transfuse with platelets if there is (are) Fresh minor hemorrhage Fever over 38°C or active infection Rapid decline in platelet count (> 50%/day) Headaches Significant gastrointestinal blood loss Presence of confluent petechiae (as opposed to scattered petechiae) Continuous bleeding from a wound or other sites Planned minor procedure such as a bone marrow biopsy
11,000–20,000/μl	Transfuse with platelets if there is more rapid bleeding or if more complicated procedures are anticipated.
> 20,000/μl	If major surgery is planned or when life-threatening bleeding occurs, the platelet count should be increased to at least 50,000/μl. For intracranial surgery, transfuse to a platelet count of at least 100,000/μl (bleeding time must be checked before surgery and must be normal). In fully anticoagulated individuals it is advisable to keep the platelet count at least 50,000/μl.

(a) **Evaluation.** Individuals who become refractory to platelet transfusion should have a laboratory evaluation for alloimmunization. They should also be evaluated for infection and DIC, as well as have all potentially offending medications stopped.

(b) **Therapy.** The therapeutic modalities for ITP (corticosteroids, intravenous immune globulin, danazol) are generally ineffective for platelet refractoriness due to alloimmunization. Two therapeutic options currently exist.

    (1) **HLA-matched platelets**

    (2) **Cross-matched platelets.** These appear to offer the best chance for regaining platelet responsiveness in the alloimmunized individual.

Either random-donor or apheresed platelets can be "cross-matched" with the recipient. The least reactive platelets can then be selected for transfusion.

b. Coagulation factor support

(1) **Fresh-frozen plasma** contains all clotting factors (but not platelets) and should be used for multiple coagulation factor deficiencies. Fresh-frozen plasma requires 20–30 minutes to thaw, as it must be thawed at 37°C or lower.

(2) **Cryoprecipitate ("cryo")** is a source of factor VIII–von Willebrand factor (vWF) complex, fibrinogen, and factor XIII. Each bag of cryoprecipitate contains the factor VIII/vWF and fibrinogen harvested from 1 unit of fresh whole blood. Cryoprecipitate is stored in a frozen state and has the advantage of concentrating the clotting factors in a small volume ($\leq$ 20 ml/unit). About 10–20 units are usually given, and the patient is evaluated to determine if the laboratory abnormalities have been corrected. The goal is to keep the fibrinogen level higher than 100 mg/dl. The usual dosage of cryoprecipitate to correct hypofibrinogenemia is 1 bag of cryoprecipitate for every 5 kg of body weight. Since 50% is recovered after transfusion, this may only raise the fibrinogen titer by approximately 50 mg/dl. Larger doses may be needed for severe hypofibrinogenemia or "flaming" DIC.

(3) **Factor IX concentrates** contain factors II, VII, IX, and X. Several precautions are worth noting.

(a) This concentrate is made from pooled plasma; therefore the risk of hepatitis is high, and the risk of contamination with human immunodeficiency virus (HIV) is significant. The dose depends on the preparation to be used. The goal is to bring the factor to more than 50% of normal.

(b) There is a small risk of DIC resulting from the use of factor IX concentrates. Patients with liver dysfunction and newborns are at increased risk.

(c) Factor IX concentrates are stored in the lyophilized state. Do not shake when reconstituting.

3. Leukocyte depletion. Patients who have not previously received transfusions and who will need long-term blood product support should receive leukocyte-depleted ($< 5 \times 10^6$ leukocytes/bag) blood products. Leukocyte depletion may prevent febrile transfusion reactions, as well as delay alloimmunization. Two methods for leukocyte depletion are currently available.

   a. Bedside filtration involves leukocyte depletion at the time of transfusion. Disadvantages include plugging of the filter, the presence of leukocyte breakdown products, bag breakage, and lack of consistency of results. Filters are available for red blood cells (RBCs) and platelets.

   b. AS-3 prestorage filtered RBCs are RBCs that have been leukocyte-depleted within 8 hours of collection. Advantages are fewer leukocyte breakdown products, ease of administration, and consistent quality (guaranteed $< 5 \times 10^6$ leukocytes/bag). The main disadvantage is the cost.

4. **Cytomegalovirus (CMV)-negative blood.** Only patients known to be anti-CMV-negative with impaired immunity should be considered for the use of CMV-negative blood. This group includes children for the most part. The use of CMV-negative blood seriously restricts the potential donor pool for these patients.

   Frozen-deglycerolized blood is considered free of CMV contamination. WBC depletion filters also remove CMV. Irradiation of blood products does not appear to render them CMV-free.

5. **Irradiated blood products.** These prevent the development of graft-versus-host disease. Irradiated blood products are expensive and should be limited to those patients with one of the following indications.

   a. Congenital immunodeficiency
   b. Premature babies/neonates
   c. Bone marrow transplantation
   d. Directed blood donations to first-degree relatives
   e. Hodgkin's disease (a relative indication)
   f. High-dose chemotherapy with growth factor or stem cell rescue
   g. Leukemia and non-Hodgkin's lymphoma (relative indication)

B. **Other forms of therapy**

1. **Desmopressin (DDAVP).** Desmopressin 0.3 μg/kg IV over 30 minutes every 12–24 hours for 2–4 days may be used to elevate factor VIII and vWF levels, as well as improve platelet function. Tachyphylaxis may occur if therapy is continued for longer periods. Intranasal desmopressin (0.25 ml bid using a solution containing 1.3 mg/ml) has been given for minor bleeding episodes.

2. **Fibrin glue.** This is a topical biologic adhesive. Its effects imitate the final stages of coagulation. The glue consists of a solution of concentrated human fibrinogen which is activated by the addition of bovine thrombin and calcium chloride. The resulting clot promotes hemostasis and tissue sealing. The clot is completely absorbed during the healing process. The

best adhesive and hemostatic effect is obtained by applying the two solutions simultaneously to the open wound surface. Fibrin glue has been used primarily in surgical settings. It has been most effective when used for surface, low-pressure bleeding. There is a small risk of anaphylactic reactions due to the bovine origin of the thrombin.

3. **Antifibrinolytic agents.** Epsilon aminocaproic acid (EACA) and tranexamic acid have been used to control bleeding associated with primary fibrinolysis as seen in patients with prostatic carcinoma and a small number of patients with refractory thrombocytopenia. Great care must be taken in the use of these agents as there may be an increased risk of thrombosis associated with their use. EACA may be used topically to control small-area, small-volume bleeding.

Selected Readings

Bauer, K. A., et al. Tumor necrosis factor infusions have a procoagulant effect on the hemostatic mechanism of humans. *Blood* 74:165, 1989.

Bern, M. M., et al. Very low doses of warfarin can prevent thrombosis in central venous catheters. A randomized prospective trial. *Ann. Intern. Med.* 112:423, 1990.

Bick, R. L. Alterations of hemostasis associated with malignancy: etiology, pathophysiology, diagnosis and management. *Semin. Thromb. Hemost.* 5:1, 1978.

Brennan, M. Fibrin glue. *Blood Rev.* 5:240, 1991.

Dzik, S. Leukodepletion blood filters: filter design and mechanisms of leukocyte removal. *Transfusion Med. Rev.* 7:65, 1993.

Esparaz, B., Kies, M., and Kwaan, H. Thromboembolism in Cancer. In H. C. Kwaan, M. M. Samama (eds.), *Clinical Thrombosis.* Boca Raton: CRC Press, 1989. Pp. 317–333.

Freedman, J. J., Blajchman, M. A., and McCombie, N. Canadian Red Cross Society Symposium on leukodepletion: report of proceedings. *Transfusion Med. Rev.* 8:1, 1994.

Fresh-frozen Plasma, Cryoprecipitate, and Platelet Administration Practice Guidelines Development Task Force of the College of American Pathologists. Practice parameters for the use of fresh-frozen plasma, cryoprecipitate, and platelets. *J.A.M.A.* 271:777, 1994.

Griffin, M. R., et al. Deep venous thrombosis and pulmonary embolism, risk of subsequent malignant neoplasms. *Arch. Intern. Med.* 147:1907, 1987.

Kunkel, L. A. Acquired circulating anticoagulants in malignancy. *Semin. Thromb. Hemost.* 18:416, 1992.

Leitman, S. F., and Holland, P. V. Irradiation of blood products: indications and guidelines. *Transfusion* 25:293, 1985.

Mannucci, D. M. Desmopressin: a non-traditional form of treatment for congenital and acquired bleeding disorders. *Blood* 72:1449, 1988.

McCarthy, P. M. Fibrin glue in cardiothoracic surgery. *Transfusion Med. Rev.* 7:173, 1993.

Mollison, P. L., Engelfried, C. P., and Contreras, C. *Blood Transfusions in Clinical Medicine* (8th ed.). Boston: Blackwell Scientific, 1987.

Murgo, A. Thrombotic microangiopathy in the cancer patient including those induced by chemotherapy agents. *Semin. Hematol.* 24:161, 1987.

Schafer, A. The hypercoagulable state. *Ann. Intern. Med.* 102:814, 1985.

Walker, P. R., and Lachant, N. A. Purpura fulminans in Trousseau's syndrome: a complication of Coumadin therapy. *Proc. Am. Assoc. Clin. Oncol.* 12:464, 1993.

Management of Acute Side Effects of Cancer Chemotherapy

Janelle M. Tipton and Roland T. Skeel

Cancer chemotherapeutic agents control tumor growth by interfering with the proliferation of cancer cells. Because cell replication is characteristic of normal cells as well as cancer cells, chemotherapeutic agents have toxic effects on normal tissue. Rapidly dividing normal cells that are vulnerable to damage include cells of the bone marrow, hair follicles, and mucous membranes. Other toxicities that are particular to the individual agents and not dependent on cell growth can occur. The side effects may be acute or chronic, self-limited or permanent, and mild or potentially life-threatening.

I. Acute reactions

A. Extravasation. Extravasation is defined as the leakage or infiltration of drug into the subcutaneous tissues. *Vesicant* drugs that extravasate are capable of causing tissue necrosis or sloughing. *Irritant* drugs cause inflammation or pain at the site of extravasation.

1. **Vesicant agents** that are commonly used include dactinomycin (actinomycin D), daunorubicin (daunomycin), doxorubicin (Adriamycin), idarubicin (Idamycin), plicamycin (mithramycin, Mithracin), mitomycin (Mutamycin), mechlorethamine (nitrogen mustard), vinblastine (Velban), vincristine (Oncovin), vindesine (Eldisine), and vinorelbine (Navelbine).

2. **Irritant agents** that are commonly used include carmustine (BCNU), dacarbazine (DTIC), etoposide (VP-16), mitoxantrone (Novantrone), paclitaxel (Taxol), and teniposide (VM-26). Case reports have also indicated that in large extravasations of concentrated solutions, cisplatin (Platinol) and fluorouracil (5-FU) may be considered irritants.

3. **Management of extravasation** is controversial, with some disagreement in the literature regarding antidotes. In addition, many of the studies concerning extravasation management have been in animals. Less than 6% of the patients receiving peripheral intravenous chemotherapy experience vesicant extravasations. The most effective management of extravasation is prevention. Nurses who administer chemotherapy need to stay abreast of extravasation guidelines in an effort to prevent or minimize the serious complications of extravasation. A complaint (e.g., pain, burning) concerning the site of vein cannulation should be considered a symptom of extravasation until proved otherwise. It is advantageous to have orders for extravasation management for common vesicant/irritant chemotherapy agents prior to administration. Extravasation kits with the

necessary drug antidotes and supplies are also helpful to have available.

    a. General procedures. If an extravasation is suspected, the following actions should be taken.

        (1) Stop administration of the chemotherapeutic agent.

        (2) Leave the needle in place and immobilize the extremity.

        (3) Aspirate any residual drug left in the tubing, the needle, or the suspected extravasation site.

        (4) Remove the needle.

        (5) Avoid applying pressure to the extravasation site.

        (6) Photograph the suspected area of extravasation according to institutional policy.

        (7) Apply warm or cold compresses as indicated for the specific drug used.

        (8) Elevate the arm.

        (9) Notify the responsible physician of the occurrence and discuss the need for further intervention or consultation with a plastic surgeon.

    b. Recommended procedures for specific agents. Antidotes and dosages for specific chemotherapeutic agents listed in Table 33-1 are based on current data in the literature. Little information is known on antidotes for other chemotherapy agents. As new investigational agents emerge, it is important to examine the literature for possible extravasation guidelines.

B. Hypersensitivity/anaphylaxis. Specific drugs with the potential for hypersensitivity with or without an anaphylactic response should be administered under the constant supervision of a nurse knowledgeable about chemotherapy and with a physician readily available. An allergy history should be documented, but may not predict an allergic reaction to chemotherapy. The drug most commonly associated with anaphylaxis is L-asparaginase. Other drugs for which hypersensitivity reactions may occur include bleomycin (with lymphoma), cisplatin, melphalan (given intravenously), paclitaxel, and teniposide. If a drug is known to have an increased incidence of hypersensitivity response, a test dose or skin test may be performed. This is generally done only with bleomycin and asparaginase. Patients may also be premedicated prophylactically with corticosteroids, histamine antagonists, or both to prevent possible reactions. Emergency equipment which should be immediately accessible includes oxygen, an AMBU respiratory assist bag, and intubation equipment. The following parenteral drugs must also be stocked in the treatment area: epinephrine (1:10,000 solution), diphenhydramine 25–50 mg, methylprednisolone (Solu-Medrol) 30–60 mg, hydrocortisone (Solu-Cortef) 100–500 mg, dexamethasone 10–20 mg, and possibly aminophylline and dopamine.

Table 33-1. Antidotes for vesicant and irritant drugs

| Chemotherapy agent | Antidote | | Method of administration |
	Pharmacologic	Nonpharmacologic	
Mechlorethamine (nitrogen mustard)	Sodium thiosulfate	Cold compresses	Inject 1–4 ml of ⅙ molar solution through existing IV line (1 ml for each ml extravasated). Inject SQ if needle is removed.
Vincristine (Oncovin)	Hyaluronidase (Wydase)	Warm compresses	Inject 1–4 ml (150 units/ml) through the existing IV line or SQ if needle is removed.
Vinblastine (Velban)			
Vindesine (Eldisine)			
Etoposide (VP-16)			
Teniposide (VM-26)			
Vinorelbine (Navelbine)			
Doxorubicin (Adriamycin)		Topical cooling (ice pack)	Cooling of the site is recommended for 24 hours after the extravasation.
Idarubicin (Idamycin)			

C. **Nausea and vomiting.** Patients who are about to begin chemotherapy are often quite concerned and apprehensive about nausea and vomiting. Nausea and vomiting can be distressing enough to the patient to cause extreme physiologic and psychologic discomfort culminating in the withdrawal from therapy. With the advent of more effective antiemetic regimens in the past 10 years, many improvements in the prevention and control of nausea and vomiting have led to a better quality of life for patients receiving chemotherapy. The goal of therapy is to prevent the three phases of nausea and vomiting: that which occurs before the treatment is administered (anticipatory), that which follows within the first 24 hours following therapy (acute), and that which occurs more than 24 hours after the treatment (delayed). It is also important to assess nausea and vomiting separately, as they are different events and may have different causes. Factors related to the chemotherapy that can affect the likelihood and severity of symptoms include the specific agent(s) used, the dose of the drug(s), and the schedule and route of administration.

1. **Emetic potential of the drug.** In order to plan an effective approach to control nausea and vomiting, the chemotherapeutic agents are grouped according to their emetic potential (Table 33-2). This type of categorization is helpful in making decisions regarding possible antiemetics to be used and how aggressive the antiemetic regimen should be for patients receiving chemotherapy for the first time or in subsequent treatments.

2. **Antiemetic drugs.** Agents that have been effective in preventing and treating nausea and vomiting (Table 33-3) come from various pharmacologic classes. They work by different mechanisms that may relate to the pathophysiologic processes causing nausea and vomiting. For many years, the mainstays of antiemetic therapy have been agents that block dopamine receptors. These agents have been somewhat effective, but have limited value for highly emetogenic agents and in escalating doses have caused problematic side effects. Recently, it was discovered that agents that block the serotonin (5-hydroxytryptamine) receptors predominantly, rather than the dopamine receptors, have greater efficacy in the prevention of nausea and vomiting. It is important to use an antiemetic regimen sufficient to prevent nausea and vomiting to the greatest degree possible to avoid the development of conditioned responses and failure of antiemetic therapy.

3. **Combination antiemetic therapy.** Several antiemetic regimens are effective but their design should be based on several general principles.

   a. **Combinations of antiemetics** have been shown to be more effective than single agents. It is very common to use two or more antiemetics to prevent or manage nausea and vomiting.

Table 33-2. Emetogenic potential for commonly used chemotherapeutic agents

I. Highly emetogenic: ≥ 75% potential for nausea, vomiting, or both

Carmustine
Cisplatin (≥ 40 mg/m^2)
Cyclophosphamide (> 1 gm/m^2)
Cytarabine (> 1 gm/m^2)
Dacarbazine (days 1, 2 only)
Dactinomycin
Ifosfamide (≥ 1.2 gm/m^2)
Mechlorethamine
Methotrexate (≥ 1.2 gm/m^2)
Mitomycin (≥ 15 mg/m^2)

II. Moderately emetogenic: 50–75% potential for nausea, vomiting, or both

Carboplatin
Cisplatin (< 40 mg/m^2)
Cyclophosphamide (200–1000 mg/m^2)
Cytarabine (200–1000 mg/m^2)
Daunorubicin
Doxorubicin
Ifosfamide (< 1.2 gm/m^2)
Methotrexate (100–1200 mg/m^2)
Mitomycin (< 15 mg/m^2)

III. Weakly emetogenic: 20–50% potential for nausea, vomiting, or both

Asparaginase
Bleomycin
Cyclophosphamide (< 200 mg/m^2)
Cytarabine (< 200 mg/m^2)
Etoposide
Fluorouracil
Melphalan
Methotrexate (< 100 mg/m^2)
Mercaptopurine
Paclitaxel (Taxol)
Thioguanine
Thiotepa
Vinblastine

IV. Minimally emetogenic: < 20% potential for nausea, vomiting, or both

Busulfan
Chlorambucil
Hydroxyurea
Vincristine

Table 33-3. Antiemetics commonly used for prevention and treatment of chemotherapy-induced nausea and vomiting

Agent	Route of administration	Dosage (adult)	Comments
Phenothiazines			
Prochlorperazine (Compazine)	PO PO sustained-release IV (slow) PR	10–20 mg q4–6h 10–30 mg q12h 2–10 mg q4h 25 mg q8–12h	Some extrapyramidal reactions. There is a potential for severe postural hypotension when the agent is given IV. Closely observe the patient and assist when getting out of bed or sitting up.
Thiethylperazine (Torecan)	PO or PR IM	10 mg q4–6h 2 mg q4–6h	Some extrapyramidal reactions.
Trimethobenzamide (Tigan)	PO IM or PR	250 mg q4–6h 200 mg q4–6h	Some extrapyramidal reactions.
Butyrophenones			
Haloperidol (Haldol)	IV	1–3 mg q2–4h for 2–3 doses	Some extrapyramidal reactions.
Substituted benzamide			
Metoclopramide (Reglan)	PO IV over 20 minutes	10–40 mg q6h 1–2 mg/kg at 2-hour intervals	Extrapyramidal reactions are common particularly at higher doses. They are worse in younger patients. Diarrhea may occur.
Benzodiazepines			
Lorazepam (Ativan)	IM, IV, or PO	1–2 mg q4–6h	Sedation is frequent. Patients are advised not to drive for 24 hours after taking.

Steroids Dexamethasone (Decadron, Hexadrol)	IV or PO	10–20 mg to start, then 4 mg PO q6h in tapering doses	Potential for agitation, delirium, gastrointestinal bleeding.
5-HT3 antagonists Ondansetron (Zofran)	IV over 15 minutes	6 mg/m^2 (0.15 mg/kg) prior to and at 4 and 8 hours after chemotherapy or 10–30 mg prior to chemotherapy	For highly emetogenic therapy. There may be a mild headache and mild transient transaminase elevations. Lower doses are effective for less emetogenic regimens.
	PO	8 mg 2–3 times in 24 hours	For moderately emetogenic therapy.
Granisetron (Kytril)	IV	0.4 mg/m^2 (10 μg/kg) prior to chemotherapy	Similar to ondansetron, for highly emetogenic therapy.
	PO	2 mg prior to or 1 mg q12h on days of chemotherapy	For moderately emetogenic therapy
Cannabinoids Dronabinol (Marinol)	PO	2.5–10.0 mg PO q6h	May be habit-forming. A controlled substance.

    b. Preemptive treatment and scheduled administration are also necessary to prevent nausea and vomiting early in therapy and to manage potential delayed nausea and vomiting for several hours or days. Table 33-4 shows examples of antiemetic regimens that may be used when the chemotherapy has a high, moderate, and low emetic potential.

    4. Nonpharmacologic interventions. Patients who may likely experience or have experienced anticipatory nausea and vomiting related to chemotherapy may benefit from the use of relaxation techniques. The use of guided imagery, music therapy, and self-hypnosis show some effectiveness in preventing nausea and vomiting. These forms of distraction assist patients in maintaining a feeling of control over their treatment effects. Patients who are able to have little or no nausea and vomiting with their first chemotherapy treatment often assert that positive thinking is helpful as well. Patients may also prepare for their chemotherapy treatments by eating foods that do not have offensive odors or spicy taste. Clear liquids, foods served at room temperature, soda crackers, and carbonated beverages are sometimes good suggestions. Some patients prefer to receive their therapy at night, so as to sleep during periods when nausea and vomiting may occur.

II. Other short-term complications related to cancer chemotherapy

    A. Oral complications. The oral mucosa is very vulnerable to the effects of chemotherapy and radiotherapy because of its rapid growth and cell turnover rate. Radiotherapy also interferes with the production of saliva and may increase oral complications because of a consequent reduction in the protective effect of the saliva. It is crucial to manage oral complications effectively as patients may experience considerable discomfort or develop secondary infections from the disruption of the oral mucosa. The likelihood of the development of stomatitis from a drug is dependent on the agent, the dose, and the schedule of administration. Continuous rather than intermittent administration is more likely to cause stomatitis with the antimetabolites.

    1. Specific chemotherapy agents that may cause stomatitis include the following.

        Antimetabolites: methotrexate, fluorouracil, cytarabine

        Antitumor antibiotics: doxorubicin, dactinomycin, mitoxantrone, mitomycin, bleomycin

        Plant alkaloids: vincristine, vinblastine, etoposide

        Others: hydroxyurea, high dose of alkylating agents

        Biologic agents: interleukins, lymphokine-activated killer (LAK) cell therapy

    2. Prevention and early detection. If oral complications are anticipated, it is important to implement

Table 33-4. Examples of regimens for antiemetic prevention and management of chemotherapy-induced nausea and vomiting

I. **Highly emetogenic chemotherapy**

Dexamethasone 10–20 mg IV 30 minutes prior to chemotherapy. Repeat dexamethasone at 10–20 mg/day on each day highly emetogenic therapy is continued. Taper over 2–3 days after chemotherapy, e.g., 4 mg PO q6h × 4 doses, then 4 mg PO q12h × 2 doses, *and*

Ondansetron 30 mg IV 30 minutes prior to chemotherapy. For a regimen where each day's therapy is expected to be highly emetogenic, this dose may be given once daily, *and*

Lorazepam 1 mg IV 30 minutes prior to chemotherapy, then 1 mg IV or PO q4–6h prn for nausea or vomiting. May wish to give 1–2 mg PO the evening prior to and the morning of therapy to avert anticipatory nausea and vomiting, *and*

Metoclopramide 40 mg PO q6h starting 6 hours after the ondansetron is given. May continue around the clock for up to 72 hours after the last dose of ondansetron.

II. **Moderately emetogenic chemotherapy**

Ondansetron 10 mg IV 30 minutes prior to chemotherapy. For a regimen where each day's therapy is expected to be moderately emetogenic, this dose may be given once daily, *and*

Dexamethasone 10 mg IV 30 minutes prior to the first dose of chemotherapy. Repeat dexamethasone 10–20 mg/day on each day moderately emetogenic therapy is to be continued. May taper over 2–3 days after chemotherapy, e.g., 4 mg PO q6h × 4 doses, then 4 mg q12h × 2 doses, *and*

Prochlorperazine 10–20 mg PO q6h or 25 mg per rectum q8–12h for 48–72 hours. May be effective to use prochlorperazine spansules, 15–30 mg PO the evening prior to chemotherapy and q12h for 48–72 hours, *and*

Lorazepam 1 mg PO or IV 30 minutes prior to each dose of chemotherapy, then 1 mg PO or IV q4–6h prn nausea or vomiting. May wish to give 1–2 mg PO the evening prior to and the morning of therapy to avert anticipatory nausea and vomiting.

III. **Weakly or minimally emetogenic chemotherapy**

Prochlorperazine 10 mg PO prior to chemotherapy, then 10 mg PO q4–6h or 25 mg per rectum q8h × 48 hours prn, *with or without*

Dexamethasone 4 mg 1 hour prior to the start of chemotherapy, *and*

Lorazepam 1 mg PO q6h prn

Notes:

1. If the patient fails to have adequate control of nausea and vomiting on regimen 2 or 3, move to the next higher intensity of antiemetic therapy on the next cycle.
2. If the patient is on a multiple-day regimen, use the highest level of antiemetics recommended on the basis of current day's therapy. However, if the previous day's regimen called for a more potent regimen, that should be preferentially followed.
3. Alternatives to prochlorperazine
   a. Metoclopramide (Reglan) 10–40 mg PO or IV q4–6h
   b. Thiethylperazine (Torecan) 10 mg PO q4–6h
   c. Trimethobenzamide (Tigan) 250 mg PO, 200 mg PR or IM q4–6h
   d. Dimenhydrinate (Dramamine) 50 mg PO q4h

a good oral hygiene program prior to the initiation of therapy. Maintaining good nutrition and dental hygiene is also a primary preventive measure. "Cryotherapy" has been used on occasion to reduce the extent of stomatitis. This is done by chewing ice chips 15 minutes prior to and during therapy. Systematic oral assessments should be integrated into the physical examination at regular intervals, e.g., 1–2 times/day. Special attention should be given to the tongue, the gingiva, the buccal mucosa, the soft palate, and the lips. It is also important to assess the patient for soreness, functional ability to swallow, and any effects on eating.

3. **Management of oral complications.** Although the primary goal is prevention, once oral complications develop, the focus of care should shift to the continuation of good oral hygiene and treatment of symptoms. Agents used for oral care are categorized according to function: cleansing agents, lubricating agents, and analgesic agents. Table 33-5 lists several commonly used agents. Commercial mouthwashes and lemon glycerin swabs are not recommended for use because of their irritating and drying effects. A common oral care agent used is chlorhexidine (Peridex) 15 ml which is swished and expectorated after meals and at bedtime. If painful ulcerations do develop, topical relief may be obtained by using a stomatitis mixture containing diphenhydramine (Benadryl) elixir 5 ml, antacid (Maalox) 30 ml, and viscous lidocaine (Xylocaine) 5 ml. Systemic pain control measures such as oral or parenteral narcotics should be implemented if topical analgesics are ineffective.

Xerostomia that follows radiation therapy to the mouth area may require treatment with artificial saliva. It may also be benefited by the administration of pilocarpine 5–10 mg PO tid before meals. Prior to the initiation of radiation therapy to the head and neck area, dental consultation is necessary to evaluate oral hygiene, the state of repair of the teeth, and the health of the gums.

Secondary oral infections should be treated promptly and as accurately as possible. Fungal infections may be treated with nystatin (Mycostatin) suspension, clotrimazole troches, or oral fluconazole. Viral infections may be reactivated following chemotherapy and are commonly treated with oral or intravenous acyclovir. The benefit of prophylactic use of antiviral agents or antifungal agents is not well established. Patients with dentures may be encouraged to remove them during the period following chemotherapy when they are at risk for infection, except at mealtime. In addition, the dentures should be cleansed prior to use. Although removal of the dentures may be detrimental to the patient's self-

Table 33-5. Agents for oral care

Oral agent	Comments
1. Cleansing agents	
Normal saline solution (½ tsp salt in 8 oz. of water)	Economical, nondamaging.
Hydrogen peroxide	Dilute with normal saline or tap water. Germicidal, debriding.
Sodium bicarbonate	Nonirritating, neutralizing acid in mouth.
Chlorhexidine (Peridex)	Antimicrobial, can stain teeth.
2. Lubricating agents	
Saliva substitutes	Decreases dryness, similar to human saliva.
Water- or oil-based lubricants	Useful emollient. Oil-based lubricants should not be used in the mouth due to danger of aspiration.
3. Analgesic agents	
a. Healing/coating agents	
Sucralfate	Binds to mucosa, forms protective coating.
Vitamin E	Protection to mucosa, healing properties.
Zilactin Gel (tannic acid)	Reduces discomfort by coating, safe.
Antacids	Enhance comfort, coat mucosa. Examples: Maalox, milk of magnesia, Kaopectate.
b. Topical anesthetics	
Lidocaine viscous	Transient pain relief, absorbed systemically.
Dyclonine hydrochloride	Transient pain relief, minimal systemic absorption.
Benzocaine	Transient pain relief, minimal systemic absorption.
c. Systemic analgesics	
Nonsteroidal anti-inflammatory drugs	
Narcotic analgesics	Taken before meals and as needed.

esteem, irritation of the dentures may lead to inflammation, ulceration, and secondary infection.

B. Alopecia. Chemotherapy-induced hair loss is not necessarily a serious physiologic complication, but psychologically it can be one of the most devastating side effects. Partial or total hair loss can contribute to a perceived negative body image due to the emphasis placed on the hair and overall appearance in society. The hair loss from chemotherapy, which often occurs suddenly about 2–3 weeks after chemotherapy, is usually temporary and hair growth returns in approximately 1–2 months after the treatment is completed. The new hair may have a different texture and/or color compared to its pretreatment characteristics.

   1. Specific chemotherapy agents with a high potential of causing alopecia include doxorubicin, cyclophosphamide, ifosfamide, vincristine, and paclitaxel. Other drugs capable of causing alopecia include bleomycin, dactinomycin, daunorubicin, etoposide, vinblastine, methotrexate, and mitoxantrone.

   2. Nursing interventions start with informing and preparing the patient for the possibility of alopecia. It is often helpful to encourage purchasing wigs and scarves before the alopecia occurs to allow the patient to adjust. It is important to encourage ventilation of feelings regarding the hair loss for both men and women and to discuss their concerns and fears. Scalp hypothermia or tourniquets have been used to aid in restricting the blood flow to the hair follicles, with the goal of minimizing alopecia. Unfortunately, these methods are not always sufficient and many times combinations of drugs are used, which decreases its effectiveness. In addition, the devices themselves and the cooling of the scalp may be uncomfortable to the patient. Scalp hypothermia is not recommended for patients with tumors with a high incidence of scalp metastases. Researchers have recently examined the use of ImuVert, a biologic response modifier, and interleukin-1 in animal models as an attempt to protect against alopecia.

C. Diarrhea. Among the many causes of diarrhea in patients with cancer are chemotherapy, radiotherapy, the cancer itself, medications, supplemental feedings, and anxiety. Infectious etiologies, i.e., *Clostridium difficile* or other bacteria-causing enterocolitis, always need to be considered in the hospitalized neutropenic patient receiving antibiotics. Prolonged diarrhea can lead to discomfort, severe electrolyte abnormalities, altered social life, and poor quality of life.

   1. Chemotherapy and biologic agents that may contribute to the development of diarrhea include aldesleukin (interleukin-2), cytarabine, fluorouracil, floxuridine, methotrexate, idarubicin, paclitaxel, and interferon alpha. When diarrhea from fluorouracil and floxuridine is present on a day of scheduled administration, the drug should be temporarily discontinued as this is a sign of toxicity that could escalate to severe levels if the drug is continued.

2. **Assessment** of a patient experiencing diarrhea should begin with a baseline report of usual elimination patterns. Presenting signs and symptoms including the frequency and volume of stools must also be determined. The history should include relevant concurrent medical conditions or previous surgeries, current treatments, and medications. The physical examination should include attention to the abdomen and signs of dehydration. Laboratory data may be obtained to assess electrolytes and blood cell counts, and stool samples should be examined for *C. difficile*, ova and parasites, and enteropathic bacteria.

3. **Management** of treatment-related diarrhea is often symptomatic and requires no alteration in cancer therapy. Agents that decrease bowel motility should not be used for longer than 24 hours unless significant infections have been excluded. Medications commonly used to treat diarrhea are loperamide hydrochloride and diphenoxylate hydrochloride with atropine sulfate. More recently, it was noted that octreotide may have some value in controlling chemotherapy-related diarrhea associated with fluorouracil regimens as well as the diarrhea associated with the carcinoid syndrome. Table 33-6 lists common

Table 33-6. Pharmacologic management strategies for diarrhea

Agent	Comments
Kaopectate	30–60 ml PO after each loose stool.
Loperamide (Imodium)	2 capsules (4 mg) PO q4h initially, then add 1 capsule (2 mg) after each loose stool. Should not exceed 16 capsules daily.
Diphenoxylate hydrochloride, atropine sulfate (Lomotil)	1–2 tablets PO q4h with prn; should not exceed 8 tablets daily. There may be anticholinergic side effects due to atropine.
Paregoric	1 tsp PO 4 times a day. May alternate with Lomotil.
Phenobarbital, hyoscyamine, atropine sulfate, scopolamine (Donnatal)	Anticholinergic, antispasmodic; may help relieve abdominal cramping. Dose: 1–2 tablets PO q4h prn.
Octreotide	May be useful for fluorouracil-induced diarrhea. Dose: 0.05–0.1 mg SQ tid.

agents used to treat diarrhea. Nonpharmacologic measures that may also assist in the prevention and management of diarrhea are a low-residue diet and increased fluids. If the diarrhea is severe, intravenous hydration is necessary to prevent serious hypovolemia and shock.

D. Constipation. In patients whose cancer has resulted in debility or immobility, or in those who require narcotic analgesics, constipation can be a particular problem. Constipation may also develop in patients who have received neurotoxic chemotherapy agents, including the vinca alkaloids, etoposide, and cisplatin, each of which may cause autonomic dysfunction. Decreased bowel motility due to intraabdominal disease, hypercalcemia, or dehydration can also contribute to constipation. Chronic constipation in patients with cancer is a problem and is more easily prevented than treated. A diet high in bulk or fresh fruits and adequate fluid intake may help to minimize constipation. Patients started on narcotic analgesics should also begin a bowel regimen, first with mild stool softeners and bulk laxatives, and then proceeding to stimulants or osmotic laxatives if the milder regimen is not effective. A bowel regimen example for a patient at risk for constipation is as follows.

   1. Docusate sodium 100 mg twice a day

   2. If no bowel movement add

      a. Senna at bedtime (dose varies with the preparation) *or*

      b. Milk of magnesia 30 ml at bedtime

   3. If no bowel movement with the above, may add

      a. Bisacodyl 1–3 tablets or one 10-mg suppository at bedtime

      b. Lactulose 1–4 tablespoons daily

   4. Other more aggressive alternatives include

      a. Cisapride 10–20 mg PO qid

      b. Fleet enema

      c. Magnesium citrate 1 bottle

      d. Tap water enema

E. Altered nutritional status. Patients with cancer often experience progressive loss of appetite and sometimes severe malnutrition during the course of the disease and treatment. Malnutrition may result from a side effect of the therapy or a direct effect of the cancer, e.g., gut obstruction or hepatic or brain metastases. The resulting effects of malnutrition are a poorer response to therapy, increased incidence of infections, and an overall worsening of patient well-being. Many times, one of the presenting symptoms that leads to the diagnosis of cancer is weight loss; therefore, the patient is most likely already experiencing some alteration in nutritional status. Malnutrition is reported to occur in 50–80% of patients with advanced disease. Nutritional management of the patient with cancer involves early intervention utilizing a supportive health care team.

   1. Effects of chemotherapy and radiation therapy on nutrition. Chemotherapy has a major impact on nutritional status because of the direct insult on the gastrointestinal tract. Among the gastrointestinal effects are anorexia, nausea and vomiting, taste changes, stomatitis, esophagitis, colitis, constipation, and diarrhea. Not only are the effects physiologic in nature, but also the psychologic impact of the disease and therapy can result in anxiety and depression which can contribute to the lack of interest in food.

2. **Nutritional assessment.** Early in the patient's treatment a thorough nutritional assessment should be completed by the health care team. The assessment should include diet history, nutrient intake, anthropometric measurements (height, weight, skinfold thickness, and midarm circumference), laboratory tests for anemia and serum albumin, and an evaluation of activity and functional status. A good nutritional assessment may help to identify patients who are already at high risk for malnutrition or those who may be prone to develop problems during the course of the illness and treatment.

3. **Nutritional intervention.** Nutritional intervention becomes very important and should be considered after the assessment. Situations that warrant nutritional intervention include involuntary weight loss (> 10% within the past 6 months, especially when combined with weakness and fatigue), history of recent physiologic stress, serum albumin level below 3.2 gm/dl, or severe immunocompromise. Nurses, dietitians, and even family members can identify problems and may be the first to act to promote weight gain. Various approaches to help increase weight gain are changes in diet; symptomatic treatment of nausea and vomiting, stomatitis, and other gastrointestinal effects of chemotherapy; and supplemental nutrition.

   a. **Nutritional supplements.** Several nutritional supplements are commercially available for oral use. One benefit of nutritional supplements is that they are a concentrated form of nutrition for protein and calories. Some of the disadvantages are the unappealing taste and the high cost to the consumer. Some patients and their families are able to develop creative high-protein and calorie supplements using household items with some suggestions from the health care team.

   b. **Tube feedings.** Enteral nutrition via a nasogastric or gastrostomy tube may be an alternative if oral intake is not possible. Enteral feedings are the recommended route if the gastrointestinal tract is functional. Advantages of enteral feedings include lower cost and fewer complications than with parenteral feedings, and maintenance of normal gastrointestinal function. Some care and maintenance is involved with feeding tubes and patients and their families need to be given information regarding available options for feeding.

c. **Total parenteral nutrition (TPN).** Parenteral nutrition should be considered in patients who are otherwise well, but who no longer have a functioning gastrointestinal tract or if the supplemental nutrition is anticipated to be needed for a short time. Patients who receive TPN usually require the insertion of a central venous catheter, which may result in other iatrogenic complications such as pneumothorax, vein thrombosis, and catheter-related infections. In many situations TPN used in the patient with cancer increases morbidity, especially from infection, without improving survival. Thus, TPN has considerable economic, ethical, and medical consequences that must be evaluated in conjunction with the patient's overall prognosis.

4. **Pharmacologic interventions.** A recent area of interest is pharmacologic appetite stimulation. Some of the agents currently under study are megestrol acetate 40–80 mg 4 times a day, cyproheptadine 8 mg 3 times a day, hydrazine sulfate, and pentoxifylline. These agents promote increased weight gain in some patients and at least a decreased rate of weight loss in others.

Selected Readings

Beck, T. M., et al. Stratified, randomized, double-blind comparison of intravenous ondansetron administered as a multiple-dose regimen versus two single-dose regimens in the prevention of cisplatin-induced nausea and vomiting. *J. Clin. Oncol.* 10:1969, 1992.

Cascinu, S., et al. Octreotide versus loperamide in the treatment of fluorouracil induced diarrhea: a randomized trial. *J. Clin. Oncol.* 11:148, 1993.

Chevallier, B. The control of acute cisplatin-induced emesis: a comparative study of granisetron and a combination regimen of high-dose metoclopramide and dexamethasone. *Br. J. Cancer* 68:176, 1993.

Hussein, A. M. Chemotherapy-induced alopecia: new developments. *South. Med. J.* 86:489, 1993.

Lindley, C. M., Bernard, S., and Fields, S. M. Incidence and duration of chemotherapy-induced nausea and vomiting in the outpatient oncology population. *J. Clin. Oncol.* 7:1142, 1989.

Oncology Nursing Society. *Cancer Chemotherapy Guidelines: Recommendations for the Management of Vesicant Extravasation, Hypersensitivity, and Anaphylaxis.* Pittsburgh: Oncology Nursing Society, 1992.

Sonis, S., and Clark, J. Prevention and management of oral mucositis induced by antineoplastic therapy. *Oncology* 5:11, 1991.

Tchekmedyian, N. S., et al. Clinical aspects of nutrition in advanced cancer. *Oncology* 49(suppl. 2):3, 1992.

Troesch, L. M., et al. The influence of guided imagery on chemotherapy-related nausea and vomiting. *Oncol. Nurs. Forum* 20:1179, 1993.

Hypercalcemia, Syndrome of Inappropriate ADH, and Other Endocrine Syndromes

Roberto Franco-Saenz

I. **General considerations.** The occurrence of endocrine syndromes secondary to the ectopic production of hormones by nonendocrine tumors has been recognized with increasing frequency over the past 25 years. Recognition of an endocrine or metabolic manifestation of cancer is most important, because in some patients the effects of the endocrine syndrome are more deleterious to the patient than the neoplasm itself. Study of the responsible hormones and related products has further significance, because they have the potential to be used clinically as markers for early detection of tumors, as indicators of the response to therapy, or as indicators of tumor recurrence.

  A. **Hormone production and clinical expression.** Production of hormone precursors is a common occurrence in malignancy. However, clinical expression of an endocrine syndrome is less common, and depends on the capability of the neoplasm to release the active hormone from its precursor. Malignant tumors may also produce subunits of the parent hormone that under normal circumstances are not released by themselves. For example, the precursors of adrenocorticotropic hormone (ACTH), calcitonin, and other peptide hormones and their subunits are usually present in all lung tumors regardless of histologic type. However, only a few patients develop clinical or biochemical abnormalities related to ectopic hormone production. The so-called oncofetal proteins, e.g., alpha-fetoprotein and carcinoembryonic antigen, and the oncoplacental proteins represent another major category of ectopic production of proteins, and although they do not cause specific endocrine syndromes, their production by tumors probably has similar pathogenetic significance.

  B. **Ectopic hormone production by nonendocrine tumors.** That nonendocrine tumors produce ectopic hormones has been documented by several lines of evidence.

    1. Arteriovenous differences in the hormone concentration across a tumor bed

    2. High concentrations of hormone precursors in tumor extracts

    3. Incorporation of radiolabeled amino acids into the hormones produced by tumors

    4. Production of the hormone by tumors grown in tissue culture

Furthermore, correction of the endocrine syndrome has followed total excision of the tumor and recurrence of the syndrome when metastases developed.

C. Mechanism of ectopic hormone production. Data indicate that most normal nonendocrine tissues synthesize and store small quantities of a variety of peptide hormones and their precursors. Moreover, when cancer develops in these tissues, they continue to produce the hormones, often in increased amounts, leading to various types of humoral syndromes.

II. Hypercalcemia

A. Causes of tumor hypercalcemia (Table 34-1)

1. **Associated tumors.** Hypercalcemia is relatively common in patients with malignancy. In fact, one study showed that the most common cause of hypercalcemia in hospitalized patients is malignancy. Hypercalcemia of malignancy can be associated with bone metastasis, or it may occur in the absence of any direct bone involvement by the tumor. Of 433 patients with hypercalcemia of cancer, 86% had identifiable bone metastasis. Breast cancer accounted for more than one-half (n = 225) of the cases, and cancer of the lung and kidneys accounted for a smaller proportion. Patients with hematologic malignancies accounted for approximately 15% of the cases. These patients usually had hypercalcemia in the presence of diffuse tumor involvement of bone, although in a small percentage there was no evidence of bone involvement.

2. **Humoral mediators.** In approximately 10% of patients with malignancy, hypercalcemia develops in the absence of radiographic or scintigraphic evidence of bone involvement. In this group of patients, the pathogenesis of hypercalcemia appears to be secondary to humoral mediators (see Table 34-1).

Table 34-1. Factors responsible for hypercalcemia of malignancy

Direct resorption of bone by tumor cells

Production of PTH-related peptide (PTHrP)

Production of osteoclast-activating factors (OAFs)
  Interleukin-1
  Tumor necrosis factor (TNF-α)
  Lymphotoxin (TNF-β)
  Colony-stimulating factor
  Interferon gamma

Production of 1,25-dihydroxyvitamin D

Production of prostaglandins (PGE$_2$)

Production of transforming growth factors (TGFs)
  TGF-α
  TGF-β

Coexistence of tumor with primary hyperparathyroidism or other cause of hypercalcemia (e.g., vitamin D intoxication, sarcoidosis)

Although for years it was thought that humoral hypercalcemia of malignancy was associated with increased production of parathyroid hormone (PTH), it has been shown that PTH levels are normal or low in patients with hypercalcemia of malignancy and that nonendocrine tumors associated with hypercalcemia do not contain PTH messenger RNA (mRNA). On the other hand, a PTH-related peptide (PTHrP) has been extracted and purified from a large number of nonparathyroid tumors associated with the syndrome of humoral hypercalcemia of cancer.

a. **PTHrP.** In 1987 a parathyroid-like humoral factor was isolated from lung and renal carcinomas. The gene for PTHrP is located on the short arm of chromosome 12, and the complementary DNA (cDNA) has been cloned and sequenced. The amino-terminal region of the PTHrP shares a similar amino acid sequence (8 of 13 amino acids) with PTH. Beyond amino acid 13, the sequence of the two peptides is completely different. PTHrP is present in very high concentrations in human milk (10,000 times higher than normal plasma), suggesting that the peptide may have a still unknown physiologic role in calcium homeostasis. A specific radioimmunoassay is commercially available for measurement of PTHrP.

b. **Osteoclast-activating factors (OAFs).** A number of cytokines with potent bone-resorbing activities have been identified. These cytokines may account for the previously designated OAF. Interleukin (IL)-1 produced by monocytes has potent bone-resorbing activity in vitro. Tumor necrosis factor-alpha (TNF-α), also produced by monocytes, and lymphotoxin or TNF-β produced by lymphocytes have potent bone-resorbing properties. Lymphotoxin plays an important role in the pathogenesis of bone destruction and hypercalcemia of multiple myeloma. Adult T cell lymphomas are frequently associated with hypercalcemia and this tumor produces several bone-resorbing factors, including lymphotoxin, colony-stimulating factor, and interferon gamma.

c. **Production of 1,25-dihydroxyvitamin D.** Hypercalcemia with increased serum calcitriol (1,25-dihydroxyvitamin D) levels in patients with malignant lymphomas was first reported in 1984. Since then, this observation has been confirmed and elevated levels of 1,25-dihydroxyvitamin D have been detected in other tumors associated with hypercalcemia such as leiomyoblastomas, Hodgkin's disease, and a large plasma cell granuloma.

d. **Production of prostaglandins (PGs).** There is evidence indicating that PGs play a role in the hypercalcemia of malignancy. PGs are potent stimulators of bone resorption. There are reports of metastatic renal cell carcinomas in which high concentrations of PGE_2 have been found in the tumor and in which hypercalcemia responded to indomethacin therapy.

    e. **Transforming growth factors (TGFs).** TGFs are small peptides characterized by their ability to stimulate cell growth and replication. TGF-α is a 5000-dalton peptide and TGF-β is a homodimer protein with a molecular mass of 24,000 daltons. Both peptides have in vitro bone-resorbing activities more potent than PTH. These peptides are produced by many solid tumors and have been implicated in the humoral hypercalcemia of malignancy.

B. Symptoms, signs, and laboratory findings. Hypercalcemia often produces symptoms in patients with cancer and, in fact, may be their major problem. Polyuria and nocturia, resulting from the impaired ability of the kidneys to concentrate the urine, occur early. Anorexia, nausea, constipation, muscle weakness, and fatigue are common. As the hypercalcemia progresses, severe dehydration, azotemia, mental obtundation, coma, and cardiovascular collapse may appear. In addition to hypercalcemia, the laboratory studies may reveal hypokalemia and increased blood urea nitrogen (BUN) and creatinine levels. Patients with hypercalcemia of malignancy frequently have hypochloremic metabolic alkalosis, whereas with primary hyperparathyroidism, metabolic acidosis is more common. The concentration of serum phosphorus is variable. PTH levels may be normal, low, or high, but marked elevations are rarely seen. Bone involvement is best evaluated by a bone scan, which is often "positive" in the absence of radiographic evidence of bone involvement.

C. Treatment. The management of hypercalcemia of malignancy has two objectives: (1) reducing elevated levels of serum calcium, and (2) treating the underlying cause. When hypercalcemia is mild to moderate (serum calcium < 12–13 mg/dl) and the patient is not symptomatic, adequate hydration and measures directed against the tumor (e.g., surgery, chemotherapy, or radiation therapy) may suffice. Severe hypercalcemia, on the other hand, is a life-threatening condition requiring emergency treatment. Therefore, for more severe degrees of hypercalcemia, other measures must be taken, including enhancement of calcium excretion by the kidney in patients with adequate renal function and the use of agents that decrease bone resorption.

    The agents used for the treatment of hypercalcemia have differences in the time of onset and duration of action as well as in their potency. Therefore, effective treatment of severe hypercalcemia requires the use of more than one modality of therapy. A suggested approach to the treatment of severe hypercalcemia is as follows.

Rehydration with 0.9% sodium chloride

Calcitonin 4–8 units/kg IV every 6–12 hours for the initial 48–72 hours

Pamidronate (Aredia) 60–90 mg in 1000 ml/0.9% sodium chloride infused over 24 hours

Saline diuresis (0.9% sodium chloride + furosemide)

1. **Rehydration.** Rehydration and restoration of intravascular volume is the most important initial step in the therapy of hypercalcemia. Rehydration should be accomplished using 0.9% sodium chloride (normal saline) and often requires the administration of 4–6 liters over the first 24 hours. Rehydration alone causes only a mild decrease of the serum calcium levels (~10%). However, rehydration improves renal function facilitating urinary calcium excretion.

2. **Saline diuresis.** After adequate restoration of intravascular volume, forced saline diuresis may be used. Sodium competitively inhibits the tubular resorption of calcium. Therefore, the intravenous (IV) infusion of saline causes a significant increase in calcium clearance. Because of the large amounts of saline that may be required to correct hypercalcemia, it is advisable to monitor the central venous pressure continuously. The infusion of normal saline (0.9% sodium chloride) at a rate of 250–500 ml/hour, accompanied by the IV administration of 20–80 mg of furosemide every 2–4 hours, results in significant calcium diuresis and mild lowering of the serum calcium level in the majority of patients. This type of therapy requires strict monitoring of cardiopulmonary status to avoid fluid overload. Also, it requires ready access to the laboratory to prevent electrolyte imbalance, since the urinary losses of sodium, potassium, magnesium, and water must be replaced to maintain metabolic balance. In some patients the infusion of saline at rates of 125–150 ml/hour plus the addition of furosemide 40–80 mg IV once or twice a day may reduce the serum calcium level until other measures aimed at inhibiting bone resorption take effect.

3. **Calcitonin (Calcimar).** This is a peptide hormone that inhibits osteocytic and osteoclastic bone resorption. Calcitonin salmon, when given by infusion, will cause a modest reduction of serum calcium levels, usually by 1–3 mg/dl, which commonly reverses after discontinuation of therapy. To avoid anaphylactic reactions, skin testing should be performed prior to the administration of calcitonin. To avoid inconsistencies in the response, it is recommended that albumin (approximately 5 gm) be added to the infusion to coat the infusion set and prevent absorption of the peptides to the walls of the set. The usual initial dose of calcitonin is 4–8 units/kg, either IV, SQ, or IM every

6–12 hours according to the serum calcium levels. Nausea with or without vomiting has been noted in approximately 10% of the patients treated with calcitonin. It is more common at the beginning of the treatment and usually subsides with continuous administration. Local inflammatory reactions at the site of SQ or IM injection have been reported in about 10% of the patients. Skin rashes and flushing occurred occasionally.

4. **Bisphosphonates (diphosphonates).** The diphosphonates or bisphosphonates are analogs of pyrophosphate in which the oxygen in the backbone of pyrophosphate (P-O-P) is replaced by a carbon (P-C-P), rendering the molecule resistant to degradation by phosphatases. The diphosphonates are potent inhibitors of normal and abnormal bone resorption and also inhibit bone formation. They bind to the surface of calcium phosphate crystals and inhibit crystal growth and dissolution. In addition, they may directly inhibit osteoclast resorptive activity.

   a. **Pamidronate disodium (Aredia).** Pamidronate (3-amino-1-hydroxypropylidene-1,1-bisphosphonic acid) is a very potent inhibitor of bone resorption and the most effective agent for the treatment of hypercalcemia of malignancy. Pamidronate has become the treatment of choice for hypercalcemia of malignancy. The hypocalcemic action of pamidronate is dose-related. In a double-blind clinical study of 52 patients with hypercalcemia of malignancy, a single IV infusion of pamidronate at 90 mg/24 hour normalized serum calcium in 100% of the patients, within 7 days of the initiation of treatment. In patients receiving 60 mg/24 hours, normocalcemia was seen in 61% of patients, whereas only 40% of those receiving 30 mg/24 hours achieved normocalcemia. The hypocalcemic action of pamidronate starts 24–48 hours after initiation of therapy and may last up to 2 weeks. In some patients normocalcemia may last for months, but in others recurrence of hypercalcemia may require repeated doses at 1–2-week intervals.

      (1) **Dosage and administration.** For symptomatic, moderate hypercalcemia (corrected serum calcium, 12.0–13.5 mg/dl) the recommended dose of pamidronate is 60 mg given IV as a single dose over 24 hours. For severe hypercalcemia (serum calcium > 13.5 mg/dl), a single IV dose of 90 mg in 1000 ml of either 0.45%, 0.9% saline, or 5% dextrose solution over 24 hours should be given. Four-hour infusions also appear safe and effective, though there is less experience with this shorter infusion schedule.

      (2) **Side effects.** Pamidronate is usually well tolerated and no serious side effects have

been reported. Mild fever with temperature elevations of 1°C was noted in 27% of patients after 24–48 hours of administration. The transient fever is presumed to be due to release of cytokines from osteoclasts. Pain, redness, swelling, and induration at the site of infusion occur in approximately 20% of patients. Hypocalcemia, hypophosphatemia, or hypomagnesemia may be seen in 15% of the patients.

Oral pamidronate has shown promising results in reducing the morbidity from skeletal metastasis in breast cancer patients. In a European study, oral pamidronate given at a dose of 300 mg/day prevented hypercalcemia and caused a significant reduction in the incidence of pathologic fractures and bone pain in 70 patients with osteolytic metastasis from breast cancer. Unfortunately oral pamidronate is not available in the United States.

b. Etidronate disodium (Didronel). Etidronate is a first-generation bisphosphonate available for oral and IV administration. Oral etidronate has been used for the treatment of Paget's disease of bone for many years. The IV preparation was the first bisphosphonate available for treatment of hypercalcemia of malignancy. Etidronate therapy is effective and well tolerated for the treatment of hypercalcemia of malignancy. IV etidronate at a dose of 7.5 mg/kg for 3 days leads to normalization of the serum calcium in 40% of patients with hypercalcemia of malignancy. Reductions in bone resorption and urinary and serum calcium levels begin to occur after 24 hours. The maximal decrease in serum calcium is observed 72 hours after the first infusion. Serum calcium level may continue to fall for several days after discontinuation of therapy and may remain normal for 2 weeks. Oral etidronate has been reported to maintain the hypocalcemic response and to prevent recurrence of hypercalcemia in some trials but not in others.

(1) Dosage and administration. The recommended dose of etidronate is 7.5 mg/kg of body weight, diluted in at least 250 ml of normal saline and administered IV over a period of at least 2 hours every day. It is important that the infusion be given slowly to minimize complications. The usual course of treatment is one infusion a day for 3 days, but some patients have been treated for up to 7 days. However, hypocalcemia may occur after prolonged treatment.

(2) Side effects. Loss of taste or a metallic

taste has been reported, but usually disappears within hours. In approximately 10% of patients a transient mild elevation of the BUN and creatinine may be observed. Hyperphosphatemia occurs frequently. In the presence of preexistent renal impairment the dose of etidronate should be reduced and renal function should be monitored frequently.

5. **Gallium nitrate (Ganite).** Gallium nitrate was shown to cause hypocalcemia and to inhibit bone resorption in patients in whom the drug was used as an antitumor agent. The drug inhibits bone resorption by reducing the solubility of bone crystals. In a recent study, gallium nitrate was more effective than calcitonin and etidronate in normalizing the serum calcium in patients with hypercalcemia of malignancy. Gallium nitrate infused at a dose of 200 mg/m^2 decreased the serum calcium level to normal in approximately 75% of patients with hypercalcemia of malignancy; normocalcemia was maintained in these patients for an average of 7–10 days. A drawback of gallium nitrate therapy is the prolonged duration of treatment necessary to normalize the serum calcium (5 days of infusion).

   a. **Dosage and administration.** The recommended dose of gallium nitrate is 200 mg/m^2 daily for 5 consecutive days. The daily dose should be diluted in 1000 ml of 0.9% saline or 5% dextrose and infused IV over 24 hours. In patients with mild symptomatic hypercalcemia a dosage of 100 mg/m^2/day for 5 days may be used.

   b. **Side effects.** Nephrotoxicity as demonstrated by rising BUN and creatinine has been seen in approximately 12% of patients treated with gallium nitrate. Simultaneous use of aminoglycosides and other nephrotoxic drugs increases the risk of renal insufficiency. Adequate hydration must be maintained during treatment with gallium nitrate. Mild to moderate hypophosphatemia occurs in up to 80% of the patients treated and severe hypophosphatemia requiring phosphate supplementation is seen in 7% of patients receiving gallium nitrate. Mild to moderate hypocalcemia was reported in 38% of patients in a clinical trial. Decreased serum bicarbonate occurs in 40–50% of cancer patients treated with gallium nitrate.

6. **Plicamycin (Mithracin).** This is a potent antineoplastic agent initially used for the treatment of some malignant tumors of the testes. Plicamycin inhibits bone resorption and causes hypocalcemia. Plicamycin at dosages of 15–25 µg/kg/day infused IV usually reverses hypercalcemia within 48 hours in patients with cancer. Plicamycin should be used only

for the treatment of hypercalcemia of malignancy that has been refractory to other modalities of therapy.

  a. **Dosage and administration.** The recommended dose is 15–25 μg/kg infused IV over 4–6 hours. The appropriate dose of plicamycin should be diluted in 1000 ml of 0.9% saline or 5% dextrose and infused IV over a period of 4–6 hours. The response of the serum calcium level and signs of toxicity should be evaluated over the ensuing 48 hours. If hypercalcemia persists, the infusion can be repeated for 3 or 4 days.

  b. **Side effects.** The most serious form of toxicity associated with plicamycin is a bleeding diathesis, which may begin as an episode of epistaxis and progress to hematemesis and generalized bleeding. The bleeding syndrome appears to be dose-related and is rarely seen after single infusions and at the dosages used for the treatment of hypercalcemia.

7. **Glucocorticoids.** Large initial doses of hydrocortisone, 250–500 mg IV every 8 hours (or its equivalent), can be effective in the treatment of hypercalcemia associated with lymphoproliferative diseases, such as non-Hodgkin's lymphoma and multiple myeloma, and in patients with breast cancer metastatic to bone. However, it may take several days for glucocorticoids to lower the serum calcium level. Maintenance therapy should be started with prednisone 10–30 mg/day PO. The mechanisms by which glucocorticoids lower the serum calcium are multiple and involve the following.

  a. Inhibition of OAFs

  b. Inhibition of phospholipase A_2, thereby blocking PG synthesis

  c. Reduction of the rate of bone turnover

  d. Reduction of the rate of intestinal absorption of calcium

  e. Reduction of the rate of renal tubular resorption of calcium

8. **Oral phosphate supplements (Neutra-Phos or Fleet Phospho-Soda).** Oral phosphate therapy is an adjunct for the chronic treatment of hypercalcemia of malignancy. Oral phosphate decreases the intestinal absorption of calcium and enhances the deposition of insoluble calcium salts in bone and tissue. Oral phosphate supplements at dosages of 1.5–3.0 gm/day of elemental phosphorus can result in mild lowering of the serum calcium levels as well as a reduction in urinary calcium excretion. Diarrhea usually limits the amount of phosphate that can be given. Phosphate supplements should never be given to patients with renal failure or when hyperphosphatemia is present, since soft-tissue calcification may occur. Monitoring of the level of calcium and phos-

phorus as well as the calcium–phosphorus ion product is important to prevent metastatic calcifications.

9. **PG inhibitors.** Nonsteroidal anti-inflammatory agents inhibit cyclooxygenase and thereby block PG synthesis. Inhibitors of PG synthesis have been effective in rare patients with metastatic renal cell carcinoma and squamous cell carcinoma of the lung. Indomethacin 50 mg tid is the most potent inhibitor of PG synthesis. Aspirin 1 gm tid has also been shown to be effective in selected patients.

III. **Hyponatremia and cancer**

A. **The syndrome of inappropriate secretion of antidiuretic hormone (SIADH) and water intoxication.** Another endocrine syndrome that frequently is associated with cancer is hyponatremia. Hyponatremia in patients with cancer can be caused by either inappropriate secretion of ADH of central origin or ectopic production of ADH by the tumor. Hyponatremia also can be caused by several drugs, including some drugs frequently used for cancer chemotherapy.

A variety of tumors have been associated with ectopic production of ADH. The material synthesized by neoplasms has been characterized and appears to be arginine vasopressin (AVP). Ectopic production of ADH has been detected in approximately 40% of the patients with carcinoma of the lung and carcinoma of the colon without clinical evidence of this syndrome. The most common tumors associated with SIADH are shown in Table 34-2.

B. **Other causes of SIADH and hyponatremia.** It is important to distinguish between ectopic production of ADH and other causes of the SIADH. Also, it is important to eliminate the possibility that the syndrome is caused by drugs that can affect water metabolism. The most common drugs that impair water metabolism and that are associated with hyponatremia are listed in Table 34-3.

C. **Spurious hyponatremia and hyperglycemia.** It must be recognized that the presence of lower than normal

Table 34-2. **Most common tumors associated with SIADH**

Small-cell anaplastic (oat-cell) and occasionally non-small-cell carcinomas of the lung

Carcinoid tumors

Pancreatic carcinoma

Esophageal carcinoma

Prostatic carcinoma

Adrenal cortical carcinoma

Bladder carcinoma

Hodgkin's disease

Acute myelogenous leukemia

Table 34-3. Drugs associated with hyponatremia

Drugs	Potentiates renal action of AVP	Potentiates release of AVP
Chlorpropamide (Diabinese)	x	x
Tolbutamide (Orinase)	x	
Clofibrate (Atromid-S)		x
Carbamazepine (Tegretol)		x
Vincristine (Oncovin)		x
Vinblastine (Velban)		x
Cyclophosphamide (Cytoxan)		x
Opiates		x
Histamine		x
Phenformin	x	
Thiazides		x(?)
Nicotine		x
Barbiturates		x(?)
Isoproterenol		x
Thioridazine (Mellaril)*		

AVP = arginine vasopressin.
*Increases thirst.

levels of serum sodium concentration does not always imply hypoosmolarity.

1. **Spurious or artifactual hyponatremia** can occur in patients with marked elevation of *serum lipids* or *serum proteins.*
2. **Severe hyperglycemia** is another common situation that can lead to hyponatremia without hypoosmolarity. With this condition, the increased osmolarity due to hyperglycemia draws water from cells and results in dilution of plasma sodium.

D. **Diagnosis of SIADH.** The important criteria for the diagnosis of SIADH are as follows.

1. Hyponatremia with hypoosmolarity of the serum
2. Inappropriate antidiuresis (urine osmolarity that is higher than that expected for the degree of hyponatremia and hypoosmolarity of the serum)
3. Normal renal, adrenal, thyroid, and pituitary function
4. Evidence of sodium wasting in the urine (urine sodium > 20–40 mEq/liter)
5. Absence of clinical signs of hypovolemia and dehydration
6. Absence of generalized edema or ascites
7. Correction of the hyponatremia and plasma hypoosmolarity by fluid restriction

Patients with mild SIADH may be asymptomatic. However, when the serum sodium levels fall to the range of 120–125 mEq/liter, loss of memory, apathy, and impairment of abstract thought may occur. When serum sodium levels fall below 115 mEq/liter, extrapyramidal signs, asterixis, convulsions, and coma may occur. Serum sodium levels below 115 mEq/liter indicate severe water intoxication and constitute a medical emergency.

E. **Treatment of SIADH.** Successful treatment of the tumor usually corrects SIADH, and reappearance of the syndrome is seen with recurrence of the tumor.

   1. **Fluid restriction.** For mildly symptomatic patients or patients whose serum sodium level has fallen below 125 mEq/liter, fluid restriction is necessary. In these patients, the major source of water loss is insensible. Therefore, to be effective in raising the serum sodium concentration, fluid restrictions to 500 ml/day or less may be necessary in some patients. Once the serum sodium level returns to normal, fluid administration should be increased to replace sensible and insensible losses plus the urine output. Unfortunately, because of the continuous production of ADH by tumors, this approach alone is often impractical and unsuccessful.

   2. **Hypertonic sodium chloride.** For severe hyponatremia and water intoxication (serum sodium < 115 mEq/liter associated with confusion, stupor or coma, muscle twitching, or convulsions), therapy should be aimed at reversing the flow of water into the cells. Such therapy may require the administration of hypertonic sodium chloride (3% sodium chloride, 514 mEq/liter). This approach requires careful monitoring of fluid and electrolyte balance and ready access to the laboratory, since hourly measurements of sodium and potassium in the urine are required. *Furthermore, rapid correction of hyponatremia may lead to permanent neurologic damage due to central pontine myelinolysis and therefore should be avoided.* To avoid neurologic complications the following are recommended.

      a. The rate of correction of hyponatremia should never exceed 1 mEq/liter/hour.
      b. The serum sodium should not be increased by more than 20–25 mEq/liter over 48 hours.
      c. The target serum sodium for correction of hyponatremia should not exceed 125–130 mEq/liter.

   The amount of sodium necessary to accomplish the desired correction can be estimated by the following formula.

   Sodium for replacement (mEq) = (desired serum sodium [mEq/liter] − observed serum sodium [mEq/liter]) × body weight (kg) × 0.6

   Use of hypertonic sodium chloride is potentially dangerous and may result in fluid and circulatory overload, especially in elderly patients. To prevent these complications, IV furosemide can be added to the regimen. Alternatively, the IV use of furosemide (1 mg/kg) as initial therapy followed by the hourly replacement of the urinary losses of sodium and potassium with 3% sodium chloride with potassium chloride added to it can correct severe hyponatremia.

3. **Demeclocycline (Declomycin).** This drug antagonizes the renal actions of AVP and therefore causes a reversible, dose-dependent nephrogenic diabetes insipidus. Demeclocycline, in divided doses of 600–1200 mg/day and combined with moderate water restriction, is successful in treating chronic SIADH associated with tumors. The most common side effects of this drug are anorexia, nausea, and vomiting. Skin rashes and hypersensitivity to ultraviolet light are also common. Because of the antianabolic effect of the tetracyclines, this drug may cause a rise in BUN. Also, when combined with fluid restriction, it may lead to sodium depletion and dehydration.

4. **Lithium carbonate.** This has also been used for the treatment of chronic tumor-associated SIADH, but it is more toxic and inferior to demeclocycline.

IV. **Ectopic Cushing's syndrome (ectopic ACTH/beta-lipotropin hormone)**

A. **Production of hormones.** ACTH-producing tumors synthesize and release ACTH, beta-lipotropin hormone (β-LPH), and beta-endorphin, which originate from the common precursor molecule pro-opiomelanocortin (POMC); γ-LPH, alpha- and beta-melanocyte-stimulating hormone (MSH), and corticotropin-like intermediate lobe peptide (CLIP) have also been found in some tumors causing the ectopic ACTH syndrome. Simultaneous production of other unrelated peptide hormones, such as vasopressin (ADH) and calcitonin, has been reported. Furthermore, production of corticotropin-releasing factor (CRF) has been documented in several neoplasms.

The tumors most commonly associated with the ectopic Cushing's syndrome are shown in Table 34-4.

Table 34-4. Tumors most commonly associated with ectopic Cushing's syndrome

Small-cell anaplastic (oat-cell) carcinoma of the lung

Thymoma

Pancreatic carcinoma (including carcinoid and islet cell tumors)

Medullary thyroid carcinoma

Pheochromocytoma, neuroblastoma, ganglioma, and para-ganglioma

Bronchial adenoma and bronchial carcinoid

Melanoma

Prostatic carcinoma

B. Symptoms and signs. The ectopic ACTH syndrome is more common in men and has a higher frequency in patients over the age of 50 years, probably because small-cell anaplastic carcinoma of the lung, which is the most common cause of the syndrome, is 10 times more common in men of this age group. Most patients with ectopic ACTH syndrome do not have the characteristic clinical appearance of Cushing's syndrome. The absence of this clinical picture is probably due to the catabolic effects of the neoplasm as well as to the sudden onset and rapidly deteriorating clinical course of patients with these malignant neoplasms. However, when the syndrome is caused by a less malignant or a benign tumor such as a bronchial carcinoid, classic cushingoid features may be found. In the more typical ectopic ACTH syndrome, anorexia and weight loss, rather than obesity, are common. Hypertension and hyperpigmentation are more common than in Cushing's syndrome of other causes. Severe muscular weakness is one of the most common manifestations of the syndrome. Edema, polyuria, and polydipsia are often seen. The course of patients with ectopic ACTH syndrome is usually more rapid and the prognosis is worse than in patients with similar tumors without the ectopic ACTH syndrome. However, cures have been reported after successful removal of bronchial carcinoids causing the ectopic ACTH syndrome.

C. Laboratory findings

1. Hypokalemic alkalosis. Severe, unexplained hypokalemia with serum potassium levels usually below 3 mEq/liter and metabolic alkalosis with venous bicarbonate levels higher than 30 mEq/liter is one of the most common findings. *Hypokalemic alkalosis when observed in a patient with cancer in the absence of diuretic use should alert the physician to the possibility of ectopic ACTH syndrome.* Severe muscle weakness, paresthesias, hyporeflexia, and muscle paralysis may occur. Cardiac arrhythmias, electrocardiographic (ECG) findings of hypokalemia, and increased sensitivity to the effects of digitalis glycosides may occur.

2. Hyperglycemia or abnormal glucose tolerance is common.

3. Hormone abnormalities. Plasma cortisol, plasma ACTH, free urinary cortisol, and 17-hydroxysteroids show marked increases. Typically, patients with ectopic ACTH syndrome caused by bronchogenic carcinoma show a lack of suppression of the plasma cortisol, plasma ACTH, and urinary free cortisol with the overnight high-dose dexamethasone (8 mg PO in the evening followed by a plasma cortisol and ACTH level the following morning) or with the 2-day high-dose dexamethasone (2 mg dexamethasone q6h for 2 days). In contrast, 20–50% of the patients with this syndrome due to bronchial carcinoids show suppression with this dose of dexamethasone.

D. Treatment

1. **Primary tumor.** The therapy of choice for ectopic ACTH syndrome is treatment of the primary tumor with surgery, radiotherapy, or chemotherapy. Unfortunately, as the most common cause of the syndrome is small-cell anaplastic carcinoma of the lung, complete removal or permanent eradication of this tumor is seldom possible. Complete removal of less aggressive tumors, e.g., bronchial carcinoids, may result in total cure of the syndrome.

2. **Correction of hypokalemia**

   a. **Oral potassium therapy.** Because of the concomitant alkalosis and hypochloremia, *only potassium chloride supplements should be employed.* The severe depletion may require that potassium 40–100 mEq/day be given. Nausea, vomiting, and gastrointestinal irritation may be important deterrents for the use of oral potassium supplementation, especially in patients who may be receiving simultaneous chemotherapy.

   b. **IV potassium administration.** IV therapy is necessary for severe hypokalemia (serum potassium < 2 mEq/liter), if the patient cannot tolerate oral potassium or in the presence of cardiac arrhythmias or extreme muscular weakness. The potassium chloride solution should be dissolved only in normal saline or 0.5% N saline solution, not in glucose-containing solutions as the availability of glucose in nondiabetic patients may cause an intracellular shift of potassium and may aggravate hypokalemia. Potassium chloride solutions at concentrations of no more than 60 mEq/liter should be used, and the rate of IV administration should never exceed 40 mEq/hour. IV potassium therapy should be monitored by frequent determinations of serum potassium. At high infusion rates (30–40 mEq/hour), continuous monitoring of the ECG is necessary. In patients with tumors producing multiple hormones (e.g., ACTH and ADH), correction of hypokalemia may restore ADH sensitivity, and hyponatremia and water intoxication may develop.

   c. **Spironolactone (Aldactone).** This is a specific pharmacologic antagonist of aldosterone that acts primarily through competitive binding of the mineralocorticoid receptors at the sodium-potassium exchange sites of the distal tubules. Doses of 100–400 mg daily may be necessary to correct hypokalemia. Spironolactone should not be used in conjunction with potassium supplements or other potassium-sparing drugs without close monitoring, as severe hyperkalemia may develop. Spironolactone may not always be effective in preventing hypokalemia and metabolic alkalosis in patients with ectopic Cushing's syndrome, but it may be used temporarily until more effective measures are established. Spironolactone should not be used in the presence of severe impairment of renal function or oliguria. The most common side effects include gynecomastia, abdominal cramping, diarrhea, dizziness, lethargy, and confusion.

3. **Management of sodium and water retention.** In patients with severe hypertension and edema, moderate sodium restriction and diuretics are indicated. Caution must be exerted with the use of diuretics in ectopic Cushing's syndrome, as hypokalemia may be aggravated by their use. A combination of thiazides with potassium-sparing drugs, e.g., amiloride or triamterine, may be effective in some patients. When severe hypertension and pulmonary congestion are present, oral or IV furosemide should be used.

4. **Treatment of metabolic alkalosis.** Metabolic alkalosis is of the chloride-resistant type and is caused by excess mineralocorticoids. This excess causes intracellular shifts of hydrogen ions and increased hydrogen ion secretion by the renal tubule, resulting in severe alkalosis. Characteristically, urinary chloride levels are less than 15 mEq/liter. Treatment consists of potassium chloride supplement, spironolactone, and more importantly, correction of the mineralocorticoid excess by the use of inhibitors of adrenal steroid synthesis.

5. **Adrenal enzyme inhibitors**
   a. **Ketoconazole (Nizoral)**
   (1) **Mechanism of action.** Ketoconazole is an antifungal, imidazole derivative agent that inhibits the production of androgens and adrenal glucocorticoids. Ketoconazole has been used successfully in the treatment of patients with Cushing's syndrome of different etiologies including ectopic Cushing's syndrome. Ketoconazole blocks steroidogenesis by inhibiting 11β-hydroxylase as well as both cytochrome P-450–dependent mitochondrial enzymes that function at the site of cholesterol side-chain cleavage. Furthermore, ketoconazole blocks androgen synthesis by inhibiting the C_{17-20} lyase enzyme. In addition, there is evidence that ketoconazole binds to glucocorticoid receptors acting as a peripheral glucocorticoid antagonist.

   (2) **Dosage and administration.** Ketoconazole has not been approved for the treatment of Cushing's syndrome. The doses employed for treatment of Cushing's vary from 400–1200 mg/day in divided doses.

   (3) **Prevention of adrenal insufficiency.** Ketoconazole in high doses may cause adrenal insufficiency and therefore monitoring of the patient for clinical and laboratory signs of

adrenal insufficiency is required. To prevent the development of adrenal insufficiency, glucocorticoids and mineralocorticoid should be replaced. Adrenal replacement therapy can be done with one of the following agents.

Hydrocortisone 40–60 mg/day in divided doses *or*
Dexamethasone 0.50–0.75 mg bid or tid

In patients receiving hydrocortisone replacement, the response to ketoconazole therapy should be monitored by measuring the plasma levels of dehydroepiandrosterone sulfate (DHEA-S). In patients receiving dexamethasone replacement, response to therapy can be monitored by measuring the levels of plasma or urinary cortisol. If hypotension or hyperkalemia develops, the patient should also receive mineralocorticoid replacement therapy with fludrocortisone (Florinef) 0.05–0.10 mg/day. Development of hyponatremia may be another indication of mineralocorticoid deficiency, but the possibility of concomitant production of ADH by the tumor has to be considered.

   (4) **Side effects.** Although the drug is well tolerated by the majority of patients, severe hepatotoxicity has been reported in some patients, including a few fatalities. Therefore patients should be instructed to report any signs or symptoms suggestive of liver disease so that appropriate testing of liver function can be done. In rare cases anaphylactic reactions occur after the first dose. Doses of 800–1600 mg/day cause testosterone deficiency and adrenal insufficiency.

b. **Metyrapone (Metopirone)**
   (1) **Mechanism of action.** Metyrapone is a synthetic compound that inhibits adrenal 11β-hydroxylase, causing a rapid reduction of cortisol production.
   (2) **Therapeutic use.** For therapeutic purposes, metyrapone can be used at a dosage of 500 mg every 4–6 hours PO (2–3 gm/day), and according to the clinical response, the dosage may be lowered.
   (3) **Effects of therapy.** Although metyrapone rapidly lowers plasma cortisol levels, it does not lower the levels of deoxycorticosterone (DOC), which is a powerful mineralocorticoid. In patients with the ectopic ACTH syndrome, the plasma levels of DOC are usually ninefold to 12-fold higher than normal. Therefore, rapid relief of symptoms caused by the excess cortisol is expected after me-

tyrapone treatment, but hypokalemia and metabolic alkalosis may not improve by treatment with metyrapone alone. The most common adverse reactions have been nausea, abdominal discomfort, dizziness, headache, sedation, and allergic reactions.

c. **Aminoglutethimide (Cytadren).** This agent is derived from the hypnotic drug glutethimide, which was formerly used for the treatment of epilepsy. Aminoglutethimide causes a reversible medical adrenalectomy, with marked reduction in the production of adrenal glucocorticoids, mineralocorticoids, androgens, and estrogens. Approximately two-thirds of the patients with ectopic ACTH syndrome treated with aminoglutethimide show clinical and biochemical evidence of improvement.

(1) **Dosage and administration.** The recommended dosage of aminoglutethimide for the treatment of Cushing's syndrome is 1 gm/day in four divided doses. In some patients, dosages of 1.5–2.0 gm/day may be necessary.

(2) **To prevent adrenal insufficiency,** hydrocortisone or dexamethasone may be used in a similar schedule as that recommended for patients treated with ketoconazole. Aminoglutethimide increases the rate of metabolism of hydrocortisone and dexamethasone, and it may be necessary to use larger doses of hydrocortisone or dexamethasone than those required for physiologic replacement.

d. **Mitotane (Lysodren, o,p′-DDD)**

(1) **Mechanism of action.** Mitotane is an oral chemotherapeutic agent known by its trivial name o,p′-DDD. It is an adrenal cytotoxic agent, although it also can cause inhibition of steroidogenesis without cellular destruction.

(2) **Dosage and administration.** Treatment with mitotane should be instituted in the hospital until a stable dosage regimen is achieved. *Signs and symptoms of adrenal insufficiency may develop in patients receiving mitotane.* Therefore, adrenal steroid replacement should be started (see sec **IV.5.a.3.**) together with the mitotane, although the effect of the drug on adrenal steroidogenesis is not immediate. Mitotane should be started at dosages of 4–8 gm/day PO in divided doses either qid or tid. If severe side effects appear, the dosage should be reduced until the maximal tolerated dosage is achieved. If the patient can tolerate higher dosages and if there is a possibility of further clinical improvement, the dosage should be increased

until adverse reactions interfere. Maximum tolerated dosages vary from 2–16 gm/day. Treatment should be continued as long as clinical benefits are observed. If no clinical benefits are observed after 3 months at the maximum tolerated dose, the drug should be discontinued. Dosages as low as 4 gm/day, when combined with metyrapone (500 mg q4h), cause complete remission of hypercorticism in patients with ectopic ACTH syndrome.

The combined administration of metyrapone, aminoglutethimide, and mitotane has been reported to be effective in some patients with ectopic Cushing's syndrome.

6. **Octreotide acetate (Sandostatin).** Ocreotide is a long-acting somatostatin analog used for the treatment of carcinoid tumors and vasoactive intestinal peptide (VIP)–producing tumors. Octreotide inhibits the release of growth hormone, glucagon, and insulin. In patients with the ectopic ACTH syndrome, octreotide (150–600 μg/day SQ) has been shown to reduce plasma ACTH and corticotropin-releasing hormone (CRH) levels and normalize urinary free cortisol excretion. Clinical improvement has been maintained for several months but tumor progression has continued. Combined therapy with ketoconazole is superior than monotherapy with either drug alone. Chronic therapy with octreotide may cause hypothyroidism.

7. **RU 486.** This experimental drug is a 19-nor-steroid glucocorticoid antagonist. RU 486 has high affinity for the glucocorticoid receptor and no agonistic effects. This drug has been used successfully to treat a patient with Cushing's syndrome secondary to ectopic ACTH secretion. Treatment with this drug produced clinical and biochemical remission of hypercortisolism despite persistently elevated levels of cortisol. The drug was well tolerated and no side effects were reported; however, at high doses it may cause glucocorticoid insufficiency, which may be difficult to recognize since cortisol levels remain elevated or even increase. Lower cost and increased availability in the future make this drug a promising therapy for the ectopic ACTH syndrome.

V. **Hypoglycemia and cancer.** A wide variety of non–islet cell tumors may be associated with hypoglycemia. Hypoglycemia may occur months or even years before recognition of the tumor, it may be present at the time of diagnosis, or it may develop after the diagnosis of malignancy has been well established.

A. **Presentation of neoplasms.** Most of the neoplasms associated with hypoglycemia are large and may present as masses in the mediastinum or retroperitoneal space. The most common non–beta cell tumors associated with hypoglycemia are shown in Table 34-5.

Table 34-5. Most common non–beta cell tumors associated with hypoglycemia

Mesenchymal or mesodermal: fibrosarcomas, mesotheliomas, neurofibromas, neurofibrosarcoma, spindle cell sarcoma, rhabdomyosarcomas, and leiomyosarcomas

Hepatocellular carcinoma

Adrenocortical carcinoma

Pancreatic and bile duct carcinomas

Lymphomas and leukemias

Miscellaneous: lung, ovary, neuroblastoma, Wilms' tumor, and hemangiopericytoma

B. **Pathogenesis of hypoglycemia.** The pathogenesis of hypoglycemia in patients with malignancy is not clear. The possible causes of hypoglycemia are production and secretion of insulin, production of nonsuppressible insulin-like protein (NSILA-p), production of insulin-like growth factor II (IGF-II), proliferation of insulin receptors, increased glucose utilization by the tumor, production of metabolites that interfere with gluconeogenesis, inhibition of glycogen breakdown, suppression of counterregulatory hormones, and destruction of the liver by tumor.

1. **Secretion of insulin by tumors is rare.** In only a few patients has an increased insulin concentration in the blood or in the tumors been reported. Such tumors include teratoma of the mediastinum, bronchial carcinoid, carcinoma of the cervix, retroperitoneal fibrosarcoma, and bronchogenic metastasis.

2. The best documented **mechanisms for hypoglycemia in cancer** are as follows.
   a. Production of the high-molecular-weight protein NSILA-p, whose action is not suppressed by insulin antibodies
   b. Production of a biologically active but not immunoreactive IGF-II
   c. Increased glucose utilization due to proliferation of insulin receptors in liver and muscle, induced by an unknown humoral substance

   There is also evidence for a high rate of glycolysis of these large tumors and this glycolysis could possibly contribute to excessive glucose utilization. It is likely that a variety of mechanisms may be responsible for the hypoglycemia in different tumors.

3. **Artifactual hypoglycemia.** In patients with hematologic malignancies and markedly elevated white blood cell counts, artifactual hypoglycemia may be seen owing to increased in vitro glucose utilization by glycolysis. In such patients plasma glucose should be measured in freshly obtained specimens to avoid possible confusion.

C. **Symptoms, signs, and laboratory findings.** The hypoglycemia that occurs with non–beta cell tumors usually occurs during fasting in the early morning or late afternoon, and its onset is usually insidious. In most patients, symptoms of neuroglycopenia predominate. They usually develop when the plasma glucose level falls below 45–50 mg/dl, at which point the patients may experience symptoms and signs that resemble a variety of neurologic or psychiatric disturbances. When the hypoglycemia is severe and protracted, generalized convulsions and coma may occur. Typically, the symptoms of hypoglycemia are relieved by the ingestion of food. The hypoglycemia caused by non–islet cell tumors cannot be differentiated clinically from that caused by insulinomas, but they can be differentiated by measuring the fasting plasma insulin and glucose levels. Whereas patients with insulinomas have fasting hyperinsulinemia in the presence of hypoglycemia, patients with non–islet cell tumors have hypoglycemia with low levels of insulin.

D. **Treatment.** Therapy of hypoglycemia associated with non–islet cell tumors is difficult because no specific agents are available. Amelioration of hypoglycemia may result from partial or complete resection of the tumor or by control of the tumor by either chemotherapy or radiation therapy.

1. **Diet.** The primary form of therapy is dietary. Frequent feedings between meals, at bedtime, and throughout the night may decrease the frequency of hypoglycemic attacks. In severe cases, it may be necessary to place an ileostomy tube for continuous feeding, especially during the night. In some patients, it is also necessary to administer continuous infusions of 10–20% glucose.

2. **Hyperglycemic hormones.** High doses of glucocorticoids (prednisone 20–80 mg or dexamethasone 10–15 mg/day) may be used in patients who do not respond to diet therapy. Also, patients may benefit from the use of long-acting glucagon (zinc glucagon) and human growth hormone. In most patients, however, the effect of these agents is only temporary.

3. **Diazoxide (Hyperstat).** This nondiuretic derivative of the benzothiadiazine group inhibits insulin secretion and thereby causes hyperglycemia. Diazoxide has been effective for the treatment of hypoglycemia associated with malignant insulinomas at dosages of 300–600 mg/day IV given in conjunction with hydrochlorothiazide (100 mg/day PO). However, in patients with hypoglycemia from non–islet cell tumors, diazoxide is frequently ineffective. Hypotension may occasionally result from the IV administration of diazoxide. Infrequently, severe hypotension and shock may be seen. Sodium and water retention after repeated injections is common but may be obviated by the simultaneous use of hydrochlorothiazide or other diuretics.

4. Phenytoin and somatostatin. These drugs are usually ineffective in patients with hypoglycemia due to non-insulin-producing tumors.

5. Streptozocin and chlorozotocin. These two drugs which may be effective in insulinomas can be tried in patients with refractory hypoglycemia, but the results have been disappointing in non–islet cell tumors.

VI. Ectopic production of gonadotropins

A. Causes and clinical observations. Ectopic production of gonadotropins can result in gynecomastia in adults and in precocious puberty in children. Increased follicle-stimulating hormone production has been documented in patients with adenocarcinoma of the lung and increased luteinizing hormone activity has been found in a hepatoblastoma from a patient with precocious puberty. In addition to carcinoma of the lung and hepatoblastoma, tumors of the testes, ovaries, pineal gland, mediastinum, adrenals, breast, and bladder and melanomas may be associated with gonadotropin production. There is no specific treatment for the ectopic production of gonadotropins other than therapy of the primary tumor. Symptomatic gynecomastia can be controlled by radiotherapy to the breast area.

VII. Ectopic thyrotropin secretion

A. Causes. Hyperthyroidism has been noted primarily in patients with trophoblastic tumors, although a similar syndrome with epidermoid cancers of the lung and mesothelioma has been reported. The hyperthyroidism in these patients is usually mild, although severe cases have been reported in association with choriocarcinomas. The nature of the thyroid stimulator in chorionic tumors has been named *molar thyroid-stimulating hormone (molar TSH),* and evidence suggests that thyrotropic activity cannot be distinguished from that of human chorionic gonadotropin (hCG).

B. Treatment. In patients with hydatidiform mole and hyperthyroidism, surgical removal is the treatment of choice and should be performed as soon as possible. If the hyperthyroidism is severe, administration of sodium iodide (0.5–1.0 gm IV q12h or Lugol's solution 8 drops q6h by mouth) effectively reduces the concentrations of triiodothyronine (T_3) and thyroxine (T_4) in the plasma. Propranolol 40–160 mg/day may be used for control of the tachycardia. In patients with choriocarcinoma, symptomatic hyperthyroidism can be treated with propylthiouracil (100 mg q8h) or methimazole (10 mg q8h) as well as propranolol. Effective chemotherapy of the tumor reduces the levels of hCG and thereby provides definitive treatment of the hyperthyroidism.

VIII. Erythrocytosis and tumors.

Erythrocytosis has been seen in association with a number of benign and malignant tumors. Because erythropoietin is normally produced in the kidney, the most common tumors associated with erythrocytosis are hypernephroma and Wilms' tumor. Other tumors associated with this syndrome are uterine fibromas, cerebellar hemangioblastomas, hepatocellular carcinoma, pheochromocytoma, and ovarian carcinoma. In contrast to patients with polycythemia vera, the plasma and urinary levels of erythropoietin are elevated and there is no splenomegaly. Patients with tumoral erythrocytosis have an elevated hemoglobin, hematocrit, red blood cell count, and red blood cell mass. Remissions are usually seen after complete removal of the tumor. For inoperable tumors, periodic phlebotomies aimed at maintaining the hematocrit below 45% may reduce the incidence of thromboembolism and decrease in cerebral blood flow.

Selected Readings

Baylin, S. B., and De Bustros, A. Hormone Synthesis and Secretion by Cancer. In K. L. Becker (ed.), *Principles and Practice of Endocrinology and Metabolism*. Philadelphia: Lippincott, 1990. Pp. 1626–1629.

Becker, K. L., and Silva, O. L. Paraneoplastic Endocrine Syndromes. In K. L. Becker (ed.), *Principles and Practice of Endocrinology and Metabolism*. Philadelphia: Lippincott, 1990. Pp. 1629–1638.

Odell, W. D. Paraendocrine syndromes of cancer. *Adv. Intern. Med.* 34:325, 1989.

Hypercalcemia and Cancer

Breslau, N. A., et al. Hypercalcemia associated with increased serum calcitriol levels in three patients with lymphoma. *Ann. Intern. Med.* 100:1, 1984.

Burtis, W. J., et al. Immunochemical characterization of circulating parathyroid hormone-related protein in patients with humoral hypercalcemia of cancer. *N. Engl. J. Med.* 322:1106, 1990.

Elomaa, A., et al. Diphosphonates for osteolytic metastases. *Lancet* 1:1155, 1985.

Gucalp, R., et al. Treatment of cancer associated hypercalcemia. Double-blind comparison of rapid and slow intravenous infusion regimens of pamidronate disodium and saline alone. *Arch. Intern. Med.* 154:1935, 1994.

Nussbaum, R. S. Pathophysiology and management of severe hypercalcemia. *Endocrinol. Metab. Clin. North Am.* 22:343, 1993.

Ryzen, E., et al. Intravenous etidronate in the management of malignant hypercalcemia. *Arch. Intern. Med.* 145:449, 1985.

Simpson, E. L., et al. Absence of parathyroid hormone mRNA in nonparathyroid tumors associated with hypercalcemia. *N. Engl. J. Med.* 309:325, 1983.

Van Holten-Verzantvoort, A. T., et al. Reduced morbidity from skeletal metastases in breast cancer patients during long-term bisphosphonate (APD) treatment. *Lancet* 2:983, 1987.

Warrell, R. P., Jr., et al. Gallium nitrate for acute treatment of cancer-related hypercalcemia. A randomized double-blind comparison to calcitonin. *Ann. Intern. Med.* 108:669, 1988.

Warrell, R. P., Jr., and Bockman, A. S. Gallium in the treatment of hypercalcemia and bone metastasis. *Important Adv. Oncol.* 205, 1989.

Ectopic ACTH Syndrome

Farwell, A. P., et al. Total suppression of cortisol excretion by ketoconazole in the therapy of the ectopic adrenocorticotropic hormone syndrome. *Am. J. Med.* 84:1063, 1988.

Nieman, K. L., et al. Successful treatment of Cushing's syndrome with the glucocorticoid antagonist RU 486. *J. Clin. Endocrinol. Metab.* 61:536, 1985.

Hypoglycemia and Cancer

Li, T. C., et al. Surgical cure of hypoglycemia associated with cystosarcoma phylloides and elevated nonsuppressible insulin-like protein. *Am. J. Med.* 74:1080, 1983.

Stuart, C. A., et al. Insulin receptor proliferation: a mechanism for tumor associated hypoglycemia. *J. Clin. Endocrinol. Metab.* 63:879, 1986.

Cancer Survivorship: Insurance, Employment, and Psychosocial Issues

Patricia A. Ganz

I. The cancer survivors

A. Survival statistics for cancer have improved dramatically during the past three decades. Patients with diseases that were once uniformly fatal (e.g., testicular cancer, Hodgkin's disease, childhood acute leukemia) now are regularly cured. Patients with other common neoplasms (e.g., breast cancer, colorectal cancer) enjoy improved disease-free and overall survival as a result of adjuvant therapy. Additional patients increasingly live with cancer that is controlled for extended periods of time, although it may not be cured. Overall, more than 50% of patients with newly diagnosed cancer can expect to survive beyond 5 years after diagnosis.

B. Cancer has become a chronic disease for many of these patients. This has occurred largely because of the more frequent use of combined-modality therapy. Unfortunately, this approach has increased the length of treatment and has prolonged the recovery period. Modern therapy requires many adjustments for patients, including often profound physical and psychologic modifications in their life-style. In addition, the careful monitoring and clinical evaluations that follow the initial phase of treatment (e.g., examinations at 3–4-month intervals) remind patients of their vulnerability to recurrence and the need for surveillance. *Once a cancer patient, always a cancer patient.*

C. The price of cure or prolonged survival sometimes includes acute organ toxicities (e.g., radiation pneumonitis, acute renal failure, sepsis), chronic toxicities (e.g., pulmonary fibrosis, congestive heart failure, graft-versus-host disease, neurologic syndromes, infertility, hypothyroidism), or serious risk of second malignancies. Comprehensive care of the cancer survivor must address appropriate health promotion and disease prevention strategies for these other medical conditions. Comprehensive care also requires that the physician understand and address social and psychologic consequences of the cancer and its therapy. Central issues for many cancer survivors are related to insurance, employment, and the availability of community resources to help deal with their social and psychologic concerns.

II. Insurance issues

A. Health insurance reform is a major issue on the public agenda today, and it is likely that important changes benefiting cancer survivors will occur. A particularly thorny problem has been the exclusion of persons with *"pre-existing conditions"* from health insurance coverage. Typically, cancer survivors have been excluded from coverage when it relates to their previous cancer, e.g., follow-up testing and physical examinations. Up until now, the only way to get around this problem had been through large group insurance plans (large corporations, federal and state governments) where the risk is distributed and a history of preexisting conditions is not considered. Individual policies and small group plans often exclude treatment and follow-up for previously diagnosed conditions. Fortunately, all of the health care reform legislation being proposed acknowledges this problem and should eliminate such exclusionary practices.

Another related problem is the *lack of portability of insurance*. If the patient or spouse who is insured changes employment, the insurance will not follow, and the patient may become uninsured as a result. This situation can lead to loss of insurance through the "preexisting condition" practices. In addition, the insured member of the family may experience "job lock"—staying in a job just to maintain the health insurance.

Cancer survivors can use several strategies to maintain their health insurance. In 1985, Congress passed the Consolidated Omnibus Budget Reconciliation Act (COBRA) health benefit provisions. This legislation contains provisions giving certain former employees, retirees, spouses, and dependent children the right to temporary continuation of health coverage at group rates. Although group health coverage for COBRA participants is usually more expensive than for active employees, it is generally less expensive than individual health coverage. Coverage through COBRA is limited to 18 months, and this time can allow an individual who is uninsured to find suitable coverage.

In a number of states, *high-risk insurance pools* have been established for individuals who have been refused health insurance or for whom the cost of an individual policy is prohibitive. In general, the applicant must demonstrate evidence of ineligibility for coverage at a reasonable charge. *Facing Forward* (see Selected Readings) lists the contact information for states with existing programs.

Other strategies for remaining insured or obtaining insurance after cancer treatment include obtaining dependent coverage under the spouse's insurance plan; joining the current company plan; joining a health maintenance organization or other insurance program during open enrollment; requesting group insurance through a professional organization or other group; applying for Medicare if 65 years or older or disabled; using Medicaid or other state or local programs; and obtaining coverage through an independent broker.

B. **Obtaining life insurance** coverage is most often a problem for childhood cancer survivors and young adult survivors. In general, these patients have not established their careers and families at the time of their cancer diagnosis. They do not face financial and life planning issues until several years after their cancer treatment. Since life insurance plans are based on an actuarial risk of death (or survival), the cancer history is often taken into account and this increases the potential risk of death at an earlier age. Some life insurance companies will not insure cancer survivors, and others will charge exorbitant premiums. Group life insurance (through employment) is a possible solution, since a health history is not usually required for such plans.

III. Employment issues

A. Work and health insurance are closely linked and will likely remain so even with health care reform. However, health insurance is not portable currently, and the loss of a job usually means the loss of health insurance (see **II.A.**). Therefore, cancer survivors or their spouses are under considerable pressure to maintain employment and adequate health insurance. As noted earlier, this situation may lead to job lock.

B. Discrimination at work may be subtle or overt. Physicians can help their patients by informing them about the protection provided to cancer patients under the *Americans with Disabilities Act (ADA)*. (Several free informational brochures are available for patients. See Selected Readings.) Under this legislation, it is illegal for an employer with 15 or more employees to discriminate against cancer patients in all employment practices, including job application procedures, hiring, firing, advancement, compensation, training, and other terms, conditions, and privileges of employment. This also applies to the recruitment, advertising, tenure, layoff, leave, fringe benefits, and all other employment-related activities. For example, an employer may not ask or require a job applicant to take a medical examination before making a job offer. The employer may not ask about the individual's health history, although the employer can ask questions about the ability to perform specific job functions and may, with certain limitations, ask an individual with a disability to describe or demonstrate how they would perform these functions. After a person starts work, a medical examination or inquiry of an employee must be job-related and consistent with the needs of the business. Information from all medical examinations and inquiries must be kept apart from general personnel files as a separate, confidential medical record, and there must be limited access to such information.

During cancer treatment, employers must provide "reasonable accommodation" to the employee. This means that patients receiving treatment might need to request a temporary reassignment or to have their work hours modified. Such accommodation is required for a "known" disability, which means that the patient must come forward to discuss the situation with the employer. Some patients may feel reluctant to do so and they should be informed about their protection under the ADA. Most often discussion with the employer will lead to accommodation; however, when it does not there are a number of approaches that can be taken. These include informal resolution of the problem through the employer's policies and procedures, use of a member of the medical team to educate the employer about the patient's situation, or seeking the support of coworkers who may have an interest in protecting their own potential for discrimination. Legal remedies should be sought if an informal solution cannot be found. Often a mediator can resolve the situation and this will prevent costly litigation.

The *physician can advocate for the patient* by systematically inquiring about the patient's current employment and work status. Informing patients about their rights under the ADA and giving proactive advice about issues related to insurance and employment can assist the patient during this critical period. Such inquiry should occur early during the treatment phase and be reviewed periodically with the patient. It is important to remember that this is usually the patient's first experience with disability, while the physician has helped many others go through this process.

IV. Psychosocial concerns

A. Establishing or continuing intimate relationships
can often become difficult for cancer survivors. The lack of a secure and healthy future, as well as the feeling of vulnerability that the cancer experience often brings about, can interfere with the establishment of new relationships. Similarly, for those survivors with a strong or supportive partner, the relationship can be enhanced by the cancer experience. If tensions in the relationship predated the cancer diagnosis, many individuals will choose to discontinue the relationship. It is rare that the cancer itself is the cause of divorce or separation. Rather, the cancer survivor is likely to reevaluate the good and bad parts of the relationship and make a decision about its continuation based on long-standing issues as well as the cancer crisis.

B. Parenting
can be challenging after a cancer diagnosis. To a certain extent, the age of the children, their life stage, and the role of the other parent during the cancer experience can modify the effects on children. Cancer is a family disease, in that everyone is affected when a member of the family has cancer. Depending on the role of that individual in the family and the severity of the disease and its treatment, a range of difficulties can occur. Early on, the physician should inquire about the welfare of the children of the patient. In many communities, there are resources for younger and older children whose parents have cancer. In general, survivors should be encouraged to be open with their children about their medical history, with a level of information that is age-appropriate. Sometimes, survivors can face difficult sit-

uations, such as during custody disputes or during adoption proceedings. It is not unheard of for the health of the survivor to be challenged and their ability to parent questioned. The physician can be supportive by providing accurate information about the survivor's status and capabilities.

C. Sexuality represents a range of issues from how one feels about one's body to the actual ability to function as a sexual being. This is a topic of considerable concern to most survivors. In spite of this fact, physicians rarely address sexual matters with survivors, assuming that all is going well if the patient is disease-free and not on treatment. In our research with breast, colon, lung, and prostate cancer survivors, issues related to sexual functioning were the most persistent and severe problems that these survivors reported. Only the most vocal or severely distressed patients will discuss these problems with their physician; yet when asked about how their sex life is, most will be pleased that the physician has inquired. Sexual dysfunction is common in the general population and can be exacerbated by cancer and its treatment. Often the sexual problems can be addressed with pharmaceutical agents or with counseling. Most often the physician can address these problems directly or refer the patient to an appropriate resource. Provision of information and reassurance are an important starting point for most patients.

D. Fear of recurrence is one of the most persistent psychologic sequelae of cancer. The intensity of this fear tends to diminish with time; however, many seasoned survivors will recount their anxiety and fear during an annual checkup decades after their cancer diagnosis. It is common for minor aches and pains to generate considerable anxiety early on in the survivorship experience. A reassuring relationship with the physician, with open discussion of how to manage and assess these aches and pains, can assure the patient that persistent pains could signal a recurrence but transient and fleeting complaints are common in everyone. Letting the patient know you are available to discuss these experiences when they occur will provide considerable reassurance. Patients vary in their anxiety, but often reaching certain landmarks (e.g., 5-year survivorship) will lead to diminishment of these fears.

V. Resources for cancer survivors and their health care providers

A. The National Coalition for Cancer Survivorship (NCCS) was established in 1986 to provide information, service, and advocacy for cancer survivors. It is a national consumer network of individuals, organizations, and institutions serving tens of thousands of cancer survivors and those who care for them. The NCCS has a number of publications relevant to employment rights and job discrimination, and communication between patients and physicians, and members of NCCS contributed to a National Cancer Institute (NCI) publication

specifically designed for cancer survivors (see *Facing Forward*, in Selected Readings). NCCS maintains a telephone inquiry service for survivors for issues related to insurance and employment. The telephone number for this organization is (301) 650-8868.
B. **The Cancer Information Service (CIS),** the NCI-sponsored hotline for information about cancer, and the American Cancer Society (ACS) local units are other important sources of information for cancer survivors. The CIS can be reached by dialing 1-800-4-CANCER and the ACS can be contacted by dialing 1-800-ACS-2345. In addition to verbal and written information, these hotlines provide information about community resources and support groups that are relevant to survivors' concerns. Examples of important referral resources include state or local vocational rehabilitation programs, or legal aid for employment discrimination issues. Survivors, family members, and health professionals should consider contacting these resources as necessary.

Selected Readings

American Cancer Society. *Sexuality and Cancer: For the Woman Who Has Cancer and Her Partner.* Atlanta: March 1991.

American Cancer Society. *Sexuality and Cancer: For the Man Who Has Cancer and His Partner.* Atlanta: May 1994.

Andersen, B. L. How cancer affects sexual functioning. *Oncology* 4(6):81, 1990.

Fobair, P., et al. Psychosocial problems among survivors of Hodgkin's disease. *J. Clin. Oncol.* 4:805, 1986.

Ganz, P. A., for the ASCO Committee on Patient Advocacy. The physician as the patient's advocate. *J. Clin. Oncol.* 11:1011, 1993.

Lacher, M. J., and Redman, J. R. (eds.), *Hodgkin's Disease. The Consequences of Survival.* Philadelphia: Lea & Febiger, 1990.

Mullan, F., and Hoffman, B. (eds.), *Charting the Journey: An Almanac of Practical Resources for Cancer Survivors.* Mount Vernon, NY: Consumer Union, 1990.

National Cancer Institute. *Facing Forward.* NIH publication no. 93-2424. Bethesda, MD: July 1990, Revised October 1992.

National Coalition for Cancer Survivorship (NCCS). *Working It Out: Your Employment Rights as a Cancer Survivor.* Silver Spring, MD: NCCS, 1993.

Schover, L. R. The impact of breast cancer on sexuality, body image, and intimate relationships. *CA Cancer J. Clin.* 41:112, 1991.

Texas Cancer Council. *Cancer and the Law.* A self-help guide for people with cancer and cancer survivors. Request through Public Information Department of the Texas State Bar, 1-800-204-222.

U.S. Department of Labor. *Health Benefits under the Consolidated Omnibus Budget Reconciliation Act.* Washington, DC: Pension and Welfare Benefits Administration, 1990.

U.S. Equal Employment Opportunity Commission and U.S. Department of Justice, Civil Rights Division. The Americans with Disabilities Act. Questions and Answers. EEOC-BK-15, revised September 1992.

Welch-McCaffrey, D., et al. Surviving adult cancers. Part 2: psychosocial implications. *Ann. Intern. Med.* 111:517, 1989.

Malignant Pleural, Peritoneal, and Pericardial Effusions and Meningeal Infiltrates

Walter D. Y. Quan, Jr.

Malignant pleural, peritoneal, and pericardial effusions and malignant meningeal infiltrates are uncommon early in the course of the malignancy. They occur more frequently with disseminated disease and often herald a poor prognosis. Although pleural and peritoneal effusions may initially have little adverse effect on quality of life, when progressive they (as well as pericardial effusions and meningeal infiltrates) can result in incapacitating disability and death. It is therefore necessary for the clinician to have a high index of suspicion for these problems and to be prepared to take appropriate action and deliver palliative treatment promptly.

I. Pleural effusions

A. **Causes.** Malignant pleural effusions arise in association with malignant cells lining the pleura, exuded into the pleural space, or blocking veins or lymphatics. The most common malignancy associated with pleural effusions in women is carcinoma of the breast, whereas in men it is carcinoma of the lung. Other causes of malignant pleural effusions include lymphoma, mesothelioma, and carcinomas of the ovary, gastrointestinal tract, urinary tract, and uterus. Malignancy is not the only cause of effusions even in patients with known neoplastic disease, and therefore it is important to attempt to rule out other possible causes such as congestive heart failure, infection, and pulmonary infarction.

B. **Diagnosis**

1. **Clinical diagnosis.** Effusions may be asymptomatic or may be suspected because of respiratory symptoms, such as shortness of breath with exertion or at rest, orthopnea, paroxysmal nocturnal dyspnea, or occasionally chest pressure or cough. The patient may feel more comfortable when lying on one side when the effusion is unilateral. On physical examination dullness to percussion, decreased tactile fremitus, diminished breath sounds, and egophony are typical signs over the area of the effusion.

2. **A chest x-ray film** should be obtained to confirm the clinical impression. If fluid appears to be present, a lateral decubitus film must be obtained to help estimate the volume of the effusion and how free it is within the pleural space.

3. **Diagnostic thoracentesis** should be performed. Ultrasonographic guidance is helpful if loculation is present. Fluid should be obtained for bacterial, acid-fast, and fungal cultures, for cytologic examination, and for determining protein concentration

(> 3.0 gm/dl in most exudates), lactate dehydrogenase (LDH) level, specific gravity, and cell count.
The cytologic examination is important because if
the results are positive, as in 50–70% of patients
with malignant effusion, the diagnosis is established. Other parameters of the pleural fluid that
may be helpful in establishing that the fluid is an
exudate and not a transudate include a specific gravity of more than 1.015, protein concentration that is
more than 0.5 times the serum protein concentration, LDH level more than 0.6 times the serum LDH
level, and low glucose level. A cytologic examination
of fluid from a newly discovered pleural effusion is
wise, regardless of whether the patient is known to
have malignancy, because for nearly one-half of all
malignant effusions this finding is the first sign of
malignancy. Analyzing pleural fluid for carcinoembryonic antigen (CEA) may be helpful in some patients. Levels higher than 20 ng/ml are suggestive of
adenocarcinoma, although they do not substitute for
a tissue diagnosis in patients who have no history of
malignancy. CEA elevations may be seen in adenocarcinomas from various primary sites, including the
breast, lung, and gastrointestinal tract. Elevated
levels between 10 and 20 ng/ml may be reflective of
malignancy or of benign disorders such as pulmonary infection. The role of assessing other tumor
markers on a routine basis has not been established.
Likewise, the utility of monoclonal antibodies and
gene rearrangement studies in patients with lymphomas to distinguish reactive mesothelial or lymphocytic cells from malignant cells has yet to be determined. The routine use of a "panel of tumor
markers" is costly and time-consuming.

4. **Pleural biopsy** may be helpful in establishing the
diagnosis in up to 20% of patients for whom the
pleural fluid cytology results are negative.

5. **Thoracotomy or pleuroscopy with direct biopsy** may be done in patients who have negative cytology and pleural biopsy results but in whom there
is still high suspicion of malignancy.

C. **Treatment.** As malignant pleural effusions are generally a sign of systemic rather than localized disease, the
best therapy is treatment that effectively treats the malignancy systemically. Unfortunately, effective systemic
treatment is often not possible, particularly when the
malignancy is commonly refractory to systemic treatment (e.g., in non-small-cell carcinoma of the lung) or in
patients who have previously been heavily treated and
systemic therapy is no longer effective. In these circumstances, local-regional therapy is required for palliation
of the patient's symptoms.

1. **Drainage.** Many malignant pleural effusions recur
within 1–3 days after simple thoracentesis; about
97% recur within 1 month. Chest tube drainage

(closed tube thoracotomy) allows the pleural surfaces to oppose each other and, if maintained for several days, may result in obliteration of the space and improvement in the effusion for several weeks to months. It does not appear to be as effective when used alone as when a cytotoxic or sclerosing agent is added, and therefore one of these agents is commonly instilled into the space while the chest tube is in place.

2. **Cytotoxic and sclerosing agents.** The most widely used agent for intrapleural administration has been the intravenous preparation of tetracycline. However, because the intravenous form is no longer commercially available in the United States, clinicians are required to use alternatives. Fortunately, there are a wide variety of available agents including talc, minocycline, doxycycline, fluorouracil, bleomycin, and interferon alpha from which to choose. Some hospital pharmacies will sterilize oral tetracycline by ultrafiltration, which provides an effective and inexpensive alternative to agents such as bleomycin. Very little in the way of prospective randomized trials has been done to directly compare these agents. In general they appear to have similar efficacy, but vary in toxicity, ease of administration, and cost. For optimal effectiveness, drainage of pleural fluid as completely as possible is required prior to instillation.

   a. **Method of administration.** The drug to be used is diluted in 50–100 ml of saline and instilled through the thoracostomy tube into the chest cavity after the effusion has been drained for at least 24 hours and the rate of collection is less than 100 ml/24 hours. Throughout the procedure, care must be taken to avoid any air leak. The thoracostomy tube is clamped, and the patient is successively repositioned on his or her front, back, and sides for 15-minute periods over the next 2–6 hours. The tube is then reconnected to gravity drainage or suction for at least 18 hours to ensure that the pleural surfaces remain opposed and to prevent the rapid accumulation of any fluid in reaction to the instillation. Some clinicians repeat the instillation daily for a total of 2–3 days. For most of the agents listed here, this has no proven benefit. Exceptions include methylprednisolone acetate and doxycycline, which appear to be more effective with additional doses. If the drainage is less than 40–50 ml over the previous 12 hours, the tube may be removed and a chest x-ray film obtained to be certain that pneumothorax has not occurred during removal of the tube. If the thoracostomy tube continues to drain more than 100 ml/24 hours after the last instillation, it may be necessary to leave it in place for an additional

48–72 hours to ensure that a maximum amount of adhesion between the pleural surfaces has taken place.

b. **Recommended agents.** One must consider efficacy, side effects, and cost when choosing a sclerosing agent. Bleomycin is probably the most widely used agent currently and, in one prospective study, was shown to be more effective than tetracycline. It is also more expensive per dose than the other agents. Talc is the least expensive, but this must be balanced against the costs of related procedures including thoracoscopy and anesthesia. Fluorouracil is relatively inexpensive, but the reported experience with this agent is notgreat. Minocycline or doxycycline may be reasonable alternatives to tetracycline, but the relative numbers of reported patients treated with these agents are small. Clearly, prospective studies of currently available agents to assess not only response but also cost and morbidity are needed.

  (1) **Bleomycin** 1 mg/kg or 40 mg/m^2 has relatively little myelosuppressive effect and is highly effective.

  (2) **Fluorouracil** 2–3 gm (total dose) may have a theoretical advantage in sensitive carcinomas, but whether that advantage is significant has not yet been established. Pain is generally minimal. Occasional patients may experience a depressed white blood cell count, especially at the higher dose.

c. **Alternative agents**

  (1) **Methylprednisolone acetate** 80–160 mg appears to be well tolerated.

  (2) **Interferon alpha** 50 million units typically causes flulike symptoms. Lower doses appear to be ineffective.

  (3) **Doxycycline** 500 mg may cause pleuritic chest pain. An injection of 10 ml of 1% lidocaine (100 mg) through the chest tube may reduce this symptom.

  (4) **Talc** has been used successfully but requires thoracoscopy and general anesthesia. Other agents include doxorubicin and thiotepa.

d. **Responses.** A combination of chest tube drainage and instillation of one of the agents discussed in sec. **I.C.2.b.,c.** controls pleural effusions more than 75% of the time. The durations of response are short, with a median between 3 and 6 months unless the patient's systemic disease comes under adequate control. In that circumstance the effusion may not recur for years or at least until the systemic disease once more emerges.

e. **Side effects** common to most agents include chest pain, fever, and occasional hypotension. These effects are usually not severe and may

be controlled by standard symptomatic management. Fever after pleurodesis is usually not due
to infection.
   3. **Thoracotomy and pleural stripping** may be tried
   subsequently for effusions refractory to medical
   treatment.
II. **Peritoneal effusions**
   A. **Causes.** Malignant peritoneal effusions usually occur in
   association with diffuse seeding of the peritoneal surface
   with small malignant deposits. The impairment of sub-
   phrenic lymphatic or portal venous flow may result in
   peritoneal effusions. Alternatively, it has been postulated that a "capillary leak" phenomenon mediated by
   tumor cells or immune effector cells could be a contrib-
   uting factor. Carcinoma of the ovary is the most commonly associated malignancy in women, whereas in men
   gastrointestinal carcinomas are most common. Other
   neoplasms that may cause peritoneal effusions include
   lymphoma, mesothelioma, and carcinomas of the uterus
   and breast. Liver metastasis by itself, unless it is far advanced, is not usually associated with symptomatic peritoneal effusions.
   B. **Diagnosis**
      1. **Symptoms and signs.** Patients may be completely
      asymptomatic or have so much fluid that they have
      severe abdominal distension, abdominal pain, and
      respiratory distress. In the presence of peritoneal
      metastases, there may be abnormal bowel motility
      that at times resembles a paralytic ileus and may re-
      sult in loss of appetite, early satiety, nausea, and
      vomiting. On examination, the lower abdomen and
      flanks bulge when the patient is supine. Confirma-
      tory signs include shifting dullness, a fluid wave, di-
      minished bowel sounds, or the "puddle sign" (peri-
      umbilical dullness when the patient rests on knees
      and elbows).
      2. **Radiographic studies.** Ascites may be suggested
      on a recumbent film of the abdomen, although x-ray
      films are less sensitive than computed tomography
      (CT) or ultrasound for detecting fluid. CT is also
      helpful for defining whether there are enlarged ret-
      roperitoneal nodes, tumor masses in the abdomen or
      pelvis, or liver metastases in association with the
      ascites.
      3. **Paracentesis** is used to distinguish malignancy
      from other causes of peritoneal effusions, including
      congestive heart failure, hepatic cirrhosis, and peri-
      tonitis. Malignant cells are found in about one-half
      of patients in whom the effusion is due to malig-
      nancy. Other tests are less reliable, and treatment
      decisions must often be based on incomplete data.
      Elevated LDH and protein levels along with a nega-
      tive Gram's stain and cultures are supportive but
      nonspecific for malignancy. The use of monoclonal
      antibodies to identify tumor cells is still experi-
      mental.

C. **Therapy.** As with malignant pleural effusions, malignant peritoneal effusions as a rule are optimally treated with effective systemic therapy. (The possible exception to this is peritoneal effusions from carcinoma of the ovary. In this circumstance, there may be advantage to intraperitoneal therapy because most systemic disease is on the peritoneal surface.) If the patient is resistant to all further systemic treatment, regional treatment should be tried, but the likelihood of success is less and the complications are greater with peritoneal effusions than with pleural effusions. Success probably is less because of the greater likelihood of loculations to areas inaccessible to therapy and the impossibility of obliterating the peritoneal space in the same way that the pleural space can be obliterated. Complications are greater because of the increase in adhesions caused by instillation therapy and the resultant increase in obstructive bowel problems.

1. **Paracentesis** may be helpful in acutely relieving intraabdominal pressure. If the ascites has caused impairment of respiration, paracentesis may thus give temporary relief. Rapid withdrawal of large volumes of fluid ($>$ 1 liter) can result in hypotension and shock, however, and if frequent paracenteses are performed, severe hypoalbuminemia and electrolyte imbalance may result. Repeated procedures could also subject the patient to increased risk for peritonitis or bowel injury. This procedure thus results in only temporary benefit.

2. **Bed rest and dietary salt restriction,** although helpful in the treatment of various nonmalignant causes of ascites, is of less benefit in malignant ascites.

3. **Diuretics** may be helpful in reducing ascites, but care must be taken not to be too vigorous in attempts at diuresis because of the possibility of dehydration and hypotension. A reasonable choice of diuretic is a combination of hydrochlorothiazide 50–100 mg daily and spironolactone 50–100 mg daily.

4. **Intracavitary therapy.** Radioisotopes, cytotoxic drugs, and sclerosing agents have been used with some benefit for treating malignant ascites; but, overall, probably fewer than one-half of patients have a satisfactory response. The utility of these agents has less to do with direct tumor cytotoxicity and more with the induction of a local inflammatory response with subsequent sclerosis. The radioactive isotopes [198]Au and ^{32}P should be used only by those with experience and appropriate certification. Cytotoxic agents such as fluorouracil are associated with less risk to the person administering the therapy.

   a. **Method.** The peritoneal fluid should be drained slowly through a Tenckhoff catheter over a 24–36-hour period. The potential distribution of the therapeutic agent can be determined by instilling ^{99}Tc glucoheptonate macroaggregated albumin in 50 ml of saline and obtaining an abdominal scintigram. Two liters of warmed 1.5% peritoneal dialysate solution is instilled, allowed to remain for 2 hours, and then drained. The chemotherapeutic agent is next mixed with 2 liters of fresh 1.5% dialysate solution containing 1000 units of heparin/liter. After warming, this solution is instilled through the Tenckhoff catheter. For some agents draining after 4 hours is recommended, but for others it is not.

  b. **Agents**

    (1) **Cisplatin** 50–100 mg/m^2 (especially for carcinoma of the ovary). Drainage is optional. Saline diuresis is recommended. Dosages higher than 100 mg/m^2 should not be used without protection by intravenous sodium thiosulfate. Cisplatin is repeated every 3 weeks.

    (2) **Fluorouracil** 1000 mg (total dose) in normal saline with 25 mEq sodium bicarbonate/liter. Drainage is optional. Treatment is given on days 1–4 monthly.

    (3) **Mitoxantrone** 10 mg/m^2. Drainage is optional. This dose has been administered on a weekly basis although white blood cell counts must be monitored.

    (4) **Interferon alpha** 50 million units (for ovarian cancer). Drainage is optional. This dose has been administered weekly for 4 weeks or longer. Patients should be premedicated with acetaminophen prior to and every 4 hours on the day of therapy.

    (5) **Bleomycin** 150 units. Drainage is recommended. The dose is repeated weekly for 3 weeks.

Other agents that have been used intraperitoneally include carboplatin, methotrexate, cytosine arabinoside, etoposide, thiotepa, and doxorubicin. High-dose interleukin (IL)-2 with lymphokine-activated killer (LAK) cells has shown activity in ovarian and colorectal cancer but at the cost of significant toxicity including peritoneal fibrosis, which in general has prevented the administration of more than one or two cycles. The use of lower IL-2 doses has not been well explored.

5. **Peritoneal-venous shunts** (Denver shunt, LeVeen shunt) may offer palliative relief for refractory ascites since recurrent paracentesis leads to infection and leakage of peritoneal fluid through the paracentesis sites. Potential disadvantages are shunt occlusion, the systemic dissemination of cancer, and disseminated intravascular coagulation (DIC).

III. Pericardial effusions. Although 5–10% of patients dying with disseminated malignancy have cardiac or pericardial metastases, far fewer have symptomatic pericardial effusion. However, although malignant pericardial effusions are not particularly common, they are of great importance because of their potential to cause acute cardiac tamponade and death.

A. Causes. The most common neoplasms causing pericardial effusions are carcinomas of the lung and breast, leukemias, lymphomas, and melanoma.

B. Diagnosis

1. **Clinical diagnosis.** Patients with developing cardiac tamponade may exhibit a variety of grave symptoms, including extreme anxiety, dyspnea, orthopnea, precordial chest pain, cough, and hoarseness. On examination, they are likely to have engorged neck veins, generalized edema, tachycardia, distant heart tones, lateral displacement of the cardiac apex, a low systolic blood pressure and low pulse pressure, and a paradoxical pulse. They may also have tachypnea and a pericardial friction rub.

2. **Electrocardiogram** (ECG) may show nonspecific low-voltage, T wave abnormalities, elevation of ST segments, and ventricular alterans or the more specific total electrical alterans. Premature beats and atrial fibrillation also occur.

3. **Chest x-ray film** typically shows an enlarged cardiac silhouette, often with a bulging appearance suggestive of an effusion ("water bottle heart"). There is frequently an associated pleural effusion.

4. **Echocardiography** can confirm the diagnosis and provide important information on the location of the effusion within the pericardium.

5. **Pericardiocentesis** reveals neoplastic cells on cytologic examination in more than 75% of patients.

C. Treatment

1. **Volume expansion and vasopressor support** is applied (if necessary) to maintain blood pressure. Adequate oxygenation must be maintained. Diuretics are contraindicated.

2. **Pericardiocentesis** under ECG and blood pressure monitoring should be done in emergent circumstances. If the patient can be stabilized or in cases of pericardial effusion without tamponade, pericardiocentesis under two-dimensional echocardiography is preferable as it significantly reduces the incidence of cardiac laceration, arrhythmia, and tension pneumothorax as a complication of the procedure.

3. **Instillation of chemotherapeutic or sclerosing agents.** Because pain may be associated with the intrapericardial therapy, lidocaine (Xylocaine) 100 mg may be administered intrapericardially as a local anesthetic. (Check with the cardiologist on the safety for each patient.) After the cytotoxic or sclerosing agent is instilled, the pericardial catheter is clamped

for 1–2 hours and then allowed to drain. One of the following agents may be used.

    a. Fluorouracil 500–1000 mg in aqueous solution as supplied commercially. This dose is generally not repeated.

    b. Thiotepa 25 mg/m^2 in 10 ml of normal saline may be preferred in tumor deemed sensitive to alkylating agents. Myelosuppression may occur. The dose is usually not repeated.

Complications of intrapericardial therapy include arrhythmias, pain, and fever.

4. Radiotherapy with radioisotopes or 2000–4000 cGy external beam therapy may help control effusions.

5. Systemic chemotherapy (with standard regimens) following pericardiocentesis is a possible alternative for newly diagnosed, potentially responsive malignancies such as leukemias and selected lymphomas. Chemotherapy, intrapericardial or systemic, or radiotherapy controls the effusion for at least 30 days in 60–70% of patients. If they are ineffective, surgical intervention to create a pericardial window may be necessary and can be effective for several months. It is not recommended, however, unless simpler measures fail.

IV. Malignant subarachnoid infiltrates

A. Causes. Leptomeningeal involvement with non-central-nervous-system (CNS) cancer is an uncommon complication of most neoplasms, although in children with acute lymphocytic leukemia who have not received prophylactic treatment the incidence approaches 50%. Of the nonleukemic diseases, breast carcinoma and lymphomas (primarily Burkitt's and T cell lymphoblastic) account for about 30% each in cases of malignant subarachnoid infiltrates. Carcinoma of the lung and melanoma account for 10–12% each.

B. Diagnosis

    1. Clinical diagnosis. Patients commonly present with headache, change in mental status, cranial nerve dysfunction, or spinal root-derived pain, paresthesia, or weakness. Any onset of change in neurologic status, particularly of cerebral, cranial nerve, or spinal root origin, should alert the clinician to the possibility of subarachnoid infiltrates.

    2. Diagnostic studies

        a. CT of the head should be done to look for any intracranial mass. If none is present, a lumbar puncture should be done.

        b. A lumbar puncture is done and the following are evaluated or performed.

            (1) Opening pressure

            (2) Cytology of centrifugal specimen for malignant cells

            (3) Total cell count and differential

            (4) Cerebrospinal fluid (CSF) chemistry, including glucose and protein

            (5) Microbiologic studies: India ink, Gram's stain,

cultures (routine, acid-fast, fungi), and special studies as indicated by the clinical situation

c. Magnetic resonance imaging or myelography with CT follow-up is performed if signs or symptoms of cord compression are present.

C. Treatment. Malignant subarachnoid infiltrates may be treated with radiotherapy, intrathecal chemotherapy, or a combination of the two.

1. Radiotherapy. The radiation field is usually limited to the most involved field (frequently the brain), and intrathecal chemotherapy is used to control the infiltrates elsewhere. This technique is used even though the entire neuraxis is usually involved because total craniospinal irradiation causes severe myelosuppression, which limits the patient's tolerance to concurrent or subsequent cytotoxic chemotherapy.

2. Chemotherapy may be administered by lumbar puncture or preferably into a surgically implanted (Ommaya) reservoir that communicates with the lateral ventricle. The latter has the advantages of being easily accessible in patients who require repeated treatments and of giving a better distribution of drug than can be obtained via lumbar puncture. The disadvantage is that of a foreign object that predisposes to infection and seizures. When the Ommaya reservoir is used, a volume of CSF equal to that to be injected (6–10 ml) should be removed through the reservoir with a small-caliber needle. The chemotherapy should then be given as a slow injection. When the chemotherapy is given via lumbar puncture, the volume of injection (usually 7–10 ml) should be greater than that of the CSF withdrawn in order to have a higher closing than opening pressure. This method facilitates distribution of the drug and minimizes post-lumbar-puncture headache. The most commonly used drugs are the following.

a. Methotrexate 12 mg/m^2 (maximum 15 mg) twice weekly until the CSF clears of malignant cells, then monthly.

b. Cytarabine 30 mg/m^2 (maximum 50 mg) twice weekly until the CSF clears of malignant cells, then monthly.

c. Thiotepa 2–10 mg/m^2 twice weekly until the CSF clears of malignant cells, then monthly.

Each of the agents is given in preservative-free saline or, if available, buffered preservative-free diluent similar to Elliot's B solution. Any subsequent flush solution should be of similar composition. Other drugs used to treat effusions, e.g., fluorouracil, mechlorethamine, or radioisotopes, *must not* be used to treat meningeal disease.

D. Response to treatment. Most patients with meningeal leukemia or lymphoma respond to a combination of radiotherapy and intrathecal chemotherapy. Carcinomas are less likely to improve, but mild to moderate improvement may be seen in up to 50% of patients.

E. **Complications.** Aseptic meningitis or arachnoiditis, seizures, acute encephalopathy, myelopathy, leukoencephalopathy, and radicular neuropathy may result from intrathecal chemotherapy with or without radiotherapy.

Bone marrow suppression is not usually severe unless the patient undergoes spinal irradiation or systemic chemotherapy as well. Oral leucovorin can be given after the intrathecal methotrexate (10 mg leucovorin PO q6h × 6–8 doses, starting either at the same time or 24 hours after the methotrexate) to prevent marrow toxicity. Serious complications are infrequent, however, and in patients with advanced metastatic disease they usually are not a major problem.

Selected Readings

Pleural Effusions

Bartal, A. H., et al. Clinical and flow cytometry characteristics of malignant pleural effusions in patients after intracavitary administration of methylprednisolone acetate. *Cancer* 67: 3136, 1991.

Bayly, D. D., et al. Tetracycline and quinacrine in the control of malignant pleural effusions: a randomized trial. *Cancer* 41:118, 1978.

Chernow, B., and Sahn, S. A. Carcinomatous involvement of the pleura: an analysis of 96 patients. *Am. J. Med.* 63:695, 1977.

Friedman, M. A., and Slater, E. Malignant pleural effusions. *Cancer Treat. Rev.* 5:49, 1978.

Goldman, C. A., et al. Interferon instillation for malignant pleural effusions. *Ann. Oncol.* 4:141, 1993.

Hausheer, F. H., and Yarbro, J. W. Diagnosis and treatment of malignant pleural effusions. *Cancer Metastasis Rev.* 6:23, 1987.

Johnson, W. W. The malignant pleural effusion: a review of cytopathologic diagnoses of 584 specimens from 472 consecutive patients. *Cancer* 56:905, 1985.

Kitamura, S., et al. Intrapleural doxycycline for control of malignant pleural effusion. *Curr. Ther. Res.* 30:515, 1981.

Mansson, T. Treatment of malignant pleural effusion with doxycycline. *Scand. J. Infect. Dis.* 53:29, 1988.

Ostrowski, M. J. Intracavitary therapy with bleomycin for the treatment of malignant pleural effusions. *J. Surg. Oncol.* (suppl. 1):7, 1989.

Ostrowski, M. J., and Halsall, G. M. Intracavitary bleomycin in the management of malignant effusions: a multicenter study. *Cancer Treat. Rep.* 66:1903, 1982.

Pavesi, F., et al. Detection of malignant pleural effusions by tumor marker evaluation. *Eur. J. Cancer Clin. Oncol.* 24:1005, 1988.

Surland, L. G., and Weisberger, A. S. Intracavitary 5-fluorouracil in malignant effusions. *Arch. Intern. Med.* 116:431, 1965.

Tamura, S., et al. Tumor markers in pleural effusion diagnosis. *Cancer* 61:198, 1988.

Van Hoff, D. D., and LiVolsi, V. Diagnostic reliability of needle biopsy of the parietal pleura: a review of 272 biopsies. *Am. J. Clin. Pathol.* 64:200, 1975.

Walker-Renard, P. B., et al. Chemical pleurodesis for malignant pleural effusions. *Ann. Intern. Med.* 120:56, 1994.

Peritoneal Effusions

Baker, A. R. Treatment of Malignant Ascites. In V. I. DeVita, S. Hellman, and S. A. Rosenberg (eds.), *Cancer: Principles and Practice of Oncology* (3rd ed.). Philadelphia: Lippincott, 1989. P. 2317.

Berek, J. S., et al. Intraperitoneal recombinant alpha-interferon for "salvage" immunotherapy in stage III epithelial ovarian cancer. A Gynecologic Oncology Group study. *Semin. Oncol.* 13(suppl. 2):61, 1986.

Bitran, J. D. Intraperitoneal bleomycin: pharmacokinetics and results of a phase II trial. *Cancer* 56:2420, 1985.

Lacy, J. H., et al. Management of malignant ascites. *Surg. Gynecol. Obstet.* 159:397, 1984.

Markman, M., et al. Phase II trial of weekly or biweekly intraperitoneal mitoxantrone in epithelial ovarian cancer. *J. Clin. Oncol.* 9:978, 1991.

Nicoletto, M. O., et al. Experience with intraperitoneal alpha-2a interferon. *Oncology* 49:467, 1992.

Papac, R. J. Treatment of Malignant Disease in Closed Spaces. In F. F. Baker (ed.), *Cancer, A Comprehensive Treatise* (Vol. 5). New York: Plenum, 1977.

Reichman, B., et al. Phase I trial of concurrent intraperitoneal and continuous intravenous infusion of fluorouracil in patients with refractory cancer. *J. Clin. Oncol.* 6:158, 1988.

Speyer, J. L., et al. Intraperitoneal carboplatin: favorable results in women with minimal residual ovarian cancer after cisplatin therapy. *J. Clin. Oncol.* 8:1335, 1990.

Steis, R. G., et al. Intraperitoneal lymphokine-activated killer-cell and interleukin-2 therapy for malignancies limited to the peritoneal cavity. *J. Clin. Oncol.* 8:1618, 1990.

Sugarbaker, P. H., et al. Prospective, randomized trial of intravenous versus intraperitoneal 5-fluorouracil in patients with advanced primary colon or rectal cancer. *Surgery* 95:414, 1985.

Pericardial Effusions

Buzaid, A. C., et al. Managing malignant pericardial effusion. *West. J. Med.* 150:174, 1989.

Callahan, J. A., et al. Two-dimensional echocardiographically guided pericardiocentesis: experience in 117 consecutive patients. *Am. J. Cardiol.* 55:476, 1985.

Helms, S. R., and Carlson, M. D. Cardiovascular emergencies. *Semin. Oncol.* 16:463, 1989.

Shepherd, F. A., et al. Tetracycline sclerosis in the management of pericardial effusion. *J. Clin. Oncol.* 3:1678, 1985.

Theologides, A. Neoplastic cardiac tamponade. *Semin. Oncol.* 5:181, 1978.

Malignant Subarachnoid Infiltrates

Gutin, P. H., et al. Treatment of malignant meningeal disease with intrathecal thiotepa: a phase II study. *Cancer Treat. Rep.* 61:885, 1977.

Olson, M. E., et al. Infiltration of the leptomeninges by systemic cancer. *Arch. Neurol.* 30:122, 1974.

Managing Cancer Pain

Charles S. Cleeland and Eduardo D. Bruera

Patients should not have to suffer needlessly from cancer pain. Most pain from cancer can be adequately controlled with analgesics given by mouth. When this is not possible, a variety of more sophisticated pain management techniques can provide good pain control. It is estimated that approximately 95 percent of patients could be free of significant pain with the techniques we have available today, at least until the last week or two of life. Unfortunately, many patients do not benefit from adequate pain control. Estimates based on surveys in the United States indicate that less than half of all patients with cancer obtain optimal pain control. Poorly controlled pain has such catastrophic effects on the patient and his or her family that proper management of pain must have the highest priority for those who take care of patients with cancer. Mood and quality of life deteriorate in the presence of pain, and pain has adverse effects on such measures of disease status as appetite and activity. Severe pain may be a primary reason why both patients and their families stop treatment. Improving the practice of anticipating, evaluating, and treating pain will benefit the majority of patients.

I. **Prevalence, severity, and risk for pain.** The majority of patients with cancer with terminal disease will need expert pain management; between 60 and 80% of such patients will have significant pain. Pain is also a problem for many patients much earlier in the course of their disease. Patients with months or years to live may be compromised by poorly controlled pain. Persistent pain is rarely a problem before metastatic cancer is present. When the cancer has metastasized, however, the percentage of patients with pain increases dramatically. In the United States, even with the availability of a full range of analgesics and other pain treatments, 60% of all outpatients with metastatic disease will have cancer-related pain, and one-third report pain so severe that it significantly impairs their quality of life. Multicenter studies indicate that approximately 40% of outpatients with cancer pain do not receive analgesics potent enough to manage their pain. Patients in minority treatment settings, female patients, and older patients are at greater risk for poorly controlled pain due to undermedication.

II. **Etiology of cancer pain.** Direct tumor involvement is the most common cause of pain, present in approximately two-thirds of those with pain from metastatic cancer. Tumor invasion of bone is the physical basis of pain in about 50% of these patients. The remaining 50% of these patients experience tumor-related pain that is due to nerve compression or infiltration, or involvement of the gastrointestinal tract or soft tissue. Persistent posttherapy pain, from long-term effects of surgery, radiotherapy, and chemotherapy, accounts for an additional 20% of all who report pain with metastatic cancer, with a small residual group experiencing pain from non-cancer-related conditions. In patients with advanced cancer, the majority have pain at multiple sites caused by multiple mechanisms. A new complaint of pain in a patient with metastatic cancer should first be thought of as disease-related, but indirectly related, manageable causes should also be considered.

The sensation of pain is generated either by stimulation of peripheral pain receptors or by damage to afferent nerve fibers. Peripheral pain receptors can be stimulated by pressure, compression, and traction as well as by disease-related chemical changes. Pain due to stimulation of pain receptors is called *nociceptive pain*. Damage to visceral, somatic, or autonomic nerve trunks produces *neurogenic* or *neuropathic pain*. Neuropathic pain is thought to be caused by spontaneous activity in nerves damaged by disease or treatment. Patients with cancer often have both nociceptive and neuropathic pain simultaneously. Neuropathic pain is less responsive to opioid analgesics and will require the additional use of other drugs.

III. **Assessment of pain.** Proper pain management requires a clear understanding of the characteristics of the pain and its physical basis. The changing expression of cancer pain demands repeated assessment, as new causes for pain can emerge rapidly and pain severity can increase quickly. In advanced-cancer patients, pain from multiple causes is the rule and not the exception. A careful history includes questions concerning the location, severity, and quality of the pain, as well as the impact the pain is having on the patient's life.

   A. **Pain severity.** Inadequate pain assessment and poor physician-patient communication about pain are major barriers to good pain care. Physicians and nurses tend to underestimate pain intensity, especially when it is severe. Patients whose physicians underestimate their pain are at high risk for poor pain management and compromised function. A small minority of patients with cancer may complain of pain in a dramatic fashion, but many more patients underreport the severity of their pain and the lack of adequate pain relief.

      1. There are several **reasons for this reluctance to report pain,** including the following.
         a. Not wanting to acknowledge that the disease is progressing
         b. Not wanting to divert the physician's attention from treating the disease
         c. Not wanting to tell the physician that pain treatments are not working
      2. **Patients may not want to be put on opioid analgesics** because of the following reasons.
         a. They do not want to become addicted.
         b. They fear psychoactive components of opioids.
         c. They are concerned that using opioids "too early" will endanger pain relief when they have more pain.

   d. They fear that being placed on opioids signals that death is near.

   e. They have accepted religious or societal norms or teachings that pain should be endured.

Presenting information that addresses these concerns in a straightforward manner will allay most of these fears and should be considered as an essential step in providing pain control. It is important that patients understand that they will function better if their pain is controlled. Patient education materials available from state cancer pain initiatives, from the National Cancer Institute (NCI), American Cancer Society (ACS), and the Agency for Health Care Policy and Research (AHCPR) can be very useful for both patients and families and should be given to patients when they develop pain.

   Communication about pain is greatly aided by having the patient use a scale to rate the severity of their pain. A simple rating scale ranges from 0 to 10, with 0 being "no pain" and 10 being pain "as bad as you can imagine." Used properly, pain severity scales can be invaluable in titrating analgesics and in monitoring for increases in pain with progressive disease. Mild pain is often well tolerated with minimal impact on a patient's activities. However, there is a threshold beyond which pain is especially disruptive. This threshold has been reached when patients rate the severity of their pain at 5 or greater on a 0–10 scale. When pain is too great (≥ 7 on this scale), it becomes the primary focus of attention and prohibits most activity not directly related to pain. While it may not be possible to totally eliminate pain, reducing its severity to 4 or less ought to be a minimum standard of pain therapy.

B. Diagnostic steps. Those who treat patients with cancer should be familiar with the common pain syndromes associated with the disease.

   1. Having the patient show **the area of pain** on a drawing of a human figure will aid identification of the syndrome. This can be particularly helpful in indicating areas of referred pain, common with nerve compression.

   2. Careful questioning concerning the **characteristics of the pain** is essential for physical diagnosis.

   3. In addition to severity, these characteristics include the **temporal pattern of the pain** (constant or episodic) and its quality. Episodic or "incident" pain is much more difficult to control than is continuous pain.

   4. Other important characteristics of pain are its relationship to physical activity and what seems to alleviate the pain.

   5. The physical examination includes examination of the painful area as well as neurologic and orthopedic assessment.

   6. Radiologic tests. Since bone metastases are a common cause of pain, and since pain can occur with changes in bone density not detectable on x-ray films, bone scans can be helpful. Computed tomography (CT) or magnetic resonance imaging (MRI) is useful in the evaluation of retroperitoneal, paravertebral, and pelvic areas as well as the base of the skull. Myelography may be necessary in determining the cause of pain if MRI cannot be performed.

7. **Diagnostic nerve blocks** can provide information concerning the pain pathway. Diagnostic blocks can also determine the potential effectiveness of neuroablative procedures that destroy the pain pathway.

C. **The impact of pain on the patient.** When pain is of moderate or greater severity, we can assume that it has a negative impact on the patient's quality of life. That impact, including problems with sleep and depression, must be evaluated. A reduced number of hours of sleep compared with the last pain-free interval, difficulties with sleep onset, frequent interruptions of sleep, and/or early morning awakening suggest the need for appropriate pharmacologic intervention, often the addition of a low-dose antidepressant at bedtime. Just as patients hesitate to report severe pain, they may hesitate to report depression. Having the patient report depression or tension on a scale of 0–10 may help overcome some of this reluctance. Significant depression should be treated through psychiatric or psychologic consultation, especially if it persists in the face of adequate pain relief.

It is important to differentiate between physical pain and psychologic stress. A very small number of patients in severe psychosocial distress will express many of their losses and concerns as a report of physical pain. While it is important to recognize severe somatization and to provide psychiatric referral or counseling to these patients, it is equally important to recognize true physical pain. Too often physicians misdiagnose true pain as depression or anxiety. Accurate pain assessment in patients who are cognitively impaired, particularly those with agitation, may be extremely difficult. These patients present with symptoms that may be attributable to either agitated delirium or pain. As a guide, patients in whom pain was well controlled before the development of delirium are unlikely to be agitated due to uncontrolled pain. Frequent discussions between various health care professionals and the patient's family will be required.

D. **The addicted patient.** Some patients with severe alcoholism or drug addiction may request analgesics for their psychologic effects. This is unlikely to occur in patients without a clear history of severe addictive behavior. Patients who are *recovered* alcoholics or drug abusers may be difficult to treat because of their resistance to taking analgesics. In any case, if this diagnosis is suspected, the issue should be discussed openly with the patient and an agreement should be reached about the use of opioids for the management of pain as opposed to mood alterations. With this group of patients, long-acting opioids or continuous infusion are preferable to short-acting opioids or patient-controlled analgesia. Prescriptions by a single physician would make the negotiation process with a patient much simpler. Although their care is more complex, patients with drug or alcohol addiction should never be denied appropriate pain medications.

IV. Treatment

A. General aspects.

All health care professionals who see patients with cancer should be familiar with the AHCPR guidelines, *Management of Cancer Pain.* The prompt relief of pain from cancer frequently involves the use of simultaneously rather than serially administered combinations of drug and nondrug therapies. Identification of a treatable neoplasm as a factor in pain production will call for appropriate radiotherapy (to bone metastases, for example) or chemotherapy or in some instances, surgical debulking. Until such treatment can be effective (this may take days to weeks), the patient's pain must be managed with analgesics. In many instances, analgesics are the only pain treatment available because of the patient's condition, the physical basis of the pain, or limited treatment options. The principles of pharmacologic management of pain are evolving through studies of analgesic effectiveness and research on the use of combinations of palliative medications.

There is a growing consensus concerning the types of drugs to use, their routes of administration, and how best to schedule them. The first step is the choice of *analgesic* drug to be used (nonopioid, opioid, or a combination of both). The second step is the choice of *adjuvant* drugs, which can increase analgesic effectiveness and can produce other palliative effects to counter the disruptive consequences of pain.

B. Nonsteroidal anti-inflammatory drugs (NSAIDs)

1. **Mechanism of action and selection of agents.**
   NSAIDs constitute the majority of nonopioid analgesics. Their effect on the inflammatory process is a key to their analgesic property. Tumor growth produces inflammatory and mechanical effects in adjacent tissues that can trigger the release of prostaglandins, bradykinin, and serotonin, which in turn may precipitate or exacerbate pain in the surrounding tissues. Prostaglandin-mediated actions on peripheral receptors probably include both direct activation and sensitization to other analgesic substances. Prostaglandins are frequently associated with painful bone metastasis because of their involvement in bone reabsorption. The NSAIDs seem to exert their analgesic, antipyretic, and anti-inflammatory actions by blocking the synthesis of prostaglandins. Table 37-1 gives the usual starting doses and dose ranges for several commonly used NSAIDs.

   By virtue of their different mechanisms of action and toxicity profiles, the NSAIDs and opioids are often administered together. Enteric-coated aspirin

Table 37-1. Starting doses and dose ranges of some nonsteroidal analgesic agents

Drug	Starting dose (mg)	Frequency	Dose range (mg)
Aspirin	650	q4–6h	Up to 1300 q6h
Choline magnesium trisalicylate	500	q6h	Up to 1000 mg q6h
Diflunisal	500	q8–12h	Up to 1500 mg daily
Ibuprofen	400	q4–6h	Up to 2400 daily
Naproxyn	250	q8–12h	Up to 1250 daily
Piroxicam	10	q12–24h	Up to 20 mg daily
Tolmetin	400	q8h	Up to 1800 mg daily

is one of the first-choice drugs for mild to moderate cancer pain. Other NSAIDs such as ibuprofen, diflunisal, naproxen, and choline magnesium trisalicylate (Trilisate) have established value in the management of clinical pain. These drugs are better tolerated than aspirin but are usually significantly more expensive. Individual differences in response to the various NSAIDs are not yet well understood.

Acetaminophen is a peripherally acting analgesic that does not inhibit peripheral prostaglandin synthesis. Therefore, it does not have anti-inflammatory effects or the side effects associated with the use of NSAIDs. Acetaminophen should be considered in patients who have contraindications to the use of NSAIDs.

Commercial preparations containing codeine or oxycodone and acetaminophen or aspirin are among the most widely prescribed scheduled analgesics and are frequently administered to patients with cancer. This is generally appropriate because of the synergistic effects of the combination. Such a combination is reported to be particularly effective for bone pain.

2. **Side effects.** NSAIDs have a number of potentially serious side effects such as gastritis and gastrointestinal hemorrhage, bleeding due to platelet inhibition, and renal failure. Most of these side effects are related to the prostaglandin inhibitory effect of these drugs and are therefore common to all these drugs. Renal failure due to the inhibition of renal medullary prostaglandins can be of particular concern in patients who might also be receiving opioids. Decreased renal elimination of active opioid metab-

olites might result in somnolence, confusion, hallucinations, or generalized myoclonus. Therefore, kidney function should be monitored in patients receiving a combination of NSAIDs and opioids.

Gastrointestinal complications include gastric pain, nausea, vomiting, hemorrhage, and in extreme cases, perforation. Gastrointestinal damage is mediated by prostaglandin inhibition. The most common form of nephrotoxicity associated with NSAIDs is renal failure, related to prostaglandin inhibition and consequent vasodilation. Hepatic injury has been reported with the use of aspirin, benoxaprofen, and phenylbutazone and less commonly, with diclofenac, ibuprofen, indomethacin, naproxen, pirprofen, and sulindac. Sulindac, however, seems to be associated with a higher incidence of cholestasis.

NSAID use is also associated with a variety of hypersensitive reactions involving the skin (rash, eruption, itching), blood vessels (angioneurotic edema, vasomotor disorders), and the respiratory system (rhinitis, asthma). In particular, aspirin may cause anaphylactic crisis, a syndrome characterized by dyspnea, sudden weakness, sweating, and collapse. Undesirable hematologic effects of NSAIDs include platelet dysfunction, aplastic anemia, and agranulocytosis. Factors often considered in the empirical selection of an NSAID for a given patient include their relative toxicity, cost, dosage schedule, and prior experience. The use of certain aspirin analogs (choline magnesium trisalicylate) has been suggested to be associated with a low incidence of gastropathy and platelet dysfunction. The effects of NSAIDs used as single agents in the management of cancer pain are characterized by a ceiling effect, beyond which further increases in dose do not enhance analgesia.

C. Opioid analgesics

1. **When to start therapy.** The choice of an opioid analgesic as opposed to a nonopioid analgesic follows from an assessment of the severity of pain. The decision is relatively easy when pain is mild (choose nonopioid) or severe (choose opioid, usually in combination with a nonopioid). The choice is more difficult when the patient reports moderate pain, especially when there is reason to suspect that the patient may be underreporting pain severity. Several studies have documented that many patients with cancer are inadequately managed because of the physician's reluctance to use opioids in dosages and with schedules known to be sufficient to relieve moderate pain.

Opioid analgesics should be prescribed promptly as soon as there is evidence that pain is not well controlled with nonopioid analgesics. Usually, nonopioid analgesics can be continued as a way of maximizing analgesia because their site of action is different from that of the opioids.

2. **Schedule of treatment and selection of dose.** Except in a minority of patients whose pain is clearly episodic, analgesics should be given on an around-the-clock basis, with the time interval based on the duration of effectiveness of the drug and the patient's report of the duration of effectiveness. There is evidence that total opioid requirement is lower when opioids are given on a scheduled basis, thereby preventing peaks of pain. Putting patients in the position of having to ask for medication or continually making a judgment about whether their pain is severe enough to take analgesics focuses their attention on pain, reminds them of their need for drugs, and allows pain to reach a severity not readily controlled by the same doses that would be effective with scheduled administration. It is important to remember that there may be large individual differences in the required dose of opioid, depending on such factors as the patient's opioid use history, activity level, and metabolism. The patient's report of pain severity and pain relief is the best guideline for opioid titration.

3. The so-called **weak opioids,** including codeine and oxycodone, usually formulated in combination with acetaminophen or aspirin, can provide active patients with good pain relief for long periods of time. As disease advances, oral administration of the more "potent" opioids provides the majority of patients with pain relief. There is considerable agreement that meperidine should not be used on a chronic basis because of its toxic metabolite normeperidine, which is a central nervous system (CNS) stimulant, has a long serum half-life, and has no analgesic properties. Oral administration is preferred, but the physician must remain flexible to changes that are dictated by the patient's ability to utilize orally administered drugs. This may include the use of opioid and nonopioid suppositories and other alternate routes of administration (transdermal, sublingual, rectal, subcutaneous).

4. **Oral morphine,** either in immediate- or sustained-release preparation, is the analgesic of choice for moderate to severe cancer pain. Long-acting morphine preparations are convenient for both the patient and the health care staff. Immediate-release morphine is much cheaper, however, and is as effective. A typical starting dose for immediate-release oral morphine is 10–30 mg every 4 hours in patients not currently receiving opioids. When a patient is switching from another opioid (usually codeine or oxycodone) to morphine, it is important to calculate the equianalgesic morphine dose as a basis for determining what morphine-equivalent doses are the thresh-

old for pain control (Table 37-2). The starting dose may not be sufficient, and relatively rapid upward titration may be needed, especially if pain is severe.

The upward titration of morphine and other oral narcotic analgesics can be done by giving a supplemental "boost" using 50% of the scheduled dose 2 hours after the scheduled dose if there is still significant pain and the patient is not overly sedated or lethargic. The scheduled dose is then set at 150% of the initial scheduled dose. Because of the time it takes to achieve a steady state, there may need to be some readjustment downward if the patient is unduly sleepy or is lethargic at the time of the scheduled dose. The supplemental dose may be given after any scheduled dose (even if there was an increase in the scheduled dose), so long as a sufficient time has passed for the drug to be absorbed from the stomach. An alternative way to titrate is simply to add 50% to the next scheduled dose, but staying with the previ-

Table 37-2. Opioid dosing equivalence

Drug	Approximate equianalgesic dose	
	Oral	Parenteral
Morphine	30 mg q3–4h[a]	10 mg q3–4h
Hydromorphone	4–8 mg q3–4h	1.5 mg q3–4h
Codeine[b]	130 mg q3–4h	
Propoxyphene[b]	See comment below[c]	
Hydrocodone[b]	30 mg q3–4h	
Oxycodone[b]	30 mg q3–4h	
Methadone	5–20 mg q6–8h[d]	5–10 mg q6–8h[d]
Levorphanol	4 mg q6–8h[d]	2 mg q6–8h[d]
Meperidine[e]	300 mg q2–3h	100 mg q3h
Transdermal fentanyl	25-μg patch = 8–22 mg/24 hours IV/IM morphine sulfate = 45–134 mg/24 hours PO morphine sulfate	

[a]Slow-release formulations of oral morphine that are available have 8–12-hour durations of analgesic action.
[b]Codeine, propoxyphene, hydrocodone, and oxycodone are often given as combination products with aspirin and/or acetaminophen.
[c]Propoxyphene is a weak analgesic; 65–130 mg is equivalent to about 650 mg of aspirin. It has a duration of action of 3–4 hours; however, its duration of action increases with chronic dosing.
[d]The duration of analgesia of methadone and levorphanol may be significantly longer than 6–8 hours in some patients.
[e]Not recommended for chronic use.
Source: From D. E. Weissman, et al. *Handbook of Cancer Pain Management* (4th ed.). Madison, WI: The Wisconsin Cancer Pain Initiative, 1993. Reprinted with permission.

ously determined schedule (usually every 4 hours).
When the doses of narcotic are higher (e.g., morphine
100 mg q4h), some clinicians will use less, e.g., 20–
30% (20–30 mg) as the boost, but will incrementally
add to the dose with each scheduled treatment until
adequate pain relief has been achieved. Depending
on the understanding of the patient and family, it is
often best to have the patient check in with a physician or nurse after every other dose increase to be
sure the treatment plan is understood, safe, and effective.

5. **Long-acting preparations.** When an effective dose
   of short-acting morphine has been established, the
   required 24-hour dose for a long-acting preparation
   can be calculated. An additional supply of short-
   acting morphine, given when necessary, will help
   the patient manage "breakthrough" pain. Consistent
   need for this additional short-acting morphine (e.g.,
   3–4 doses daily) will dictate an upward adjustment
   of the dose of sustained-release drug. Orders for immediate-release morphine should allow for some upward titration of dose by the patient or by the
   nurse. Each dose of short-acting morphine for breakthrough pain is usually 15–25% of the 24-hour dose
   of long-acting morphine. If more than this is required, it is usually an indication for increasing the
   dose of the long-acting preparation.

6. While the **opioid agonist-antagonist analgesics**
   have established their effectiveness in the control of
   acute (especially procedurally related) pain, their
   use in chronic cancer pain is limited by the possibility of precipitous withdrawal in the patient who has
   been taking morphine-type drugs, by their analgesic
   ceiling effect (when the drug does not provide more
   pain relief), and by the lack of an oral form of administration (with the exception of pentazocine, which
   yields a relatively high proportion of patients reporting disturbing psychotomimetic effects).

7. **Alternative potent opioids** may sometimes have
   less side effects than morphine. Methadone is an agonist opioid analgesic that has the advantage of extremely low cost and lack of known active metabolites. However, because of its long and unpredictable
   half-life and relatively unknown equianalgesic dose
   as compared to other opioids, methadone should only
   be used by pain specialists who are experienced in
   its use. Other alternatives are levorphanol, which
   has a longer half-life than morphine, and hydromorphone, which has a half-life similar to morphine.
   Equivalent starting doses can be selected from Table
   37-2, but if the patient has been on high doses of
   morphine, care must be taken not to switch cava-
   lierly to proportionally higher doses of the alternative, as unexpected side effects may occur.

8. **Alternate routes.** Approximately 70% of patients
   will benefit from the use of an alternate route for

opioid administration sometime before death. The duration for which patients need these routes varies between hours and months. While intermittent injections can be effective for a brief period of time, this method is painful for the patient, time-consuming for the nursing staff, and difficult to manage at home.

a. **Intravenous infusion.** A number of studies have shown that intravenous infusions of opioids produce stable blood levels of drug and that they are safe and effective for treating both postoperative and cancer pain. Intravenous infusion using a patient-controlled analgesia pump may be very effective in gaining rapid control over pain that has gotten out of hand. It may also be of value when the patient cannot take medications orally and does not wish to take suppositories. The main problem associated with continuous intravenous infusions is the prolonged maintenance of an intravenous line. Patients may need to be subjected to numerous venipunctures when peripheral intravenous lines are used. Totally implantable intravenous catheters represent a major improvement, permitting long-term intravenous access. However, these catheters are expensive and need to be surgically implanted, and their maintenance requires considerable nursing expertise and patient teaching. If such a catheter is already available in a patient with advanced cancer who has pain, it certainly could be used for the administration of opioids. Starting doses of morphine for severe pain are 2–3 mg hourly as a continuous infusion with patient-controlled boosts of 1 mg every 15 minutes. At the end of 24 hours, 50% of the patient boosts can be added to the total 24-hour dose of the continuous infusion until the patient is requiring less than one boost hourly. At that time, a shift to oral analgesics can be started, if the patient is able to take oral medications. If the doses of intravenous morphine are high, the shifting to appropriate oral doses may take several days. It is usually safe and effective to give a 24-hour dose of long-acting morphine orally that is equal in milligrams to the 24-hour requirement intravenously, and simultaneously to reduce the intravenous dose (continuous infusion rate) by one-half. Boosts can be given by mouth, but the patient should have the intravenous boost option as reassurance. The next day, the 24-hour intravenous dose required (continuous plus boosts) can be added orally to the previous day's oral dose (long-acting plus short-acting) and the infusion further reduced. The same process is repeated until the patient is getting adequate pain relief with the oral morphine. The infusion can usually be stopped and needed boosts given orally by the third or fourth day.

b. Subcutaneous route. This route has been found to be safe and effective for the administration of morphine, hydromorphone, and levorphanol. Subcutaneous opioids can be administered as a continuous infusion using a portable or nonportable pump (use as small a volume as possible, e.g., < 5 ml/hour) or as an intermittent injection. A butterfly needle can be left under the skin approximately 7 days, making both intermittent injections and continuous infusion painless. The needles are frequently inserted in the subclavicular region, anterior chest, or abdominal wall. This allows patients to have free limbs.

c. Rectal route. The majority of the experience reported in the literature is with the short-term use of rectal opioids for the management of acute pain. Both solid and liquid solutions have been used. While there is considerable interindividual variation in the bioavailability of rectally administered morphine, there is generalized consensus that this drug is well absorbed following rectal administration. A number of authors have treated terminally ill patients with cancer with rectal morphine, with good pain control until death. Advantages of the rectal route include the absence of the need for the insertion of needles and the use of portable pumps. However, rectal administration can be uncomfortable; absorption may be decreased by the presence of stool in the rectum, by diarrhea, or simply by normal bowel movements; and progressive titration may be difficult because of the limited availability of different commercial preparations.

d. Transdermal route. The recent development of a transdermal preparation of fentanyl citrate has revitalized an interest in this route. Pharmacokinetic data suggest that transdermal fentanyl is well absorbed, although there is considerable delay in reaching steady-state blood levels and a slowly declining plasma concentration after removal of the patch. These characteristics are potential obstacles for its regular clinical use, particularly in unstable patients. Although clinical experience is still very limited, treatment appears to be well tolerated. Future research will need to focus on comparisons between the transdermal route and long-acting morphine preparations and continuous subcutaneous infusions of opioids.

e. Spinal route. Some patients suffering from localized pain syndromes might benefit from intraspinal administration of opioids. The advantage of this route is the lack of systemic side effects of opioids and the fact that a relatively very small dose of drugs is necessary. The disadvantage is the need for the insertion of catheters into the epidural or intrathecal space, the need for expensive infusion pumps, and in many patients the rapid development of tolerance to the analgesic effect of different opioids. To overcome this rapid development of tolerance, some clinicians have used a combined infusion of opioids and local anesthetic. Because of the complexity associated with this route, it should only be considered in selected patients and after an adequate trial of systemic opioids and adjuvant drugs. The insertion of the catheter and the maintenance of the spinal analgesic regime should be under the control of a pain specialist.

9. **Adverse effects of opioids.** Fear of the inability to manage side effects is one of the main reasons cited by oncologists for why they limit their use of opioids. Yet, most of the agents used in chemotherapy are associated with more potent side effects than the opioids. The analgesic and side effects of opioid agonists are not identical for all patients. Some patients may require a higher equivalent dose of a certain opioid agonist in order to achieve adequate analgesia. This higher equivalent dose may result in a higher incidence of side effects such as nausea or sedation. Therefore, when significant toxicity occurs in a patient treated with a certain opioid agonist such as morphine, it may be appropriate to change to another opioid such as hydromorphone. In addition, after prolonged treatment, very high dosages, or renal failure, patients may experience the accumulation of active metabolites of opioid agonists. Active metabolites have been identified for both morphine and hydromorphone. This accumulation results in CNS side effects such as sedation, generalized myoclonus, confusion, and in some patients, agitated delirium or grand mal seizures. In these patients, it is also useful to change from one opioid to another.

It is important to understand the side effect liability of these analgesics and be prepared to deal with side effects prophylactically or when they do occur. *Most patients develop tolerance for side effects much more rapidly than they develop tolerance for the analgesic effects of the opioids.*

   a. **Sedation.** This occurs in the majority of patients during the beginning of opioid treatment or after a major increase in dose. Most patients develop rapid tolerance to this side effect and while the sedation disappears within 3–5 days, the analgesic effect persists. When sedation occurs in patients with cancer receiving a stable dose of opioid, it is necessary to suspect the potential accumulation of active opioid metabolites such as morphine-6-glucuronide. This occurs more frequently in patients who are receiving high doses of opioids or who present with renal failure. It is also important to suspect other non-opioid-related causes since these patients are frequently very ill. Opioid-induced sedation can be managed by opioid rotation (some opioids have a higher ratio of analgesic effects to sedation than others) or by the addition of amphetamine derivatives such as methylphenidate, starting with 5 mg PO bid daily, or dextroamphetamine/amphetamine 5 mg bid (last dose no later than 3 P.M. to avoid insomnia).

b. Nausea and vomiting. Most patients present with these symptoms after initial administration or a major increase in dose. Some authors propose the use of prophylactic antiemetics on a regular basis during the first days of treatment since in most patients, nausea disappears after that period. The mechanism for the nausea is central. These side effects can be well antagonized by antidopaminergic agents such as metoclopramide 10 mg PO qid. Dexamethasone 2–4 mg PO qid is also a useful antiemetic that potentiates metoclopramide in these patients, but has significant side effects when used for more than a week or two. As with sedation, nausea is a multicausal syndrome in patients with cancer who are receiving opioids: Severe constipation, cancer-induced autonomic failure, gastritis, increased intracranial pressure, and opioid metabolite accumulation are all possible causes of nausea.

c. Constipation. This is probably the most common adverse effect of opioids, and it is necessary to anticipate constipation when opioid therapy is started. Opioids act at multiple sites in the gastrointestinal tract and spinal cord. The result is decreased intestinal secretions and peristalsis. While tolerance to both sedation and nausea develops quickly, it develops very slowly to the smooth muscle effects of opioids so that constipation will persist when these drugs are used for chronic pain. At the same time that the use of opioid analgesics is initiated, provision for a regular bowel regimen including stimulants and stool softeners should be instituted to diminish this adverse effect. (See Chap. 33.)

d. Respiratory depression. This is the most serious adverse effect of opioid analgesics. Opioids can cause increasing respiratory depression to the point of apnea. In humans, death due to overdose of opioids is nearly always due to respiratory arrest. At equianalgesic doses, the morphine-like agonists produce an equivalent degree of respiratory depression. When respiratory depression occurs, it is usually in opioid-naive patients following acute administration of an opioid and is associated with other signs of CNS depression including sedation and mental clouding. Tolerance quickly develops to this effect with repeated drug administration, allowing the opioid analgesics to be used in the management of chronic cancer pain without significant risk of respiratory depression. If respiratory depression occurs, it can be reversed by the administration of the specific opioid antagonist naloxone. In patients chronically receiving opioids who develop respiratory depression, naloxone diluted 1:10 should be titrated carefully to prevent the precipitation of severe withdrawal syndromes while reversing the respiratory depression. Long-acting drugs such as methadone, fentanyl patches, or slow-release morphine are likely to cause a higher incidence of respiratory depression. The accumulation of active opioid metabolites and the simultaneous use of other depressants such as benzodiazepines or alcohol are risk factors for respiratory depression. While this is the most feared side effect of opioid analgesics, it occurs very seldom in patients receiving chronic opioid therapy for the treatment of cancer pain.

e. **Allergic reactions.** These occur very infrequently with opioids. However, it is very common that patients will be described as "allergic" to a number of opioid analgesics. This commonly occurs due to a misinterpretation by the patient or clinician of some of the common side effects of opioids such as nausea, sedation, vomiting, or sweating. In most instances, a simple discussion with the patient is enough to clarify this issue.

f. **Urinary retention.** The increase in the tone of smooth muscle of the bladder induced by opioids results in an increase in the sphincter tone leading to urinary retention. This is most common in the elderly patient. Attention should be directed to this potential transient side effect, and catheterization may be necessary for management.

g. **"Newer" side effects.** During recent years, as a result of increased education in the assessment and management of cancer pain, patients have been receiving higher doses of opioids for longer periods of time than ever before. This more aggressive use of opioids is associated with additional side effects, usually only seen in patients with late-stage disease receiving very high doses of opioids.

(1) **Cognitive failure.** Patients can experience a transient decrease in concentration and psychomotor coordination after starting opioids or after a sudden increase in the opioid dose. In some patients, the opioid-induced cognitive failure can be permanent.

Some of the cognitive effects can be reversed by the administration of amphetamine derivatives such as methylphenidate. Screening tools such as the Mini-Mental State questionnaire are useful in patients receiving high doses of opioids.

(2) **Other central effects.** Organic hallucinations, myoclonus, grand mal seizures, and even hyperalgesia hve been observed in patients receiving high doses of opioids for long periods. These effects are likely due to the accumulation of active opioid metabolites. Improvement is frequently seen after a change in the type of opioid.

(3) **Severe sedation—coma.** When coma occurs in patients receiving a stable dose of opioids for a long period of time, it should be suspected that accumulation of active opioid metabolites has occurred. These patients usually improve quickly after discontinuation of opioids.

(4) **Pulmonary edema.** While noncardiogenic pulmonary edema is a well-recognized complication of narcotic overdose in addicts, it had not been recognized until recently as a potential complication of cancer pain treatment. Pulmonary edema usually occurs when patients have undergone rapid increases in dose, usually as a result of severe neuropathic pain. While the mortality of the syndrome is very low among patients presenting with acute opioid overdoses, because of the conservative nature of the treatment of terminally ill patients with cancer, the mortality of pulmonary edema is much higher within this population.

(5) **Myoclonus.** Myoclonus may occur in patients who are on opioids for long periods, particularly with higher doses and toward the end of life when metabolic problems may also be present. While it is often not disturbing the patient, if it does become a clinical problem, it can be treated with clonazepam 0.5 mg PO bid to start, with titration every 3 days up to a maximum daily dose of 20 mg.

V. Adjuvant drugs. Opioid analgesics are the most important drugs for the treatment of cancer pain. Although these drugs can, in most patients, control severe pain even when they are used appropriately, they may produce new symptoms or exacerbate preexisting symptoms, most notably nausea and somnolence. This aspect of treatment with opioid compounds is particularly problematic in patients with advanced cancer. The combination of severe pain, anorexia, chronic nausea, asthenia, and somnolence is a frequent finding in patients with advanced cancer. The term *adjuvant drug* has been used in a variety of ways, even in the context of cancer pain management. For the purposes of the following paragraphs, an adjuvant drug meets one or more of the following criteria.

Increases the analgesic effect of opioids (adjuvant analgesia)

Decreases the toxicity of opioids

Improves other symptoms associated with terminal cancer

Most symptomatic patients with cancer receive more than one or two adjuvant drugs. Unfortunately, there is still very limited consensus as to the type and dose of the most appropriate adjuvant drugs.

Claims have been made for the adjuvant analgesic effect of many drugs, but unfortunately, most of the evidence for these effects is anecdotal. Controlled clinical trials are needed to better define the indications and risk-benefit ratios. These agents, some of which have the potential to produce significant toxicity, can aggravate the toxicity of opioids.

A. **Tricyclic antidepressants.** Despite the frequent use of these agents in British hospices and South American and European cancer centers, the use of tricyclics in North American cancer centers has been infrequent. Tricyclic antidepressants have been found to be useful for a variety of neuropathic pain syndromes, especially when pain has a prominent dysesthetic or burning character. Both amitriptyline and desipramine have been found to be effective in the management of postherpetic neuralgia, diabetic neuropathy, and other neurologic conditions. There is, however, only very limited evidence for a significant analgesic effect in cancer pain. Clinical experience and expert consensus suggest that tricyclics should be tried for the management of pain of central, deafferentation, or neuropathic origin. The optimal drug and dosing regimens are unknown. The effects of newer analgesics such as the selective serotonin uptake inhibitors (SSRIs) or specific monoamine oxidase (MAO) inhibitors on pain control have not been clearly established. Until further evidence is available, the more traditional tricyclics should be used as adjuvant analgesics. The toxic effects of these drugs are mainly autonomic (dry mouth, postural hypotension) and centrally mediated (somnolence, confusion). Because their use may contribute to symptoms already present in debilitated patients, they should be administered cautiously in those who are very ill.

B. **Anticonvulsants.** Carbamazepine, phenytoin, valproic acid, and clonazepam, alone or in combination with the tricyclic antidepressants, have been used successfully to treat neuropathic pain. Based on the well-documented efficacy for the treatment of trigeminal neuralgia, considerable experience and expert consensus suggest the use of these agents for neuropathic cancer pain syndromes, including neural invasion by tumor, radiation fibrosis or surgical scarring, herpes zoster, and deafferentation. Based on clinical observations, improvement can be expected in a proportion of patients whose predominant complaint is pain of a shooting, lancinating, burning, or hyperesthetic nature. Side effects of therapy are potentially serious, particularly in patients with advanced cancer, and can include bone marrow depression, hepatic dysfunction, ataxia, diplopia, and lymphadenopathy. Periodic monitoring of complete blood cell count and liver function is recommended.

C. **Corticosteroids.** Controlled studies suggest that the administration of corticosteroids to selected patients with advanced cancer results in decreased pain and improved appetite and activity. Unfortunately, the duration of the effects is probably short-lasting. The mechanism by which corticosteroids appear to produce beneficial symptom effects in patients with terminal cancer is unclear, but may involve their euphoriant effects or the inhibition of prostaglandin metabolism. The optimal drug and dosing regimens have not been established. For the treatment of painful conditions, prednisone or dexamethasone are often administered in doses totaling 30–60 mg PO daily and 8–16 mg PO daily, respectively. As soon as symptomatic relief is obtained, attempts should be made to progressively decrease the dose to the minimally effective dose. Although long-term side effects are not an important consideration in many patients with advanced cancer, treatment may produce limiting side effects in these patients, particularly immunosuppression (candidiasis will occur in most patients), proximal myopathy, and psychiatric symptoms. The incidence of psychologic disturbances ranges from 3 to 50%, with severe symptoms occurring in about 5% of the patients. The spectrum of disturbances ranges from mild to severe affective disorders, psychotic reactions, and global cognitive impairment.

VI. **Neuroablative procedures.** Evaluation of the physical basis of the pain may indicate that a neuroablative procedure, where the pain pathway is destroyed, would be of benefit for pain control. As aggressive opioid analgesia becomes more accepted, the great majority of patients with cancer do not require these neuroablative interventions. Destruction of the pain pathway can be accomplished surgically or through destructive nerve blocks using an agent such as phenol. The major barrier to the more widespread application of these techniques is the limited number of persons expert in their use. The most frequently used neurosurgical procedure is the anterolateral or spinothalamic cordotomy. This is often performed as closed percutaneous cordotomy by stereotaxically placing a radiofrequency needle in the anterolateral quadrant of the cervical spinal cord. Unilateral pain control can unmask significant pain on the opposite side of the body. For pain of head and neck cancer, procedures such as percutaneous radiofrequency coagulation of the glossopharyngeal nerve may be used. Pituitary ablation via injection (hypophysectomy) has been reported to be of benefit for diffuse pain. It is important to remember that performance of such procedures does not eliminate the need to administer and monitor the effectiveness of analgesics. Because of afferent regeneration, destructive procedures have had their greatest application in patients whose expected life span is only a few months.

Destructive anesthetic block of the celiac plexus had been used for several decades in the management of pain in the abdominal region. This block, which can be preceded by reversible diagnostic block, is a boon to many patients suffering from the severe pain accompanying cancer of the pancreas and may also be helpful for pain from cancers of the liver, gallbladder, or stomach. If success is achieved with the diagnostic block, lasting disruption of the pain pathway can be achieved using alcohol or phenol. Pain from rib metastases or tumors of the chest wall can be relieved with intercostal nerve blocks. Intrathecal and epidural nerve blocks have provided pain relief, but those procedures carry a risk of sensory and motor deficit.

VII. **Coping or behavioral skill techniques.** Teaching the specific skills to manage pain can be of help to a majority of patients, especially those who face pain for months to years. Evaluation and prescription of the specific skills most beneficial to the individual can often be obtained through consultation with a behavioral psychologist, psychiatrist, or pain nurse specialist. Such techniques should never be used as a substitute for appropriate analgesia. The skills include relaxation, self-hypnosis, and other distraction and cognitive control techniques. These measures can affect the sensation of pain by reducing muscle tension on pain-generating lesions, as well as by maximizing the patient's ability to cope with the pain and remain as active as the disease permits.

Selected Readings

Agency for Health Care Policy and Research. *Management of Cancer Pain.* Rockville, MD: U.S. Department of Health and Human Services, 1994.

Bruera, E., and Ripamonti, C. Adjuvants to Opioid Analgesics. In R. Patt (ed.), *Cancer Pain.* Philadelphia: Lippincott, 1992. Pp. 142–159.

Bruera, E., and Ripamonti, C. Alternate Routes of Administration of Opioids for the Management of Cancer Pain. In R. Patt (ed.), *Cancer Pain.* Philadelphia: Lippincott, 1992. Pp. 161–184.

Cleeland, C. S., et al. Pain and its treatment in outpatients with metastatic cancer. *N. Engl. J. Med.* 330:592, 1994.

Eisele, J. H., Jr., Grigsby, E. J., and Dea, G. Clonazepam treatment of myoclonic contractions associated with high-dose opioids: a case report. *Pain* 49:231, 1992.

World Health Organization (WHO). *Cancer Pain Relief and Palliative Care.* Geneva: WHO, 1990.

Emotional and Psychiatric Problems in Patients with Cancer

Kathy S. N. Franco-Bronson

I. **General principles.** Clinical psychiatric disorders occur in up to 50% of patients with cancer at some point during their treatment. Delirium, depression, and anxiety are those most frequently seen and may coexist in the same patient. Careful monitoring for the early symptoms of psychiatric distress is important to the care of these patients. The clinician should inquire regularly about symptoms in the affective and cognitive domains. Symptom clusters help differentiate anxiety, depression, and organic brain syndromes from other psychiatric disorders. Once an accurate diagnosis is made, appropriate treatment that may include medication can be planned for the target symptoms. More than one psychiatric diagnosis may be present requiring a hierarchical approach. For example, if both delirium and depression are present, the etiology of the delirium should be determined and treated before starting antidepressant therapy (which could worsen the delirium). Once organicity has improved, treatment for the depression can be considered. When major depression and an anxiety disorder coexist, treatment for the depression is started first and may adequately manage both disorders.

II. **Acute confusional states**

   A. **Precepts.** Psychiatrists are often asked to assist in the care of "agitated" patients. The initial request may be for medication advice, but prescribing psychotropic drugs without understanding the cause of the patient's distress can have serious consequences. Delirium is characterized by fluctuating levels of alertness/consciousness, shortened attention and concentration, rapidly changing moods, irregular sleep–wake cycles, garbled or slurred speech, hypervigilance, and behavior not consistent with good judgment. The delirious patient may also have delusional ideas or hallucinations. Visual, auditory, tactile, and occasionally olfactory hallucinations can be present. The more sensory modalities that are involved in the hallucinations, the greater is the likelihood the patient is experiencing an acute confusional state.

   B. **Etiologies**

   1. **Medications** remain the most common reason for acute confusional states. The most frequently identified medications to cause delirium are sedatives, narcotics, analgesics, anxiolytics, anticholinergic drugs, and corticosteroids.

   2. **Metabolic causes** are often seen in patients with cancer and include hyper- and hyponatremia, hyper- and hypothyroidism, poorly controlled diabetes mellitus, and hypercalcemia.

3. **Infections** of the respiratory, urinary, central nervous, and other systems are common, especially in immunosuppressed patients.
4. **Chemical withdrawal** from benzodiazepines, alcohol, and others can induce delirium.
5. **Vitamin deficiencies** (B_{12}, folate, thiamine), tumors, cardiac arrhythmias, congestive heart failure, liver disease, trauma, strokes, renal failure, and a variety of other conditions can cause acute changes in mental status.

C. **Therapeutic approach.** Once an acute confusional state is identified, the primary therapeutic approach is to treat the cause. Antipsychotic medications may be helpful for managing symptoms such as hallucinations, delusions, and extreme agitation, but they do not treat the cause of the delirium.

1. **Orientation** aids in the reduction of confusion.

   a. It is helpful to frequently orient the patient to place, time, and why they are at the hospital, and to give current explanations of procedures. This routine should be done once or more per shift when the delirious patient is awake. Because patients' attention, concentration, and recent memory are often impaired, they often do not recall instructions given to them earlier. Leaving a large, legibly written note card with the patient's name, date, hospital name, and so on is beneficial in some instances.

   b. A large calendar, a clock, and family pictures or mementos can assist the patients in feeling less estranged from their environment.

   c. Some patients are reassured by a small night light in their room, which cuts down on illusions or misinterpretations. Individuals with compromised vision or hearing are particularly distraught when they are even less able to discern what is happening around them.

2. **Medication** helps to control hallucinations, delusions, and psychotic agitation. The lowest dose to control symptoms is usually preferable.

   a. **Haloperidol** (Haldol) (Table 38-1) is a butyrophenone, antipsychotic agent with potent dopamine blocking action. It is less likely to produce cardiovascular, respiratory, gastrointestinal, and general anticholinergic side effects than many of the other antipsychotic medications. However, moderate doses may cause extrapyramidal symptoms. The starting dose in a patient with an acute confusional state is 0.25–2.00 mg PO or IM, on an "as needed" or regular dosing schedule every 4–6 hours. A marked advantage of haloperidol is that sedation is minimized while controlling agitation. There are exceptions to the usually preferred low doses of antipsychotic medications. For example, if patients tolerate higher doses with few side effects, they may benefit by having improved

Table 38-1. Antipsychotic medications: prominent characteristics and dosage for patients with cancer

Agent	Starting dose (mg)*	Characteristics
Phenothiazines		
Chlorpromazine (Thorazine)	10–25	Significant hypotension risk, lowers seizure threshold, highly sedating, anticholinergic
Thioridazine (Mellaril)	10–25	Similar to chlorpromazine but more likely to alter ECG; not available IM
Mesoridazine (Serentil)	10–25	Similar to chlorpromazine and thioridazine
Perphenazine (Trilafon)	4	Moderate sedation and hypotension
Trifluoperazine (Stelazine)	2	High frequency of extrapyramidal side effects
Fluphenazine (Prolixin)	2	High frequency of extrapyramidal side effects
Prochlorperazine (Compazine)	5–10	Weak antipsychotic; used more as an antiemetic
Others		
Haloperidol (Haldol)	0.5–2.0	High frequency of extrapyramidal side effects
Thiothixene (Navane)	1–2	High frequency of extrapyramidal side effects
Loxapine (Loxitane)	10	Moderate in most side effects noted above
Molindone (Moban)	5–10	Less weight gain
Pimozide (Orap)	1–2	Used in monodelusional disorders and Tourette's syndrome
Clozapine (Clozaril)	Little experience with the physically ill patient, except in Parkinson's disease	Recommended for patients who have chronic schizophrenia or evidence of tardive dyskinesia
Risperidone (Risperidol)	Little experience with the physically ill patient	Recommended for patients who have chronic schizophrenia or evidence of tardive dyskinesia

*Dose generally can be repeated every 4–6 hours, either on an as-needed or a regular schedule (e.g., qid).

pain control. Intravenous (IV) haloperidol has not been approved by the U.S. Food and Drug Administration (FDA), although it is commonly used in the seriously agitated patient. Half the oral dosing is prescribed when the medication is given IV. Some patients require larger IV doses to control symptoms. Avoid very high doses in patients with alcohol cardiomyopathy, those prone to torsades de pointes or similar arrhythmias, and those with an excessively long Qt_c interval. Extrapyramidal side effects are minimal with IV administration.

b. Additional **high-potency, low-sedation options** include thiothixene (Navane), trifluoperazine (Stelazine), and fluphenazine (Prolixin).

c. **A delirious patient** with vision or hearing impairment is likely to hallucinate during periods of excessive sedation.

d. If the patient demonstrates a **predictable period of confusion,** e.g., early evening ("sundowning") when there is less environmental activity, a once-a-day dose at that time may be adequate.

e. **When increasing the dose of antipsychotic drugs,** muscle spasms, restlessness, or pseudo-parkinsonian symptoms may occur. Adding a small amount of trihexyphenidyl (Artane) 1–2 mg bid, benztropine (Cogentin) 1 mg bid, or diphenhydramine (Benadryl) 25 mg bid can often reduce the side effects. However, increasing the level of anticholinergic activity with these choices may cause an atropinic-like psychosis. Constipation, urinary retention, dry mouth, tachycardia, and increasing confusion are warnings of this potential problem, especially when multiple anticholinergic medications (e.g., antiemetics, analgesics) are being prescribed. Therefore antiparkinsonian drugs are not prescribed prophylactically but only if clearly indicated.

f. **Benzodiazepines,** e.g., lorazepam (Ativan) 0.5–2.0 mg q8h, are sometimes given in small doses to a patient who needs some sedation without added anticholinergic activity or whose cardiac status is at risk (i.e., heart block) if the antipsychotic medication is increased. Using both benzodiazepines and antipsychotics is sometimes helpful. One pattern might be 0.5–2.0 mg haloperidol at 4 p.m., 1–2 mg of lorazepam at 8 p.m., and so forth if the patient is agitated.

g. **Increasing delerium.** Too much medication may have been given if the patient's level of agitation increases with higher doses.

h. **Hypotension.** Avoid adding other antipsychotics, e.g., thorazine, as they predispose to hypotension and shock. If the blood pressure does drop significantly, norepinephrine bitartrate (Levophed) or a similar choice may be necessary because the antipsychotic medications block the action of dopamine. The half-life of the antipsychotic is generally 24–48 hours.

III. Depression. Patients with cancer have various emotional responses to their diagnoses. The mourning period for some is brief, does not inhibit their ability to interact with family and friends, and does not hinder participation in their own treatment. Support from others, acceptance of their feelings, and time may be all that is necessary for them to continue the emotional work ahead. However, approximately one-fourth of patients with cancer develop longer, more severe depressions. The greatest risk of depression is at the time of first relapse. There are many variables that influence this process, including emotional conflicts with loved ones, disproportionate guilt, previous losses that were never resolved, long-standing debilitating illness, some personality characteristics such as dependency, and inadequate support systems. Any of these factors, along with a family history of depression, are warnings for the physician to heed.

A. Therapeutic approach

1. Emotional support at frequent intervals from the physician is generally needed. Some patients explore old emotional conflicts, whereas others just need a safe person to whom they can express their feelings. It is important for patients to be able to hold on to hope. A degree of "denial" is acceptable, normal, and upheld. Only when this denial makes it impossible for a patient to make informed treatment decisions is it necessary to probe into the denial.

Psychotherapy of a supportive nature is often provided by the primary care physician, oncologist, psychiatrist, clergy, nurse, family, or friend individually or in any combination. For patients who wish to explore ambivalence, a professional psychotherapist trained in psychodynamic or interpersonal therapy is a good option. Cognitive therapy is helpful in letting go of detrimental interpretations while increasing one's ability to deal with emotional pain.

2. Psychiatric care may be particularly instrumental when the patient's other physicians are struggling with how much of the patient's preexisting personality style is interfering with treatment. Anniversary responses to previous losses, important family events, or past hospitalizations may have a great impact on the presentation of the depression and deserve exploration by a psychotherapist if a pattern is found. If there is a designated psychiatric consultant, this individual must work closely with the rest of the oncology team, communicating in a helpful way to the patient, family, and staff.

If a patient has felt depressed, distressed, or irritable for some time or describes a loss of pleasure from formerly enjoyable relationships or activities,

Table 38-2. Characteristics of commonly used heterocyclic antidepressants

Antidepressant	Sedation[a]	Anticholinergic effect[b]	Other characteristics
Amitriptyline (Elavil, Endep)	+4 to +5[c]	+4 to +5	Also available IM
Clomipramine (Anafranil)	+1	+1	Blocks dopamine (has antipsychosis effect, but can cause extrapyramidal symptoms including tardive dyskinesia)
Desipramine (Norpramin)	+2 to +3	+3	Recommended for obsessive-compulsive disorders
Doxepin (Sinequan, Adapin)	+4	+4	Highest appetite increase
Imipramine (Tofranil)	+3	+3	Also available IM
Maprotiline (Ludiomil)	+2	+2	Lowers seizure threshold significantly
Nortriptyline (Pamelor, Aventyl)	+2	+3	Less likely to cause orthostasis than other TCAs
Protriptyline (Vivactil)	+1	+3 to +4	More activating; less pulmonary suppression
Trimipramine (Surmontil)	+4	+4	

TCA = tricyclic antidepressant.
[a] Associated with histaminergic blockade; appetite increase follows somewhat similar trends.
[b] Constipation, dry mouth, urinary retention, and so on.
[c] Scale of 1–5, where 1 is least and 5 is most.

inquiry about the following symptoms is necessary: insomnia or hypersomnia, alteration in appetite with expected weight change, reduced interest in family, sexuality, work, or hobbies, increased guilt, low energy level, poor concentration, thoughts of death or suicide, frequent crying episodes, and psychomotor hypo- or hyperactivity. When the diagnosis of depression in the medically ill patient is being made, the emphasis is placed on psychologic features as opposed to physical ones. These include rumination or repetitive negative thoughts, increased tearfulness, withdrawal from family or friends, and anhedonia. These symptoms are characteristic of a major depressive disorder for which antidepressant medication in addition to psychotherapy is recommended.

3. **Medications.** Patients with cancer are often undertreated for major depression that has been mistaken for simple grief. Evidence is beginning to accumulate that psychosocial adjustment and improved life adaptation, in general, occur when patients with cancer and major depression are treated with antidepressant medications.

   a. **Selection of agents and their side effects.** An antidepressant medication should be selected on the basis of its tendency to sedate or activate, cause orthostatic changes, or produce anticholinergic effects. Medication selection should also be tailored to the patient's symptom cluster, such as the need for sedation or weight gain versus the need for activation (Tables 38-2 and 38-3). Route of metabolism and elimination may also figure into a choice as well as the medication's tendency to cause seizures.

   Highly anticholinergic medications frequently produce dry mouth, blurred vision, tachycardia, and constipation. They can also produce urinary retention, ileus, and acute confusion. The drugs that are also antihistaminergic can increase sedation, appetite, and hypotension. Medications that produce alpha-adrenergic receptor blockade are associated with increased orthostatic hypotension, dizziness, and reflex tachycardia.

   b. **Dosages** (Table 38-4). Weak, debilitated, or elderly patients need protection from many of these side effects. Starting out with small doses and gradually increasing the dose is prudent. Splitting doses may also be helpful for minimizing side effects and maximizing pain relief from these medications.

   If a patient has a personal history, family history, or previous drug response that reflects mania or hypomania, it is necessary to proceed carefully, perhaps with lithium alone or an alternative mood stabilizer (Table 38-5).

Table 38-3. Characteristics of commonly used nonheterocyclic antidepressants

Antidepressant	Sedation[a]	Anticholinergic effect[b]	Other characteristics
Amoxapine (Asendin)	+2 to +3[c]	+2 to +3	Blocks dopamine (has antipsychosis effect, but can cause extrapyramidal symptoms including tardive dyskinesias)
Bupropion (Wellbutrin)	+1	+1	Increases seizure risk, especially if organic brain pathology or eating disorder is present; more activating; less weight gain
Fluoxetine (Prozac)	+1	+1	May cause restlessness and gastrointestinal upset; more activating; less weight gain; safe in patients with renal disease, but may accumulate in those with liver disease

Trazodone (Deseryl)	+4	+1	Least anticholinergic of sedating options; priapism rate increased
Fluvoxamine (Luvox)	+1	+1	Similar to fluoxetine
Sertraline (Zoloft)	+1	+1	Similar to fluoxetine
Paroxetine (Paxil)	+1	+1	Similar to fluoxetine
Venlafaxine (Effexor)	+1	+1	Both serotonin and norepinephrine reuptake inhibitor; increases blood pressure at higher doses

[a]Associated with histaminergic blockade; appetite increase follows somewhat similar trends.
[b]Constipation, dry mouth, urinary retention, and so on.
[c]Scale of 1–5 where 1 is least and 5 is most.

Table 38-4. Dosages for antidepressant therapy

Drug	Starting daily dose (mg)	Average daily dose for patient with cancer (mg)
Amitriptyline	10–25	75–150
Amoxapine	25	75–150
Bupropion	75–150	300
Clomipramine	25	75–150
Desipramine	25	75–150
Doxepin	25	75–150
Fluoxetine	10–20	20
Fluvoxamine	50	100
Imipramine	10–25	75–150
Maprotiline	25	75
Nortriptyline	10–25	50–100
Paroxetine	10–20	20
Protriptyline	5–10 qA.M.	20 (10 mg A.M. & noon)
Sertraline	25–50	100
Trazodone	50	150–300
Trimipramine	10–25	75–150
Venlafaxine	25	75 mg (37.5 mg bid)

    c. Monoamine oxidase inhibitors (MAOIs) (Table 38-6) may be used to treat major depression or panic disorder but are somewhat inconvenient in that tyramine dietary restrictions and medication interactions require much attention. They are often tried as an alternative when other choices have failed if the depression is accompanied by phobic and histrionic features or if the individual was effectively treated with an MAOI for an earlier depression.

IV. Anxiety

  A. Approach to the problem. As grieving is described as normal, so is anxiety in patients with cancer. However, this anxiety varies in its etiology, severity, and treatment. A detailed history of the onset, characteristics, and length of distress is important. Knowledge of the patient's previous symptoms, current and past physical illness, and chemical and medication usage is essential to the evaluation process. Antianxiety agents may be helpful for alleviating patients' distress and helping them to cope with other problems associated with their cancer (Table 38-7).

  B. Problems that present as anxiety. The duration of the symptom is one of the first factors to assess in the anxious patient.

1. **Suspect an adjustment disorder** when maladaptive anxious symptoms have persisted less than 6 months and apparently represent an adjustment to learning the diagnosis or reactions to the treatment. This kind of anxiety may benefit from supportive therapy, relaxation therapy, or benzodiazepines.
2. **Generalized anxiety.** If the anxiety has been present for more than 6 months, continuing no matter what environmental alterations occur, and is accompanied by signs of physical tension or poor attention to conversation or other daily activities, the patient is likely to have generalized anxiety. Supportive therapy, relaxation tapes, biofeedback, buspirone, and benzodiazepines are useful.
3. **Brief, isolated episodes of anxiety** that come and go lead the examiner to consider other diagnoses.
   a. **Panic attacks.** If the patient has repeated "attacks" that have a rapid onset and last 20 minutes to a few hours, and if they are accompanied by tachycardia, palpitations, hyperventilation, sweating, dizziness, and the wish to flee without a physical or chemical explanation, they are most likely panic attacks that often preexisted. They are best treated with benzodiazepines such as clonazepam and alprazolam, antidepressants such as tricyclics, or MAOIs. Beta blockers to block autonomic symptoms may be tried if performance anxiety around specific activities is identified.
   b. **Organic etiologies** are often responsible for the anxiety.
      (1) **Hypoxia.** Repeating episodes of anxiety accompanied by alterations in intellectual functioning, poor orientation, reduced judgment, shortened attention, a rapidly fluctuating mood, and difficulty with memory suggest hypoxia. When anxiety is induced by hypoxia, it is wise to reduce central nervous system (CNS) depressant medications and give small doses of an antipsychotic drug if the anxiety is accompanied by delirium. Antipsychotic medications, however, often produce akathisia, an extrapyramidal restlessness that anxiety mimics. Alternating the antipsychotic drug with small doses of a short-half-life benzodiazepine is one option for organically induced anxiety—if respiratory status or arterial blood gases (ABGs) measurements do not worsen.
      (2) **Liver disease and other physical disorders.** If anxiety is associated with liver disease, start by reducing CNS depressant medications. When needed, small, infrequent doses of a short-acting benzodiazepine that requires conjugation but not oxidation in the liver are prescribed. These include lor-

Table 38-5. Other medications used to treat affective disorders

Drug	Starting dose	Average dose for cancer patients	Disorder	Pretreatment work-up	Follow-up studies	Comment
Stimulants[a]						
Methylphenidate (Ritalin)	2.5–5.0 mg qA.M. + noon	5–20 mg qA.M. + noon	Medically ill patient with depression	CBC	CBC	
Pemoline (Cylert)	18.75 mg qA.M.	37.5 mg qA.M. + noon	Medically ill patient with depression	Liver function tests	Liver function tests	
Dextroamphetamine (Dexedrine)[b]	2.5 mg qA.M.	5–20 mg qA.M. + noon	Medically ill patient with depression			
Lithium carbonate (Eskalith, Eskalith-CR, Lithobid)	300 mg qhs	300 mg tid	Depression[c] (may need to add an antidepressant) Mania[c] (may need to add clonazepam or an antipsychotic)	ECG, electrolytes, UA, BUN/ creat., thyroid (T₄, TSH), CBC (including differential)	Lithium level initially 2 ×/wk. Gradually lengthen to q3mo. Thyroid studies q6mo or earlier if indicated. UA/BUN/creatinine, CBC if infection	Monitor blood level 12 hours after evening dose. 0.8– 1.0 mEq/liter *is* most effective. Watch for hypothyroidism, diabetes insipidus, nephropathy, dehydration.
Anticonvulsants						
Carbamazepine (Tegretol)	100 mg bid	200 mg tid	Depression or mania	CBC, reticu- locytes, serum iron, liver	CBC, thyroid studies, blood level	Watch for leuko- penia, throm- bocytopenia,

Drug	Starting dose	Dosage	Use	Monitoring	Monitoring	Comments
Valproic acid (Depakene, Depakote)	15 mg/kg/day	500–750 mg/day (divided into tid doses)	Mania	Liver function tests, UA, BUN	Liver function tests, CBC, blood level	hepatotoxicity, decreased effect of warfarin. Watch for hepatotoxicity, especially in young children.
Benzodiazepines						
Clonazepam (Clonopin, Klonopin)	0.5 mg qhs	2 mg or higher	Mania	CBC, liver function tests	CBC, liver function tests	Do not withdraw rapidly. Impaired renal function and respiratory distress require extremely cautious use.
Alprazolam (Xanax)	0.5 mg qhs	1 mg tid or higher	Depression			Do not withdraw rapidly (reduce daily dose by 0.25 mg weekly). Use cautiously if respiratory impairment.

CBC = complete blood cell count; ECG = electrocardiogram; UA = urinalysis; BUN = blood urea nitrogen; TSH = thyroid-stimulating hormone.

[a] Checks on weight, pulse, and blood pressure. Tolerance may develop, and doses may require adjustment.
[b] Caution required because of multiple drug interactions.
[c] Natural or corticosteroid-induced.

Table 38-6. Antidepressants: monoamine oxidase inhibitors

	Starting dose (mg bid)	Average dose (mg)	Characteristic
Tranylcypromine (Parnate)	10	20–60	More activating
Phenelzine (Nardil)	15	30–90	More sedating

Avoid

Foods: Tyramine-containing foods: aged cheeses, flat, broad beans, sausage, pickled herring, chianti or other red wine, beer, yogurt

Drugs: Meperidine; phenylethylamine compounds including stimulants, appetite suppressants, decongestants, bronchodilators; large doses of aspartame sweeteners

azepam, oxazepam, and temazepam. Many other physical disorders can also produce anxious symptoms, including various brain tumors, pheochromocytoma, carcinoid, hyperthyroidism, cardiac arrhythmias, drug or alcohol withdrawal, and hyperparathyroidism.

    (3) Medications such as theophylline, corticosteroids, antidepressants, and antipsychotic drugs can produce anxiety.

  C. Precipitants can be identified in patients with cancer that initiate the previously discussed adjustment disorder lasting generally no longer than 6 months. Posttraumatic stress disorder, less often seen in patients with cancer, follows a distressing event outside the range of usual human experience. More frequently observed, however, are individuals who describe intense fears of needles, radiotherapy rooms, or confined-space scanning devices. Often the history unfolds to describe previously existing phobias. These patients, like those with anticipatory anxiety about procedures or chemotherapy, may be assisted with relaxation or desensitization techniques, imagery, antianxiety medications, and reassurance. If patients begin to experience procedures, treatments, or interpersonal situations as being particularly stressful, anticipatory anxiety intensifies the requirement for larger doses of as-needed medication to attain some relief. Therefore regular scheduling of antianxiety medication similarly to that of pain medication is in order.

V. Insomnia

  A. Principles. An inability to fall asleep may be associated with anxiety, whereas awakening in the middle of the night is generally more closely related to depression. In

Table 38-7. Antianxiety agents and nighttime sedatives

Agent	Half-life (hours)	Onset	Starting dose (mg)
Benzodiazepines			
Triazolam (Halcion)	1.5–3.5	Rapid	0.125 (qhs)
Oxazepam (Serax)	8–20	Moderate	10 (tid)
Lorazepam (Ativan)	10–20	Rapid	0.5 (tid)
Temazepam (Restoril)	12–24	Rapid	15 (qhs)
Alprazolam (Xanax)	12–24	Moderate	0.25 (tid)
Chlordiazepam (Librium)	12–48	Moderate	10 (bid or tid)
Clonazepam (Klonopin)	20–30	Rapid	0.5 (bid)
Diazepam (Valium)	20–90	Rapid	2–5 (bid)
Clorazepate (Tranxene)	20–100	Rapid	7.5 (bid)
Flurazepam (Dalmane)	20–100	Rapid	15 (qhs)
Imidazopyrine			
Zolpidem (Ambien)	1.5–4.5	Rapid	5 (qhs)

Antidepressants (for panic disorder)
  See Tables 38-2, 38-3, 38-4, 38-5, 38-6. May use lower doses than for depression; i.e., an imipramine starting dose of 10 mg tid.

Beta blockers (for autonomic symptom control)
  Propranolol (Inderal) 10–20 mg tid
  Atenolol (Tenormin) 25–50 mg daily

Antipsychotics (for anxiety associated with delirium)
  See Table 38-1.

Antihistamines
  May be safer in some cases when respiratory impairment is a complication; also used for insomnia.

  Diphenhydramine (Benadryl) 25 mg; starting doses bid or tid
  Hydroxyzine (Vistaril) 25 mg; starting doses tid or qid

  Note: Elderly or extremely debilitated patients should be given lower doses. Caution should be taken when prescribing long-acting sedating medications, as they have been associated with a high incidence of falls and hip fracture.

addition, there are a variety of physical disorders that cause sleeping irregularities. The sleep–wake cycle is almost always disturbed in a delirious patient, no matter what the etiology. Pain often awakens a patient with cancer. Medications can awaken some patients directly (e.g., fluoxetine) or indirectly (e.g., diuretics). Aside from sorting out these influences, the physician must take into account the environment. Is the patient too hot or cold? Is the ward too brightly lit or too noisy? Do the patients awaken each time they are checked by the night staff? When any or several of these concerns are corrected, sleeping medication may not be necessary, although the need for sedatives remains in some patients.

B. Benzodiazepines (see Table 38-7). This class of drugs is most often prescribed if a patient needs nighttime sedation. The shorter half-life benzodiazepines (i.e., triazolam or temazepam) with a rapid onset produce less daytime grogginess than those with a longer half-life. Short-acting ones tend to accumulate less and are safer for patients with liver disease. On the other hand, longer half-life drugs (i.e., diazepam or flurazepam) with a rapid onset produce less rebound insomnia or unwanted awakening during the very early morning.

C. Antihistamines (see Table 38-7). These medications may be chosen if physicians are hesitant to prescribe benzodiazepines, e.g., for patients with respiratory disease. A disadvantage may be the higher anticholinergic potential of these drugs compared to the benzodiazepine family.

D. Others. Chloral hydrate (500–1000 mg), an old standby hypnotic, can still be used so long as patients are free of gastrointestinal or liver disease. Barbiturates, e.g., amobarbital sodium, are occasionally used to treat some refractory sleeping disturbances for a short time but are not routinely used because they induce respiratory depression and have addictive potential.

Selected Readings

Adams, F., Fernandez, F., and Anderson, B. Emergency pharmacotherapy of delirium in the critically ill cancer patient. *Psychosomatics* 27(suppl. 1):33, 1986.

Anderson, B., Adams, F., and McCredie, K. High-dose neuroleptics for acute brain failure after intensive chemotherapy for acute leukemia. *Acta Psychiatr. Scand.* 70:193, 1984.

Bernstein, J. G. *Handbook of Drug Therapy in Psychiatry* (2nd ed.). Littleton, MA: PSG Publishing, 1988.

Bezchlibnyk-Butler, K. Z., Jeffries, J. J., and Martin, B. A. (eds.), *Clinical Handbook of Psychotropic Drugs* (4th ed.). Seattle: Hogrefe and Huber Publishers, 1994.

Cassileth, B., et al. Psychosocial correlates of survival in advanced malignant disease. *N. Engl. J. Med.* 312:1551, 1985.

Endicott, J. Measurement of depression in patients with cancer. *Cancer* 53:2243, 1984.

Evans, D. L., et al. Treatment of depression in cancer patients is associated with better life adaptation: a pilot study. *Psychosom. Med.* 50:72, 1988.

Holland, J. C., and Rowland, J. H. (ed.). *Handbook of Psychooncology.* New York: Oxford University Press, 1989.

Lecrubier, Y., and Puech, A. Neuropharmacology. In J. E. Costa e Silva and C. C. Nadelson (eds.), *International Review of Psychiatry* (Vol. 1). Washington, D.C.: American Psychiatric Press, 1993. Pp. 441–482.

Maguire, P., and Faulkner, A. How to improve the counseling skills of doctors and nurses in cancer care. *B.M.J.* 297: 847, 1988.

Massie, M. J., and Holland, J. C. Depression and the cancer patient. *J. Clin. Psychiatry* 51(suppl. 7):12, 1990.

Perry, P., Alexander, B., and Liskow, B. *Psychotropic Drug Handbook* (4th ed.). Cincinnati: Harvey Whitney Books, 1985.

Spiegel, D., et al. Effect of psychosocial treatment of patients with metastatic breast cancer. *Lancet* 2:1447, 1989.

Zonderman, D. B., Costa, P. T., and McCrae, P. R. Depression as a risk for cancer morbidity and mortality in a nationally representative sample. *J.A.M.A.* 262:1191, 1989.

Principles of Oncology Nursing and Safe Handling of Antineoplastic Agents

Janelle M. Tipton

Cancer nursing continues to grow as a recognized specialty in nursing. With the ongoing advancements in cancer care, nurses must provide care that reflects an understanding of the complexity of cancer and its treatments. Oncology nurses are challenged with the task of providing very sophisticated care, education, and emotional support in a changing health care environment. Nurses must continually use their skills and creativity to meet the needs of patients with cancer and their families.

Chemotherapy administration is an aspect of cancer nursing care that requires the skill and responsibility of the professional registered nurse. In this chapter, several aspects of chemotherapy administration including safe handling practices are discussed.

I. **General guidelines.** Antineoplastic agents are administered by nurses in a variety of settings, including hospital inpatient units, outpatient clinics, physician offices, and patient homes. The Oncology Nursing Society, a professional organization for oncology nursing, has developed qualifying criteria for the registered nurse to administer chemotherapy, to promote the safe delivery of antineoplastic agents in the various settings.

A. The nurse must be designated as **qualified to administer chemotherapy** by a variety of routes after educational preparation as outlined by the individual institutional policies and procedures.

B. The nurse must have a **current license to practice** as a registered nurse in the state of employment.

C. The nurse should have **cardiopulmonary resuscitation (CPR) certification and intravenous therapy skills** prior to participating in chemotherapy administration.

D. The nurse should **demonstrate knowledge and skills** in the following areas.
1. Pharmacology of antineoplastic agents
2. Handling, preparation, and disposal of antineoplastic agents
3. Principles of chemotherapy administration
4. Chemotherapy-related intravenous (IV) therapy skills (e.g., venipuncture and vascular access device management)
5. Chemotherapy-related side effects and their nursing management
6. Common problems encountered by patients and families
7. Educational strategies and knowledge of resources for patients and families

E. **Evaluation** of knowledge and skill in chemotherapy administration on an annual basis may be established by the administrative authorities of the institution.

F. Participation on a regular basis in **continuing education** offerings on chemotherapy or oncology-related care is recommended to maintain knowledge base.

The Nurse Practice Act of individual states may also have requirements for practice.

II. **Informed consent to administer chemotherapy.** It is recommended that individual institutional policies regarding informed consent be reviewed, prior to the administration of chemotherapy. All patients receiving chemotherapy, either investigational or noninvestigational, should receive information and appropriate explanation prior to receiving the drug(s). When a patient is participating in a research study, written consent is necessary and this document is considered a permanent part of the patient's medical record. Many institutions also have consent forms that help to ensure that patients understand the procedures, risks, and benefits of standard, noninvestigational treatment. One copy of the document is given to the patient for reinforcement of the informed consent educational process, while the other copy goes into the patient record for documentation of the information exchange and consent to therapy. The physician has primary responsibility for obtaining informed consent, but the nurse shares in this responsibility by providing supplemental information and discussing the treatment, anticipated benefits, and side effects. All education and evaluation of the patient and family's understanding should be documented in the patient's chart.

III. **Routes and methods of chemotherapy administration**

A. **Oral route.** Although oral administration of chemotherapy is usually straightforward and can be done at home, it is very important to be certain the patient is clear about correct dosing and scheduling. Patients and their families must also be educated on possible side effects and assessment of the side effects, as oral chemotherapy has potential toxicities similar to parenteral chemotherapy. It is generally best not to give a patient a prescription for more than one cycle of chemotherapy. If a patient does not understand the dose and schedule or is not clear about the necessity to have blood cell counts checked prior to a new cycle of therapy, potentially fatal overdose may occur when prescriptions are written for more than one cycle of therapy at a time. This caveat may be modified for experienced patients who have a clear understanding about the importance of holding the start of a new cycle until after adequate blood cell counts have been verified by the nurses or physicians.

B. **Subcutaneous and intramuscular routes.** Chemotherapy agents administered by these routes must not be vesicants and should be given only if they cause minimal irritation to the tissues. Many of the biologic response modifiers are also given by the subcutaneous route. The smallest-gauge needle possible should be used, depending on the viscosity of the medication. Sites of administration should be rotated if the medication is given frequently, to prevent tissue irritation and the development of induration and fibrosis. The subcutaneous route is also used for the administration of slow-release pellets or depots. Because of the large-gauge needle required for these applications, the needle puncture site and tract should be anesthetized with a local anesthetic. Patients may complain of irritation at the injection site from the alcohol, the diluent, or the medication itself. The intramuscular route is generally avoided in thrombocytopenic (platelet count < 50,000/µl) or neutropenic (absolute neutrophil count [ANC] < 1000/µl) patients.

C. **IV administration.** This method is the most common route for the delivery of chemotherapy agents. IV administration can be by push, sidearm, "piggyback," or continuous infusion. An IV bolus could be given by any of the first three methods. Which is used depends on the volume of administration (push for small volume, piggyback for large) and the necessity to avoid infiltration (sidearm).

1. **IV push** is a method used for the administration of nonvesicant drugs only. After a small butterfly needle is inserted into a vein, a flush syringe with normal saline solution is attached and 2–3 ml is infused to establish patency. The flush syringe is detached, the medication syringe is attached, and the medication is pushed into the vein at an appropriate rate for the medication. The flush syringe is then reattached, and 3–5 ml of flush solution is used to clear the line. The IV push method is a very quick method to administer chemotherapy in the outpatient setting.

2. **IV sidearm** is the preferred method to administer vesicant agents. A needle is placed in a vein, and IV tubing is attached with solution freely flowing. A medication syringe is inserted or attached into the lowest Y site of the tubing closest to the insertion site. The medication is infused while the IV fluid is freely flowing at a wide open rate, to ensure continual dilution of the medication and to minimize the irritation to the vein. The person administering the chemotherapy is able to observe the site at all times during the infusion and to monitor for potential extravasation. It is important to flush the line with 20–30 ml of the IV solution between the administration of each agent to ensure the medication has completely been given, and to prevent the mixing of incompatible agents.

3. **IV piggyback** administration of chemotherapy is useful for medications that require dilution and administration over a longer period of time than the other IV methods allow. This method is not usually used for the administration of vesicant agents (except with a central venous access device), as the nurse may not be in constant view of the IV site and

extravasation may occur unnoticed. After venous access has been established, an IV solution is infused to establish patency. The chemotherapy medication is placed in a smaller bag of solution, generally 50–250 ml. IV piggyback tubing is inserted into the smaller bag, and attached to the upper Y site of the main IV tubing. The primary flush solution bag should be lowered to allow for easier infusion of the chemotherapy. The piggyback medication is infused over a specified period of time and on completion, the primary flush solution that was first started flushes the line.

4. **Continuous IV infusion (CIV)** is a method used to administer chemotherapy agents over a prolonged period of time, commonly 24–96 hours. Chemotherapy medications are added to an infusing solution, and are administered over a specified period of time. Vesicant agents may be administered by this method, but must be administered via a central venous access device. Continuous infusions of chemotherapy can be carried out in the home or elsewhere outside of the hospital using portable ambulatory infusion pumps or implanted pumps.

D. **Intraarterial therapy.** This may be given by means of an arterial catheter. Chemotherapy is given by this route to allow for regional delivery of drug via a vessel that supplies the tumor. Intraarterial chemotherapy administration often involves use of the femoral artery or the brachial artery. Systemic anticoagulation may be necessary to prevent clotting of the vessel during infusions that last several days. When the hepatic artery is selected, medications can be given by an implanted or external infusion pump.

E. **Intrathecal therapy.** This is given by injecting antineoplastic agents directly into the cerebrospinal fluid (CSF). Intrathecal therapy can be administered by a physician performing a lumbar puncture and injecting the chemotherapy into the intrathecal space. The chemotherapy agent is injected 1–2 ml at a time; patency of this route is ensured and mixing of the chemotherapy agent with the CSF is facilitated by withdrawing and reinjecting 1.0–1.5 ml from the CSF each time 2 ml of the agent has been injected until the entire volume of drug has been injected—usually 6–10 ml. The entire process of injection will usually take 0.5–2.0 minutes. Specially trained nurses may administer intrathecal therapy with the use of an Ommaya reservoir, a surgically implanted device with a catheter that is inserted into one of the lateral cerebral ventricles or the lumbar subarachnoid space. The reservoir is implanted subcutaneously in the scalp or lumbar area. For this method of chemotherapy administration, sterility is critical throughout the procedure. The skin is cleansed with an iodine-povidone (Betadine) solution and wiped with alcohol. The reservoir is accessed obliquely with a 23- or

25-gauge butterfly needle to ensure the self-sealing capacity of the reservoir diaphragm. Approximately 3 ml of CSF is withdrawn, and this sample may be set aside to flush the reservoir after the drug is instilled. Other CSF specimens may be obtained for cytologic or microbiologic studies. The medication is then administered slowly, over at least 5 minutes. The medication must be mixed in a preservative-free solution to minimize meningeal irritation. Following injection of the medication, the CSF flush is administered. On removal of the needle, the reservoir is gently pumped or compressed 3–5 times to facilitate flushing of the medication from the reservoir into CSF or the lateral ventricles.

F. **Intraperitoneal therapy.** Intraperitoneal therapy is the delivery of chemotherapy directly into the abdominal cavity, which allows for the delivery of high concentrations of drug to the tumor site. This method requires the insertion of a catheter or implantable port attached to a catheter into the peritoneum. A Tenckhoff catheter similar to that used for peritoneal dialysis is often used. Sterile technique is necessary when manipulating the catheter or administering chemotherapy via this route. The chemotherapy agent is administered in 1–2 liters of fluid and is allowed to dwell into the abdomen for a specified period of time. The fluid may or may not be drained off the abdomen, and some of the medication may be systemically absorbed. (See Chap. 36.) The patient may experience temporary discomfort or cramping from the solution and potential systemic side effects.

G. **Intrapleural therapy.** This is usually administered through a chest tube. (See Chap. 36.) Fluid that has accumulated in the pleura is drained, and medication is instilled through the tube. The chest tube is temporarily clamped and the patient is encouraged to change positions frequently to distribute the medication for 1–2 hours. The tube is then unclamped and connected back to suction or a water seal. This procedure is the responsibility of the physician, but the nurse may assist in the position changes and in monitoring the patient for side effects.

H. **Intrapericardial therapy.** This form of therapy is administered via a catheter placed into the pericardial cavity surrounding the heart. (See Chap. 36.) This therapy is given to patients who develop malignant pericardial effusions. Following the drainage of the excess fluid in the pericardial cavity, the chemotherapy agent may be instilled by a qualified physician using appropriate cardiac monitoring. The medication is often not drained and is systemically absorbed. The nurse's responsibility is to monitor for any complications associated with the administration, including changes in cardiac or respiratory status.

IV. **Vascular access**

A. **Insertion of IV needles.** For many patients with difficult venous access, this procedure can be one of the most anxiety-provoking events of the treatment. The skill and experience of the nurse in venipuncture and the ease in insertion can have a considerable impact on the comfort and anxiety level of the patient to receive chemotherapy.

1. **Site of venipuncture.** Proper selection of veins for chemotherapy administration is quite important to the process. The upper extremities are the sites of choice due to easier access, patient mobility, and decreased risk of thrombophlebitis. Limbs with compromised circulation due to mastectomy, fractures, or superior vena cava syndrome should be avoided. Veins that are sclerosed or inflamed are also to be avoided. The best site for venipuncture is controversial. The antecubital fossa is generally avoided for the following reasons.

   a. Arm mobility is restricted.

   b. It is difficult to assess for extravasation due to the large amount of subcutaneous tissue.

   c. If extravasation occurs, increased tissue damage could follow because of the extensive reconstruction area and joint structures.

   d. If venous fibrosis occurs due to the caustic effects of the drugs, drawing blood from that vein could be difficult. In addition, smaller veins distal to the obstruction are then rendered useless because of poor drainage.

   Those who favor use of the veins in the antecubital fossa do so because of the large vein size, which allows for a more rapid infusion of the drugs and permits the agents to reach the circulation sooner, thus decreasing the irritation to the vein. Distal veins, such as those in the dorsum of the hand, are preferred by some nurses because of their easy access and allowance for additional venipuncture when necessary.

2. **Needle size.** This is another controversial area in administering chemotherapy agents. The use of a 19- or 21-gauge needle may allow for a more rapid infusion and could minimize potentially irritating agents from affecting the vein. Smaller-gauge needles (e.g., 22 or 23 gauge) may be easier to insert, produce less scar tissue, be less painful, and cause less mechanical phlebitis. A 23-gauge butterfly needle is frequently used in the outpatient setting for ease of insertion and minimal vein irritation. Larger Teflon-type catheters are used for longer infusions and administration of high volumes of fluid.

3. **Problem veins.** Persons with cancer often have frequent needle sticks for chemotherapy or diagnostic procedures, which results in scarring, irritation, and sclerosing of veins. Finding veins large enough to access may become difficult. Applying moist heat to allow for vein dilatation may be necessary. A general rule is to limit venipuncture attempts by one nurse (or physician) to three when trying to start an IV infusion. It is wise to have another colleague attempt

the venipuncture or to call the phlebotomy service if several attempts are to no avail. Successful venipuncture is very important in reducing patient anxiety, discomfort, infection, and thrombosis, and to safely deliver the medication.

B. Venous access devices. Due to the frequent peripheral vein problems associated with chemotherapy administration, the development of venous access devices has been beneficial for cancer care. Potential advantages of the use of venous access devices include prevention of extravasation, increased patient comfort, promotion of self-care, and facilitation of continuous infusions. If the need for a venous access device is anticipated early, the patient may receive the treatment on schedule and without the anxiety of frequent venipunctures.

    1. Long-term central venous catheters. The Silastic right atrial catheters (e.g., Hickman, Broviac, or Groshong catheters) are tunneled under the skin and inserted into a large vein, with the tip resting in the right atrium. The exit site is usually on the chest wall. The catheters are available in single, double, and triple lumens. The clinical utility increases with the number of ports; unfortunately the risk of phlebitis also increases with the increasing catheter diameter. These catheters can be used for drawing blood, as well as for administering blood products, antibiotics, chemotherapy agents, and total parenteral nutrition. Involvement of the patient or family is required for dressing changes and flushing of the catheter.

    The frequency of dressing changes and the cleansing agents used for the dressing changes vary according to institution. When the catheter is first placed, it is my practice to change the dressing daily. Hydrogen peroxide and iodine-povidone (Betadine) solution are used around the catheter at the entry site which is covered by a sterile gauze (2 × 2 inches). Clear plastic dressings (Opsite) are not used as they tend to hold moisture and cause skin irritation in warm weather. Usually by 3–4 weeks after placement, no dressing is required. The patient and family are taught home care of the device by the nursing staff at the time of implantation.

    The frequency of flushing the catheters also varies in the literature. My practice has been to flush the catheters daily with 2 ml of heparinized saline solution (100 units/ml). Saline may be substituted for heparinized saline in the daily irrigations of the Groshong catheter. It is important, however, to flush with heparinized saline after a treatment has been given or a blood sample drawn. Further research needs to be done to standardize the care of these catheters.

    2. Implanted vascular access ports. Another type of long-term central venous access device is the implanted port. This port is implanted under the skin (commonly on the chest wall) and is attached to a catheter, which is inserted into a large vein (usually the subclavian) and threaded down to the right atrium. Common brand names include Port-a-cath, Infus-a-port, Mediport, Lifeport, and Omegaport. Each device has a self-sealing septum and silicone catheter. The port itself may be metal or plastic. They are also manufactured as single- or dual-lumen devices. The latter allows two different fluids to be administered simultaneously. These devices are used for the same purposes as the long-term central venous catheters. A special Huber point needle must be used to access the port to prevent damage to the port septum. These "solid point" needles prevent coring of the septum by standard hollow-point needles. Right-angled Huber needles and butterfly Huber needles are available for use. Very little care is required for ports, with the exception of a heparin flush of 5 ml (100 units/ml) following each use and every 4 weeks when not in use. Some patients prefer the ports because of the better cosmetic appearance, ease in use, and minimal care required. When medications are given via a port, blood return should be obtained to ensure proper placement of the catheter and external needle. When vesicant chemotherapy agents are administered through a port, caution should be taken to obtain a good blood return and to prevent extravasation.

3. **Temporary catheters.** Smaller-gauge catheters, such as the peripherally inserted central catheters (PICC lines), may be placed for patients requiring less than 2 months of therapy. These catheters are placed nonsurgically and can be used for infusion of some types of chemotherapy. Care similar to that used for the long-term central venous catheters is required for flushing and dressing changes.

V. **Safe handling of chemotherapeutic agents.** The potential risks involved in handling cytotoxic agents have become a concern for health care workers. The literature reports various symptoms such as eye, membrane, and skin irritation, as well as dizziness, nausea, and headache experienced by health care workers not using safe handling precautions. In addition, increased concerns regarding the mutagenesis and teratogenesis continue to be investigated. Many chemotherapy agents, the alkylating agents in particular, are known to be carcinogenic in therapeutic doses. Due to the potential hazards and the controversies regarding chemotherapy effects on those exposed, the Occupational Safety and Health Administration (OSHA) developed guidelines for proper workplace practices in 1986. Many institutions have based policies and procedures on the recommendations of OSHA, although many health care workers do not comply with the guidelines. The OSHA recommendations are summarized here.

A. Personnel

1. Personnel who handle cytotoxic agents, cytotoxic waste, or both should receive adequate education and training prior to assuming their responsibilities.
2. Individuals should document any acute exposure to antineoplastic agents.
3. Personnel should be provided with periodic health examinations. Employee health departments should keep a current list of employees who are routinely involved in handling cytotoxic agents, cytotoxic wastes, or both.
4. Women who are trying to conceive, are pregnant, or are breast-feeding should be informed of the potential hazards of exposure. Institutional policies should be established to address this issue.
5. All chemotherapeutic agents should be mixed in an approved class II biologic safety cabinet (BSC) with a high-efficiency, particulate-air (HEPA) filter and vertical laminar flow hood.
6. Syringes and IV tubing should contain Luer-lock fittings.
7. Disposable, lint-free, nonabsorbent gowns with cuffed long sleeves should be worn when antineoplastic agents are handled. Surgical latex gloves are also recommended for use.
8. Handwashing should be done before gloves are put on and again when they are taken off, as all gloves have some permeability.
9. When no biologic safety cabinet is available, a hydrophobic filter is recommended to vent the drug vials.
10. IV tubing should be primed with a noncytotoxic solution.
11. Sterile gauze should be wrapped around the chemotherapy needles and syringes when removing them from injection ports.
12. Syringes should not be recapped, as needle sticks are a risk.
13. The person cleaning up small spills should wear a gown, two pairs of surgical latex gloves, and eye protection.
14. Smoking, eating, drinking, and applying cosmetics are not recommended in the preparation or administration areas.
15. All antineoplastic agents should have a chemotherapy hazard label.
16. Gloves and gown should be worn when handling blood, vomitus, or bodily excretions of persons who have received antineoplastic agents in the past 48 hours. Linens contaminated with body fluids should also be handled with precautions.

B. Disposal procedures

1. All equipment used for the administration of chemotherapeutic agents should be placed in a closed, leak-proof, puncture-proof container labeled "hazardous waste."

2. When handling hazardous waste containers, housekeeping personnel should receive instruction on safe handling procedures and should wear surgical latex gloves and gowns with cuffs and back closure.
3. If chemotherapy is administered in the home, the leak-proof container should be taken to a designated area for disposal.
4. The two major methods of safe disposal of antineoplastic drugs are incineration at temperatures of 1000°C (1800°F) and placement in a landfill. Both methods should be done at places with Environmental Protection Agency approval. The nurse who is working with antineoplastic agents is encouraged to maintain current knowledge of safe handling practices. The institutional policies and procedures should be reviewed on an annual basis ideally, to promote safety among all personnel exposed to antineoplastic drugs.

Selected Readings

Oncology Nursing Society. *Cancer Chemotherapy Guidelines, Module I: Recommendations for Cancer Chemotherapy Course Content and Clinical Practicum.* Pittsburgh, PA: Oncology Nursing Society, 1988.

Oncology Nursing Society. *Cancer Chemotherapy Guidelines, Module II: Recommendations for Nursing Practice in the Acute Care Setting.* Pittsburgh, PA: Oncology Nursing Society, 1988.

Oncology Nursing Society. *Safe Handling of Cytotoxic Drugs: An Independent Study Module.* Pittsburgh, PA: Oncology Nursing Society, 1989.

OSHA Work Practice Guidelines for Personnel Dealing with Cytotoxic Drugs. OSHA Instructional Publication 8-1.1. Washington, D.C.: Office of Occupational Medicine, 1986.

Rogers, B., and Emmett, E. A. Handling antineoplastic agents: urine mutagenicity in nurses. *Image J. Nurs. Scholarship* 19:108, 1987.

Valanis, B., et al. Antineoplastic drug handling protection after OSHA guidelines: comparison by profession, handling activity, and work site. *J. Occup. Med.* 34:149, 1992.

Wainstock, J. M. Making a choice: the vein access method you prefer. *Oncol. Nurs. Forum* 14:79, 1987.

Vascular Access, Infusion, and Perfusion

Hollis W. Merrick

The ability to gain reliable access to the vascular system is an important part of the management of patients with cancer. Progressive loss of peripheral veins makes subsequent treatments increasingly more difficult and dangerous; thus, fear of needle sticks during intravenous therapy often becomes one of the most traumatic aspects for patients undergoing chemotherapy. Fortunately, there have been significant advances in vascular access with the introduction of new devices, and increasing numbers of patients are gaining benefit from these devices early in the treatment of cancer. These devices spare the patient discomfort, preserve the remaining peripheral venous sites, and prevent major problems such as drug extravasation and resultant tissue slough. Similar devices that have been developed permit administration of chemotherapeutic agents into arteries and the peritoneal cavity, facilitating these important routes of regional therapy.

I. **Venous access.** The use of Silastic right atrial catheters is simple and safe, even in leukopenic and thrombocytopenic patients. Complications associated with the insertion of these catheters are uncommon, and the incidence of problems associated with their use (e.g., phlebitis, thrombosis, and infection) is lower than that associated with peripheral venous access sites. Right atrial catheters are easy for nursing staff to use, since these catheters are essentially central lines with which nurses have had much experience. Use of these catheters avoids the need for repetitive venipuncture, and the ensured access facilitates timely blood testing and adherence to chemotherapy scheduling.

Dual-lumen catheters should be used in most instances. They are particularly useful for patients who are hospitalized and require continuous (and often logistically difficult) administration of blood products, multiple antibiotics, chemotherapy, and hydration. They are also useful for patients whose therapy requires uninterrupted administration (e.g., infusional therapy or hyperalimentation) in addition to other medications. Patients can resume normal activities, including showering and swimming, with the catheter in place. The newer devices are available in smaller diameters so that virtually all patients can have double- or if needed, triple-lumen catheters.

A. **Types of devices**
1. **Percutaneous devices.** In 1971 Broviac described the use of a permanent central venous catheter for hyperalimentation, and during the late 1970s the catheter began to be used for chemotherapy. In 1979 Hickman described an improved version of this catheter that had a larger diameter to facilitate infusion of drugs and fluids as well as sampling of blood.

Dual-lumen catheters that have been developed allow flexibility in administering fluids and drugs and in taking blood samples simultaneously. The first dual-lumen catheters were simply two Hickman catheters or a Hickman and a Broviac catheter attached side to side. They required placement by a direct operative approach to the internal jugular vein. More modern dual-lumen catheters are round with a septum in the lumen. They are small enough to be introduced by the subclavian approach using a "peel-away" sheath introducer. Table 40-1 outlines the characteristics of percutaneous vascular access devices currently available.

2. **Implantable devices.** A subcutaneously implantable right atrial catheter and injection port is also available. These devices are introduced into the subclavian vein by a peel-away catheter, and the port is then placed in the same incision in a subcutaneous pocket. These devices are entirely under the skin and therefore are more cosmetically appealing and less susceptible to infection. They are usually irrigated monthly. The subcutaneous ports and catheters offer the same advantages as the percutaneous catheters but require a percutaneous needle stick with a special atraumatic Huber needle for access into the port. Nursing staff must be trained to use these devices and to recognize when the needle is not positioned properly. If the needle is not securely docked in the port, subcutaneous infusion of drugs occurs, and with vesicants this occurrence can be hazardous. Currently, several types of implantable devices are available. They are listed in Table 40-2.

Table 40-1. Percutaneous central vascular access devices

Catheter	Description
Right atrial single-lumen catheters	
Broviac[a]	Pediatric age group; 2.7–6.6 French
Hickman[a]	Adult patients; 9.6 French
Groshong[a]	Slit-valve end; requires less frequent irrigation; 3.5–9.5 French
Hemed[b]	4.0–14.0 French
Dual-lumen catheters	
Broviac[a]	
Hickman[a]	
Groshong[a]	
Quinton[c]	Temporary hemodialysis and apheresis catheter
Permacath[c]	Permanent hemodialysis catheter

[a]Davol, Inc. (C.R. Bard, Inc.), Cranston, RI.
[b]Gish Biomedical, Inc., Santa Ana, CA.
[c]Quinton Instrument Co., Seattle, WA.

Table 40-2. Implantable vascular access devices

Device name	Manufacturer
Infus-a-port	Infusaid Corp. (Norwood, MA)
Mediport	Cormed (Medina, NY)
Port-a-cath	Pharmacia (Piscataway, NJ)
Lifeport	Strato (Beverly, MA)
Hickman port	Davol (Cranston, RI)
Groshong port	Davol (Cranston, RI)
Omega port	Norfolk (Skokie, IL)

B. **Important aspects of catheter placement.** The catheters are usually placed by way of the subclavian or internal jugular vein. Placement must be performed in the operating room under fully sterile conditions. Proper placement of the catheter tip in the right atrium must be confirmed by fluoroscopy or chest film after the procedure. Placement of the catheter tip in the upper superior vena cava or subclavian veins may result in an inability to draw blood samples or in thrombosis due to infusion of irritating chemicals in lower-flow vessels.

The most frequent complications of the procedure are pneumothorax and hemothorax. A postoperative chest film is essential to rule out the presence of either complication. Rarely, a pneumothorax will not be present immediately but will appear after several hours. If there is any suspicion of this being the case, a repeat chest film is necessary. The insertion tunnel should become less tender with time. An increase in tenderness should be considered a probable sign of infection.

C. **Management of access devices.** Management of these devices varies considerably. Our practice has been to flush the catheters daily with 2 ml of heparinized saline solution (100 units/ml). Saline may be substituted for heparinized saline in the daily irrigations. It is important, however, to flush with heparinized saline after a treatment has been given or a blood sample drawn. The subcutaneously implantable devices are flushed monthly.

The dressings are changed daily. Dilute hydrogen peroxide and iodine-povidone (Betadine) solution are used around the catheter at the entry site, which is covered by a sterile gauze (2 × 2 inches). Clear plastic dressings (Opsite) are not used as they tend to hold moisture and cause skin irritation in warm weather. Usually by 3–4 weeks after placement, no dressing is required. The patient and family are taught home care of the device by the nursing staff at the time of implantation.

D. **Blocked devices.** Catheters that become blocked can usually be cleared by flushing with heparinized saline solution. If this step is not successful, infusion with urokinase can be effective in unblocking the catheter. Urokinase (500 IU in 1-ml ampule) is injected into the catheter, left in place for 5 minutes, and then withdrawn. This will unblock most catheters. If this procedure is unsuccessful, a second administration, left in place for 30 minutes, may be used; it is even more effective to leave the urokinase in place overnight.

Frequently, it becomes difficult to draw blood from a catheter despite the fact that substances can be easily infused through it. This difficulty is due to either the position of the catheter tip against the vessel wall or the presence of a small thrombus or fibrin sheath at the catheter tip. Forceful flushing with heparinized saline, a change in patient position (including Trendelenburg), or infusion with urokinase may be successful in reopening the catheter. A chest film is helpful to verify satisfactory positioning of the catheter, as the tip may have been accidentally moved from its original position. If these maneuvers are unsuccessful, the catheter usually must be replaced surgically.

Implantable ports may become blocked by sludge if the blood is not completely evacuated from the port after use. Blood tends to become lodged at the angles of the base and with subsequent infusions may actually throw off microemboli. This problem is minimized with newer designs which eliminate corners and angles in the chamber. Multiple authors have reported lower rates of thrombosis and infection with the use of ports rather than Hickman-type catheters.

Low-dose warfarin (1 mg/day) should be started after catheter insertion to decrease the risk of catheter or port clotting and the likelihood of venous thrombosis resulting from catheter irritation.

E. **Catheter infection.** Infection, as manifested by subcutaneous inflammation or fever, remains one of the most persistent problems with the use of venous access devices.

1. **Subcutaneous infection.** The patient may show signs of infection with inflammation or drainage around the catheter at the skin exit site or along the catheter tunnel. The subclavian incision may break down, and the catheter or cuff may become visible. The wound should be sampled for cultures and treated with warm compresses and antiseptic dressing changes; the patient should be given appropriate antibiotics. Depending on the severity of the infection and the status of the patient and therapy, the catheter is usually not removed unless the infection does not clear after an extended course of therapy.

2. **Fever.** The patient may show no local signs of catheter infection and may demonstrate only a fever. Blood cultures are commonly positive when fever occurs during the nadir leukopenia due to chemotherapy. Culture samples should be taken from the catheter and a peripheral vein, and appropriate antibiotics then administered. If the patient's condition deteriorates, the catheter should be removed. In

most circumstances, however, a catheter infection can be cleared with the catheter still in place.

   3. Treatment. As discussed in Chapter 31, in catheter-related sepsis, staphylococcal infections predominate. Removal of infected indwelling intravascular devices is optimal, but not always possible. Eradication of infection often can be accomplished with long-term antibiotics alone. There is approximately a 70–80% chance of curing a gram-positive infection (e.g., *Staphylococcus epidermidis*) with 3–4 weeks of antibiotics. The antibiotic administration should be rotated through each port of the device. The chance of success drops to 30–50% for gram-negative infections. Fungal infection or infection with *Corynebacterium jeikeium* requires immediate removal of the catheter. Tunnel infections (but not exit site infections) generally also require catheter removal, though one may wish to defer a decision until a trial of antibiotics has been completed, if the catheter is critical to patient care.

   Patients who are neutropenic will have a diminished response to subcutaneous infection. They will have tenderness but less swelling and redness. Close examination by "walking your fingers" over the tunnel on a daily basis, looking for tenderness and other signs of infection, is useful.

F. Catheter repair. Damaged catheters can be fixed easily with a repair kit from the particular manufacturer. The individual repair kits, however, vary considerably in the technical details. It is advantageous to use a practice kit to refresh your memory before possibly fumbling the repair in front of the patient.

G. Catheter removal. A catheter is easily removed in the clinic or the patient's hospital room using a simple cutdown set. The position of the cuff of the catheter is established by gentle traction on the catheter, and a cutdown is made over this point. The cuff is mobilized, and after placing clamps over and below it, the cuff is removed from the catheter. The upper end of the catheter can then be withdrawn from the central tract and the lower portion withdrawn through the catheter entry site. Simple pressure over the venous tract is all that is necessary to control bleeding. It is essential to obtain material for culture from the tip of the catheter (rather than the tunnel) at the time of removal to determine if potential bloodstream infection from the catheter exists. Culture of the tunnel does not suffice, as it is invariably contaminated.

H. Peripherally inserted center catheters (PICCs). PICCs have become widely used. They permit bedside insertion for central access via a peripheral vein. Better results are obtained, however, when this is done under fluoroscopic control.

I. External iliac vein approach. In patients where the superior vena cava is occluded, central access is not possible. Use of the femoral vein has been considered hazardous; however, a recent report by Mathur indicates that this can be a useful approach, although with a relatively high incidence of catheter-related sepsis.

II. **Arterial access.** Intraarterial chemotherapy has become increasingly popular for the treatment of localized malignant disease in the extremities, head and neck, abdomen, and liver.

A. **Hepatic artery infusion.** There is renewed interest in the treatment of hepatic tumors by infusion. Access to the hepatic artery has been gained with both percutaneous and implantable devices. Whichever technique is used, it is vitally important to obtain preoperative arteriograms to verify the vascular anatomy of the liver, as it is highly variable. Catheterization of the hepatic artery by way of the gastroduodenal artery provides full infusion coverage of the liver in only 60% of patients. The reason is that the major right hepatic artery arises from the superior mesenteric artery in 12% of patients, and the major left hepatic artery arising from the left gastric artery supplies the left lateral segment of the liver in 25% of patients. Catheterization of these additional arteries may be necessary to gain complete coverage of the arterial system of the liver. Complete coverage of the hepatic circulation is essential for successful infusion therapy. Infusion by implantable and percutaneous devices can be carried out by placing a Hickman or other similar catheter in the appropriate vessel(s). The percutaneous infusion can then be carried out with a portable external infusion pump, such as that manufactured by Cormed.

B. **Implantable devices.** The Infusaid pump is currently available for permanent implantation by placement in the subcutaneous tissue of the abdominal wall. The catheter is brought through the abdominal wall and placed in the appropriate vessel. This pump allows continuous infusion without external catheters. Its use has eliminated many of the technical problems associated with the use of external pumps and catheters. However, the response rate of tumors is similar to that achieved by percutaneous infusion, and no improvement in survival has been proved. Publications have reported a significant incidence of biliary sclerosis that was not found in previous studies using percutaneous infusion. Recent controlled studies indicate no significant improvement in overall survival; however, patients who responded to treatment had extended survival.

C. **Percutaneous devices.** Percutaneous devices have been utilized for arterial or portal vein infusion. Catheters can be placed by a radiologist in the main hepatic artery by way of the femoral or brachial arteries. These catheters can then be used for continuous or intermittent percutaneous infusion.

III. **Cavitary access intraperitoneal chemotherapy**

A. **Rationale.** Direct instillation of chemotherapeutic agents into the peritoneal cavity offers the advantage of increasing drug levels at the site of disease compared to those that could be achieved by systemic therapy. Drugs with a low lipid solubility and high molecular weight have low peritoneal clearance and thus have a pharmacologic advantage with this route of administration. The rate of clearance from the peritoneal cavity is controlled by the peritoneal membrane permeability and by the size of the peritoneal surface area. After systemic absorption, the drug is cleared by the usual mechanisms. The ideal drug must have a slow peritoneal clearance, a steep dose-response curve, and acceptable local peritoneal toxicity.

The initial clinical use of this method has been for cancers of the ovary and colon. When ovarian carcinoma is primarily confined to the abdominal cavity, combinations of IV chemotherapy give a 60–80% response rate, but complete remission is achieved in only 10–15% of patients. Intraperitoneal (IP) chemotherapy may offer the means to improve these results. IP spread of colon cancer is a common feature of advanced disease. Ninety percent of IP flu-orouracil can be extracted from the blood as it passes through the portal system; consequently, IP chemotherapy offers the potential for high drug levels in the peritoneal cavity as well as the liver.

B. Technical considerations. IP chemotherapy has been administered by means of a temporary or a semipermanent peritoneal dialysis catheter such as a Tenckhoff catheter (Table 40-3). The optimal means of delivering IP chemotherapy has yet to be established. Peritoneal dialysis catheters have been demonstrated to function well with an acceptable incidence of complications. They can be used both for drug administration and for assessment of response by peritoneal cytology or computed tomography scans of the abdomen following instillation of contrast medium. A small number of peritoneal catheters become blocked with a fibrin sheath that prevents complete evacuation of the infusate. Patients may experience abdominal pain due to peritonitis secondary to chemotherapy instillation. The use of a totally implantable system for peritoneal therapy has also been reported. Recent reports demonstrated the use of a Groshong catheter, as well as catheters placed percutaneously under fluoroscopic control.

Table 40-3. Cavitary catheters

Device type	Manufacturer
Percutaneous peritoneal catheters	
Tenckhoff	Davol (Cranston, RI)
Trocath	McGaw (Puerto Rico)
Implantable peritoneal catheter	
Port-a-cath	Pharmacia (Piscataway, NJ)

Selected Readings

Abi-Nader, J. A. Peripherally inserted central venous catheters in critical care patients. *Heart Lung* 22:428, 1993.

Abraham, J. L., and Mullen, J. L. A prospective study of prolonged central venous access in leukemia. *J.A.M.A.* 248:2868, 1982.

Balch, C. M., et al. A prospective phase II clinical trial of continuous FUDR regional chemotherapy for colorectal metastases for the liver using a totally implantable drug infusion pump. *Ann. Surg.* 198:567, 1983.

Broviac, J. W., Cole, J. J., and Scribner, B. H. A silicone rubber atrial catheter for prolonged parenteral alimentation. *Surg. Gynecol. Obstet.* 136:602, 1973.

Cardella, J. F., Fox, P. S., and Lawler, J. B. Interventional radiologic placement of peripherally inserted central catheters. *J. Vasc. Intervent. Radiol.* 4:653, 1993.

Cohen, A. W., and Wood, W. C. Simplified technique for placement of long term central venous silicone catheters. *Surg. Gynecol. Obstet.* 154:721, 1982.

Groeger, J. S., et al. Infectious morbidity associated with long-term use of venous access devices in patients with cancer. *Ann. Intern. Med.* 119:1168, 1993.

Gyves, J., et al. Totally implanted system for intravenous chemotherapy in patients with cancer. *Am. J. Med.* 73:841, 1982.

Hayward, S. R., Ledgerwood, A. M., and Lucas, C. E. The fate of 100 prolonged venous access devices. *Am. Surg.* 56:515, 1990.

Henriques, H. F., III, et al. Avoiding complications of long-term venous access. *Am. Surg.* 59:555, 1993.

Hickman, R. O., et al. A modified right atrial catheter for access to the venous system in marrow transplant recipients. *Surg. Gynecol. Obstet.* 148:871, 1979.

Hohn, D., et al. Biliary sclerosis in patients receiving hepatic artery infusion of floxuridine. *J. Clin. Oncol.* 3:98, 1985.

Hurtubise, M. R., et al. Restoring patency of occluded central venous catheters. *Arch. Surg.* 115:212, 1980.

Kemeny, N. E. Is Hepatic Infusion of Chemotherapy Effective Treatment of Liver Metastases? Yes! In V. T. DeVita, S. Hellman, and S. A. Rosenberg (eds.), *Important Advances in Oncology.* Philadelphia: Lippincott, 1992. Pp. 207–227.

Kirk, I. R., et al. Intraperitoneal catheters: percutaneous placement with fluoroscopic guidance. *J. Vasc. Intervent. Radiol.* 4:299, 1993.

Linos, D. A., and Mucha, P. A. A simplified technique for the placement of permanent central venous catheters. *Surg. Gynecol. Obstet.* 154:248, 1982.

Markman, M., et al. Intraperitoneal chemotherapy with high-dose cisplatin and cytosine arabinoside for refractory ovarian carcinoma and other malignancies principally involving the peritoneal cavity. *J. Clin. Oncol.* 3:925, 1985.

Mathur, M. N., et al. Percutaneous insertion of long-term venous access catheters via the external iliac vein. *Aust. N.Z. J. Surg.* 63:858, 1993.

Myers, C. E. The use of intraperitoneal chemotherapy in the treatment of ovarian cancer. *Semin. Oncol.* 11:275, 1984.

Naumann, R. W., et al. The Groshong catheter as an intraperitoneal access device in the treatment of ovarian cancer patients. *Gynecol. Oncol.* 50:291, 1993.

Niederhuber, J. E., et al. Totally implanted venous and arterial access system to replace external catheters in cancer patients. *Surgery* 92:706, 1982.

Niederhuber, J. E., et al. Regional hepatic chemotherapy for colorectal cancer metastatic to the liver. *Cancer* 53:1336, 1984.

Ozols, R. F., Myers, C. E., and Young, R. C. Intraperitoneal chemotherapy. *Ann. Intern. Med.* 101:118, 1985.

Raaf, J. H. Two Broviac catheters for intensive long-term support of cancer patients. *Surg. Gynecol. Obstet.* 158:173, 1984.

Sariego, J., et al. Major long-term complications in 1,422 permanent venous access devices. *Am. J. Surg.* 165:249, 1993.

Savage, A. P., et al. Complications and survival of multilumen central venous catheters used for total parenteral nutrition. *Br. J. Surg.* 80:1287, 1993.

Shivnan, J. C., et al. A comparison of transparent adherent and dry sterile gauze dressings for long-term central catheters in patients undergoing bone marrow transplant. *Oncol. Nurs. Forum* 18:1349, 1991.

Sugarbaker, P. H., et al. Prospective randomized trial of intravenous vs intraperitoneal 5-FU in patients with advanced primary colon or rectal cancer. *Surgery* 98:414, 1985.

Tyburski, J. G., et al. Delayed pneumothorax after central venous access: a potential hazard. *Am. Surg.* 59:587, 1993.

Wade, J. C., et al. Two methods for improved venous access in acute leukemia patients. *J.A.M.A.* 246:140, 1981.

Appendix

Nomogram for Determining Body Surface of Adults from Height and Mass*

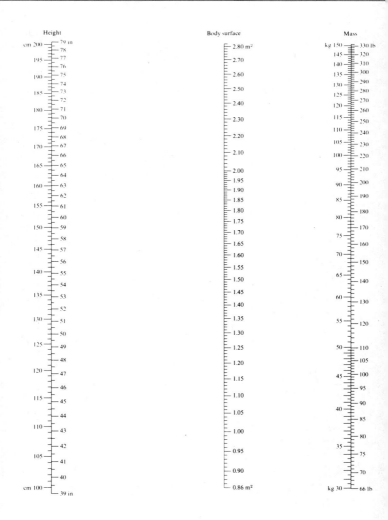

Height	Body surface	Mass

*From the formula of Du Bois and Du Bois. *Arch. Intern. Med.* 17:863, 1916 [$S = M^{0.425} \times H^{0.725} \times 71.84$, or $\log S = \log M \times 0.425 + \log H \times 0.725 + 1.8564$ (S = body surface in cm²; M = mass in kg; H = height in cm)]. Source: C. Lentner (ed.), *Geigy Scientific Tables* (8th ed., Vol. 1). Basel, Switzerland: Ciba-Geigy, 1981. P. 227.

Nomogram for Determining Body Surface of Children from Height and Mass*

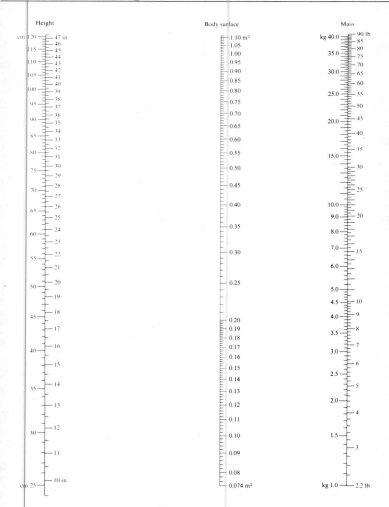

Height	Body surface	Mass

*From the formula of Du Bois and Du Bois. *Arch. Intern. Med.* 17:863, 1916 [$S = M^{0.425} \times H^{0.725} \times 71.84$, or $\log S = \log M \times 0.425 + \log H \times 0.725 + 1.8564$ (S = body surface in cm^2; M = mass in kg; H = height in cm)]. Source: C. Lentner (ed.), *Geigy Scientific Tables* (8th ed., Vol. 1). Basel, Switzerland: Ciba-Geigy, 1981. P. 226.

Index

Index

Note: Page numbers followed by f indicate figures; page numbers followed by t indicate tables. When used in regimens, individual drugs are indexed by regimen names.

Endocrine disorders. *See also*
Ectopic Cushing's
syndrome; Hyperglycemia
chemotherapeutic agents
causing, 114
erythrocytosis, 611–612
Endocrine syndromes, 590–612.
See also Hypercalcemia;
Syndrome of inappropriate
secretion of antidiuretic
hormone
ectopic gonadotropin
production, 611
ectopic thyrotropin secretion,
611
hormone production and
clinical expression of,
590–591
islet cell carcinoma and,
261–262
Endocrine therapy, for breast
cancer, 273, 275, 281–282,
283. *See also* Hormones;
Hormone therapy; *specific
hormones*
Endometrial cancer, 293–298
adjuvant chemotherapy for,
295–296
advanced disease, 296
diagnostic tests in, 294
histology of, 293
papillary serous carcinoma,
297
patterns of spread of, 293–294
preservation of fertility and,
298
radiotherapy for, 295, 296
recurrent, 296–298
risk stratification for, 294–295
staging of, 294, 295t
surgery for, 295
Enterobacter aerogenes, antibiotic
resistance of, 540
Enterobacter cloacae, antibiotic
resistance of, 540
Enzymes, 128. *See also*
Asparaginase
EOC. *See* Epithelial ovarian
cancer
EPI. *See* Epirubicin
4'-Epi-doxorubicin. *See*
Epirubicin
Epinephrine, for anaphylaxis,
525, 574
Epipodophyllotoxin. *See*
Etoposide

Epirubicin, 125t, 159–160
Epithelial ovarian cancer, 299.
See also Ovarian cancer
EPOCH regimen, for non-
Hodgkin's lymphoma,
low-grade, 469t
Epoetin alfa. *See* Erythropoietin
Epogen. *See* Erythropoietin
EP regimen, for lung carcinoma,
small-cell, 230t
Epsilon-aminocaproic acid
for hemorrhage, 571
for promyelocytic
coagulopathy, 422
Ergamisol. *See* Levamisole
Erythrocytosis, 611–612
Erythropoietin, 37, 160–161
for agnogenic myeloid
metaplasia, 446
for anemia, 492
for myelodysplastic syndromes,
448
Escherichia coli, antibiotic
resistance of, 540
ESHAP regimen, for non-
Hodgkin's lymphoma, low-
grade, 469t
Eskalith. *See* Lithium carbonate
Eskalith-CR. *See* Lithium
carbonate
Esophageal carcinoma, 236–240
advanced disease, 238–239
clinical manifestations and
pretreatment evaluation
of, 237, 238t
combined-modality therapy for,
239–240
epidemiology of, 236–237
prognosis of, 237–238
staging of, 237, 238t
Essential thrombocythemia,
444–445
Estramustine, 124t, 161
for prostatic cancer, 327–328
Estrogen antagonists, 129
Estrogens, 129, 162
for prostatic cancer, 326
receptors for, in breast cancer,
275
thromboembolism associated
with, 556
Ethical considerations, 71–79.
See also Informed consent
decisions at end of life and,
77–79
refusal of treatment, 76–77